Sexual Paradox

Complementarity,
Reproductive Conflict
and
Human Emergence

Christine Fielder
&
Chris King

Sexual Paradox

Complementarity, Reproductive Conflict and Human Emergence

Christine Fielder & Chris King © Feb 2004

christine@sexualparadox.org   chris@sexualparadox.org

Further supplements, and updates online at:
http://www.sexualparadox.org

ISBN: 1-4116-5532-X

Genotype 2.5.3, 30-1-2006.

Cover: Cranach © Courtauld Institute Gallery, London

Contents

Introduction: Sex, Paradox and Existence

This book is about sexual paradox, the nemesis of our pretensions, yet the genesis of our living destinies. It demonstrates that sexual paradox is at the core of all descriptions of reality, lurking in the quantum realm and in the relationship between body and mind as much as in our hormone-steeped bodies and rising pulses. Sexual paradox is not just as an inscrutable icon for the vagaries of sexual intrigue, but a cosmic principle spanning the widest realms, from physics, through biology to our social futures - an ultimate tension between contraries and complements, out of which verdant complexity emerges.

Without Contraries is no progression. Attraction and Repulsion, Reason and Energy, Love and Hate, are necessary to Human existence.

William Blake - The Marriage of Heaven and Hell

The nature of sexual paradox is portrayed in the Maori creation (Alpers R11): The primal pair, Papa and Rangi, Earth Mother and Sky Father, are unwillingly pushed apart by the very complexity generated by their primaeval complementation, to let light permeate, enabling their children to multiply, amidst the ramifying prisoners' dilemma of betrayal:

At the beginning of time stood Te Kore, the nothingness - Io.
Then Rangi the sky, dwelt with Papa tu a nuku the Earth,
and was joined with her, and land was made.
But their numerous offspring lived in darkness,
for their parents were not yet parted,
Tane mahuta, god and father of the forests
and all things that inhabit them answered
"Let the Sky become a stranger ,
but let the Earth remain close to us as our nursing mother."
Over vast time, the Kauri tree pushed them apart.
With heavy groans and shrieks of pain, the parents cried
"Why did you do this crime, why did you slay your parents' love?"

But then we find the root paradox of biological sexuality becomes the nemesis of death itself. In an archetypal portrayal of the descent from parthenogenetic immortality, to sexual transgression and the individual mortality that comes from sexual reproduction and diversity, we find that *incest* - the primal auto-sexual encounter - becomes the source of death and the contrast between an eternal male mind sky and the uterine life-giving yet Kali-like death-taking natures of the earthly feminine:

Tane was without a female companion. First he turned to his mother, Papa, who rejected him. Then he united with several different beings, but each time their offspring were things like mountain streams, reptiles and stones. This did not satisfy Tane, who bore the likeness of a man and he longed to have a partner to match himself. At last he took his mother's advice and formed the shape of a woman out of the soft red sand on the sea shore of Hawaiki. He breathed life into her nostrils, ears, mouth and eyes. Hot breath burst from her mouth and she sneezed. She opened her eyes and she saw Tane. Her name was Hine-hau-one, the Earth-formed-maiden. Their first child was called Hine-titama, the Dawn maiden. After a while Tane took the Dawn maiden as his wife. The girl did not know that Tane was her father as well as her husband. When she asked who her father was, she was told to "...ask that question of the pillars of the house". Hine did so but the housepost did not answer nor did the side panel. Then the Dawn maiden realised the truth. She fled in shame from Hawaiki to the darkness of Po, the under-world. When Tane tried to follow her, she cried out to him that she had "...cut the cord of this world" and that he must return to look after their children in the world of light while she remained in the world of darkness to drag their children down. This was the origin of death. Hine-titama, Dawn maiden became Hine-nui-te-po, great-goddess-of-darkness. Hine is both the first woman and a goddess who is guardian of the land of the dead. She is both a life-giver and a destroyer of life. (http://www.janeresture.com/polynesia_myths/newzealand.htm).

Maui the phallic Polynesian hero was then crushed between her thighs when he sought immortality by crawling into her vagina and the fantail laughed alerting her.

Sex and Paradox: Founding Aspects of a Complementary Reality

For all the trappings of civilized society, and our attempts to restrain and civilize it, sex remains forever the chaotic vital force, eclipsing our hearts and capturing our minds, winging on the airwaves in the throbbing beat of rock and roll, ensnaring all, in love's enticements and torments, from our founding creation myths, to our greatest dramatic performances. Its mountains of spice span the great divide between divine comedy and stark tragedy. It is *sine qua non* our universal, mortal, yet fertile condition, celebrated in the seclusion of bedrooms and boudoirs, in the back seats of drive-ins, in thatched huts, behind bushes, in the wilds of nature, and even under the lurid neon of red-light districts.

Although the sexual quest is seemingly a simple act of fertilization in a reproductive dance shared by even the simplest organisms, its consequences for our lives and culture are profound and inescapable. 'Falling in love' epitomizes the devastating way the psychic power of sexual love lays subterranean claim to our hearts and minds, to our very sense of being, and to our life directions, in the twists of fate our relationships entwine us into. Lubricious sex is the animal force of 'defilement' that religion and conventional morality seek to tame, sometimes through dire punishments, from stoning to infibulation. It is both the ultimate transgression and our liberating fulfillment. Just as sex divides us, so it unites us in our moments of 'splendour in the grass', being both the source of mortality and our vital quest to the ultimate mysteries of existence, with promise of endless regeneration.

This work is not just about sex (p 328), orgasm (p 361), or sacred love (p 468), but the cosmic paradox, which is itself a sexual paradox. Just as sexuality is at the foundation of our continued biological existence, so sexual paradox is at the foundation of our existential condition. Sexuality at the very root of cosmology might seem a contradiction in terms. Sexual reproduction (p 334) is a recent development in the evolution of higher organisms (p 323), themselves ephemeral and fragile in a universe of annihilating energies, whose origin is far more ancient and mysterious (p 298). Yet it is not just biological reproductive sexuality we are describing here, but cosmic complementarity. The cosmic condition manifests, from its source, as an implicitly sexual paradox - between subjective experience and objective reality, wave and particle, chaos and order, each dependent on the other for their existence, in a way which makes the 'other' both the ultimate genesis and nemesis of each, in the dance out of which climax diversity (p 327) emerges.

The core idea of sexual paradox is an extension of complexity theory (p 506) to deal with the paradox that arises when a division occurs into two domains of order that can neither resolve their outcomes fully by cooperation, nor by conflict. Complexity theory suggests they will achieve optimal complexity in a state of instability in strategic paradox between the two regimes. This is a different form of complexity theory from 'edge of chaos' ideas (p 506) but is very well established in evolutionary game theory and is manifest both in the prisoners' dilemma game matrix (p 13) and the cusp catastrophe (p 14), when neither conflict nor cooperation can be resolved determinately - hence the paradox.

A paradox is "a statement, doctrine or expression seemingly absurd or contrary to common notions or to what would naturally be believed, but in fact really true" (p 451). Thus paradox may be counter-intuitive, but is yet a root truth which remains integral to our condition. By contrast with paradox, a contradiction is to specifically 'speak against'. The contradiction often implied by paradox is implicitly sexually co-antagonistic in that it arises from a logical division between two conditions, true and false, each of which denies the other. But paradox can come in more subtle forms than contradiction. For example the wave and particle aspects of the quantum are not contrary, so much as interdependent. A quantum can manifest only as a wave, or a particle, but not both at the same time. However any attempt to mount a description based on one aspect implicitly involves the other.

Division is itself implicitly sexual (p 451), expressed in the occurrence of sexuality among all 'dividing' life forms, from bacteria (p 329) to higher animals (p 329). Such 'sexual' division is not necessarily into two dyadic classes alone, even with reproductive sexuality. It may include many classes (p 336). In Eden we see it in Eve's cleaving from an 'androgynous' Adam and their ensuing 'concupiscence' (p 208). It may even be simply the primal distinction from the unified 'background' in which the undivided whole - the uncarved block (p 456), or *tohu vohu* (p 498), as primordial feminine is partitioned by masculine 'distinction', in the primaeval division of existence, or manifestation. The very act of distinction leads to an endless regress into a plethora of sub-division. By contrast, the undivided whole remains a totipotent matrix for new form, possessing attributes of chaotic entanglement in so far as it resists, or complements, the intrusion of discriminating order:

I am a tree whose leaves are trees
you are the endless colours of the night
you forever dissolve me, I slice through you
endlessly dividing your eddies of eddies.

We have two key ways of diverting ourselves from the depths of sexual paradox. On the one hand we cling to an identification with a monadic cosmic 'self', or godhead - an all-encompassing singular identity, providing sanctuary from the uncertainty of the abyss, in a fatherly or motherly creator deity. At another extreme, we seek to dispel all such myths, in a purely physical description of ourselves, as biological machines in a material world, where selfishness and expedience are as real and enticing as any notions of ethics, or altruism. However, mind and body cannot be so easily separated. Our actual relationship with the universe, and with existential reality, is a paradox of complementarity, which is sexual in its very essence.

We can see manifestations of sexual paradox in all the ultimate complementarities. At the core is the dyad of subjectively conscious mind and an objectively physical organism, sometimes projected into dualities of body and soul, earth and heaven, nature and the divine. From the point of view of objective science, only our brain states are verifiable phenomena, and our subjective experience seems to be merely an internal model of reality constructed by our chemical brains. But our conscious experience is the only direct *veridical* 'data' we have access to. All our knowledge of the physical world comes via our subjective experience, so it appears to have an existential status complementary to the physical universe. Subject-object complementarity is also a key to our capacity to take responsibility for our actions in the form of free-will. It is this principle of autonomous choice on which law and personal accountability are founded. Despite the ephemeral nature of mind, the root complementation between subjective experience and objective reality implies that our consciousness is also, in some sense, a founding cosmic aspect.

The patriarchal paradigm leans to the mind-sky perceiving mind (p 364) as 'finer' (above gross particulate matter) or 'indivisible' (suggesting a feminine wave like character). This is a frank sex reversal between 'particulate' sperm and an 'engulfing' egg. At the same time the feminine is assigned to be physical, divided existence an inferior world of mortal 'slime', typified by menstrual taboos (p 198), *maya* or illusion (p 460), Eve's earthly sin (p 210), and Wisdom of Proverbs (p 208) diminished to mere common sense by comparison with the higher realms.

Fundamental to the quantum world of physics we have wave-particle complementarity, which is also the source of quantum uncertainty (p 299). In the dynamical world we have the complementation of order and chaos (p 498), whose mutual interaction has recently been discovered to be key to generating climax complexity (p 506). This is reflected again in thermodynamics, where the equilibrium condition we associate with the inexorable growth of entropy, or disorder, to a maximum does not have to occur in open thermodynamic systems, which exchange energy or material with their environment.

Only then do we come to the conventional evolutionary manifestations of biological sexuality and engendering, with which we are familiar, in our conventional notions of sex as reproduction, and its symmetry-breaking into masculine and feminine genders (p 334). With the advent of the egg and sperm, we see again the shadow of wave and particle aspects in a huge enveloping ovum with it's lightning wave of membranous excitation - the cortical reaction, selecting one from a multiple, essentially particulate collection of DNA-bearing sperm.

Although each of these complementarities differ fundamentally in their basis, all share key features of sexual paradox, summarized as follows:

1. **Sexual Division:** Nature, cosmology, biogenesis, evolution, reproduction, consciousness and existential reality all present as dichotomies, rather than mechanisms composed of clearly defined parts, atoms or elements.
2. **Symmetry-Breaking:** The divided aspects are asymmetric, or qualitatively distinct.

3. **Complementarity:** The aspects are mutually complementary. Neither can be eliminated from the process, resulting in a double-bind of mutual interdependence.
4. **Paradox:** Any description based on only one aspect of such a complementarity results in incompleteness, logical paradox, contradiction, conflict, or death.

Only then do we come to the additional features we traditionally associate with biological sex, (5) **genetic recombination**, (6) **fertilization**, and (7) **sexual reproduction.** The result is a sexual prisoners' dilemma (8), from which permanent escape in an outright win is generally impossible, and the best strategy available is co-evolution in strategic paradox (9).

Paradoxes of Fidelity and Deceit in Sexual Evolution

In Section A we develop the central thesis, that sexual paradox, is the basis of cultural complexity. Evolution depends on sexuality to generate genetic variety through the vast opportunities for structured mixing and selection resulting from genetic crossing over's almost unlimited capacity to generate new combinations of viable genome (p 330). Ultimately it is this aspect of sexuality which has made multicellular organisms possible. In this process reproductive sexuality became central to the evolution of higher organisms. While certain organisms can defer reproductive sexuality for a while, sexual genetic exchange of various types is ubiquitous to organisms, from simple bacteria to humans. We find, beginning with a viral form of pan-sexual promiscuity between bacteria (p 329), a new form of complementary sexuality emerged, making an almost endless variety of viable recombinations possible. This began firstly with identical sex cells called isogametes then becoming engendered into a large egg and multiple sperm competing to fertilize it (p 334), representing in molecular terms a subtle expression of the complementary between a single wave-manifesting membranous egg and multiple particulate packets of DNA.

All multi-celled animals depend on engendered symmetry-broken complementation to be able to evolve the complexity we see across the metazoan realm, and in the development of higher plants as well, but it has come at a cost through a tortuous arms race (p 336). The sperm, and with it all males, have inherited a sneaky smaller investment in reproduction than the egg and with it the massive out-front 'honest' investments female animals and particularly mammals make, in gestation, lactation and child-rearing (p 340). Consequently virtually all males down to the human line have inherited a reproductive strategy of sewing wild oats by many partners, while females have been choosy about whose genes will impregnate their valuable and scarce eggs, thus retaining their own reproductive rights to covert betrayal in the amatory race of love (p 29). The extremes of sexual polarization occur in mammals, where the female has inherited the hugely significant investments of internal gestation of live young, lactation, and early child care, leaving the males more than in any other group, to seek sexual favours as their prime reproductive investment (p 28). Humans in many ways have carried this polarization to it utmost limit (p 83).

This leads us to a unique paradoxical game of fidelity and deceit, which is sometimes referred to as the 'prisoners' dilemma' (p 13), in which each participant is 'tempted' into mutual betrayal because the payoffs of deceit are great enough to make the win-win of mutual cooperation a mere consolation prize, leading to the nemesis of mutual defection. However, in the prisoners' dilemma game, fidelity and betrayal remain founding co-contributors to the complexity arising from the mutual paradox, leading to transgression of orthodox morality in a liberation, in which the outlawed aspects of affair and intrigue are as essential to our evolutionary survival as primal chaos *tohu vohu* is to the 'order' of creation. This makes a paradoxical tale for the morality of sexual commitment, for fidelity and deceit are forever two faces of the one sexual paradox. While fidelity is the 'desired condition', to maintain genetic selection, reproductive choice and hence covert 'deceit', remains essential, inescapable, and central to successful evolution (p 18), with men sewing wild oats and women covertly engaging strange affairs - all in a ground swell of public declarations of at least temporary monogamy (p 83). The prisoners' dilemma in its varied two and many person forms spans a variety of situations rearing their heads in the evolutionary process, the diversity of genetic and ecosystemic life, and in human society. Crowning this foray, we have biological sexuality as we know it, and the paradox of sexual selection, with its extensions into gender and its diverse and contradictory manifestations in human society and culture. Although the genetic process and with it the reproductive strategies of each sex in a given species are partially independent and even in conflict, neither sex can escape the double-bind of mortality in the immortal dance of reproduction.

In the Red Queen hypothesis (p 26), sexual species are in an irresolvable arms race with their parasites, and each sex with the other, in a permanent state of prisoners' dilemma running while standing still to out adapt and hence survive one another. It is this which has generated the diversity of our immune systems and tissue recognition histocompatibility proteins. Sex has evolved to be not only a quintessential expression of the prisoners' dilemma in genetics, but permeating our very molecular architecture, our reproductive immortality and all our displays of culture, society and politics both revered and tabooed. This dyadic sexual relation extends to more complex forms of the prisoners' dilemma in ecosystemic relationships (p 15), to climax diversity and to all evolutionarily stable strategies of inescapable coexistence in survival in the biosphere. It also extends to many ways in which this delicate paradoxical relationship breaks down, in 'tragedy of the commons' (p 15), rape of the planet (p 419), the boom and bust (p 420)so characteristic of unmediated male reproductive investment, and many other forms of dominion and oppression.

All's Fair in Love and War

Despite male pretensions to charismatic 'sexual conquest' of the female, mesmerized by the turgid charms of an all too unpredictable member, and the hopefully not too premature heights of thrusting climax, a careful look at female orgasm leads to some very stark and dangerous conclusions - that despite some women having a tamer, or equivocal experience in our male-dominated culture, women's sexual energies are, to quote Mary Sherfey (R624): "insatiable even in the face of the highest degree of sexual satiation". Energies that ride wild over the most hopeful pretensions to 'conquest' any male can assume. A woman's endowment of clitoral, G-spot, and uterine orgasms (p 361), amid a propensity for multiple, repeated, or continual climax, all in a context of beguiling sexual privacy (p 74) amid almost permanent sexual receptiveness, ever-so-inscrutably coloured by subtle hormonal shifts at ovulation towards sexual adventure, launch female eros into a sustained stratospheric territory, which no man alone can lay claim to, nor be sure of sustaining, in his 'own right'.

In our primate relatives, including bonobos (p 66) and chimps (p 63), female sexual incitement, particularly during estrus, (which ironically means 'gadfly') is at peak time of fertility, a play for the best male genes available, and to either side of the peak, a more general all-comers insurance that as many males as possible will be inveigled into the 'paternity net' and will thus be encouraged to support, rather than injure or kill, the ensuing offspring. No male can thus be sure he is not 'the father of the child' and will be drawn into protecting more offspring than his own and refraining from eliminating small competitors, as males are want to do, as harbingers of hunting and death as opposed to gathering, birth and life. On the side, out of sight of others, there are also covert matings with an undisclosed partner 'on safari'. A degree of 'infidelity' is also essential to optimize a female's mating with a male with complementary histocompatibility and thus superior disease resistance. Ape females also solicit sex when they are not ovulating, for socially 'manipulative' reasons, which run from such maternity insurance to heterosexual, or lesbian erotic 'love' - social bonding, easing competition, even at the sight of food. In one short sentence - female sexual ecstasy serves to strategically reduce paternity certainty (p 85), just as male ejaculation serves to increase it.

The advent of pair-bonding in humans has overlaid a more 'partnered' theme to this open sport, with the female's almost perpetual sexual receptiveness, enticingly curvaceous form, concealed ovulation, sexual privacy and hormonal 'incitement' during ovulation - otherwise known as 'female reproductive inscrutability' - only adding to the intrigue. Our most central and basic social mental faculties are consequently to do with detecting cheating and betrayal, with sex at the emotional centre of the cyclone. Biologists are frank that 'monogamy' as they use the term is not equatable with genetic or sexual fidelity, but social bonding, for increased reproductive gain and that females in monogamous species also do 'time on the side' with the best studs they can find, as genetic testing has confirmed human females do to a similar degree. Seventy percent of married women over 35 admit to marital infidelity in the US, confirming that this astute and inscrutable pattern continues. Hence all the archaic manifestations of male jealousy and violence, which even in socially monogamous prairie voles, with all their oxytocin and vasopressin bonding, still cause males to become aggressive and suspicious of other males the moment they have sexually 'bonded' with a female.

Given that small, exclusive female territories, amid female reproductive competition (p 33), rather than all-embracing sisterly love is the best indicator of mammalian and primate monogamy, rather than paternal parental resourcing as in birds, we have an interesting paradox. Female espousal of monogamy thus looks as much the 'two-faced' resourcing gambit, albeit for genuine reproductive investment, as is men claiming 'their' women as patrilineal 'property' in our human version of mate guarding, while also sewing wild oats far and wide. The only situations where we find what we might call loosely egalitarian female coalitions are in the decidedly bisexual bonobo, where females make love passionately together in *hoka-hoka* (p 66) and spend seven times as much time together as with males, and in baboons and monkeys a single matriline's kin altruistic affinities.

The clitoris is no dependable organ of biological fertility, like the penis, but a fickle and yet precocious discriminator of male attention - the intimate diviner of genuine indicators of fitness (p 85). The impetuous nature of female orgasm, inaccessible as an enclosed garden one minute, and an overflowing chalice the next, does not serve well the monotonous security of monogamous pair-bonding, but the intrigue, thrill and the novelty of the chase, the young buck, fine as an apple tree in the orchard, seduced by 'fatal attraction', amid our all too brief fallings in love, ephemeral as a spring breeze, incessant as the eternal triangle.

Mortal Fear and Violent Oppression

As discussed in Section B, given this perilous heritage, it is no wonder the patriarchy fears female sexuality like primal chaos, and attempts to anathematize it, to cauterize it, to cut it out, , by circumcision (p 283), subincision (p 170) and infibulation (p 283), or to bottle it up in chastity belts, or hide it, by sequestering and veiling (p 201), in burkas and chadors (p 276), in closed rooms with high windows, and every form of control and repression, from stoning (p 269), to drowning (p 191), to burning alive (p 292) and throwing acid in the face of the beloved, or in more 'sexually liberated' times to tame it into a milder subservient domesticity, with nubile pornographic appeal on the side.

Our creation myths and religious imperatives are disguised attempts by diverse peoples to mark out the boundaries of sexual transgression between women and men, rather than the innocent creation and ordering of the universe they pretend. Deities, from Yahweh condemning Eve's lubricity (p 210) decreeing her husband 'shall rule over her'; through the incestuous enticement of the Sun by Venus (p 161), highlighting the intoxicating nature of female sexuality at the root of sexual antagonism among the Amazon's 'fierce people' (p 161); to the excoriating Dogon primal conflict of sexual energies between God and Mother Earth (p 139), resulting in female circumcision (p 283), are all projections of central male sexual and reproductive anxieties, and stratagems of male control over female sexuality.

A quick look at the few existing matrilocal, quasi-matrilineal societies such as the Canela (p 168) attests precisely to this theme. Here, women are expected to share their sexual favours as widely as possible, just as chimps and bonobos do, until they become pregnant and settle into the matriarchal network of motherhood and the familial ties of child rearing. Marriage is only a token in partnership to ensure paternal care of any infant a woman gives birth to. The role of the father is secondary to the mother's maternal uncles, and males are expected to show no jealousy over their 'wives' affairs. Men are expected to be 'forbearing' and women abide no conventions of emotional control.

This is a close parallel to the *beena* marriage of the Old Testament (p 189), which Jacob rejected in leaving Laban's fold with Rachel and Leah. Conflicts over such sexual motifs are reflected in Lilith's mythical refusal to lie under Adam, rising up to the wild heavens in her own ecstasy (p 211); the whoring ways of the Queen of Heaven (p 214); the fertility rites, on every high hill and under every green tree; and the strange woman of Proverbs, her lips dripping with honey comb, but her ways going right down to Sheol (p 211).

At the opposite extreme, the polygynous, patrilocal, patrilineal Dogon summarily chop the clitorises off their women folk (p 138) so they, won't be led to stray into surreptitious affairs by their all-to-precocious genitals. They confine them to menstrual huts in full view of the men's houses (p 137), so that the men folk in the village can readily observe just who is going to be ready to be fertilized by their reproductive 'owners' and when they can best achieve it, threatening them with cosmological calamity if they break the rule.

Similarly, throughout the central arenas of our cultural emergence (Lerner), from Sumeria and Egypt, through Babylon (p 195), Assyria (p 200), Greece (p 202), Rome, Israel, Vedantic India (p 286), Islamic Arabia (p 263) and Confucian China (p 205), a consistent theme of patriarchal dominion amid confinement of women and fear and repression of their sexual nature, the abduction and capture of women (p 195) and their exploitation as slave concubines (p 195), their assignment to marriages, nunneries and brothels, along with male rights of exclusive patriliny (p 196), primogeniture, and paterfamilias (p 206) often in the name of patriarchal religions, has led to a distorted, violent and unstable cultural paradigm. These diverse sources confirm our worst fears: The sex wars are the foundation of our entire human social and cultural edifice.

Sexuality in Biology and Complementarity in the Physical Universe

In Section C, we investigate in full detail the most complete expressions of complementarity, in the complex entwining of the sexes in biology, as already noted many times in this introduction. We explore the genetic, hormonal, and developmental aspects of biological sexuality, the counterpoint of male and female investments in the symmetry-broken egg and sperm (p 334), X and Y chromosomes (p 340), genetic imprinting, hormonal influences (p 348) and developmental pathways of the sex cells (p 355), the emergence of gonads and external sex organs (p 358). We then investigate the entwined manifestations of sexuality in the brain (p 374), in terms of emotions (p 375) and hormones (p 379), sexual orientation (p 382) and the gatherer-hunter cortex (p 388).

We also show in detail how complementarity becomes central in quantum cosmology, and how biology takes us more deeply into sexual paradox than ever before in the scientific description of the universe and nature. Quantum reality (p 298) is founded on *wave-particle complementarity*. All quanta display wave and particle aspects in a way which comes in a sexual paradox - we cannot measure both these properties at the same time. This complementarity is central to the distinction between the quantum and classical world. Every quantum manifests either as a wave or as a particle at a given time but never both at once. We experience the colour of light, interference patterns, lasers and holograms from its wave properties, but depend on its particle properties both to generate light and to perceive it or capture it on film or tape, and to exist in a molecular world of electromagenetic bonding. Any description in terms of either wave or particle aspect comes with an implicit use of the complementary aspect in the process. Neither can be fully eliminated in the physical description. The *uncertainty* intrinsic to all quantum phenomena (p 299) is a direct consequence of the indeterminacy of the particle within the extensive wave function which determines only probabilities.

Wave-particle complementarity is succeeded by an almost endless procession of ensuing dyadic sexual complementarities. Space and time have complementary roles, along with energy and momentum. All quanta are divided into two complementary types. The integer-spin *bosons* (p 310), such as photons, constitute all forms of radiation and mediate the forces of nature. The *fermions*, such as electrons and protons, with half-integer spin, can co-exist in one wave function only as opposed pairs and thus constitute incompressible matter. In supersymmetry, there is one *boson* for each type of *fermion*, although they appear quite different in the everyday world. We also have binary divisions between the emitter and absorber of an exchanged particle, and between the virtual and real particles (p 304) that mediate forces and radiation. We finally have a complementarity between the *advanced* and *retarded* solutions of special relativity travelling in forward and backward directions in time. Many other manifestations of sexual paradox and complementarity occur in quantum *entanglement* (p 305) and and the match-making handshaking between emitters and absorbers in the *transactional* interpretation (p 308), like a chain of entwined scarves pulled endlessly out of a magicians top hat. .

In the realm of dynamics, the complementation of chaos and order is also critical (p 498). Chaos is found to be essential to the genesis of new order and to contain within it complex fractal structures (p 500). Virtually all complex systems in nature either occur at the edge of chaos (p 506), or as a result of transitions between chaos and order. In thermodynamics, open systems, which exchange energy or material with their environment, the equilibrium condition we associate with the growth of entropy to maximum disorder does not have to occur. The most outstanding example of this is the growth of complexity of the biosphere as a 'negentropic' far from equilibrium open system, whose entropy is decreasing and complexity increasing (except in periods of mass extinction) through the photosynthetic fixing of incident solar radiation to induce chemical reactions.

We now understand the universe, and with it time and space, appear to have had a common 'origin' in the 'big bang' some twelve billion years ago (p 298). Many aspects of this origin display sexual paradox at work. In the inflationary model (p 310), the universe appears to have emerged from its own wave function as a quantum fluctuation. Trapped in an artificial low energy false vacuum, it expanded exponentially until a profound *symmetry-breaking* occurred, resulting in the highly engendered asymmetric forces of nature we experience today. Gravity then became attractive and the complex interactional process which gave rise to galaxies, stars and planets began. Throughout this process, wave-particle complementarity and interaction between order and chaotic processes have molded the shape of cosmic evolution to the planetary context in which we find life.

The establishment of life leads to a second type of interactive process, at 'the edge of chaos' in which selection and mutation give rise to endless transformations of new living form. Like the individual particles and wave amplitudes of the quantum realm, evolution is a partly ordered process molded by natural or sexual selection, and partly an intermittent discrete, seemingly random mutational process. Single mutations function like single particles reflecting quantum uncertainty, while selection operates as the superposition of many particles, reinforcing many mutations along consistent avenues. Evolution is thus a phenomenon which is not fully classical and displays quantum paradoxes in action. This is reflected in the contrast between key developments like the camera eye, which results from a continuous invagination and idiosyncratic molecules produced only by one or a few species (p 324).

Cultural Visions of Sexual Complementarity and Fusion

Rabbi Akiva who committed the Song of Songs "Shir HaShirim," (שיר השירים) to the Torah said: "Heaven forbid that any man in Israel ever disputed that the Song of Songs is holy. For the whole world is not worth the day on which the Song of Songs was given to Israel, for all the Writings are holy and the Song of Songs is the Holy of Holies." The mystery beyond mysteries of the Holy of Holies is that the deepest metaphor and nature of our 'relationship with God' lies in the teeming fertility, love and comingling of the sexual union and the intimacy, caring, playfullness, ravishing beauty, mystical insight and creative flowering that this subtle sacro-sexual condition brings about. Sexual Paradox is thus the key to the Judeo-Christian *mysterium tremendum*.

Appendix A, investigates cultural traditions in which complementarity is implicit in the cosmology. One of the best known is the Tantric cosmic origin (p 459). Unlike the patriarchal idea of a beneficent Vishnu dreaming the universe as a lotus emerging from his navel, the Tantric origin begins in intimate conjugal embrace between two complementary manifestations, Shiva as eternal, subjective, cosmic consciousness, and Shakti, the dynamic feminine force, which motivates the universe, and all material phenomena, in time. Although she is sometimes depicted as a mere projection of the male cosmic Self (p 466), an Eve emerging from Adam's rib (p 209) in a Brahmanic patriarchal twist, Shakti's origins lie in the untamed powers of the black planter goddess Kali, creatrix and destructress of time, whose roots, are far more ancient, lying at the source of the pre-Vedic Indus valley civilizations, whose images also spawn Shiva in yogic posture, as Lord of the Animals, (p 463) a gatherer-hunter name he still bears at Pashupatinath, among the burning ghats of Katmandu.

The Tantric origin begins in a state of deep coital fusion - an annihilating ecstasy of cosmic union (p 463). Then, as the complements step back from this conjugal communion, subjective mind becomes distinct from and complementary to the objective phenomena of the physical universe. Mind becomes aware of itself, freeing Shiva from passive inertness, and Shakti dances the dance of maya or illusion, in which the unity embracing self and world becomes endlessly divided and multiplied into the full complexity of all natural manifestations and we each become fragmented into separate conscious selves. This is portrayed as a love dance, spawning and eventually destroying the worlds. Once again the patriarchal will to order attempts to assert dominance in the form of mind being finer than the gross nature of matter, but the message is clear - climax diversity and the magical complexity of the sentient universe arises from sexual paradox between two cosmic aspects acting in complementary relationship, to evoke the dance of life's abundance.

The Chinese philosophy of the *Tao*, or 'way' of nature (p 452) brings to the surface other aspects of this fundamental cosmic sexual paradox, perceiving all natural phenomena as arising from the mutual interaction of two cosmic principles, *yin*, a receptive dark, fecund, principle identified as feminine and *yang* a shining, active creative principle identified as masculine. Each also contains the germ of the 'other'. Again here however there is an ancient deference to the feminine as the mother, matrix of time, beyond being and non-being, source of all natural diversity in the uncarved block. The Tao teaches that the universe is a product of impersonal forces and that the role of humanity is to keep the balance in nature. It is in the sexual relationship and its consequences that we engage in a participatory process of taking responsibility for the future of life, having already assumed the capacity for annihilation. Taoistic thought invokes continual transformation and change and decries any attempt to hierarchically organize or analyze into ordered categories, as flawed in this cosmology of flowing interdependence (p 453). Pivotal to Taoist philosophy is the notion of chaos as a primal progenitor of natural form and diversity, manifest in vibration, in eddies, in streaming clouds, the gnarled shapes of trees and fungi and the forms of naturally eroded objects. It notes that chance, life and consciousness are three common manifestations of the Tao, identifying uncertainty, life and consciousness as a fundamental part of the creative process. Central here is the idea that in transformation nothing repeats itself, despite the immense totality of this transformation being itself an invariant. In the I Ching oracle (p 457), the *yin-yang* division is multiplied into 256 x 256 archetypal transformations, representing the diversity of existential conditions.

Such dyadic creation myths span many cultures, from Sumeria, to the 'Elohistic origin of Genesis 1, male and female in 'Our' likeness (p 208) and the Maori creation myth (p 1). We can see these ultimate complementarities in the source Judeo-Christian tradition in the creation out of chaos, or *tohu vohu*, 'without form or void' like the 'nothingness' of Io (p 1). We again have the idea of god in the plural as 'Elohim, with humanity female and male in *their* likeness, implying both a feminine and masculine presence, confirmed in the exhortations of Hochmah, or Wisdom, in the proverbs:

The Lord possessed me in the beginning of his way, before his works of old.
I was set up from everlasting, from the beginning, or ever the earth was.

This motif continues in the complemention between the tree of life in the centre of Eden (p 209) and the binary division of the tree of knowledge of good and evil, whose two realities together would make us even 'as god' - forming a complementarity between life-giving synthesis and an analytical knowledge, whose supremacy in dominion has led inexorably to our Fall from paradise. A complementation as fundamental as the binary division between a pregnant, vaginal, encircling 0 and a discriminating, divisive, penile 1 (p 489).

Unraveling the Gordian Knot

Section D deals with the planetary consequences. What do we do about the violent consequences of breakdown of sexual paradox? Exert some form of social control? This is exactly what the patriarchs have done to women, violently to the occlusion of feminine nature, the detriment of human nature, and our future viability, resulting in multiple, repeated and continual warfare, genocide, apocalypse, mutually-assured nuclear (p 427), chemical and biological destruction, overpopulation (p 420), the rape of the Earth (p 419) and the entire diversity of life (p 423), climatic crisis (p 425), and boom and bust economies with no long-term stability of future (p 429), all in the spermatogenic (p 419), venture-risk, winner-take-all, competitive paradigm of the patriarchal imperative. However, real or repressed sexual conflict is neither inevitable, nor is it a fatal flaw in the human species. The complexity of human culture appears to have emerged from the creative amatory race sexual selection induces in a state of sexual paradox (p 53). Our founding genetic and cultural archetypes in the Bushmen and Pygmy Forest Peoples, such as the !Kung (p 106), Sandawe (p 118), Biaka (p 124) and Mbuti (p 120) exist in a state much closer to sexual paradox and egalitarian cooperation between the sexes than many more 'highly evolved' societies. Our gatherer-hunter origins are a manifestation of an interdependence, despite differing sexual strategies, coinciding with the deepest in female and male nature, in the resourcing of life's continuity in motherhood, and the death culling performed by the all-too-mortal male hunter-warrior.

Those anthropologists, sociologists and cultural feminists who assert the human psyche is a 'blank slate' (p 40) which has left behind its biological origins need to consider the deleterious consequences of the patriarchal cultural adventure, when cultural prerogatives are imposed in denial, or even in affirmation, of our sexual sociobiology, particularly when applied to the role of mothering, so critical for human survival (p 35). Our genetic nature is not deterministic and remains adaptive, both to individual emotional and intellectual responses, and to social and cultural forces. However society and culture prosper and ultimately survive only in constructive relationship with our biological nature, not in spite of it, or imposed upon it. Rather than psychological pathology, fear of the power of female life-giving (p 178), testosterone poisoning (p 379), or the consequences of a fundamentally violent species (p 47), the rise of patriarchy appears to be a natural product of primate sociobiology, and the gatherer-hunter division of labour, driven into male dominance by many factors - inter-group conflict by male coalitions (p 44), need for intra-group moral cohesiveness in response, resulting social stress and resource uncertainty (p 143), paternity uncertainty, and the rise of urban class and property with large-scale agriculture (p 176).

Sexual complementarity cannot be unraveled overnight and may be integral to the cosmic design. Subjective mind and physical reality present as inextricable complements (p 364) as do wave and particle (p 299). The relationship between our sexes is as polarized as the primally-broken symmetry of the universe, let alone that between a single enveloping ovum, ripe with cytoplasmic fecundity, and the myriads of particulate sperm competing to fertilize it, only to be capriciously chosen by the shock 'neurological' awakening of the egg's cortical reaction (p 337). Failing to understand the depth of this relationship between the sexes is the root ignorance that has caused war and genocide and could bring our utopian pretensions in the genetic age crashing down, if we fail to recognize our ancient, immortal reproductive quest in sexuality and depend only on cultural fantasies and technological fixes.

IVF techniques (p 398), which already include direct injection of immature sperm nuclei incapable of fertilization into the egg (p 403), conserve deleterious mutations perpetuating and amplifying infertility in the human population. Sperm counts have been falling (p 404), partly as a result of the feminization of nature from industrial estrogen contamination (p 406), putting further pressure on this technology. Experiments are under way to see if a human embryo can be engineered from two sperm nuclei and an enucleate egg (p 407), or from two egg nuclei to satisfy the cultural desire of homosexuals of both sexes to have offspring who are children of both partners (p 409). These techniques could render sexual fertility obsolete. Massive over use of Caesarian delivery (p 398) also has the potential to make natural birth unviable by removing natural selection at a principal point of difficulty in human evolution. Contraceptive techniques, while essential to control a burgeoning population and provide sexual freedom of choice, particularly for women, have divorced our sexuality from the reproductive quest, cutting sexuality off from its biological motivation in fertility. Consequently extreme cultural imbalances are developing in the reproduction rate. While paternity testing and the sexing of unborn infants provides valuable information to and about parents, it is both exposing our innate sexual strategies, and potentially exacerbating existing trends to cull offspring of one sex or another for cultural or personal reasons.

At the same time there are pressures to engineer the germ line (p 414) to remove genes for deleterious conditions, or undesirable characteristics, with neither a clear idea of the evolutionary implications nor the ethical implications. Proposals are afoot to begin across the board IVF combined with genetic testing as an avenue of choice for all births to screen for and avoid a variety of genetic defects (p 401). In such a brave new world scenario we know neither how interactive this process may be not what grotesque directions runaway cultural and sentimental interference in our genetic identity could become. Both sickle cell and cystic fibrosis which many would love to eliminate confer disease resistance in heterozygous form against malaria and typhoid respectively two major world killers. The consequence of these changes for sexuality and our reproductive future are profound and can't be properly understood and debated while, despite our apparent sophistication, we remain naively in a state of cultural and personal denial about our sexual and sociobiological roots. We risk circumcising - lobotomizing, the very paradox of nature at the root of maleness and femaleness and life itself, and with it our sustainability as a species.

Our two natures carry, hidden within their diversity, not only our sex wars, but imprints of ancient genetic wars of attrition, including cytoplasmic incompatibility between isogametes (p 335), which first consumed the cytoplasm of one sex to form the sperm, causing the male to become the 'sneaky' low-investment sex (p 340) and which carry with them all the tangled history of life between. A history of mutual genetic pot-shots that have molded our X and Y-chromosomes (p 340) and sometimes attack one sex or another with infertility or death (p 336), in a mutual, perilously unstable arms race of sexually-antagonistic coevolution (p 16). A genetic struggle between male genes which would force the female to invest all her reproductive energy immediately in his offspring, expressed in the invasiveness of the placenta itself. The female's resistance to this is also indelibly marked in our genome, in a precarious 'balance' between opposing male and female forces, in genetic imprinting which may govern the development of our emotional and intellectual brains (p 346), and can cause pathological conditions, or fetal abnormalities, when either opposing influence is disrupted.

The gender polarization of internally fertilizing (p 334), gestating, lactating mammals (p 29), where sexual and parental investment is as one-sided as it can be, has evolved to an even more radical extreme in the full-blown 'travail' and voluptuous pregnancy of the human female (p 83), with her pendulous sequelae in lactation, and her unique dilemmas of maternal care amid ambivalence (p 35) at such a huge investment in time, effort and resources in the face of fluctuating male support. Women have solved this dilemma, both in partnership with males, and in allo-parenting (p 88) with older daughters, post-menopausal grandmothers, female friends and others, in cooperative familial and tribal networks. We thus cannot expect to reduce this tangled tale to a convenient androgynous erotic simplicity, devoid of reproductive meaning. The only viable answer is to accept and reflower the paradox of sexuality for what it is - the sweetest yet most devastating prisoners' dilemma of immortality, fertilized between mortal sexual beings, where we will always, like the Red Queen (p 26), be running while standing almost still, treading water while putting the very best of our creative potential into a seemingly unwinnable race of culture, art, music, and the music of love and lust - not 'against the opposite sex', but 'with the complementary one'.

Males should accept the rewards that come from flying like a moth into the flame of female sexual desire, revering menarche as sacred, and as good husbands, resting content if some four out of every five offspring sired by our partner are our own progeny, accepting in love those that may not be, while sewing the wild oats we can, as the male sex has striven to do since time immemorial, just as serial monogamy has indeed become a form of 'moderate' polygyny in the US, due to differences in remarriarge and subsequent fertility rates between divorced, or separated men and women. Until we bring our two natures together, life, and human society, even the biosphere, raped and exploited, will remain forever in the valley of the shadow of death, that great shadowy vagina that swallowed Maui when the fantail cried out, which all men fear, but which is also the source of life renewed. Our two orgasms, one 'a mere shot in the dark', and the other 'the perfect wave', contain an oracle - the unveiling, the key, the coda, the tattoo and taboo, the nemesis and genesis, the Song of Songs, the belonging and the longing, and the future destiny of our immortally entwined human sexes. The emergence of cultural complexity appears to be a result of human evolution in a condition of reproductive sexual paradox in which neither sex has had the upper hand, driven by sexual selection and displays of cultural prowess as genuine indicators of fitness. This selection involved both sexes in mutual mate choice but predominantly through the female reproductive choice common to many species despite attempts by males to preempt this through male competition and domination.

Ultimately we come back to the conscious mind and to the balance between the analytical thought often prized by men and 'feminine' intuition - between empathy and analysis and the paradoxes of how 'eureka' can emerge from the neurodynamic chaos of an unsolved problem. We are thus brought back to square one, coming now from the 'feminine' side of physical nature, looking at consciousness as an 'internal model of reality' made by the brain - potentially a mere illusion of matter, thus counterbalancing the mind-sky emphasis on primal cosmic mind of and the philosophy of the primacy of 'self' and 'soul' and again right into the abyss of cosmic sexual paradox. Here the problem lies, waiting for our apocalyptic unveiling to reveal all, no longer as through a glass darkly, but face to face - in the 'naked awareness' of sexual paradox itself. Thus we come to the present context and find ourselves as sentient conscious beings inhabiting a biological genetic organism, with a sappy biochemical brain, whose electrochemical excitations evoke the most puzzling unsolved mystery of modern science, that of subjective conscious experience and the enigma of free-will. Although materialistic views of science have endeavoured to finesse consciousness away as an epiphenomenon and free-will as an illusion, the development of consciousness research attests to the fact that subjective consciousness remains a founding phenomenon lying qualitatively outside the confines of objective description. Although mind states can be correlated with brain states they are qualitatively so different that we are brought full circle to the question "Is subjective consciousness a complementary manifestation to all objective phenomena, as fundamental as the cosmic origin itself?

Although human culture appears to have flowered through runaway aspects of sexual paradox in human evolutionary origins among gatherer-hunter clans, a male reaction has subsequently occurred from the earliest foundings of Jericho and Sumeria with the growth of militarized urban societies, through the great civilization of the East and West to the present day against sexual paradox, and its implicit paternity uncertainty. Patriarchal human cultures have endeavoured since to assert paradigms of order over these primal contradictions. A continuing trend throughout our cultural history has been for the climax diversity of sexual paradox to become undermined, or made degenerate, by patterns of male sexual domination, which lead to breakdown of the complexity and verdant instability, into ordered patterns of control, and often of repression, violence, and genocide which lead to planetary rape and exploitation and compromise the living genesis and emergence in complexity sexual paradox evokes. We shall thus explore, along with sexual paradox itself, all the many ways in which its breakdown leads to double jeopardy and how sexual paradox is a koan and oracle for our social transformation to a sustainable society.

The Inescapable Game of Life

"All's fair in love and war" leads us to a point of no return. To all intents and purposes, love is the uniting force of empathy and requital, and war is the ultimate Armageddon, conflict run amok on a collective scale. How can the two ends of the spectrum be so indistinguishably entwined? What does this spell out about our striving for unity in the face of disunion? What hope do we have of reaching a resolution, if love and war are so equatable - indeed equitable - as if dark and light were simply faces of one another? And what does it mean to say that ALL is fair, as if every position we could take, from integrity to deceit, from faithfulness to betrayal, are all legitimate players of a summer game? And how do we successfully negotiate these paradoxically entwined paths, one of which leads to a wasteland of attrition, wounding and death and the other to paradoxical reunion, completion, abundance and life? This is the answer to the Prisoners' Dilemma in sexual paradox.

Of course, life is a game we can never escape except in death. The evolutionary struggle is no better, doomed to a purgatory of survival amid conflict and cooperation, so long as our genes mutate and survive. The only culmination of this game is extinction. The outright wins all animals have, in the predatory process of feeding, are merely another step on the road of survival, staving of the hour of final reckoning.

The Prisoners' Dilemma as a classical game matrix. Payoffs for each player are such that each is 'tempted' into defection, resulting in mutual nemesis. Attempts to resolve the devastating simplicity of the matrix may involve conditional strategies (e.g. I'll do what you do) or mixed strategies playing both strategies with probabilities. Real tournaments also involve repeated and sequential exchanges, which encourage cooperation, at least until the last round or two.

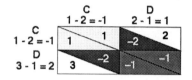

The Prisoners' Dilemma

The Prisoners' Dilemma is a universal contradiction of betrayal in game theory in which mutual defection leads to the 'double jeopardy' of collective downfall. In the classic case, two criminals are to be tried for a joint offence. If one betrays the other and becomes an informant, they will get protection, but the other will go down as the ringleader with no parole. If they both stay silent, they will only get done for a minor offence, but if both defect and spill the beans they will get a jail term for conspiracy. If the game is played only once, any rational player will defect. If they cooperate in silence they will at best get a minor felony and worst no parole, but if they defect, they might get sprung with a middle term, or they might get off with a non-custodial sentence. However an astute player facing repeat encounters will be much more canny and cooperate, at least until the last round's high noon.

Joseph Heller's "Catch 22" (R300), describes a classic form of the Prisoners' Dilemma as a logically paradoxical double bind. With a growing hatred of flying, Yossarian pleads to be grounded on the basis of insanity. His appeal is however useless because, according to army regulation Catch-22, insane men who ask to be grounded prove themselves sane through a concern for personal safety. The only truly crazy people are those who readily agree to fly more missions. The only way to be grounded is to ask for it, yet this act demonstrates sanity and thus demands further flying. Crazy or not, Yossarian is stuck.

The Prisoners' Dilemma is a root paradox permeating all areas of knowledge, from the stability of rational assumptions of best interest in economics (R101) to the fractal complexity of climax forests (p 506). It's status has been acknowledged by economists and utopian thinkers, from Hobbes to Rousseau. All its diverse forms involve the splitting of a process, under increasing polarization into competing domains leading to nemesis - any situation in which the participating entities are 'tempted' into a course of action which would bring disaster if everyone did the same thing. The game applies in a chilling manner to the risks of nuclear war and the knife-edge advantage of first strike.

Ironically one of the first people to introduce the concept of cooperation into a view of nature as a pitiless "war of each against all" as Thomas Huxley described it in Hobbes' words, was the Russian anarchist Prince Petr Kropotkin (Ridley R565), who had himself escaped prison in a daring ingenious feat of cooperative insurrection. In 'Mutual Aid' (R385) he rejected the notion that selfishness is an animal legacy and morality a civilized one, claiming that supportive species were fitter than those endlessly at war, challenging a long tradition, going back through Malthus and Machiavelli to Augustine, shared today in the stress on competition as a motivating force for the free market. We can see in Kropotkin's twist of fate just how conducive to 'inscrutable cooperation' in a Machiavellian context, the Prisoners' Dilemma can be. Kropotkin's work emphasizing the role of cooperation and his intuitive opposition to an exclusive focus on competition has recently received recognition from authors as diverse as Ridley (R564) and de Waal (R161).

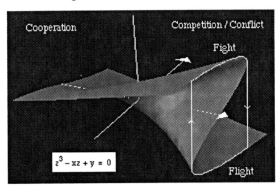

The cusp, the first of Rene Thom's classical catastrophes (R673) enters criticality, causing the process to bifurcate between competing regimes. As x passes through 0 the surface folds, causing cooperation to move into competition, and behavior to flip between fight and flight. Prisoners' dilemma games attempt to resolve the disparity between these two conditions and their varying payoffs.

The Prisoners' Dilemma became transformed into the battleground of the genetic arms race by the work of evolutionary biologists George Williams and William Hamilton in the 1960s epitomized by Richard Dawkins (R150) infectious phrase "the selfish gene". This shifted the pendulum from collective concepts, such as 'survival of the species' and 'group selection' to a detailed analysis of how genes act as agents of their own selection in a way which leaves even the poor organism little more than a doomed collection of apparently selfish genes, barely held in check in a common, yet shifting genome. While group selection and the capacity for social selection has not been entirely extinguished, George Williams in 1966 demonstrated that it is unstable to individual defection. The primacy of genetic selection shone a new spotlight on the exact processes of selection providing stable strategies in evolution, which are robust to defection.

The Red Queen hypothesis of sexuality (p 26) with its paradoxes between parasite and host and between female and male genetically and more particularly sexual evolution, both of which we shall examine next, are outstanding examples of the Prisoners' Dilemma. In the sexual context the Prisoners' Dilemma genetic race between female and male is also bifurcated between the differing strategies of female out-front long-term investment and the male strategies of sneaky short term fertilization and direct male-male reproductive conflict. Thus not only do we have male and female locked in a genetic race from which neither can escape, but the male strategy is prone to natural flight and fight of its own accord. This male tendency to conflict is liable to a break down of the game into a male dominance over the female, profoundly exaggerating the tendency to violence and war. Thus while the male and female are both strategic players of the game, they also represent relative extremes of the energy landscape in terms of cooperation or conflict. The emergence of patriarchal dominance in human society has been explained as a response to ecological stress (Sanday R596 181) in terms entirely consistent with a symmetry-breaking of the Prisoners' Dilemma between male and female into a protracted impasse involving crisis and instability.

The arms races that result from the Red Queen process extend via the Prisoners' Dilemma to all forms of competitive arms race, such as the mutually assured destruction from nuclear holocaust we have all continued to face since the beginning of the Cold War despite symbolic efforts at nuclear arms reduction, the knife-edge cooperator-defector zero-infinity dilemmas of launching a first strike and all runaway militarization races between competing powers, who could also cooperate to their mutual but less successfully exploitative benefit. It also applies to mediation between intergroup competition, protection from aggression and the consequent need for cooperation within groups in evolving the kinds of systems we come to associate with morality, ethics and the rule of law. Richard Alexander (R6) in "The Biology of Moral Systems" has given an in-depth analysis of the relationship between these two phenomena which has been widely applied by many researchers (p 44). Key here is the interaction between inevitable competition between groups which are large in the case of humanity and the complementary ensuing need to evoke systems of social selection which ensure the group is internally cooperative enough to remain competitive or even dominant. The theory thus explains the emergence of moral systems and ethics based on principles of natural selection, rather than cultural constructs alone. The breakdown of such moral conventions often involves the breaking of a common pact for individual gain, as when a ring of hunters joining to encircle a deer is broken by one person or another diving off after a rabbit he is sure to catch, as noted originally by Rousseau. A similar analysis by Turchin (R693) examines cycles of cooperative foundation, empire, growth of inequality, disaffection on the turbulent perimeter, and rebellion.

The Prisoners' Dilemma also comes in more complex ecosystemic forms than the one-on-one arms races of host-parasite and sexual relations . The complexity of a climax forest is the result of a prisoners dilemma relationship between many plant species competing for light. It also permeates animal species in the natural competition between the members of a population for reproductive, and food resources and for personal power and fortune. Nowak and Sigmund (R499) point out that evolutionary game theory places the usually presumed constant fitness landscape of natural selection in a feedback process, in which payoffs can be reversed by population changes, leading to rare strategies being reinforced (p 60), amid stable coexistence or unstable oscillation, or punctuated equilibrium.

A graphic illustration of the diversity of life as a Prisoners' Dilemma game caught midway between cooperation and defection is given by the diversification into plants and animals, (p 327). Plants are broadly cooperative although there is always competition for limiting resources since they fix their energy from sunlight rather than depending on consuming one another. Animals defect by directly consuming plants, subsequently bifurcating into second order defections in the form of predatory carnivores who also eat other animals. The earliest life forms were either phototrophs, or converted free mineral energy such as that in hydrothermal vents, so the evolution of life into diversity is a movement from initial cooperative exploitation of an external energy source, subsequently filling sufficient defection niches to provide ever-increasing diversity to climax and the pyramidal populations of food webs.

The evolutionary tree of life is our richest example of the Prisoners' Dilemma. The survival of every gene of every species is a Prisoners' Dilemma. Each gene, organism and species lives as long as its Prisoners' Dilemma of coexistence as parasite and host, predator and prey, symbiotic, saprophytic and reciprocal interactions with others of its kind. As long as we survive, we remain locked in the Prisoners' Dilemma mediation of cooperative and competitive forces that we call life. Death is a loss. The only hope is to remain in the game. This however condemns each species to evolutionary adaption through mutation. This brings in the issue of genetic algorithms and the entire concept of gene as a fundamental response to the Prisoners' Dilemma in molecular terms.

A paradigm-defining example of Prisoners' Dilemma is the 'tragedy of the commons', which Gareth Hardin (R283) used as the title of his renowned paper on the exploitation of the commons in economics (p 439). In this form of the paradox, it always pays off exploiters of the commons better to claim the competitive certainty of exploitation than the 'altruists' who cooperate to preserve the common wealth. The end result is multiple jeopardy, the commons is destroyed and every one loses out. Various forms of the tragedy of the commons underlie all of the major forms of human exploitation on the planet, from depletion of non-renewable resources to causing the mass extinction of biodiversity.

Puccini's opera Tosca well illustrates how deeply related the Prisoners' Dilemma is to sex and sexual betrayal. Tosca's lover Cavaradossi has been condemned to death by the police chief Scarpia. He offers her to tell the firing squad to use blanks if she will sleep with him. She resolves to pretend to agree to lie with him only to stab him to death as soon he has given the order. He gives a coded order to use live bullets and she stabs him, instead of submitting to his advances, only to find he has also betrayed her and executed her lover regardless. She commits suicide in despair. Double betrayal. Triple jeopardy.

The sexual relationship is from beginning to end a permanent state of Prisoners' Dilemma paradox. The two sexes are reproductively entwined, so neither can escape the other. Even parthenogenesis is only a temporary fix, until evolving circumstances, such as disease, require sexual adaption for survival. For this reason sex has remained an essential feature of higher organisms. Although the interests of the female and male coincide in reproductive fertilization, their overall reproductive strategies and genetic 'drives' are competing in significant ways, both reproductively and genetically.

In describing the dilemma of female chimps mating promiscuously with every male to avert the threat of infanticide from the males, Sarah Hrdy (R324) notes the cutting truth of William Rice's term "sexually antagonistic coevolution" (R562), emphasizing the Prisoners' Dilemma of the interaction for each sex. Increasing female choosiness in relation to the lengthening peacocks tail is an example of sexually-antagonistic coevolution, as is the race between an increasingly turgid penis and an increasingly discriminating clitoris.

Darwin noted somewhat chauvanistically: "man has ultimately become superior to woman. It is indeed fortunate that the law of equal transmission of characters to both sexes prevails with mammals. Otherwise it is probable that man would have become as superior in mental endowment to woman as the peacock is in ornamental plumage to the peahen". The fallacy of this position is itself an irony - the attribution of reproductive choice principally to females and runaway sexual selection principally to males . The realities of human sexual evolution, while they do support sperm competition and moderate polygyny speak strongly of a more complex pattern of mutual mate selection, something Darwin also recognized was possible as Geoffrey Miller has noted. It is this very complexity that we shall claim is at the centre of our cultural emergence.

William Rice's cogent commentary comes from his experiments into the mating habits of flies, where male semen reduces the subsequent fertility of the female at the expense of rearing the current male's progeny, either by plugging her, inserting digestive enzymes, or affecting her hormonally. For this reason a female house fly mates only once, because her partner's poisons are so potent she can never mate again (Jones R340). In other species of fly, where multiple mating occurs, an arms race sets in between male toxins and female resistance. Consequently these genes are the most rapidly evolving in insects. This process is accentuated when mating is frequent but diminishes when mating occurs only rarely or once in a lifetime. During fruit-fly sex, the proteins in the semen enter the bloodstream of the female and migrate to, among other places, her brain. There they have the effect of reducing the female's sexual appetite and increasing her ovulation rate. The male's seminal fluid redirects her behaviour to that end. After breeding generations of increasingly 'super-macho' male flies while allowing the females' resistance to diminish, Rice found the semen had become toxic to the point of being lethal (Friedman R225 235, Ridley R566). Hrdy (1999 41) comments that this demonstrates the way in which not only female reproductive choice but its curtailment can have profound consequences.

A fundamental characteristic of modern mammals - the birth of live young - is another extreme example of this phenomenon. The placenta is controlled by rapidly evolving paternal genes. As noted a double Y induces a placental pregnancy called a hydatidiform mole. David Haig (Ridley R566) considers the placenta to be a parasitic takeover of the mother's body by paternal genes in the fetus. The placenta tries, against maternal resistance, to control her blood-sugar levels and blood pressure to the benefit of the fetus. By contrast X-inactivation in female embryos is skewed from a random process in cells inside the embryo towards inactivating the paternally-imprinted X in the placenta (p 346). Boys also impose a greater strain on the mother, causing her to have a longer lapse until her next child, possibly increasing the chances of abnormalities in subsequent pregnancies and reducing the mothers life expectancy by about 6 months. By contrast a girl child slightly increases it. The male determining gene SRY and the female pathway driven by DAX are similarly in a state of sex-determining conflict. One SRY defeats DAX giving our usual male profile but an accidental two DAX in the genome overwhelm SRY resulting in a female (p 358). Intriguingly, endogenous retroviruses or ERVs, transmitted down the germ line of every mammal, may have also played a starring role in the evolution of mammalian life and its crowning achievement-live birth. ERVs which bloom on the placental tissue, appear to be critical to the emergence of the placental membrane and the mechanisms that protect the fetus from pathogens and the mother's immune system. Without ERVs, humans might still be laying eggs (p 333).

Ridley (R566) notes that communication itself becomes an informational pawn in the game: "Rice and Holland come to the disturbing conclusion that the more social and communicative a species is, the more likely it is to suffer from sexually antagonistic genes, because communication between the sexes provides the medium in which sexually antagonistic genes thrive. The most social and communicative species on the planet is humankind. Suddenly it begins to make sense why relations between the human sexes are such a mine field, and why men have such vastly different interpretations of what constitutes sexual harassment from women. Rice now believes that sexual antagonism is at work in an sorts of environments. It leaves its signature as rapidly evolving genes." Consistent with this, Dawkins has pointed out that 'information' serves the 'giver' only if it includes a component of self-serving deceit. This is not however true of genuine indicators of fitness, such as the peacock's tail, which have to be costly to be effective in the sexual race.

We may have genetic conflict to thank for the fact that we have feelings toward other people at all. One might at first think that evolution would endow a species in which the genetic interests of two mates were identical, with a blissful perfection of sexual, romantic, and companionate love, but, Donald Symons argues the relation between the mates would then evolve to be like the relation among the cells of a single body, whose genetic interests are also identical. There would be no falling in love, because there would be no alternative mates to choose among, and falling in love would be a huge waste. You would literally love your mate as yourself, but - you don't really love yourself, you *are* yourself. The same is true for our emotions toward family and friends: the richness and intensity of the feelings in our minds are proof of the preciousness and fragility of those bonds in real life. In short, without the possibility of suffering, what we would have is not harmonious bliss, but little or no emotional consciousness (Pinker R532 268).

This kind of conflict between complexes of genes does not just apply to sex but to all forms of deceit and detection of cheating the Prisoners' Dilemma game implies. A gene that increases the telling of lies might thrive by making its possessors successful con-artists. But then any set of genes that improves the detecting of lies would thrive to the extent that it enabled its possessors to avoid being taken in. The two would evolve antagonistically, each gene encouraging the other, even though it would be quite possible for the same person to possess both. Rice and Holland call this 'interlocus contest evolution' (R563). If the conflicting genes are on different chromosomes or not closely linked they can both evolve. The signature of such genes is rapid evolution and in comparing human and mouse genomes, such genes are notably found in immunity and sex determination.

Ridley notes: "Exactly such a competitive process probably did indeed drive the growth of human intelligence over the past three million years. Most evolutionists believe in the Machiavellian theory that bigger brains were needed in an arms race between manipulation and resistance to manipulation. In Rice and Holland's words: "The phenomena we refer to as intelligence may be a by-product of intergenomic conflict between genes mediating offense and defense in the context of language".

However in spite of competition, sexual destinies are inextricably entangled. Two male imprinted genes in mice , Mest and Peg-3 are both involved in good mothering in daughters (p 346). Peg-3 affects neurons that react to oxytocin, inducing lactation and mediating maternal behavior. Mice with defective Peg were slower to build a nest and gather stray pups, losing 9/10ths rather than the normal 2/10ths of their first litters. It is difficult to interpret good mothering in daughters as selectively benefiting male genes.

Sexual selection by the opposite sex, particularly the female is pivotal in evolutionary viability. We need sex to survive, while sacrificing half our genetic endowment to another and suffering the ultimate penalty - mortality - in seeking the variety sex produces. We can ultimately succeed at playing this Prisoners' Dilemma game only through producing viable offspring and in this the investments and strategies of men and women are clearly as different as our haploid manifestation as sperm and ovum. A man's investment can be as small as a few drops of semen, but a woman's is as overwhelming as pregnancy, as needful as lactation and as enduring as childhood. Men marry and sew wild oats, while women seek a resourceful monogamous partner and have secretive affairs. Neither is strictly faithful overall, nor could they be and fully protect their own genetic heritage. There is thus no escape from the paradox of sexual betrayal either, just temporary respite in fidelity and love's sweet embrace. The downfall of the Prisoners' Dilemma game in marital discord, jealousy, divorce, violence and desertion is a frequent cause of murder and suicide.

The sexually paradoxical nature of the mind-body relationship brings with it the implicit risk of 'double jeopardy'. The root of the existential dilemma is to experience consciousness through a physical body suffering inevitable decay and mortality. Yet the physical world and with it our body and sensory organs are our gateway to conscious experience (p 364). In the breakdown of this paradox into conflict comes the notion of light and dark forces and the mortal combat of god and satan. This has led religious thinkers, from the first gnostics, through Augustine, all the way to modern Western culture to perceive conscious existence as a spiritual, godlike self or soul trapped in lustful, fallible, flesh (p 242). A flesh that both condemns us to mortality through its frailty and robs us of our freedom through sexual desire. The penis, which is the source of future life for mankind, then becomes an agent of the devil's work. In turn, lubricious sexual intercourse with demons became a central fantasy in the witch hunts. This degenerate view of sex as evil exploitative lust still pervades Western society's views. It continues to surface in diverse forms of perversion, pornography and prostitution.

Given the universal nature of the Prisoners' Dilemma, it is of little surprise to discover that humans are innately attuned to distinguishing cheating, deceit and betrayal. In many experiments Leda Cosmides and John Tooby have shown that we can far more easily solve a logical puzzle if it is presented as a question of detecting betrayal. To detect proof of unmitigated altruism is far more counter-intuitive. Matt Ridley (R565) illustrates this in the following story. Chief Kiku, who demands his followers are tattooed, tells four hungry villagers "If you get a tattoo on your face you will get a cassava root in the morning". A visiting economist wonders "Will he keep his word?", while an anthropologist, thinking he is bluffing says "Surely he would not refuse food to a man just because he didn't get a tattoo!" Kiku's reply is "Tell me this or I will tattoo your faces myself. The first got a tattoo, the second had nothing to eat, the third did not get a tattoo and the fourth I gave a large cassava root. Now tell me which of them you must ask of to answer your question." This is an example of the "Wason test", which is counter-intuitive as a logical puzzle unless it is presented as a test of breaking a social contract. Three quarters of Stanford students get the answer to economist's puzzle right, but most flunk the anthropologist's test.

The paradox underlying the Prisoners' Dilemma has a kind of physical realization in the form of a 'spin glass - a material in which a set of embedded spins, acting in the same way as molecular domains in a magnet, are coupled by a random, normally distributed linkage. Unlike a ferromagnet, where all the spins line up in one dominant, polarized minimum energy state, a spin glass has a large number of potential energy minima in which cooperation between some spins results in frustration between others. The medium partitions into zones of cooperation punctuated by interfaces of defection. This displays a deep relationship between symmetry-breaking, complexity, instability, and the Prisoners' Dilemma.

The intractable nature of the Prisoners' Dilemma in the 1960s made it a cause celebre in the burgeoning area of game theory in economics. At first theorists believed there was no escape from the implications that the game equilibrium favoured selfishness because the relative payoffs of the strategies of each meant that defection remained a strategic equilibrium for both players. Human generosity thus seemed an aberrant and foolish deviation. But then a new generation of game tournaments set a stage for a more realistic appreciation for a way out. In the first of these, it was noted that real humans playing repeated Prisoners' Dilemma games are much nicer to one another than the single game payoffs would suggest. Knowing the rules of the game they generally cooperated till the end of the tournament when they would stage final defections to secure a terminal advantage.

In the 1970s there came a convergence with evolutionary biology in the form of John Maynard-Smith's concept of an 'evolutionarily stable strategy' - a product of natural selection which would arrive at a game theoretic strategic equilibrium and hence be sustainable in evolutionary terms because no strategy of an opponent could lead to break down of the selected trait. Towards the end of the decade the rise of computers made strategic tournaments possible and the political scientist Robert Axelrod, exploring the logic of cooperation, catalyzed the first strategic answer to the Prisoners' Dilemma. He invited all comers to submit computer programs to a repeated tournament of 200 games. The astounding result was that a simple strategy in the form of 'tit-for-tat', submitted by Anatol Rapoport, another political scientist, with an interest in problems of nuclear confrontation, proved the decisive winner. We all know tit-for-tat in the form of the Biblical invocation of 'an eye for an eye and a tooth for a tooth'. We also know tit-for-tat is forgiving in cooperation, doesn't seek to defect, but punishes defectors by retaliation. However it does have one serious flaw - intractable bouts of revenge retaliation. Following on from this discovery emerged a whole series of challenges in a development of the game in which strategies could compete and proliferate according to their success in the manner of an artificial life experiment. While 'tit-for-tat' was singularly effective at driving out the hawks of defection, even 'nicer' strategies which broke the impasse of retaliation surfaced. Upon his discovery, Axelrod contacted William Hamilton and a further expansion of understanding occurred. Evolutionary genetics was at this time in full retreat from the notion of group and species selection, with the realization that selection was predominantly on an individual, not a species basis, and that it was genes and certain genetic traits which were being selected for, not the welfare of the organism or the species as a whole. Richard Dawkins' notion of 'the selfish gene'(R150), although a clichéd oversimplification, carries a root truth - that it is *genes* which are being selected, even if the vast majority do so under the constraints of co-residing in a given organism, which must itself survive under social, and environmental, conditions, including running the gauntlets of sexual enticement, and good parenting, shared by a species.

This pendulum has now swung back from the brink of extreme genetic selfishness, in a recognition that group social selection can also play an important role in shaping individual traits. If battery hens are selected for individual laying capacity they tend to compete, become stressed, and not to lay well in cages. However selecting for good laying cages results in socially more compatible chickens which lay better over all. More generally, forms of social selection, from ostracism to violence, do have selective evolutionary effect. Nevertheless genetic selection is the key to the whole mechanism of mutation and selective advantage, so biologists have ever since sought with ingenuity to elucidate ways in which genetic selection could give rise to the altruism we find in human interactions.

A key step was Hamilton's discovery of 'kin selection' - the idea that organisms will evolve not just to preserve and reproduce their own genes but will also invest in the protection of the common genes they share with their relatives and offspring. This relation is neatly expressed in the inequality $C < Br$, where C is the cost, B the fitness benefits and r the relatedness of the benefited relative. We thus expect raw genetic considerations to favour strategies where an organism will invest around half as much effort in protecting immediate offspring and siblings as in one's own livelihood. A host of examples confirm these principles in nature, from the honey bee to chimpanzees. As Hamilton (R279) put it: "a gene causing altruistic behavior towards brothers or sisters will be selected only if the behavior and the circumstances are generally such that the gain is more than twice the loss

... to put the matter more vividly, an animal acting on principle would sacrifice its life if it could thereby save more than two brothers, but not for less" (Hrdy R323 64).

Robert Trivers (R689) then introduced the wider arena of reciprocal altruism. De Waal (R162 24), in exploring friendship and mutual aid, notes the outstanding characteristics of reciprocation: "Rather than simplifying the relations between genes and behavior, [Trivers' article] pays full attention to the intermediate levels such as emotions and psychological processes. It also distinguishes different types of cooperation based on what each participant pus into and gets out of it. For example cooperation for immediate reward does not qualify as reciprocal altruism. ... Because of the instant payoff, this kind of cooperation is widespread [and could be viewed as mutual self-interest]. Reciprocal altruism on the other hand costs something before it delivers benefits. It has the following three characteristics: (a) the exchanged acts, while beneficial to the recipient are costly to the performer, (b) there is a time lag between giving and receiving, (c) giving is contingent on receiving."

Hamilton was struck by the correspondence of Axelrod's results with Trivers' idea of reciprocal selection. This would require each to punish cheating by reciprocating only with individuals who had fulfilled their part of the reciprocation bargain, and would thus require careful social discrimination and recognition. During the 1980s, field evidence of such reciprocation began to emerge. Vampire bats, who roost together in hollow trees, can generally get more than a meal for themselves if they do score a hapless victim in the night. They can only survive a day or two without blood and roost together so they have evolved an elaborate system of reciprocation to feed their neighbours, who are not necessarily genetically related. They have evolved to vomit excess blood to their co-residents on a reciprocal basis. These 'neighbours' have relatively stable roosting places although they are not necessarily related individuals. Reciprocation requires careful score keeping, rewarding cooperators and punishing defectors. To do this it needs stable long-term relationships without frequent mixing of individuals or the tally cannot be kept. Notably Vampire bats have the largest brains of bats, consistent with the relative complexity of such social discrimination. They also groom one another closely in the stomach region, which could be a giveaway for cheating. African vervet monkeys are similarly reciprocal in getting aid in fights. Cleaner fish on reefs are in a mutually reciprocal relationship with those they clean of parasites, who never seem to take advantage and eat the cleaners. Although this doesn't involve strict reciprocation, it clearly has reciprocal advantages.

However reciprocation is actually quite rare in the natural world, apart from a handful of additional examples from dolphins, monkeys and apes. Miller (R464 301) notes "Evolution appears to avoid reciprocity whenever possible". For example lionesses investigating a potential threat do not enforce reciprocal favours. Some lead the counter-threat and though they may look balefully at their laggardly sisters who slink behind, do not punish them for their cowardice even when it is repeated, or fails when most needed. In many situations, the payoffs may be too indifferent, the populations too mobile and the score keeping too cumbersome to maintain reciprocity. In addition the tit-for-tat nature of reciprocity, as we have noted, leads to intractable cycles of revenge punishment. De Waal notes "this process is evidently a lot more complicated than simultaneous cooperation. There is for example the problem of the first helpful act - a gamble since every partner does not follow the rules. ...Reciprocal altruism does not work for individuals who rarely meet or who have trouble keeping track of who has done what for whom: It requires good memories and stable relationships, such as are found in primates. De Waal then explores the evolution of what we might call 'morality' in "Good Natured" in the variety of mutual 'friendship' behavior in apes based on the similarity principle - contemporary individuals (particularly females) sharing mutual interests in a similar life situation and social ranking.

Game theorists such as Martin Nowak were quick to pick up on tit-for-tat's weaknesses and an artificial life contest ensued between different strategies under a variety of conditions. Probabilistic strategies now came into play which could vary their response a proportion of the time. In addition, learning from mistakes and successes were now allowed to take place. Out of this milieu came new strategic variants which could engulf 'tit-for-tat', such as 'generous', which forgives single defections about a third of the time but rejects them sufficiently to repel 'always defect'. Thus 'turning the other cheek' becomes part of astute Machiavellian behaviour. Among 'generous' players, 'always cooperate' can now thrive, but this again becomes susceptible to 'always defect', resulting in a complex system with no fully effective strategy, leaving a solution to the Prisoners' Dilemma again beyond reach. This cyclic ambiguity caused consternation until 'simpleton', a game originally invented by Rapoport, with a , with a 'win-stay; lose-shift' strategy, called 'simpleton' or 'Pavlov', once discarded because it was a 'sucker' to 'always defect' now proved to be able to trounce 'tit-for-tat' once 'always defect' was eliminated. Essentially tit-for-tat is an extrovert, who does what the opponent did last, and simpleton is an introvert who switches if they get punished. There is evidence for such behaviour in nature. In the alternate leading and following of stickleback scouting parties testing the reaction of predatory pike, which superficially looks like tit-for-tat reciprocation, the scout fish will alternate between defection and cooperation, when faced with persistent defection.

By introducing alternating moves, as in reciprocation, Marcus Frean established 'firm-but-fair' as a winning strategy. Like 'simpleton', this cooperates with cooperators, returns to cooperating after a mutual defection and punishes a sucker by further defection, but it also continues to cooperate after being the sucker in the previous round. This accords with the common sense of giving a good impression if you want others to act in your example. Even lowly guppies have complex scouting strategies, preferring reliable colleagues in scouting parties, ostracizing laggers, and being more tolerant of defections in consistent cooperators. Grim (R265) has noted that the sequence of such strategies results in the ultimate winner of the Prisoners' Dilemma becoming an undecidable proposition (p 491).

Prisoners' dilemma games can readily be played as cellular automata (p 510), leading to and complex and punctuated equilibria (p 21). Nowak et. al. (R495) have run such competitions with genetic algorithms for mutation and natural selection of strategies for millions of generations. Outcomes even for fixed automata may become formally undecidable (p 492) because they can only be modeled by a computational simulation.

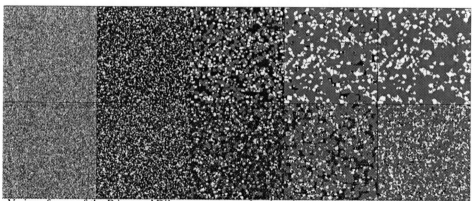

Various forms of the Prisoners' Dilemma game can be played as cellular automata, (p 510), which display complex punctuated equilibria between defectors (black), cooperators (red), tit-for-tatters (purple), 'simpletons' using win-stay lose-shift (green) and random strategies (cyan) (ex. Flake R212). Players on the grid play in pairs for several rounds and then each cell adopts the most successful strategy in its neighbourhood. The top row shows the 1st, 2nd, 5th, 10th and 50th tournaments. An initial wave of defection is taken over by reactive strategies. The system stratifies in a state dominated by tit-for-tat and 'simpleton' with a few islands of cooperators and the odd defector. The bottom row includes 10% mutation and noise and is in dynamic flux. Such interactions can help explain how reciprocal altruism can emerge without complex memory, if nearest neighbours remain stable, for example because of fixed territories in a given habitat (Nowak et. al. R495, R499).

Of course, in a real world, defection is the 'criminal' element that can never be fully eliminated once and for all. Mutation and selection are always throwing up such strategies in evolution in a manner which can never be eliminated. Parasites and disease are an inextricable part of the tooth and claw of the evolutionary endowment. Furthermore the realities of population movement allowing cheaters to drift to new victims and the varying payoffs each life situation provoke make it difficult or impossible for any single strategy to prevail. The ineradicability of defecting strategies is as signal of human society as it is of the evolutionary paradigm. Most people will learn to take advantage of flagrant opportunities foolishly presented. While criminality can be contained through a mix of penalties and good social policy, only in a naive world would it be expected to disappear entirely. Moreover in real situations, rare strategies often invoke equally high payoffs which guarantee no escape. In a promiscuous society of deceiving whores, a single faithful wife can command a king's ransom and will become at an inestimable advantage reproductively. By the same token in a monotonously monogamous society, a single scarlet woman can command the affections of every man to the highest station. Evolutionary geneticists comment that for this reason, pure genetic monogamy is not an evolutionarily stable strategy, always liable to invasion by 'fast' females and 'philandering' males. Thus the real games of life often tend to an equilibrium between cooperating and defecting strategies, making the Prisoners' Dilemma a permanent feature of natural and social survival. The Red Queen evolutionary arms race between parasites and prey is likewise a perpetuating prisoners dilemma, giving high enough payoffs to maintain sexuality, despite the halving of each parent's genetic endowment.

In mammalian evolution we also have the emergence of emotions and the effects of emotional reactions on the whole question of genetic determinism, selfishness and altruism. Rather than following instinctual or imprinted genetic strategies, mammalian brains have evolved a meta-strategy providing an emotional spectrum of reactions, from flight to fight, from love and close intimate bonding to hate, and the violence of hunting play, within which the direct simplicity of kin and reciprocal altruism become a complex emotional dynamic only partly genetically based. Instances abound, not just of seemingly irrational human generosity, which cannot be interpreted to benefit the individual directly or indirectly, but irrationally altruistic emotional reactions of mammals. A hippopotamus may repeatedly rescue a wounded gazelle from an alligator, or a lioness raise a young ungulate. We need to explain how evolution could have arrived at such an indirect emotional process as a universal win-win, given the raw constraints of natural genetic selection.

Even in human society, where we have large brains, and abundant capacity to detect cheating and punish defection, neither kin, nor reciprocal altruism, fully explain our behaviour. In differing circumstances, we may retaliate like the vampire, or endure laggards like the lioness. We also have an innate capacity to respond to the plight of others, who may be unrelated, or not even of the same species, with acts of compassion, for which no reward can be gained, or expected. Although human societies have imposed Draconian punishments for criminal defection and sexual betrayal, our life relationships are motivated by the unbounded quest for love and belonging as by astute judgement of character.

A good indication of the degree to which human societies respond to the general issue of egalitarian cooperation comes from the ultimatum bargaining game, where a player is offered a financial reward which they can keep only if they give sufficient to a second player for them to accept the bargain. The second player thus receives either the offered portion, or nothing if they refuse and one might expect them to accept only a small portion. However they also know the first player will receive nothing either if they do so they can quickly punish for perceived 'cheating' on a fair bargain. Even when players play anonymously, so do not suffer a retaliatory round, the experienced players in many cultures from Los Angeles (48%) to Yogyakarta and Tokyo (45%) end up offering only a little less than half - with the most frequent amount being a half share, reflecting the keen eye humans in many cultures have for not accepting a second-class treatment. The people of Jerusalem were a little more stingy at 36% and the Machiguenga of the upper Amazon were a notable exception, offering only a meagre 24% of the booty (Henrich R301).

In the Dictator game, the proposer simply divides the sum between the two players and there is nothing the respondent can do about it. With no fear of reprisal, the proposer makes a far stingier offer. The offer still tends to be more generous than it has to be, because the proposer worries about getting a reputation for stinginess that could come back to bite him in the long run. We know this because of the outcome of the Double-

Blind Dictator game, where proposals from many players are sealed and neither the respondent nor the experimenter knows who offered how much. In this variant, generosity plummets; a majority of the proposers keep everything for themselves (Pinker R532 256).

Another game which aptly demonstrates tendency to a winning defection by a dominant group and has major implications for first past the post election, majority democracy and the consequent 'tyranny of the majority' is illustrated as follows. Seven people are given anonymous numbers and connected by computer network. If they are asked to reach consensual agreement to gain a reward, they will negotiate to do so. However, if they are told simply to find a majority to get the reward, they will quickly engage the minimum number of four at random or by pattern, e.g. 1,2,3 and 4 or 1,3,5, and 7, and go straight for the booty, cutting the other three out of the bargain. Majority 'defection' against the whole becomes the rule.

In the 'public good' game, everyone makes a voluntary contribution to a common pot of money, the experimenter doubles it, and the pot is divided evenly among the participants regardless of what they contributed. The optimal strategy for each player acting individually is to be a free rider and contribute nothing, hoping others will contribute something and he can get a share of their contribution. Of course, if every player thinks that way, the pot stays empty and no one earns a dime. The optimum for the group is for all the players to contribute everything they have so they can all double their money. When the game is played repeatedly, however, everyone tries to become a free rider, and the pot dwindles to a self-defeating zero. On the other hand, if people are allowed both to contribute to the pot and to levy fines on those who don't contribute, conscience doth make cowards of them all, and almost everyone contributes to the common and profitable good (R532 257).

Left: Real play in the prisoners dilemma game between pairs of women involves high levels of mutual cooperation until the last few rounds. Right: Play against a computer engaging tit-for-tat results in reciprocal defection (R570).

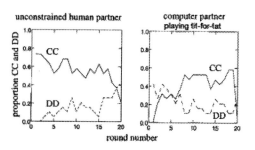

People do more for their fellows than return favors and punish cheaters. They often perform generous acts without the slightest hope for pay back, ranging from leaving a tip in a restaurant they will never visit again to throwing themselves on a live grenade to save their brothers in arms. Trivers, and economists Robert Frank and Jack Hirshleifer, have pointed out that pure magnanimity can evolve in an environment of people seeking to discriminate fair-weather friends from loyal allies. Signs of heartfelt loyalty and generosity serve as guarantors of one's promises, reducing a partner's worry that you will default on them. The best way to convince others that you are trustworthy and generous is to be trustworthy and generous. Indeed many players of the prisoners dilemma game choose to cooperate consistently until the last few rounds and altruistic punishing of defectors even at high cost to the perpetrator is another paradoxical sign of 'moral' defection for the common good.

Simple virtue cannot be the dominant mode of human interaction or we could dispense with the deliberate financial and legal processes designed to keep exchanges fair and base our economy on the honor system. At the other extreme, people also commit acts of outright treachery and deceitful or criminal exploitation. Machiavellian traits are a central part of human nature, with most people displaying mixtures of, pure generosity, reciprocity and expedience (R532 259). Brain experiments (p 378) have verified that the common emotional basis of both cooperation and altruistic punishment stems from anticipation of social satisfaction associated with pleasure - hence the term 'revenge is sweet'.

We thus need to look more deeply for sources for the natural goodness we associate with social altruism, emotional bonding and human agreeableness and love. It is here that Geoffrey Miller's ideas of sexual selection (p 53) come into their own. Miller notes that all forms of social selection are weak and indirect by comparison with the inescapable powerful positive feedback provided by sexual selection. Every organism has to both survive and reproduce to run the evolutionary gauntlet. To reproduce, we must pass the test of mating selection by the opposite sex, a positive feedback process with capacity for runaway and complexity. Furthermore it is in sexual selection that detecting cheating comes to the knife edge of betrayal, requiring genuine indicators of fitness such as the peacock's tail, the male guppy's orange stripes, and with it, human generosity in love. In Miller's terms the complexity of human society is a product of such fitness indicators, elaborated in response to runaway discerning partner choice, and along with it our innate capacity to detect cheating, while retaining a generosity of heart necessary to entice the other sex into choosing us as worthy mates.In conceiving the complexity of human society and its teeming Prisoners' Dilemmas of social coexistence and competition, sexual paradox thus remains central as the gateway through which all our intellectual and cultural pretensions go down the plug hole to the next generation. It is also our heart centre, our *raison d'etre* motivating our passion and our jealousy in a way which all the other panoply of social interactions from hard nosed business to internecine strife serve as a resourceful backdrop. We thus need to strike a creative balance between the dictates of reciprocation and its manifestations in social game theory and sexual selection as a generator of cultural complexity.

The Prisoners' Dilemma does not have to lead to dissonance and a war of attrition. It its fully contradictory form, the paradox it contains leads to sexual interdependence and climax diversity. The fulfillment of sexual paradox is constructive engagement with the opposite sex in choices which abet successful child rearing, trading off the nemesis of deceit and betrayal with the sexual freedom of choice each gender must needs retain to fulfill their own reproductive design. The solution to the existential Prisoners' Dilemma of conscious existence is likewise constructive engagement with the living universe, through realizing love in the passage of the generations, assuming personal responsibility for ones willed actions and their cumulative affect on the future world around us. This is essentially the sustainable reproductive solution - evolutionary sustainability. But it is also the psychic resolution in mature interdependence, rather succumbing to mutual defection in the face of the win-lose strategies of submission and dominion, with their consequent tragedy of planetary destruction and the loss of future quality of life for the generations to come.

The success of reality TV shows such as "Survivor" depend on human interest in Machiavelian strategies in a Prisoners' Dilemma trial in which one person from a group wins a million dollars in a succession of eliminations in contests and tribal councils in which coalitions and betrayals are climaxed by a final vote of the eliminated members for the victor.

Many of the crises and tragedies of human 'civilization' arise from the loss of sexual paradox through prisoners dilemma betrayal by one party or another, leading to a degenerate process of domination, exploitation and atrophy. Rather than coming to the conclusion that humanity is a sick or dangerous species, which through its implicit violence poses a threat to the future of the living planet, our answer here to these maladies will be to restore the state of sexual paradox and with it our evolutionary and cultural sustainability as a species.

'Don't get even, get mad': Why Emotions Matter

Studies of brain function attest to emotional responses being central to how humans respond to issues of fidelity, and deceit, trust, cooperation altruistic punishment (p 378) and revenge (p 391).

Attempts to make game theory applicable to real life date back to the 1950s, when mathematicians used it to advise the US Air Force on Cold War strategy. Even then, it was obvious that most real-life problems aren't remotely like zero sum games where what is good for one is bad for the other and in which game theory recommends choosing the highest scoring tactic in the worst situation. What is bad for one 'player' can often be equally bad for the other, as the Prisoners' Dilemma shows. A classic is the game of Chicken, immortalized in James Dean's 'Rebel Without a Cause'.

As with zero-sum games, there's a rule for finding optimal strategies for these more complex games, which won RAND mathematician John Nash a share of the 1994 Nobel Prize for Economics. Nash's theorem says that it is always possible for a player to choose a strategy that is best for him or her when all the other players are also following their best strategies. In this 'equilibrium', no player can improve his or her prospects by choosing an alternative strategy. But there is no single state of equilibrium for a game like Chicken. There are two: you can decide to swerve, while the other person plans to keep driving, or vice versa. In either case, neither you nor your opponent can improve your score by unilaterally changing your mind, reflecting the cusp catastrophe's two states (p 14).

Enter the role of emotions. Only truly irrational players can credibly threaten to drive on no matter what - and so a rational strategy is to be completely irrational. Such 'paradoxes of rationality' dogged game theorists through the 1970s and 1980s. A huge effort was made to find rules for selecting the most 'rational' strategy in every game; none really worked. Nigel Howard, a veteran game theorist who had advised the US government in the Strategic Arms Limitation Talks during the 1960s was well used to applying game theory in real-life situations - and well aware of its limitations and called a meeting of game theorists at Sheffield University in 1991 in which 'drama theory' or 'soft game theory' was born (R439). He points out that the effects of rationality can be dire, recounting the following story. Two economists are taking a taxi to their hotel in Jerusalem. Worried that they are going to be overcharged, they decide not to haggle about the price until they reach the hotel. But the driver is so outraged at their conduct that he locks the taxi doors, drives them back to where they started, and dumps them on the street. "What we were really dealing with here weren't just games," recalls Howard. "They're dramas, where the beliefs and values of the characters evolve as the plot unfolds." At its heart is the idea that games are not static, one-shot deals decided by rationality, but dynamic situations that can be utterly transformed by the emotions of the players.

During the 1960s, Howard himself had developed 'metagame theory', which focused on the role of paradoxes in determining the outcomes of games. In the game of Chicken, for example, it seems pretty rational for Jimbo to want to win. Yet to do this, he must convince Buzz that he will not swerve, no matter how much Buzz insists he won't either. But coming from a rational person, Jimbo's threat is hardly credible: no sane person would declare a determination to follow hell-bent Buzz clear off the edge of the cliff. There's a way out of this 'credibility paradox', however: Jimbo should stop acting rationally, and instead behave as if he is crazy before he goes anywhere near his car. Suddenly, his threat to keep on driving becomes all too credible. Irrational behaviour thus sometimes pays, although it seems to be more to impress male mates and become a popular hero than to directly impress the girls (p 55). Howard has showed that the idea of credibility paradoxes gives a firm mathematical basis for drama theory (R321). "The basic idea is that paradoxes have an emotional effect on the characters and the reason these emotions emerge - like anger and fear, or affection and goodwill - is that they have a drama-theoretic role. They shake the characters out of old ways of thinking, allowing them to see a new way forward."

Chicken involves an 'inducement paradox', in which Jimbo must use an irrational threat to induce Buzz to swerve. Others, including the Prisoner's Dilemma, involve a 'cooperation paradox'. For each prisoner as an individual, Nash's theorem gives a unique, rational solution: accept the police offer, and start talking. But for the pair as a team, both spending a month in prison is preferable to one being locked away for years. But the only way of achieving this is for both prisoners to put their trust in each other and stay silent. This creates a cooperation paradox: each must convince the other that they will act as a team despite the fact that each could do better for themselves by defecting. For long-standing partners in crime emotional bonds will come to the fore when they face the cooperation paradox. But if one of the prisoners has always been an unwilling accomplice, the cooperation paradox will trigger anger and distrust and he'll act to save his own skin.

The Red Queen on the Origin of Sex

In "The Red Queen" (Ridley R564) explains the origin of sex (p 334) in a way which makes it effective, even in a single generation, despite losing half the genes transferred to the next, an acid test for the process having evolutionary stability at the outset:

"Sex is not about reproduction, gender is not about males and females, courtship is not about persuasion, fashion is not about beauty and love is not about affection. It is about getting your genes into the next generation, and trumping the Terrible Three: predators, parasites, and the neighbors. Of that trio, parasites rank as the greatest foe."

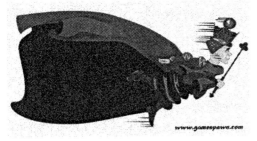

The idea is that sexuality evolved from an immediate potent advantage in the first generation that results from confounding parasites and predators because of genomic diversity that results from sexual recombination (p 329). Parasites and hosts are locked in a genetic arms race in which sexuality provides a potent advantage in generating variety, making it difficult for a parasite to adapt to varying individual hosts. It gives the clearest and most powerful explanation for the widespread occurrence of sex in higher organisms. There has to be at least a twofold advantage to make up for transmitting only fifty percent of our genes per generation sexually rather than the hundred percent transmission in parthenogenesis. It answers the bootstrap question in a way which doesn't makes sense otherwise. Although we now know that sexual recombination is a powerful source of variety, enabling complex organisms to evolve, this goes no way to explaining how the process could get going in the first place. It's really no use trying to explain this in terms of an evolutionary advantage of greater adaptability if this only emerges very gradually in the long-term over a large number of generations. We need a powerful immediate effect in the first generation, otherwise sexual game theory will say we still have a better chance of survival to invest all our genes in parthenogenesis than only half in a sexual exploit that would take up to a hundred thousand years to come to fruition. We would all die waiting, swamped by our parthenogenetic predecessors. The answer to this is that sex provides an immediate answer to the epidemic cataclysm awaiting a parthenogenetic organism when parasites or diseases adapt to a single genotype. The Red Queen is thus the 'scarlet woman' in sexual evolution. A similar one-generation advantage will accrue if an organism is subjected to any form of stress which compromises survival of daughter offspring of the current clone (p 336).

The "Red Queen" hypothesis has itself evolved historically through a sequence of based on coevolution. The original idea is that in tightly coevolved interactions, evolutionary change by one species (e.g., a prey or host) could lead to extinction of other species (e.g. a predator or parasite). Van Valen (R702) named the idea "the Red Queen hypothesis," because, under this view, species had to "run" (evolve) in order to stay in the same place. The next idea is that coevolution, particularly between hosts and parasites, could lead to sustained oscillations in genotype frequencies (Bell R53). In species where asexual reproduction is possible, coevolutionary interactions with parasites may select for sexual reproduction in hosts as a way to reduce the risk of infection in offspring. The idea of the Red Queen hypothesis as a founding strategy leading to sexuality has been given a compelling case by Ridley (R564).

In Alice's dream (Carroll R108) about the looking glass house, she first finds that things appear left-to-right, as if shown in a mirror. She then finds that chess pieces are alive. Alice decides that it would be easier to see the garden if she first climbs the hill, to which there appears to be a very straight path. However, as she follows the path, she finds that it leads her back to the house. When she tries to speed up, she not only returns to the house, she crashes into it. Hence, forward movement takes Alice back to her starting point (Red Queen dynamics), and rapid movement causes abrupt stops (extinction). The flowers tell Alice that someone like her often passes through, and Alice decides to seek the Red Queen. She begins moving toward her, but, the Red Queen quickly disappears from sight. Alice decides to follow the advice of the rose: "walk the other way". Immediately she comes face-to-face with the Red Queen (Lythgoe and Read R418). Already, in this world, straight can become curvy, and progress can be made only by going the opposite direction; now, according to the Red Queen, hills can become valleys and valleys can become hills (a peak in a sexually reproducing host population leads to a coevolutionary peak in parasites and a subsequent valley in the hosts). At the top of the hill, the Red Queen begins to run, faster and faster. Alice runs after the Red Queen, but is further perplexed to find that neither one seems to be moving. When they stop running, they are in exactly the same place. Alice remarks on this, to which the Red Queen responds: "Now, here, you see, it takes all the running you can do to keep in the same place". And so it may be with coevolution. Lewis Carrol's Red Queen is running while standing still, just as we end up as sexual species running while standing just about still with respect to our parasites and diseases in a paradoxical arms race with no final resolution. Evolutionary change may be required to stay in the same place. Cessation of change may result in extinction. We may find it hard to accept that we are evolving and evolved sexuality just to evade our parasites, but we nevertheless acknowledge that parasitism and infectious disease is a principal cause of death, even in the age of modern technology.

A basic feature of both immune system genes and the histocompatibility genes that make each individual's tissue unique is the existence of a large library of variant genes in individually unique combinations. A single mammalian species contains over a hundred different histocompatibility genes. The immune system is even more complex combining the effects from several light and heavy chain gene libraries and further induced mutations at the variable binding site, to generate millions of different antibodies. Sex acts as an agent to promote the diversity required to evolve such libraries. It also recombines them genetically each generation in a way which makes it difficult for pathogens to adapt to more than one generation of host. Sex gives a doubly powerful first-generation advantage because the descendents of each individual have both different immunity and different idiotype.

An outstanding example, which illustrates the dynamic nature of intermittent sex occurs in freshwater snails in Africa which are hermaphroditic in a self-contained way. Whenever the nematode parasite *Bulinas truncatas* strikes with the rains, the snail responds by growing penises and sexually recombining (Blum R65 8). In many species, evolution of sexual genes is very rapid as a result of a Red Queen arms race between male and female. This is true of the abalone, where the sperm secretes lysins which dissolve the egg membrane admitting parasites, so there is a genetic immunity arms race between the egg and the sperm (Jones R340 133). It is also true of the human Y chromosome where maleness genes are evolving rapidly. Ursula Goodenough also sees in such rapidly evolving sex genes the capacity to induce speciation, and believes this is happening between the Cuban and American ocean populations of the single-celled alga *Chlamydomonas* (R65 11). Likewise social patterns of promiscuity in higher apes are reflected in increased rates of evolution of the SEMG2 gene which makes semen thicken after ejaculation (R756).

There are intriguing indications of an arms race in humans between sperm production and cancer resistance. The genes most rapidly evolving between humans and chimps are immune defense genes - a classic Red Queen race between parasites and hosts, and cell apostosis genes programming cell death. Protection against cancer resulting from apostosis may compete with the need for sperm to evade apostosis in competitive reproduction (Nielsen R491). There is a similar evolutionary arms race in the SEMG2 gene coding the thickness of semen correlating with promiscuity in differing ape species (Wyckoff R756).

The result of sex is profound. Once established, sexual recombination makes possible the most powerful means of creating genetic diversity known. Genetic crossing-over in meiosis and the careful sorting of the DNA this entails (p 329), enables a precise and complete genetic combination of the genes of each parent, crossing the sister alleles so perfectly that virtually every sexual offspring contains a fully viable genome when the sex cells merge again in fertilization. It is this almost endless variety and the powerful selection it provides that has made the evolution of higher organisms possible. Hence all higher organisms have evolved from sexual species and the vast majority are obligately sexual.

Species which have both sexual and asexual reproduction tell us a lot about what causes the equilibrium to shift between the two. Asexual reproduction is good at rapidly multiplying to invade a habitat, as with aphids and vegetative reproduction of the Nile lotus. In the freshwater minnow *Pocillopsis* asexual individuals are good at populating extreme environments, where sexual recombination would dilute adaptive characteristics. But sexual individuals are better at populating varied, fluctuating and evolving environments.

Sexual recombination has the capacity for eliminating undesirable mutations which are continually accruing, by concentrating them in only some offspring, where natural selection can effectively eliminate them - a process cryptically called 'Muller's ratchet'. If we reproduced clonally, all our offspring and their offspring would inevitably suffer the random mutations of entropy. Selection cannot necessarily keep all these in line and prevent gradual degradation of a complex genome, despite selection unless there are some forms of recombination as insurance of error protection. We already have sophisticated error-correcting enzymes which read off one strand of DNA to correct the non-complementary or damaged bases on the complementary strand. But even these processes cannot distinguish which strand is a mutation and which is the original, so error correction also involves keeping and comparing variants and allowing these a chance of survival. If we are sexual beings, our children each contain half our genes in a unique combination. If each of us have only one or a few mutations at the tolerable load per generation, some of our children may have two mutations but others will be free of any. This ensures some individuals are carrying unmutated genomes. Lynn Margulis has suggested that a similar error-correction process may have driven bacterial pan-sexuality. Notably asexual rotifer species have a much smaller load of transposable genetic elements (p 331) consistent with a mutational basis for sexual recombination. For eucaryotes existing before life generated the oxygen atmosphere and the protective ozone layer, a solid reason for sexual recombination, again consistent with the Red Queen, would have been to protect the genomic information of small exposed single-celled organisms from the ravages of ultraviolet mutagenesis.

The Red Queen hypothesis also naturally leads naturally to a partially competitive genetic and evolutionary race with the opposite sex, an amatory arms race, genetically interdependent, yet with conflicting reproductive strategies and modes of genetic selection. These arms races are evident in the natural world. A male fly may introduce toxins into the female which cause her to invest more energy in the current offspring than her natural investment spread evenly among all her offspring, thereby maximizing her investment in his offspring (p 16). These have other effects, reducing the females capacity to eject sperm and her capacity to mate successfully with other males. She responds by developing immunity. Repeated fertilization can become poisonous to the female. The Red Queen can thus be extended directly to the genetic arena in the form of 'interlocus contest evolution' between competing genetic influences, for example antagonistic genetic selection between opposing sexual characteristics in males and females, characteristic of sexually antagonistic co-evolution.

A stunning extreme of this conflict between the sexes occurs in the little fire ant, where the haplo-diploid sexuality where workers are produced by normal sexual reproduction, but daughter queens are clonally reproduced. Although clonal reproduction increases the queen's relatedness to reproductive daughters, it can potentially reduce the male reproductive success to zero. To compensate the males have also evolved to reproduce clonally from father to son in a sexual standoff, probably by expelling the maternal chromosomes, which leaves their gene pools entirely separate and selected only through the workers although it remains possible that males may occasionally mate with a top queen (R218).

The Red Queen is an instance of the Prisoners' Dilemma. Both parasite and host and male and female are running a treadmill in evolutionary terms while standing still in an arms race from which in the case of the sexual arms race neither party can escape.

Sexual Selection, Reproductive Fitness and Sexual Paradox

"The idea that females are discriminating and can actively choose with whom to mate was controversial from its inception - perhaps because male-male battles can be quite spectacular. ... In comparison female choice is much more subtle. Over the past 25 years, a considerable body of evidence for female choice has accumulated. Females actively choose their mates in a large variety of species." (Dugatkin and Godin R176).

Even 'lowly' guppy fish display a complementation of genetic 'nature' and social 'culture' in female reproductive choice. Although female guppies prefer larger, brighter orange, daring males who closely explore predators, a test of both their metabolic (carotenoid pigments are costly to make) and physical fitness and alertness, they will also follow a previous female's choice in 'social copying', and favour a less-orange mate, provided the differences in orange colouration between two males are less than 25%. However if a female is living under genuinely threatening conditions, she may prefer to mate with a less showy male who provokes less direct risk and genes which carry this lower risk. Her sexual choices are thus a subtle mix of genetic and social and involve both natural and sexual selection. Although people are more complex than guppies and lekking sage grouse, the same mate-choice rules apply to human mating. According to popular wisdom, it is human females who are the choosier sex when it comes to selecting a mate. As a species, humans meet the criteria for female choice: men for the most part, will avoid fighting to the death for the hand of a maiden. And females distinguish between various males on the basis of their characteristics.

Sexual choice can lead to runaway sexual selection, particularly in birds, which have flashy males partly due to the ZW sex chromosome system (p 342). The peacock's tail is a genuine indicator of fitness because, although mesmerizing to females, it makes the peacock vulnerable to predators. There is a runaway selection happening here between the peacock's tail and the choosy genes of pattern discrimination in the female brain. Song birds have partially evaded this penalty by choosing ultra-violet markings. Birds have four colour vision, but song birds push one colour receptor up into the ultra-violet where mates see it stands out but out of the visual range of predatory birds which use a lower wavelength receptor (R14). Sperm are a scarce resource which invites sophisticated social strategies. Male fowl devote considerably more sperm to their first encounter with a new mate than with a familiar one. They will also increase sperm if rival males are around. An attractive hen with a large comb will receive more sperm. Cockrels will even seduce regular partners with sperm-free mountings which trick the female into fidelity even though they would expel the sperm of an inferior mate within seconds of copulation (R535, R536).

Humans are no exception to the rule that variance in reproductive fitness is greater in males than in females. While a significant number of males have no children at all, a few sire hundreds or even thousands of children. In biological terms, humanity is moderately polygynous, regardless of cultural mating systems. It holds as true in serially-monogamous America as it does in polygamous Africa.

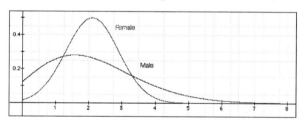

The sexes are intrinsically polarized in their reproductive investments (p 334), with females contributing cytoplasmic eggs and the males only contributing DNA, becoming the 'sneaky' sex (p 335). Females can bear offspring by any fertile male, but males must compete to fertilize females, or their larger less abundant eggs, to reproduce. This greater female investment tends to make the female more choosy about her mate and gives female sexual selection a primary role in sexual evolution . This polarization is extreme in mammals, where internal fertilization, gestation, live birth and lactation cause the female investment to be maximally different to the male. It is particularly true of the human female with her vulnerable enormity of pregnancy (p 83). Trivers (R690) first laid out the impacts of the differing investments made by males and females in reproduction and their consequences for sexual selection (Hrdy R323 37). Mating investment has a large fixed cost to succeed at all, so males tend to invest primarily in mating, tending towards competitive polygyny (Low R416 42), while females invest primarily in parenting. Males thus look for reproductive value in females, while females look more to resourcing value.

At an extreme of choosiness, female Californian fiddler crabs, *Uca cernulata*, will investigate up to 100 male burrows, beckoned inside by the males' large waving claws, to find a burrow of just the right size which will hatch their progeny just in time for them to be spread by the peak outward night time flow of the bi-weekly tidal cycle.

Measures of polygyny are biologically related to the differential variance in reproductive efficacy which is generally higher in males. The means of the two are always the same since it takes a male and a female to reproduce sexually. Thus by biological measures human societies are moderately polygynous, even though we are predominantly socially monogamous. This manifests in a variety of ways. 85% of human societies permit polygyny and in these about as many males as can resource two partners at once do so. Some males engage despotic sexuality. Moulay Ismail the Bloodthirsty of Morocco had 888 offspring and 40 sons in a single month (Hrdy R323 84). Ghengis Khan's Y-chromosome occurs in about one in 200 people as a result of several generations of polygynous descendents and 1 in 12 Irish men are descended from Niall of the Nine Hostages. Wandering males seducing women also contribute, through the standard mammalian strategy of simple sexual courtship. Although we call many human societies 'monogamous' this is clearly a biological misnomer. Most societies with one-spouse-at-a-time rules are called polygynous in a biological definition: more men than women fail to marry, and more men than women remarry after death or divorce, producing more offspring in these later unions. The most reproductive men have many more children than the most fertile women. All of these phenomena increase the variability of men's reproductive success compared to women's, making us polygynous by a biologist's definition (Low R416 54).

The larger divergence in male reproductive opportunity in humans at first caused sociobiologists to concentrate on male evolutionary selection by females, assuming females all reproduced close to the maximum feasible rate. Sarah Hrdy (R322) in "The Woman that Never Evolved" set out to correct this anomaly, noting that real reproductive differences and competition exist in females, particularly in the central issue of successful parenting.

On the other hand, female choice also implies that females will not necessarily remain faithful to a socially monogamous pair bond. A female in socially monogamous species which seek paternal support will seek a resourceful partner but also engage other sexual liaisons in up to 20% of her sirings. Females in polygynous species with dominant males also covertly seek non-alpha partners. This pattern of female 'infidelity' is as true for colonial birds as it is for humans. The principal reason is as insurance so her large parental investment in eggs and in mammals pregnancy and lactation are not entirely bound up in an inferior set of genes. However there are more complex reasons. Females need not just to find a male with the best genes but the most compatible complementarity to hers. Smells of MHC histocompatibility proteins give mammals sensitive indications of sexually attractive mates with good immuno-complementarity. Females also mate with many males to confuse paternity and invite more paternal support and less infanticide. Finally they may mate with non-alpha males to avoid being forced into a undesirable decision by the forces of male competition

Trivers and Willard (R691) went on to establish the relation between such variation and sex ratios: *"wherever variation is greater in reproductive success for one sex than the other, and where the reproductive success of individuals of that sex depends on maternal effects, then mothers in good condition should favour the sex with the greatest variance in reproductive success"*. It has been confirmed in species as diverse as deer, baboons and rodents. Broadly speaking, we expect mothers in poor condition to have more girls and those in good condition to have more boys, possibly mediated by hormonal mechanisms such as testosterone (Grant R251). Women who expect a long life (and are thus likely to be in good condition) have more boys (Johns R334) and Gibson and Macey (R235) showed that rural Ethiopian women with low levels of nutrition are more likely to give birth to girls (p 96). It applies also to human dowry and bride price, where low ranking families save for a dowry to 'marry up' daughters and high ranking families favour only sons and may kill their infant daughters (p 286). Such 'hypergamic' marriage patterns become pronounced under conditions of environmental stress, where upper class families are better protected against famine and can afford males, while lower class families may starve (Low R416 70, Hrdy R323 338) and whose best reproductive prospects over time involve 'marrying up' daughters, in what is called hypergamy.

The rule applies when sexual selection, (access to females) is the dominating factor, but may be reversed when other factors, such as female dominance limit resources. When daughters remain within the group and resources are scant, as in savannah baboons, high ranking mothers produce daughters, but low ranking ones sons who can at least migrate (Hrdy R323 333-5). When daughters can be harnessed for allo-parenting, this advantage can determine the sex ratio, as in Seychelles warblers. Such sex imbalances tend to return to Fisher equilibrium of equality (R211) when the driving factors are mitigated, because the rarer sex gains a strategic advantage. Each sex thus has its own distinct and often conflicting strategy of reproduction. To fulfil a given sex's reproductive imperative requires also fulfilling the reproductive strategy and choice of the opposite sex. Male competition is subject to the paradox of female reproductive choice because it is the most powerful agent of sexual selection in most species. Even in species with pronounced male conflict, female choice remains a prominent selector of male fitness.

Sexual selection is prone to runaway feedback, as for example the outgrowth of the peacock's tail as a genuine indicator of fitness which can't be faked and imposes a significant cost on the bearer in terms of predation. This in turn is driven by the ever-more-choosy retinas and visual areas of the peahen. The balance of these forces and the actual state of strategic advantage one or other sex enjoys varies from species to species. For example in non-monogamous birds where the male contributes only his genes, the prominent display of the peacock's tail and the bower bird are driven by precocious female sexual selection. To be a genuine indicator of reproductive fitness these ornaments are often chosen to be costly, as the peacock's tale is, as well as being a sensitive indicator of highly tuned developmental symmetry indicative of good genes. Experiments have shown that females in displaying avian species will continue to prefer artificially enhanced ornaments and mate with males possessing them confirming runaway selection. The male has little choice here but to make the best job of capitalizing on its runaway evolutionary burdens, which may give it a good chance of siring offspring, but bring costs in vulnerability to predators as a bulky and garish genuine indicator of fitness. This is partly a reflection of the minimal investment made by such males and the incapacity of the males to monopolize female reproduction except through enticement.

Human beauty is has been found to be linked with more perfect symmetry, and mor erecently in an experiment reducing dancing performances to identical computer mannequins, it has been found that, the best dancers are also those who are the most symmetrical and beautiful (Brown R90). The effect was stronger for women watching male dances than for men watching women and the dances performed by men scored more highly overall than those by women, consistent with male display of fitness and female choice.

Even alpha males, who would prefer to engage male competition to win a harem, rather than submit to female choice, find themselves subject to genuine indicators of fitness. An alpha male gelada baboon has a highly visible red chest mark, which indicates his condition. This is probably a sign that also tells others that females are sexually bonded in a way which will be harder to break into. Coalitions of bachelor males will confront a leader of a harem and try to take it over only if his genuine indicators of fitness are lacklustre.

In monogamous species which have mutual mate choice, pronounced sexual differences of display are reduced or non-evident, however as Darwin noted mutual mate choice can still drive selection and consequent evolution, albeit without such strong or polarized sexually selective forces operating. Humans are mildly sexually dimorphic, with testicle size and sperm competition suggesting pair-bonding in a climate of moderate polygyny with mutual mate choice skewed somewhat towards female reproductive choice. Male reproductive variance is greater than that of females. Sexual strategies are complex and mixed with a considerable number of medium to long-term pair bonds, a minority of polygynous associations, serially 'monogamous' partnerships which tend to favour male reproductive polygyny, overlaying a shifting pattern of covert female affairs and sometimes blatant male philandering, all contributing to varying reproductive strategies and outcomes.

At an opposite extreme, the bull elephant seal appears to have caught the female in a not too tender trap as a result of male resource guarding. Because seals often breed in low temperature climates, the females have evolved to have a counter-cyclical pregnancy and lactating season and gather on sheltered warmer beaches where they can nurse the pups often without feeding, using their blubber alone to keep both mother and offspring alive, at the same time becoming pregnant for the next season. A dominant male secures these spots before the females arrive and thus can guard a large harem (Low 2001 44). The much greater size of the male is a reflection of the harem size and male competition. How efficient this counter-cyclical nursing has evolved to become is shown by the hooded seal who gives birth on ice flows and whose creamy milk with 60% fat can cause a pup to gain fifty pounds in a matter of days (Hrdy R323 129).

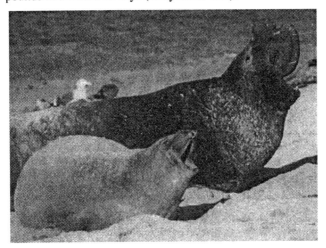

Sexual dimorphism: Elephant seals (Maier R420).

We should note that this form of male domination only exists because of the relative success of the female strategy of counter-cyclical pregnancy and breast-feeding. Females do secure superior genes for their pups, but at the cost of having some trampled by the bull and having to endure being raped and bitten by sub-dominant males should they leave the colony to fish (Low R416 45). A dominant male elephant seal can sire up to 90 pups and a female 10. Complementing the male strategy, it has been proposed that elephant seal females signal their receptivity to a broad array of males specifically to incite competition among the bulls to apply female choice genetically (Cox and LeBoeuf R134). Females apparently take advantage of this situation to actively pursue smaller subdominant males on the side, partly because they run a small risk (1/1000) of being suffocated by a large dominant male. Female choice between herding and time on the side is acting to keep the hugely larger male size in equilibrium (Sparks R641 13). In some seal species such as Weddell seal, dominant males may die from exhaustion at the end of a season. In others thy are simply overtaken exhausted by younger fitter males. On the other hand when a female seal leaves the colony she is liable to assault and rape by sub-dominant males who bite her if she doesn't submit. In some senses these patterns are not too different from human male dominant warrior societies trading their women as reproductive tokens where a Yanomamo village head such as 'Shinbone' sired 43 children by 11 wives (Chagnon R110 150). Much larger sirings have been made by human potentates who have clearly established the largest harems of any species. One in 200 people today carry the Y-chromosome of Ghengis Khan. One can only speculate where this would take human dimorphism, continued over evolutionary time scales.

Orangutans have pronounced dimorphic male phenotypes. Degrees of phenotypic dimorphism may be very important in maintaining diverse mating strategies which enable a species to adapt rapidly to changing circumstances with now socialization patterns by altering the frequencies of the corresponding alleles in the population. Female coho salmon display a similar form of two phase female choice, in which there are two dimorphic forms of male, hooknoses which are fighting fit but took two seasons to mature and younger leaner jacks which came up river the first year. Contrary to expectations, females prefer the jacks, possibly because they are showing early fitness. Jacks just wiggle to signal an invitation and the females comply. By contrast they face a conflict of interest with the aggressive hooknoses who will bite them if they don't have sex (Mason R437). Roughgarden (R580) suggests that in polyphenic fish species there is reproductive cooperation between dominant male 'controllers', and the sub-dominant male phenotype which he calls 'cooperators', however the viability of this idea remains to be established. It is also doubtful that 'sneaker' male crickets, which sit silently behind a singing alpha male, assist the alpha, rather than exploit his efforts. Male cuttlefish are even known to become transvestites, assuming the form and colouring of a female to trick a dominant male and the female he is guarding into allowing his sperm to intervene in about a third of fertilizations (R282).

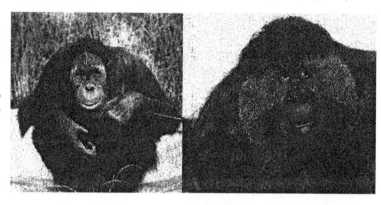

Male orangutans are called 'polyphenic' because there are two distinct male phenotypes, one a gangling 'peter pan' who tries to insidiously sidle up to and rape females, even when they are out of estrus, and the other an alpha male who beats his chest and roars through the forest enticing estrus females to his call (Hrdy R323 74).

The difference in reproductive investment strategies between the sexes, with males investing less causes the vast majority of animals to be polygynous. This applies consistently to invertebrates, fish and mammals. Only birds which uniquely are both egg-laying and warm-blooded are commonly monogamous because hatching the egg requires the cooperation of both partners. But even then, monogamy is social, rather than genetic and there are frequent clandestine affairs. Monogamy in the biological sense is social mating and does not imply sexual fidelity. Only 10% of 180 socially monogamous bird species are sexually faithful. Both monogamous birds and mammals clandestinely 'outsire' up to 20% of the offspring due to individual reproductive choice by either or both sexes to spread or extend their genetic investment.

Only about 3% of mammals are socially monogamous and only two monkeys, the marmoset and the tamarin, are truly monogamous. In mammals, where females both gestate live young and lactate, mating patterns are primarily determined by the way females distribute themselves, e.g. in relation to the food resource. Males will responsively distribute themselves in such a way as to guard either scarce resources (e.g. special territory) to monopolize females using them, or groups of females themselves (mate guarding) if they are wandering freely, foraging in wide areas in groups. At an extreme, if there are no means to monopolize female fertility, a few mammal species also resort to the lekking well known in birds, where males competitively display to the females for sex on an arbitrarily chosen stomping ground. Variations in how spread apart the females are in relation to plant food distributions in apes are believed to determine the spread from monogamy in gibbons through fission-fusion promiscuity in chimps to harem building in gorillas. Although the advantages of paternal help with child-rearing as well as widely spread females have been cited as factors predisposing to mammalian monogamy, the key factor appears to be simply how females use space (Komers and Brotherton R376). In many of the monogamous mammal species monogamy results not from male parental investment, but from males being forced to guard a lone female with a small exclusive range. In monogamous marmosets and tamarins, for example, females compete to pair with quality males and drive off competing females (Miller R464 185).

Prairie voles have become renowned for their pair-bonding based on the neuropeptides oxytocin and vasopressin (p 352). But their monogamy is unusual in that the founding pair are the sole breeders in a wider family group whose other females remain sexually immature and help to rear the young until they eventually mate with and form a pair bond with another outside male, causing the onset of ovulation and a new dynasty. Monogamous hibernating marmot mothers similarly engage aggressive displays towards their daughters as winter sets in causing them to fail to ovulate and remain with the nest, adding enough warmth to tide the next round of her infants through the cold spell. Noting its correspondence to human history Hrdy (R322 173) calls one female forestalling reproduction in another "the Hagar phenomenon". The coincidence of social monogamy and allo-parenting 'day care' is a common feature of mammal species in which the mother is adapted to produce a greater load in offspring than she can care for on her own. Cotton-top tamarins likewise depend on cooperative child rearing and give multiple birth to enable rapid population increase when the conditions are right. Mothers routinely give birth to twins and rely on the father or other group members to help rear them, or the babies may be abandoned within 72 hours of birth (Hrdy R323 180). In humans even one slow growing relatively helpless infant is more than a mother can easily care for and gather food for at the same time, so both pair-bonding and allo-parenting are readily evoked in a manner exceptional for other apes. The titi monkey is also monogamous. A couple regularly sit together on a branch, tails entwined. The mother is so engrossed with the father that she appears to pay marginal attention to her offspring, who drink from the mother, but cling to the father when she pushes them off. Nevertheless extra-pair couplings were observed in titis before female philandering in monogamous birds caused a sensation. Her attention to her partner makes perfect sense, because if he strays his resourcing commitment may be lost. As with tamarins and marmosets the female drives away females who enter her territory to avoid dividing her partner's attentions (R323 213). Infidelity in monogamy applies even to prairie voles: "What we say about prairie voles is that they'll sleep with anyone but they'll only sit by their partners" (Blum R65 95). It's no surprise that as soon as a prairie vole mates, he becomes more suspicious and aggressive of other males (R65 241).

Evolution towards extremely rapid increase in complexity, as exemplified by human cultural emergence, is consistent with a state of paradox in which neither sex is fully dominant over the sexual choices of the other, rather than any state of sexual dominion where the strategy of only one sex is brought fully into play. The emergence of culture is an abrupt process consistent with powerful sexual selection. The state of sexual paradox entices each sex to strive to gain the choice of the other through genuine indicators of fitness, involving both prowess and social astuteness as well as kindness and generosity to one's partners. These are all features characteristic of human emergence.

Key and Aiello (R349) has applied the prisoners dilemma game in detail to sexual relations in human emergence and concluded that "when male reproductive costs are less than female reproductive costs, males cooperate with females even when females do not reciprocate" entitling this 'non-reciprocal altruism' - an investment in a female and her offspring. The game showed that as costs increase, females will begin to help one another . Key notes: "That's because females have the same interests, such as food and child care". While it was to females' advantage to put all their effort into raising a small number of offspring, the best strategy for males was to attempt to father as many offspring as possible and not stick around to watch them grow up. However the model showed that males and females will cooperate when two conditions are met: first, when female reproductive costs are much higher than those of males, and second, if females can somehow punish uncooperative males. This associates with human emergence and the increasing head size of a larger and more complicated brain, motifs in which human females may have cooperated and applied forms of sexual enticement or even cooperative coercion to ensure male cooperation, possibly phased with the lunar and menstrual cycle (p 77). Noting that females are frequently more sexually active in socially monogamous species Enquist and Rodriguez-

Girones (R194) developed a game-theoretic model to establish the idea that male 'fidelity' is driven by female 'deceit' in the form of concealed ovulation and opportunistic extra-pair couplings because the advantages to male philandering are reduced.

Parental Investment and Mother-Child Conflicts of Interest

Sarah Hrdy (R323 42) points out that selection of mothering traits is central to the equation of sexual evolution, particularly in mammals. "Over the course of her life, a female bound for fitness is required to make a series of physiological and developmental 'decisions' about how big to grow, when to mature, how soon to reproduce, and how much time to allow between offspring. One of the biggest challenges for understanding selection pressures on mother that confronted sociobiologists in the early years was getting the balance right between considering traits that are sexually-selected (for example through female choice or male choice) and equally important, if not more important, female traits that are naturally selected because they increased survival of the mother and her offspring." Females are thus applying a variety of skills in raising and caring for their offspring, all of which are critical and subject to natural selection for successful mothers in addition to sexual selection. In considering the question of reproductive sexual paradox we have to understand it not just in terms of sexual selection, but in terms of the overall reproductive strategies of each sex and their combined mating and parental investments. Sexual paradox is not thus a paradox of sexual selection but complete reproductive investment.

Although the female, particularly in gestating, lactating mammals invests more directly in parenting, the male's overall reproductive success is measured in offspring survival as well. Although a male elephant seal is primarily making a mating investment, his actions are part of a successful reproductive strategy in which his efforts are also indirectly parental. By providing a large harem with a warm relatively safe nursing space and driving off potentially infanticidal male competitors, and even ironically by killing off other males' competing offspring, he is furthering survival of his own progeny and hence his genes.

In "Mother Nature" Sarah Hrdy (R323) sets out a monumental account of why maternal ambivalence is a central evolutionary feature of the human condition with a long set of parallels shared in various forms by diverse primates and mammals. Many of these relate closely to the predominantly parental reproductive investment a female mammal makes and the trade-offs involved in dealing with limited resources, insufficient reserves, infanticidal males and the lack of condition and experience of a first time mother. In addition to the conditional mothering we have seen in the monogamous species such as tamarins and titi monkeys, she documents a variety of cases of maternal discretion, from absorbtion of a pregnancy in many rodents when an alien male makes an incursion which signals the threat of infanticide (R323 89), to maternal infanticide. In the monogamous California mouse a mother who loses her partner may kill the pups rather than try to rear them alone. This species is reputedly also monogamously faithful reflecting the fact that a bonded pair can raise four times as many offspring as a lone mother. Likewise to abandonment or even participatory cannibalism occurs in about one in ten prairie dogs when a pregnancy results in a newborn for whom the mother has insufficient resources (R323 93). Weddell seals likewise often abandon their first set of pups because they have not accumulated enough fat to support them through the nursing season, where they have little opportunity to feed.

Hrdy exposes a litany of forms of frequently resource-based maternal ambivalence in human practices of exposure, infanticide, and very large scale abandonment in European societies during the Christian era, which run completely counter to our idealistic notions of maternal devotion to the ultimate blessing of helpless dependent lovable yet demanding infants. Hrdy (R323 345) suggests that fixed strategies in other mammals such as reabsorbing a litter in mice and the biasing of sex ratios, for example in wasps are transferred to a discriminating maternal ambivalency in humans which leaves a decision whether to keep an offspring of a given sex to the last feasible moment, allowing for greater responsiveness to ecological and social contingencies. The consistent theme of this work is that, despite two conflicting views one of 'essentialist maternal instinct' and the other a cultural 'blank slate', human mothering responses are contingent, varied and a natural consequence of Hamilton's rule. "The cost function of Hamilton's rule calls [mother-infant harmony] into question. Instead of viewing it as an abnormality, a pathology to be treated , sociobiologists accept some degree of maternal ambivalence as inevitable. ... For as designed by Mother Nature, the delectability of infants seduces to quite different ends [from consuming them] ... to be consumed by them, to give up bodily resources, and time ... so that we could all (more or less) take our place at posterity's table" (R323 539).

In 1972 Robert Trivers (R690) extended Hamilton's rule of kin altruism to child-parent conflict. A child naturally shares all their own genes but only a quarter to a half those of their maternal siblings, depending on whether they have a common father. A child will thus settle for shared resources or attention only if it benefits a full sibling twice as much as the cost to themselves. Hence the apparent selfish greed of the squalling toddler vying for the attention of the mother makes genetic sense (Hrdy R323 427). It also applies to discriminating maternal responses to keep or abandon an infant based on its condition and potential impact on the viability of older offspring (R323 365), something Western society, still under the influence of patriarchal religions and social mind set, has great difficulty coming to terms with. In mammals, Haig's work shows the demands of the child in everything from placental invasion to relative size are partly a function of paternal influences.

Humans with massive pregnancies, difficult births and long periods of lactation and immediate infant care take an excessive toll on the mother. Hrdy (R323 175) expresses this succinctly as "a tooth for a child." Thus the prisoner's dilemma between mother and child is a direct extension of the sexual tug of war between sexually antagonistic paternal and maternal influences. One can cast this dilemma more generally in terms of parent-child conflict, but in most mammals the male reproductive investment is primarily in mating, rather than parenting and even in strongly pair-bonding humans the mother's child-care investment is primary. In the case of the male we, move from ambivalence to discriminating infanticide. In a large number of mammal species, males will immediately kill any offspring of a female they gain access to as a potential mate. Langurs are cautious and kill only infants which couldn't be theirs, both removing genetic competition and triggering early ovulation and pregnancy of their own offspring (ibid 34). Chimps are less conservative and kill infants who might not be sired by the troop. Male mice have a biological clock which is primed to inhibit infanticide just long enough for a female they have impregnated to come to full term (R323 89).

It is the mother-child relationship and its implications for female autonomy that became the deepest evolutionary affront to feminist sensibilities. On the one hand we have a traditional patriarchal view, exacerbated by 19th century social Darwinism, of woman as merely a 'reproductive human' destined to be a mother rather than an innovator and expected to possess an unqualified maternal 'instinct' in response to the profound needs for love and security in the human infant, the absence of which is assumed to be a pathological condition. On the other we have a cultural view shared by many feminists, and a generation of anthropologists and sociologists that maternal reactions are culturally determined and that infants have no specific attachment needs but only desires.

Simone de Beauvoir pivotally expressed the concern that biological stereotypes would lead to the "enslavement of the female to the species and the limitations of her various powers". Reacting to attachment theory - the idea that human infants have an innate need for a primary attachment figure in the first years of life - a role that mothers are uniquely qualified to fill caused feminists to define female biological roles as 'essentialist' and to deny that biology is relevant to human affairs or that infants have innate needs for any personalized care on the basis that the human brain and our capacity for culture make us so different from other animals that humans can learn to be anything they choose.

Hrdy (R323 24) however notes that, although humans can learn a lot, this does not apply without biological restraint to such ancient emotional domains as those involved with 'love'. Nevertheless, the idea took on that maternal love was a socially-constructed sentiment without any biological basis." (R323 308):

"Decades before the sudden-infant-death-syndrome scandals surfaced in the 1990s, or before data on foundling homes started to be quantified in the 1970s, psychiatrists, historians, and social scientists all noted the poor match between real-life mothers and nineteenth and early twentieth century stereotypes of instinctively nurturing mothers. Feminists in particular had long ago lost patience with Darwinian perspectives that struck them as essentialist and which patently disregarded womens felt experience. They were eager to discount biological explanations, and had little incentive to keep up with what was going on in reproductive ecology or sociobiology. They continued to project on to those fields their own worst assessments about essentialist and determinist assessments of 'female nature' even after biologists had themselves abandoned these types of explanations. The result was that feminist theorists were producing models to explain what was essentially a biological phenomenon (namely the failure of an infant to elicit nuturing responses from its mother) but without any reference to biology. They used the evidence of the high numbers of non-nurturing mothers as a tool to jettison altogether the confining stereotype of the instinctively nurturing mother that had long been used to prescribe social roles for women ... Instead of taking a closer, critical look at the original biologically-based explanations to see if perhaps something had been left out, feminists (along with other social scientists who were trying to explain the widespread practice of abandonment by mothers) patently rejected evolutionary explanations. The biological basis of motherhood was replaced by a new environmentalism. The way a mother feels toward her infant must be solely determined by her cultural milieu. - epitomized by Elizabeth Badinter's comment 'I am not questioning maternal love - I am questioning maternal instinct'."

This is echoed archetypally in Gerda Lerner's (R397 52) reaction to Freud's statement that for women "anatomy is destiny". "What Freud should have said is that anatomy *once was* destiny. This statement is accurate and historical. What once was, no longer is so, nor should it be so." Yet this biological destiny remains true for both men and women, so long as we reproduce naturally on the planet. Hrdy continues:

"Growing numbers of women were coming to regard attachment theory, [the idea that a growing infant had strong needs for a close mother] as an anathema. Rarely mentioned in feminist circles, [John] Bowlby's name, when it did come up, was uttered with derision. Why might women have a stake in discrediting research ostensibly focussed on infant well-being? Having panicked often enough myself over whether I could live up to the stiff responsibilities of motherhood I understand why" (R323 489).

Just how sensitive this issue became is etched out by Hrdy (R323 406):

"Compared with Darwin's 'dangerous idea' the evolutionary philosophy that Daniel Dennett has termed 'universal acid' because it cuts so deeply into human conceits about our place in the universe, Bowlby's intellectual acid was less corrosive. Yet for psychoanalysts, for feminists and for any woman with ambitions, it burns very deeply indeed. ... By situating the mother (or primary care taker) at the center of each developing infant's universe, Bowlby's theory of attachment stings most smartly where it pricks the conscience of every mother who is aware of her infant's needs but who aspires to a life beyond bondage to them".

Hrdy notes that the debate over whether or not women have 'maternal instincts' has taken decades to unravel to the point where the patriarchal assumptions of earlier generations of moralists have been corrected and 'Darwin's evolutionary paradigm widened to both sexes. But by this time, feminists, social historians and philosophers were convinced that what evolutionists had to offer was essentially flawed, determinist and uninsightful. Natural selection, and with it the most powerful and comprehensive theory available for understanding the basic natures of mothers and infants was rejected, as feminists and social scientists took a path, rejecting biology and science, constructing their own version of wishful thinking about socially constructed men and women, and infants born with merely a 'desire' for mothers rather than a 'need'. Maternal love could then safely be interpreted as a 'gift' consciously bestowed, or a by-product of changing fashions and sentiments. The more multifaceted view of mothers, being developed by biologists, featuring flexible actors whose responses were contingent on circumstances went largely unheeded. "Lost in the shuffle over what it was natural for mother to do and dust ups over bonding and mother love was the infant's often noisy two cents worth "No matter who gives it, I need it. And need it now."

Hrdy (R323 535) notes that Bowlby provided scientific legitimacy to the anxiety, distress terror and finally desolation that infants experience when they fail to detect 'the meeting eyes of love' and that although many of the dangers turn out to be different from those he initially envisioned, his central explanation of how and why infants become attached to their caretakers was on target. He was correct that primate infants, including humans, are born immobile and vulnerable. He rightly pointed out that they respond very poorly to being left alone, or otherwise being made to feel insecure. Human infants have a nearly insatiable desire to be held and to bask in the sense that they are loved. To this extent the needs of human infants are enormous and largely non-negotiable. The question that remains is, what are the implications of this for their mothers? Part of the problem is that there is little agreement about whose interests are to be maximized in a world where conflicting self-interests, are endemic between parents and offspring, between mothers and fathers, within families, between families. Hrdy comments:

"Understandably, perhaps, those most threatened by acknowledging infant needs - mothers with aspirations to do things other than mother - were the ones who felt most compelled to down play infant needs" (R323 493).

We see in this a succinct expression of Hamilton's rule and the extension of sexually antagonistic coevolution striking home directly to the feminist reaction to the mother-child issue in a strategic attempt by mothers, if not to entirely gain control over the infants their reproductive investment depends on, by a culturally relativistic finesse, at least to regain from moralizing males the freedom of choice for that very maternal ambivalence that lies at the root of the Prisoners' Dilemma of long-term survival between mother and offspring.

This discussion of the mother-child relationship raises a further question about the role of the father. Hrdy has proposed that much of the child-rearing effort in early humans was done by allo-mothers or allo-parents - other helpers, such as older daughters, sisters, relatives such as aunts and uncles and reciprocal female friends in addition to or in spite of the father's role, which in most societies does not come anywhere to a near match to the mother's at least in the early years. This follows a mammalian pattern in which mothers who need extra help do so from several sources even in many socially monogamous species. It is notable that in Sandays' (R596) survey of human societies that in most societies fathers were involved only rarely or occasionally with child care.

This leads to another interesting hypothesis. Judith Rich Harris (R286, R287) has all but demolished the socialization theory of parental molding as a process of reward and punishment, however the genetic links between the personalities and many aspects of the mental life of parents and children do have a manifest genetic basis. Her alternative hypothesis - that the peer group forms the major influence on the socialization of the growing child also has a basis in evolutionary sociobiology. As Ridley (R567 259) points out the peer group provides a context for niche diversification and specialization of a growing individual to find skills and specialities a growing person discovers are appreciated and sought after by the group they will spend their early adult life with. The formative influences on children during human emergence are likely to have been a fluid mix of influences from their mother, father, allo-parents, extended family and peer/play group in a small band of gatherer-hunters, rather than a rigid nuclear family structure. We are thus likely to see young humans genetically kin with their parents sharing a vertical affinity across the generations while engaged in a struggle of partial conflict of interest. At the same time they have an adaptive horizontal social orientation towards the peer groups which will also be essential in their social survival.

The major theme of Ridley's (R567) "Nature via Nurture" is that the biological role is not one of genetic determinism, but of genes adaptively influencing and not rigidly determining a complex conscious neurodynamic response to circumstances. However nature via nurture also implies the nurture needs only to be sufficiently responsive and diverse to allow the natural genetic potentials to emerge. Hrdy (R323 378) concurs "Every human mother's response to her infant is influenced by a composite of biological responses of mammalian, primate and human origin. These include endocrinal priming during pregnancy, physical changes (including changes in the brain) during and after birth, the complex feedback loops of lactation, and the cognitive mechanisms that enhance the likelihood of recognizing and learning to prefer kin. But almost none of these responses are automatic. To survive in evolutionary time all of these systems had to pass through the evolutionary crucible so well summarized by Hamilton's rule ... probable costs or benefits are factored in. In humans whose infants are so costly and for whom conscious planning (thanks to the neocortex) is a factor, maternal investment in offspring is complicated by a range of new considerations: cultural expectations, gender roles, sentiments like honour or shame, sex preferences, and the mother's awareness of the future. ... We are still far from understanding how genetically influenced receptors in the brain, thresholds for responding to different chemical signals hormone levels, and feelings of anxiety and contentment interact to produce the myriad 'decisions' that continuously affect maternal development."

The Naturalistic Fallacy, Human Nature, and Evolutionary Ethics

Alexander (R6 167) and others (Hrdy R323 23) highlight the importance of the 'naturalistic fallacy' - that what sometimes *is* in evolution tells us what *ought* to be in ethics and morality - in understanding pitfalls in applying evolutionary ideas to culture and morality. This has been used to claim a variety of positions later critiqued as fallible. A classic example which has reverberated down the decades was Herbert Spencer's division of labour by sex - 'men produce but women reproduce' - the founding tenet of 'social Darwinism' - on the basis that there was too little variation among females for proper selection to occur, precluding the evolution in women of higher 'intellectual and emotional' faculties which are the 'latest products of evolution'. Darwin noted "whether requiring deep thought, reason or imagination, or merely the use of the sense and the hands, [man will attain] a higher eminence ... than can woman" (Hrdy R323 15-19) basing his notions squarely on sexual selection "man [could] have become as superior in mental endowment to women, as the peacock is in ornamental plumage to the peahen" (Jolly R338 361).

Gerda Lerner (R397 19) brands the entire sociobiological position as traditionalist.

> "E.O. Wilson's sociobiology has offered the traditionalist view on gender in an argument which applies Darwinian ideas of natural selection to human behavior. Wilson and his followers reason that human behaviors which are 'adaptive' for group survival become encoded in the genes, and that they include in these behaviors such complex traits as altruism, loyalty and matenalism. ... Mothering is not only a socially assigned role but one fitting women's physical and psychological needs. Here once again biological determinism becomes prescriptive, in fact a political defence of the status quo in scientific language. Feminist critics have revealed the circular reasoning absence of evidence and unscientific assumptions of Wilsonian sociobiology. From the point of view of the non-scientist, the most obvious fallacy of sociobiologists is their ahistoricity in disregarding the fact that modern men and women do not live in a sate of nature".

When some sociobiologists argued that rape among humans, though undesirable, is really quite understandable because, after all, the males perpetuating it are merely trying (however unconsciously) to spread their genes (Symons R665; Thornhill and Thornhill R676), Anne Fausto-Sterling (R201 5), noted what a short step it would be from this line of thinking to the legal defense of a male rapist on the grounds that 'his genes made him do it'.

Linda Stone (R654) notes: "Other sociobiologists have contrasted human male and female 'reproductive strategies' ... moreover, they say, because women want to improve their children's fitness by increasing the parental investment of their mate, they devise ways of keeping a man around as provider and protector; and in trying to hold on to the man, they become 'coy' and 'clinging' females. Understandably, this line of argument drove many women to distraction. Criticism of this form of sociobiology has come from within the field as well as from outside it. Sarah Hrdy (1981), complained that previous sociobiologists had either ignored or misinterpreted females and female sexuality in their study of primate behavior and evolution ... that female primates, far from being sexually passive, could be active, competitive, and aggressive and that their roles in human evolution were important". Hrdy (R323 24) quips that David Buss's "Evolution of Desire" throws similar sops to Spencer's idea of beauty as a signal of fertility and genetic quality: "all women today are unique, distinctive winners of a five million year Pleistocene beauty contest of natural selection. Every female ancestor of the readers of these words was attractive enough to obtain enough male investment to raise at least one child to reproductive age".

Into the centerpiece of this debate we find Edward O. Wilson (R737) the founder of sociobiology takes an ambiguous position. Although he claims "the naturalistic fallacy has not been erased by improved biological knowledge, which still describes the *is* of life but cannot prescribe the *ought* of moral action", he then demurs "An understanding of the roots of human nature now seems essential to ethical philosophy. Any judgement concerning whether an act is natural or abnormal depends on such information, through behavioral categories as diverse as cousin marriage, homosexuality, territorial prerogatives and cannibalism. All attempts to define 'natural law' by unaided intuition are dangerously incompetent. This is equally true whether applied to such personal matters as the wisdom of contraception or to the supposedly inevitable trajectory of economic history."

Wilson's point here is valid. Our future viability is not just a function of cultural or economic expectations which are notoriously unstable and in the absence of an understanding of sociobiology prone to self-deceptive pitfalls which could be lethal. The evolutionary evidence both from our past and form other species, all who have had to pass the evolutionary test over cumulative lifetimes is the best indication we can hope to avail ourselves of in assessing our own directions and course of action in future. Neither does this determine any social course of action based on biological grounds, but rather gives a wider deeper context in which to understand culture and our own evolutionary decisions.

Central here is the vexed question of whether there is in fact such a thing as human nature. This argument has woven back and forth throughout the last few centuries and theories of evolution have only served to up the ante between the conflicting proponents of nature versus nurture, evolution versus morality, and genetic determinism versus cultural relativity.

Steven Pinker (R532) mounts a systematic case against the sociological notion that human nature is essentially a *tabula rasa* or 'blank slate' on which we can superimpose cultural or social imperatives without regard to our evolutionary heritage. His concerns are highly justified. Social paradigms that assume the right to dictate and reshape human nature rapidly veer into totalitarian agendas. "Skinner was a staunch blank-slater and a passionate utopian. His uncommonly pure vision allows us to examine the implications of the 'optimistic' denial of human nature. Given his premise that undesirable behavior is not in the genes but a product of the environment, it follows that we should control that environment-for all we would be doing is replacing haphazard schedules of reinforcement by planned ones. Why are most people repelled by this vision? Critics of Skinner's Beyond Freedom and Dignity pointed out that no one doubts that behavior can be controlled; putting a gun to someone's head or threatening him with torture are time-honored techniques. Even Skinner's preferred method of operant conditioning required starving the organism to 80 percent of its free-feeding weight and confining it to a box where schedules of reinforcement were carefully controlled. The issue is not whether we can change human behavior, but at what cost" (169).

Like Hrdy, Pinker (R532 171) applies this criticism specifically to the culturally relativistic positions of 'glass body' feminism:

"Nothing in the concept of human nature is inconsistent with the ideals of feminism ... But some feminist theoreticians have embraced the Blank Slate and with it an authoritarian political philosophy that would give the government sweeping powers to implement their vision of gender-free minds. In a 1975 dialogue, Simone de Beauvoir said: 'No woman should be authorized to stay at home to raise her children. Society should be totally different. Women should not have that choice, precisely because if there is such a choice, too many women will make that one.' Gloria Steinem was a bit more liberal; in a 1970 Time article she wrote: 'The [feminist] revolution would not take away the option of being a housewife. A woman who prefers to be her husband's housekeeper and/or hostess would receive a percentage of his pay determined by the domestic-relations courts.' Betty Friedan has spoken out in favor of 'compulsory preschool' for two-year-olds. Catharine MacKinnon (who with Andrea Dworkin has pushed for laws against erotica) has said, 'What you need is people who see through literature like Andrea Dworkin, who see through law like me, to see through art and create the uncompromised women's visual vocabulary' -oblivious to the danger inherent in a few intellectuals' arrogating the role of deciding which art and literature the rest of society will enjoy. In an interview in the New York Times Magazine, Carol Gilligan explained the implications of her (preposterous) theory that behavior problems in boys, such as stuttering and hyperactivity, are caused by cultural norms that pressure them to separate from their mothers: Q 'You would argue that men's biology is not so powerful that we can't change the culture of men?' A: 'Right. We have to build a culture that doesn't reward that separation from the person who raised them'.... Q: 'Everything you've said suggests that unless men change in fundamental ways, we're not going to have a sea change in the culture'. A: 'That seems right to me'. An incredulous reader, hearing an echo of the attempt to engineer a 'new socialist man,' asked, 'Does anyone, even in academia, still believe that this sort of thing turns out well?' He was right to be concerned. In many schools, teachers have been told, falsely, that there is an 'opportunity zone' in which a child's gender identification is malleable. They have used this zone to try to stamp out boyhood: banning same-sex play groups and birthday parties, forcing children to do gender-atypical activities, suspending boys who run during recess or play cops and robbers . In her book The War Against Boys, the philosopher Christina Hoff Sommers rightly calls this agenda 'meddlesome, abusive, and quite beyond what educators in a free society are mandated to do.'

Pinker (R532 172) sees an urgent need for biological feminism:

"Feminism, far from needing a blank slate, needs the opposite, a clear conception of human nature. One of the most pressing feminist causes today is the condition of women in the developing world. In many places female fetuses are selectively aborted, newborn girls are killed, daughters are malnourished and kept from school, adolescent girls have their genitals cut out, young women are cloaked from head to toe, adulteresses are stoned to death, and widows are expected to fall onto their husbands' funeral pyres. The relativist climate in many academic circles does not allow these horrors to be criticized because they are practices of other cultures, and cultures are superorganisms that, like people, have inalienable rights. To escape this trap, the feminist philosopher Martha Nussbaum has invoked 'central functional capabilities' that all humans have a right to exercise, such as physical integrity, liberty of conscience, and political participation. She has been criticized in turn for taking on a colonial 'civilizing mission or (white woman's burden,' in which arrogant Europeans would instruct the poor people of the world in what they want. But Nussbaum's moral argument is defensible if her 'capabilities' are grounded, directly or indirectly, in a universal human nature."

Anne Campbell (R102) defends human nature in similar terms:

"The denial of human universals is central to the liberal agenda because of critics' erroneous acceptance of the naturalistic fallacy and their mistaken belief that biology is destiny. If something is universal it may reflect a fundamental human nature and if such a thing exists at a biological level then attempts to ameliorate the status quo are doomed". However she notes: "Critics often seem confused about just what is meant by human nature. Consider the following quote from Sandra Bem (R56 21) 'As a biological species, human beings do not have wings, which once meant that it was part of universal human nature to be unable to fly. But now human beings have invented airplanes, which means that it is no longer part of human nature to be unable to fly'. Now the idea that sitting in a seat a few thousand miles above the ground [Anne is a very high flyer] constitutes an alteration of 'human nature' is an odd distortion of the concept. ... Do we seriously suppose that aeroplane passengers have a [fundamentally] different psychology or physiology from those who have not flown? ... It is equally hard to know what to make of Fausto-Sterling's (R201 199) claim that 'there is no singly undisputed claim about universal human behavior (sexual or otherwise).' Presumably even the most ardent cultural relativist would accept that everywhere people live in societies, that they eat, sleep and make love, and that women give birth and men do not. The problems seem to arise when we move from basic biological functions to behavior. Though everywhere women are the principal caretakers of children, the fact that there may be variation in how that task is fulfilled leads some anthropologists to conclude that mothering is not universal".

At issue is not just the question of whether humans have an evolutionary heritage, including sexual differences, or whether human culture can be modeled on natural and particularly evolutionary principles, but whether there can be considered to be any universals characterizing humanity. This is itself a paradoxical situation, because humanity has clearly evolved in a way which places itself in a universal position. We have become a meta-species creating and discovering as many niches within the burgeoning complexity of human culture and its many vocations as a diverse ecosystem in a tangled bank. We have achieved this through an adaptive trend in the brain towards universality of perception, emotion and conception, which has made it possible for philosophers to contend we are a *tabula rasa* - a blank slate upon which the diversity of the cultural record can be imposed freely. It is thus a deep contradiction for cultural relativists to deny human universality, even if of an evolutionary ilk.

Donald Brown (R83) in 'Human Universals' has documented ethnographically the extent of such universals, including gossip, lying, verbal humour, story telling, metaphor, distinction between mother and father, kinship categories, logical relations (not, same, equivalent, opposite), interpreting intention from behavior and recognition of six basic emotions. In regard to gender we find binary distinctions between men and women, more aggression and violence by men, acknowledgment of the differences between male and female natures and domination by men in the public political sphere. In 1973 Stephen Goldberg (R243) wrote documenting the universality of patriarchy, with upper positions in hierarchies occupied by males across even ostensibly matrilineal societies. Despite a showering of claimed exceptions his second work (R244) in 1993 continues to insist the thesis stands.

The Western tradition proceeds from a cultural background in which nature has been regarded as a lower realm subject to animal lust and the violence of tooth and claw in opposition to the purity of God's commands, despite the pristine beauty of Genesis 1's creation. The basic notion that we have been given the power to choose good and evil over natural instincts leads inevitably to a potential conflict between evolution and higher motives in which morality plays an enigmatic role.

The naturalistic fallacy is neatly expressed in David Hume's 'A Treatise of Human Nature' (R325): "In every system of morality, which I have hitherto met with, I have always remarked that the author proceeds for some time in the ordinary way of reasoning, and establishes the being of God, or makes observations concerning human affairs; when of a sudden I am surprised to find, that instead of the usual copulation of propositions, *is* and *is not*, I meet with no proposition that is not connected with an *ought*, or an *ought not*. This change is imperceptible; but is however, of the last consequence. For as this *ought*, or *ought not*, expresses some new relation or affirmation, it is necessary hat it should be observed and explained; and at the same time that a reason should be given, for what seems altogether inconceivable, how this new relation can be a deduction from others, which are entirely different from it." This distinction between *is* and *ought*, which Hume found so mysterious, may not be a mark of moral conscience so much as the capacity to semantically distinguish past and future in the emergence of semantic language.

Proponents of biology have taken a variety of views about the relation between evolution and morality. Darwin (R147 500) developed the first complete theory of morality and ethics, in the following words: "Ultimately our moral sense or conscience becomes a highly complex sentiment-originating in the social instincts, largely guided by the approbation of our fellow men, ruled by self-reason, and confirmed by instruction and habit. It must not be forgotten that although a high standard of morality gives but a slight or no advantage to each individual man and his children over the other men of the same tribe, yet that an increase in the number of well-endowed men and advancement in the standard of morality will certainly give an immense advantage to one tribe over another. A tribe including many members who, from possessing in a high degree the spirit of patriotism, fidelity, obedience, courage, and sympathy, were always ready to aid one another, and to sacrifice themselves for the common good would be victorious over most other tribes; and this would be natural selection. At all times throughout the world tribes have supplanted other tribes; and as morality is one important element in their success, the standard of morality and the number of well-endowed men will thus everywhere tend to rise and increase".

Interestingly, this is a group selection model reflecting Darwin's lack of knowledge of exact genetic mechanisms. Since George Williams' argument that which alleles survive depends primarily on reproductive successes and failures of individual organisms, rather than of groups, group selection has become a more complex proposition to assert, however it does have particular application when dealing with the group competition and social fluidity that is concomitant with the emergence of moral systems. Darwin's model depends on confluences of interests within groups and does not deny the existence of countering conflicts of interest within groups in a manner predictive of Alexander's ideas below.

Julian Huxley (R326 132) states clearly that morality must be founded on evolution:

"the evolutionist is able to provide new general standards or criteria for ethics ... contributions from ... [other] fields have been either incomplete (as in theology) or limited in extent. It is only in relation to the evolutionary process as a whole that our ethical standards can be fully generalized, and the system be rounded out to completion."

He goes further setting an evolutionary paradigm for a valid ethic: (142)

"evolutionary ethics must be based on a combination of a few main principles: that it is right to realize ever new possibilities in evolution, notably those which are valued for their own sake; that it is right both to respect human individuality and to encourage its fullest development; that it is right to construct a mechanism for further social evolution which shall satisfy these prior conditions as fully, efficiently, and as rapidly as possible".

By contrast, in the same work, Thomas Huxley, (83) coming from a pessimistic view of violent nature argues, as Augustine might have, that the imitation of 'the cosmic [evolutionary] process by man is inconsistent with the first principle of ethics':

"Let us understand, once for all, that the future depends, not on imitating the cosmic process, still less in running away from it, but in combating it ... the practice of that which is ethically best - what we call goodness or virtue - involves a course of conduct which, in all respects, is opposed to that which leads to success in the cosmic struggle for existence. Ethical nature may count upon having to reckon with a tenacious and powerful enemy as long as the world lasts."

However he footnotes this statement with an evolutionary qualification:

"Of course, strictly speaking, social life, and the ethical process in virtue of which it advances toward perfection, are part and parcel of the general process of evolution, just as the gregarious habit of innumerable plants and animals which has been of immense advantage to them, is so. A hive of bees is an organic polity, a society in which the part played by each member is determined by organic necessities ... Even in these rudimentary forms of society, love and fear come into play, and enforce a greater or less renunciation of self-will. To this extent the general cosmic process begins to be checked by a rudimentary ethical process, which is, strictly speaking, part of the former, just as the 'governor' in a steam-engine is part of the mechanism of the engine".

In this statement Huxley too seems to see moral systems as an outcome of the 'general cosmic process' as well as something that combats, or opposes it.

There are major questions here about what is 'good' in terms of nature, amicability or sustainable survival. Many evolutionary arguments are not made on agreeableness or non-violence but an appeal to the innate principles of viability contained in evolutionarily stable strategies and their ecosystemic relationships. Society may thus need to learn to incorporate paradigms of violence and conflict in its ethical models to ensure its own survival. Indeed capitalistic free market models are based on overweening competition of a kind not even found in living ecosystems.

This means that some critiques of the so called 'naturalistic fallacy' are themselves fallacies. Steven Pinker (R532 162) critiques environmentalist conservation of predators: "We have already met the naturalistic fallacy, the belief that whatever happens in nature is good. One might think that the belief was irreversibly tainted by Social Darwinism, but it was revived by the romanticism of the 1960s and 1970s. The environmentalist movement, in particular, often appeals to the goodness of nature to promote conservation of natural environments, despite their ubiquitous gore. For example, predators such as wolves, bears, and sharks have been given an image makeover as euthanists of the old and the lame, and thus worthy of preservation or reintroduction." There is clearly a confusion here between 'good' in terms of a viable ecosystem, which generally does need predators (p 507) to avoid population boom and bust, and 'good' in the social sense of non-violent.

Pinker noting its converse, exacts the fallacy from the feminist movement:

"It would seem to follow that anything we have inherited from this Eden is healthy and proper, so a claim that aggression or rape is 'natural,' in the sense of having been favored by evolution, is tantamount to saying that it is good. The naturalistic fallacy leads quickly to its converse, the moralistic fallacy: that if a trait is moral, it must be found in nature. That is, not only does 'is' imply 'ought,' but 'ought' implies 'is.' Nature, including human nature, is stipulated to have only virtuous traits (no needless killings, no rapacity, no exploitation), or no traits at all, because the alternative is too horrible to accept. That is why the naturalistic and moralistic fallacies are so often associated with the Noble Savage and the Blank Slate. Defenders of the naturalistic and moralistic fallacies are not made of straw but include prominent scholars and writers. For example, in response to Thornhill's earlier writings on rape, the feminist scholar Susan Brownmiller wrote, 'It seems quite clear that the biologicization of rape and the dismissal of social or 'moral' factors will ... tend to legitimate rape.... It is reductive and reactionary to isolate rape from other forms of violent antisocial behavior and dignify it with adaptive significance.' Note the fallacy: if something is explained with biology, it has been 'legitimated'; if something is shown to be adaptive, it has been 'dignified'."

Edward O. Wilson the founder of Sociobiology (R738) advances some curious evolutionary arguments, accepting homosexuality as having a possible offshoot genetic advantage in uncle parenting (such a tendency has by no means been demonstrated in gay men) and condemning incest as genetically deleterious, while introducing some intriguing personal moral interpretations of sexuality: "The primary functions of sexual behavior are pair bonding and the creation of genetic diversity, rather than reproduction per se. Thus the sexual revolution, but not promiscuity, is in concert with the innate learning rules." Alexander (R6 169) comments: "One is led to believe that he is implying by this that promiscuity somehow violates a 'natural law.' When asked following his oral presentation of this material if he meant that promiscuous people cannot be happy, he hesitated, but responded affirmatively, stating that in regard to questions of monogamy and fidelity he was conservative. After denying the validity of the naturalistic fallacy, Wilson is suggesting there are natural laws governing what is right and wrong about human behavior, and that only biologists, or those with extensive biological knowledge, are able to discover them".

This debate has manifest political dimensions. In supporting the purity of racial blood, Hitler quotes providence: "God having created races, it is therefore the noblest and most sacred duty for each racial species of mankind to preserve the purity of the blood which God has given it.' At the same time he practised eugenics and evolutionary amorality "the most cruel methods are humane if they give a speedy victory" (Alexander R6 167).

Critical in human universals is innate violence. In 1963 Konrad Lorenz added, in his influential 'On Aggression' (R415) that our species unfortunately has not had time to evolve the same inhibitions we see in 'professional' carnivores, such as lions and wolves. As a result, we are dangerous to our own kind. This pessimistic view soon met with resistance. Social psychologists and anthropologists demonstrated that aggressive behavior can be learned, and they questioned the universality of human violence by cultures believed to be peaceful. However it later became clear that Chimpanzees, rather than being peaceful vegetarians, also shared characteristics of human violence, including predation on monkeys, lethal intercommunity aggression, infanticide and even occasional cannibalism. Richard Wrangham and David Peterson in 'Demonic Males' (R750) put it this way "That chimpanzees and humans kill members of neighbouring groups of their own species is ... a startling exception to the normal rule for animals. Add our close genetic relationship to these apes and we face the possibility that intergroup aggression in our two species has a common origin. This idea of a common origin is made more haunting by clues that suggest modern chimpanzees are not merely fellow time-travellers and evolutionary relatives, but surprisingly excellent models of our distant ancestors. It suggests that chimpanzee-like violence preceded and paved the way for human war, making modern humans the dazed survivors of a continuous 5-million year habit of lethal aggression."

De Waal (R163) notes that both our subsequent experience of bonobos, for which we have no evidence for intercommunity raiding, infanticide, cooperative hunting or any of the other lethal activities, stressed as the hallmark of our species, and the greater flexibility and processes of reconciliation we now associate with ape aggression, which are quite distinct from predation, means our ideas are no longer dependent on the Lorenzian drive concept and the killer ape myth, which did little justice to the complexity of our species and its many distinct features other than aggressiveness. Bonobos particularly associate sex with reconciling aggression, where chimpanzees would merely kiss and embrace (p 66). Inter-male aggression is also reduced by the cooperative attitude of female bonobos when two groups meet.

Group Cooperation and Social Competition

Alexander (R6 79) and others have developed the idea that human evolution and in particular the morality of intra-group cooperation, has been guided to some large extent by intergroup competition and aggression, which we shall explain in detail because it is the basis of some of De Waal's views and it neatly explains many aspects of the sexual paradox between cooperation and competition inherent in the Prisoners' Dilemma.

Group living entails automatic costs to individuals, which must be compensated by specific benefits if group living is to evolve. Larger groups involve greater costs to individuals. Even if cooperative group hunting was the original context of human grouping, it cannot explain much of the history of human sociality. As hunting weapons and skills improved, group sizes should have decreased. Cooperative group hunters among nonhumans tend to live in small groups (canines, felines, cetaceans, some fish, and pelicans).

Large groups are typically what Hamilton called 'selfish herds', whose evolutionary *raison d'etre* is security from predation. Even groups evidently evolved to cooperate against predators are typically small (chimpanzees, baboons, musk ox). The only adequately significant external threat is other groups of humans. This can explain any size of group (as results of balance-of-power races). It accords with recorded human history. It is consistent with the fact that humans alone play competitively group-against-group on a large and complex scale. It also accords with the ecological dominance of humans as a species. In effect, organized in competitive groups, humans have become their own principal 'hostile force of nature.' Most of the evolution of human social life and the human psyche, may thus have occurred in the context of within- and between-group competition, the former resulting from the latter. Without the pressure of between-group competition, within-group competition would have been mild, nonexistent - or else dramatically different - because groups would have been smaller and would have required less unity and cooperativeness. Strate (R656) has concluded from a cross-cultural study that defense against other human groups accounts for variations in social organization better than any alternative. No other sexual organisms compete in groups as extensively, fluidly, and complexly as humans do. No other organisms play competitively group-against-group. So far as we know, in no other species do social groups have as their main jeopardy other social groups of the same species - hence the unending selective race toward greater social complexity, intelligence, and cleverness in dealing with one another.

To make the above argument requires some way of distinguishing primary causes of social grouping and secondary responses to it. On the other hand, one must also consider that any cooperative cause of group living cannot be expected to last and be elaborated unless it leads to increased reproductive success among all participants, which by definition means in relation to members of other groups, thereby establishing at least an indirect intergroup competition. Although indirect reciprocity may be unique to humans, we cannot ignore the possibility that there may be a parallel to morality in many nonhuman social groups that cooperate. Rudimentary moral systems (indirect reciprocity) would thus be expected to appear where outside threats most powerfully dictate group cohesion, when such threats are combated best by complex social organization within the group, and when the actions of single individuals or small subgroups can threaten, from within, either the group as a whole or its most powerful elements.

Alexander's theory has the following key features: (1) Individuals seek their own interests. (2) Their interests are ultimately reproductive , so include the interests of relatives and other shared relationships such as partners (3) Interests of individuals can be furthered by cooperating with others (4) The mechanisms are direct and indirect reciprocity, the latter involving a very complex significance of reputation or status. (5) The rules consist of restraints on particular methods of seeking self-interests that impede the efforts of others to seek their own interests. What is new in this theory is that (a) interests are seen as reproductive, not as individual survival, and, accordingly, pleasure and comfort are postulated to have evolved as vehicles of reproductive success, and (b) the mechanism of indirect reciprocity is made explicit as the central feature. These are not trivial refinements, since together they can account for aspects of beneficence that have perplexed philosophers, theologians, and students of morality.

A variety of research results lend confirmation to the thrust of Alexander's theory as an explanation for why human altruism extends far further and in much larger groups than kin and reciprocal altruism would allow for alone. Ernst Fehr, in developing the concept of 'strong reciprocity' (R204) notes: "many people are willing to cooperate and to punish those who don't even when no gain is possible". Robert Trivers has suggested that small group cooperation might have been a feature of regular interactions between known parties based on reciprocal altruism, which might have become maladaptive and be dying out in our larger social structures, where one shot interactions have become more common. Gächter and Falk (R228) have demonstrated that repeated play more than doubles cooperation levels. However Joseph Heinrich has noted that one-shot versus repeated interactions would have also occurred in gatherer-hunter times (Buchanan R92). Rilling et. al. (p 378) have demonstrated cooperation activates areas involved in emotional rewards and de Quervain et. al. (R157) similarly demonstrate that altruistic punishment of defectors also stimulates reward centres in an emotional form of 'sweet revenge'. Boyd et. al. (R72) using computer simulations have demonstrated that group competition encourages cooperation - punishing cheats increases the size of cooperative groups from 10 up to 30 the size of gatherer hunter bands. In a key extension of this idea, Fehr and Fishbacher (R203) have noted that punishing those who fail to punish cheats can increase cooperative group size to hundreds of individuals, effectively explaining in one stroke both large scale human social cooperativity and punitive moral codes. In another cumputer model Pamchanathan and Boyd (R516) have shown that such selection can be based more generally on coveting good reputations and punishing the bad.

Both the essential components of Alexander's theory of conflict between and within groups are manifest features of ape societies. Inter-group conflict is matched by mechanisms of reconciliation and mediation of aggression in intra-group conflict, noting that moral systems are produced by tension between individual and collective interests. Reconciliation is essential to maintain group cohesion against splinter defection and is widespread in animals societies, most often initiated by the 'victim' towards the 'aggressor' (p 67), as noted in "Natural Conflict Resolution" (Aureli and de Waal R27). The authors point out that reconciliation is even more important to individuals who have a long-standing cooperative relationship - the valuable friendship model. It is also worth a dominant individual reconciliating to avoid debilitating stress at the top (Dugatkin R175).

In "Good Natured" De Waal (R161 38) notes "Philosophers tell us that there is an element of rational choice in human morality, psychologists say there is a learning component, and anthropologists argue that there are few if any universal rules. The distinction between right and wrong is made by people on the basis of how they would like their society to function. It arises from interpersonal negotiation in a particular environment, and derives its sense of obligation and guilt from the internalization of these processes. Moral reasoning is done by *us* and not by natural selection" . However he then goes on to make the argument that "Evolution has produced the requisites for morality: a tendency to develop social norms and enforce them, the capacities of empathy and sympathy, mutual aid and a sense of fairness, the mechanisms of conflict resolution, and so on. Evolution has also produced the unalterable needs and desires of our species: the need for the young for care, a desire for high status, the need to belong to a group, and so forth. How all these factors are put together to form a moral framework is poorly understood, and current theories of moral evolution are no doubt only part of the answer." In the remainder of 'Good Natured' De Waal investigates the extent to which aspects of morality are recognizable in other animals, and "how humanity may have moved from societies in which things were as they were to societies with a vision of how things ought to be" bringing to the surface instances of sympathy and empathy, guilt and shame, giving and taking, reconciliation, peacemaking and just getting along.

Evolutionary Foundations of Original Sin and the Cultural Fall

The concept of original sin and its relation to free-will leads to major questions of the origin of good and evil and social responsibility, which have wracked religious thinking and moral imperatives throughout the millennia. There is no such thing as natural evil in any meaningful sense. Nature survives by tooth and claw. Homicide is natural as predation itself is an extension of the primary division between autotrophic plants and heterotrophic animals which must survive by consuming other life forms (p 325). This division leads in turn to herbivores and carnivores. Even parasites and diseases are an integral part of an ecosystem and must adapt to survive. Although some animals kill mercilessly, or toy with their injured victims for skill, predators and prey are in a dynamical sense interdependent (p 507). Too few predators and the herbivores may eat and reproduce themselves to starvation and population crisis. We need to learn from nature what are the true universals before attempting to exert moral or religious ideas of good and evil. We are taught "Thou shalt not kill" but every man woman and child was reputedly slaughtered in the fall of Jericho and Hazor, illustrating that this injunction was for the Hebrews but not apparently for the

Canaanites or Philistines. Our ideas of social evil are thus relative.

Left: The tooth and claw of predator and prey is a delicate dynamic which often helps preserve both. Too few predators and the prey may become epidemic and eat themselves to catastrophic extinction. Stragglers may die quickly from suffocation or a neck bite, although hunting play can become torment. Right: Crocodile guards its young in its mouth (R30).

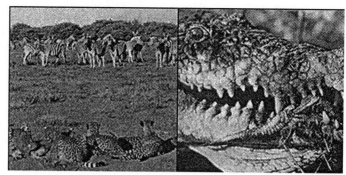

However there is another dimension of human evil which in the development of culture and utopian visions and the capacity of psychopathic individuals to gain disproportionate power, can become unhinged from nature and diabolical in their manifestations, from the programmed genocide of Shoah through the nuclear insanity of MAD - mutually assured destruction of the Cold War. One can draw the similar conclusions about an expedient George Bush stoking the fires of industrial pollution while every man woman and child in the US uses up to 150 times more non-renewable resources than a person in a developing country, strategically denying symptoms of climate change, when a mass extinction of biodiversity caused by human impact is in full swing.

We also have growing examples of genetic influences on criminality that lead to inferences that in some cases at least, anything from individual violence to compulsive gambling could be regarded as 'original sin' inherited in our genomes. Steve Jones' 'In the Blood' notes: "The law's basic assumption is that of autonomy: that everyone is liable for their deeds and is obliged to pay the price if they misbehave", based on the philosophy of the Greek Stoics of 300 BC who saw everyone as equally imbued with virtue and equally accountable for their misdemeanors. This makes a key distinction between the absence of natural evil in violent acts such as the predatory behaviour of carnivores, since this conforms to the natural processes of evolutionary selection and the human expedience of violence that comes from the exercise of free-will. This in turn is an affirmation for the pivotal role free will begins to have when sentient beings come of 'cosmic age' and begin to recognize how their intentionality can come to shape beneficent futures of abundance or agonizing unholy futures. of betrayal, attrition. competition and violence.

However the balance between nature and nurture is sensitive. Wild rhesus monkeys with low serotonin and aggressive behaviour were found to become socially adjusted when given supportive mothering (see Stephen Suomi Biological Psychiatry). A similar result has been found in the New Zealand serial study of the fate of 1037 children born in 1972 in Dunedin, New Zealand. They found that children were much more likely to grow up to be aggressive and antisocial if they had inherited a 'short' version the MAOA gene, which makes monoamine oxidase A, an enzyme which helps to break down neurotransmitters suchas serotonin, and was less efficient in the individuals with the 'short' version. But carriers only went off the rails if they had had an abusive upbringing. Carriers with good mothering were usually completely normal (R466).

The classic view of accountability must have exceptions when the culprit's soundness of mind is compromised, genetically or otherwise. Just as genes can give us the power to love, some genetic 'profiles' predispose to depression, psychosis, or psychopathic behaviour. In a climate of genetic predisposition this predispositions can and do lead to the defence that the actions were genetically caused, effectively citing original sin as a plea of individual 'innocence' or at least mitigation. For example there are up to 100-fold variations in the activity of the monoamine oxidase A enzyme involved in processing neurotransmitters such as serotonin, associated with emotional confidence. The short-arm versions of the MAOA gene results in individuals much more likely to suffer from depression, apprehension under stress (Ridley 2002 267). Chaotic behavior of people, particularly males, at the bottom of the social hierarchy, resulting from emotional dysphoria, may tend to give them more of a chance to break out of an invidious reproductive position and such 'delinquent' genes could thus be selected for. Schizophrenia also appears to have genetic correlates (Ridley 2002 109) raising a further spectre of original genetic 'evil' causing insanity, but here again there may be a trade-off in creative genius being associated with borderline insanity. Corballis (2002 178) also considers 'magical thinking' to be a social adaption, possibly associated with reduced cerebral dominance, reinforced by a form of reproductive advantage.

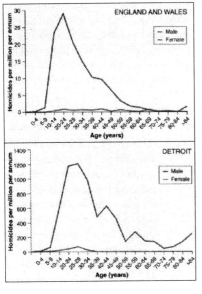

Genetic and environmental factors interpenetrate in non-relative homicide. Detroit has a 40 times higher murder rate than the UK. However men commit about 30 times as many murders as women. Genes and cultures are not mutually exclusive explanations, but the trend towards male violence is incontestable. Genetic and cultural factors of family disintegration may combine here. Limiting weapons is an obvious social measure (Jones R339 213).

From an evolutionary point of view, the leading cause of violence is maleness. "Men have evolved the morphological, physiological and psychological means to be effective users of violence" - Daly and Wilson. Some Darwinists such as Randy Thornhill (1983, 2000) contend that rape may be a 'natural' and even effective means to the male reproductive imperative. In fact, rape *is* more likely to get a female pregnant than intercourse with a partner. Rape is also clearly to get women pregnant in times of war as in Bosnia, so the simple idea of sex an non-reproductive naked power ignores key realities. In a light and shade debate, Robin Dunbar suggests rape is an evolutionarily viable reproductive strategy for a less attractive man, while Robin Baker counters this 'loser' theory stating that a woman selects for a rapist's genes because they have 'above average [reproductive] potential' (Taylor R670). However all human social actions are also influenced by social responses to them.

Feminists such as Anne Fausto-Sterling (R201) object that such work opens the door to frivolous exonerating pleas in the criminal justice system ('I beat my wife because it is man's nature to experience extreme sexual jealousy because of internal fertilization') (Campbell A R102 19). Robert Wright (R754) notes: "Of course, to call these things 'natural' isn't to call them beyond self-control, or beyond the influence of punishment. And it certainly isn't necessary to call them good. Evolutionary psychology might even be invoked on behalf of the doctrine of Original Sin: we are in some respects born bad, and redemption entails struggle against our nature". It is only by men understanding the biological roots of their violence and tendency to dominion over nature that society can become whole and the environment can survive. The key to undoing the negative endowment of the Fall is understanding ourselves and adopting an ethic which induces the unity of purpose required to coexist in a closing circle of life. Wright (R755) continues:

By Darwinian lights, the classic sins, such as gluttony, lust, greed and envy, are the unchecked expression of impulses that arose by natural selection, or worse still the calculated use of them in a newly unfeeling, menacing and expedient way. More than a century ago, Thomas Huxley, Darwin's popularizer, lamented the fact that evolution has given all children "the instinct of unlimited self-assertion - their dose of original sin." However as we shall see, evolutionary psychology asserts that our "ethical sentiments" likewise have an innate basis. Such impulses as compassion, empathy, generosity, gratitude and remorse are genetically based. These impulses, with their checks on raw selfishness, helped our ancestors survive and pass their genes to future generations.

Patriarchy is still a major force in informed human society, especially in the upper echelons of academia (New Scientist 2 Oct 2004 45). Compare fig (p 392).

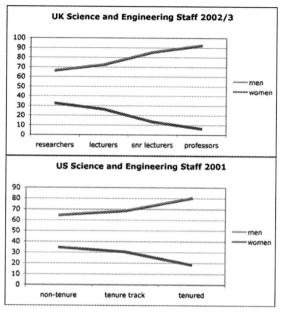

The U.S. Centers for Disease Control and Prevention reported in 2005 that homicide is a leading cause of traumatic death among new and expectant mothers, accounting for 31% of maternal injury deaths, second, after auto accidents (44%), other unintentional injuries (13%) and suicide (10%) among trauma deaths of pregnant women and new mothers. Black women had a maternal homicide risk about seven times that of white women. At ages 25 to 29, black women were about 11 times as likely as white women to be killed, although the age factor is more prominent. Using 617 cases, the CDC calculated a ratio of 1.7 homicides per 100,000 live births, but Chang, the lead author, acknowledged the ratio is understated because homicides are so poorly tracked. In Maryland, researchers found 11.5 homicides per 100,000 live births. In two other state studies, the figures were much higher in other studies. These figures suggest male jealousy is a significant factor in the pregnant female death rate.

Some human societies, such as the Yanomamo (p 148) and Jivaro (p 156) are avowedly violent and practice levels of warfare lethal to 25% to 60% of adult males (p 149), in pursuing practices of wife capture and abduction driven by clearly reproductive imperatives. Martin Daly and Margo Wilson (R143) have also found suggestive evidence that male infanticide of competitors seen in apes (p 65) also exists among humans. Surveying crime statistics, they noted that when an adult male murders a child he is 65 times more likely to be a stepfather or live-in boyfriend than the child's biological father.

In an analysis of 25,000 studies involving 8 million people, Susan Fiske concludes (Science 306) that almost anyone was found to be capable of torture, not just psychopathic people, if a peer group and/or commanding figures of authority were also condoning it. Stress of war, and alienation towards the 'other', were also factors conducive to torture. It is notable that even in such situations the study also found there was often a moral, defecting whistle blower who bucked the trend. Culture thus acts strongly enough on the average human genetic makeup to be capable of generating acts of atrocity. This is not a genetic form of 'original sin' but rather a cultural product of the 'fall'. To a large extent, it is culture which has to be accountable for many aspects of human violence, and patriarchy is human culture's classic alienation, across the sexual divide. Unlike genes, which are conserved over many generations and thus both trustworthy and slow to change, culture can be creatively transformed for the better by an informed act of choice.

Geoffrey Miller (R464) claims our propensity for generosity is also a product of selection, albeit sexual, rather than natural, leading to compassion for others and agreeable good nature. When starving people watch on television, the public respond and are often moved with great emotion by their empathy with situations of human plight. Throughout the world organizations like Amnesty International and Greenpeace receive their grass roots vitality from an emotional force that flows like a river towards an altruism which underlies our very will to survive in a world of light and life. It is clearly within the power of human communication to give a common sense of purpose to the human family, so that in reaching to the desire of humanity to live "creatively, intensively and successfully in the world" we all gain a measure of the blessing of fulfillment. The need to balance forgiveness with firm but fair responses to exploitation and aggression is part of our evolutionary endowment. To "Love your enemies, bless them that curse you, do good to them that hate you, and pray for them which despitefully use you, and persecute you", is conducive to mutual coexistence but not practiced in a one-sided way that let's them hang us accursed on a tree, or more innocent blood will flow. Evolution appears to have struck this balance well.

Original Virtue and the Evolution of Love

In "The Origins of Virtue", Matt Ridley (R565) explores what causes moral sentiment and social altruism, given an organism which, at the genetic level, might appear to be a bundle of selfish genes. Pivotal to this idea is the common role of emotion. Ridley casts moral sentiments in the practical light of reciprocal exchange and cites the work of Cosmides and Tooby as portraying the deep role detecting cheating has in maintaining commitment and transactional 'trust' in social groups. The great sensitivity of humans to tests defined in terms of deceit and fidelity such as the Wason test tends to emphasize how sophisticated our social sense of long-term commitment is in the shifting interplay of human liaisons.

The pendulum having swung away from notions of group selection and survival of the species towards survival of genes we have to investigate all forms of social altruism in a genetic context. We have already discussed Hamilton's concept of kin altruism (p 19). Because we share our genes sexually, most species display forms of kin altruism in which for example crocodiles will carefully protect their offspring in their mouths. Obviously if each of our offspring contains half our genes, our genes' survival is furthered by making a 50% investment in each of our offspring of that we make in our own survival. The same argument applies to our siblings. The extension of this by Trivers to reciprocal altruism (p 20) still falls within strict guidelines of reciprocal exchange, which is initially detrimental to the initiator, eliminating simultaneous mutual cooperation as potentially self-serving.

This leaves a heritage, which at face value falls short of the universal love expressed in the notion of divine union. It abets a society where unrelated competing individuals may take the expedient route and try to do away with their competitors, or take advantage of them in hard-nosed competition. It does not immediately lead to humanitarian compassion for the unrelated 'other' in plight. Defection always emerges as a competitor to cooperation in any game theoretic situation. However humanity has also evolved in ways which promote a resolution of this social dilemma. Much of human social evolution has been to do with learning when people in our immediate personal lives are trustworthy and distinguishing deceit from sincerity. We are also endowed with a strong urge for meaning and a place in life and for partnership. We are emotional and yearn for sexual and filial love.

Emotions are a common currency of declaring commitment and revealing about our personal situations and intentions sufficiently enough to facilitate cooperation socially, which is conducive to a common interest which compensates for the supposed selfishness at the level of the gene and to a certain extent also in the genetic competition between individuals. Emotions themselves thus form a central arena where moral sentiments gain credible biological meaning and explain why, despite a twenty times higher level of violence in males than females, humans are nevertheless far less violent to one another on an individual footing then many animal societies. The discovery of 'mirror neurons' (p 379) puts this universality of emotions, and along with it the capacity to make strategic choices about the way other individuals are behaving on to a sound physiological footing.

The idea that we have original virtue is central to this perspective. Although organisms act to conserve and replicate their genetic identities, the evolution of the mammalian emotional 'limbic' system has set the stage for the evolution of love. Although we further our own personal and family interests, we have evolved to be emotionally responsive in a way which gives us all an evolutionary advantage through constructive social cooperation. It is from the development of universal algorithms in the mammalian emotional system that our emotional view of the world and society derives and our paradoxical mix of freedom of choice, guilt, compassion, empathy and expedience. This system is also closely coupled with one which links peak emotional experiences with spiritual feelings of great significance in the links between the limbic system and temporal lobes, suggesting the religious imperative may be a social expression of a genetic trait towards coherent societies with a sense of common meaning and destiny, illustrated by seemingly paradoxical acts such as altruistic punishment o f defectors at cost to the individual (p 378).

As we have noted, evolutionary game theorists have drawn attention to the need to realistically picture the evolutionary stability of any strategy to test questions of altruism and survival in an environment of cooperators and defectors (p 13). Many of these games bear very directly on the central moral teachings of Judaism and Jesus. A very effective game strategy is tit-for-tat. This manifests in cooperative and retributive forms "an eye for and eye and a tooth for a tooth". For a significant initial period, tit-for-tat was extolled as an evolutionarily stable strategy, but it is prone to wasteful internecine strife and costly vendettas. So there are strategies which are more compassionate but don't go so far as saying if you slap me I will always turn my cheek. For example firm-but-fair makes sorties out of tit-for-tat loops to see if cooperation might be insightful to the 'opponent'. This is taking us to territory right in the grey area between Jesus frank "love your enemies even to the point of martyrdom" and Leviticus' "love your neighbour as yourself", or Jesus' "do unto others as you would they should do unto you", or as Hillel said more protectively before him "Do not do unto others as you would they should not do unto you".

The idea of fair punishment has been found to help maintain altruism in human groups (Fehr and Rockenbach R205). An egalitarian sense of fair play is shared by chimps and capuchins as well as humans, with a similar sense of justification for gains and protestation at discrimination (R81). Strategic bluffing is also characteristic of such large brained primates. People playing an investing game with real money rapidly abandoned their altruistic behaviour if they felt the punishment given for selfish acts was unwarranted, suggesting that groups of our ancestors who found the best strategies to promote altruism prospered, and bequeathed their behaviours to us. In an anonymous investing game, the 'investor' can invest up to 10 'dollars' with a 'trustee', requesting a specific rate of return. The trustee receives triple the investment put in by the investor and then can choose how much, if any, to return. Even though anonymous trustees could have just kept the investment without being identified, 19 out of 24 of them returned some money. And the more money invested - implying faith in the trustee by the investor - the more they returned. Next, the researchers gave the investors the option of setting a punishment for the trustee in advance, if they did not return the amount asked for - a fine of four 'dollars' . Choosing not to impose any punishment went down well with the trustees - they gave back 50 per cent more money on average. They feel an obligation to pay back, because they have been treated nicely by the investor. But, crucially, trustees make a distinction between fair and unfair punishments. When the requested return is low, meaning the trustee will make more than the investor, imposing a fine did not significantly change the payback. However, if the investor is more greedy and asks for a large return that leaves the trustee worse off, then an additional threat of punishment makes trustees slash their payouts by nearly two thirds. If people feel the punishment is fair, they cooperate, but defect against an unfair punishment.

Intriguingly hormones can alter the whole strategic basis of the game. In a variant of the trustee game (Kosfeld et. al. R380, R144), 45% of those sniffing oxytocin (p 352) entrusted all their funds to the trustee while only 12% of those on a placebo did so, probably because it helps overcome avoidance behavior and helps cement emotional bonding.

Geoffrey Miller (R464) proposes an antidote to the dilemma of selfishness, ingenious in its explanation at a single stroke of the ultimate origins of compassionate generosity beyond any form of kin or reciprocal altruism. This is the positive filter of sexual selection for generosity as a genuinely costly indicator of genetic fitness which is also conducive to social harmony and affectionate loving nature. If our potential sexual partners choose tokens of fitness which result in uncheatable expressions of generosity, not only will we choose a fit resourceful partner but we will have a fulfilling partnership whose offspring have an excellent chance of survival. From this source original virtue flows like an eternal spring.

In this context, mammals have evolved a new type of evolutionary response to the question of genetic altruism through the limbic emotional brain. By endowing us with emotions it has become possible for us to respond with an emotional kinship which is far more subtle than instinctual genetic responses. We can respond fully to one another as devoted friends, not just because we further direct reciprocal altruism but because the emotional landscape of friendship is a type of resource made possible by emotional bonding, which is a win-win situation for survival and for coexistence. Although mammals do display shocking behaviour such as a cat playing with a mouse, or killer whale batting a baby seal to death for sport, these generally have a survival explanation in maintaining good hunting prowess and motivation, so that they do not constitute the evil of tooth and claw, but life attuned to the hunt. The limbic system is capable of experiencing all the states of emotion from the heaven of divine ecstasy, to the hell of fear at impending doom. Within this magnificent and terrifying spectrum lie all the colours of emotion from true love, through to heated infatuation, jealousy, and guilt to anger, hate and mortal dread. We have thus been fully-equipped to experience the entire ecosystemic condition as sentient beings.

We have evolved to be capable of universal love through wisdom, through the coevolution of the limbic system and neocortex. This love is not locked in endless battle with hate, it is the win-win healing of the mortal dread of hate in peaceful coexistence. Through our wisdom we can heal the human condition to make the human passage of incarnation a loving and sacred experience of minimal pain and maximal fulfillment. This does not require moral conditioning and the rule of law and punishment alone to achieve, but an appreciation for the integrating power of love as a consensual integrative process by which we can come to be able to experience the universe in a way which promotes constructive harmony and compassionate responsibility for our actions.

The transition to love is however an act of choice for each of us. We are all capable of selfishness and calculated unfeeling expedience, particularly when we can exercise winner-take-all advantage by stealth and greed. This is the 'evil' within that we need stand firmly but fairly against in ourselves and in our dealings with others, so that we can fulfill the collective unfolding of cooperative emotional love. In this sense we can say that god is really love. The 'evil' within is not an active satanic force, but a form of defection which we have the free choice not to exercise - our powers of selfish or unfeeling exploitation or pleasure at the expense of others. The universe has evolved so that we have the free will to love and are genetically-endowed to be capable of love as the fabric of the continuity of life.

The universe has thus evolved to make us capable of love, destined even. One can argue that powerful evolutionary selection for both sensual and compassionate love, and with it what William Blake called 'incarnational jouissance' - the whole panoply of sexual and emotional pleasure - has occurred because, given our increasingly self-conscious freedom of choice, it is only beings endowed with such richly motivating emotional experiences who have the innate capacity to evoke a comprehensive and coherent tenacity for survival amid the vagaries of an existence caught in the mortal coil.

Being of good character, agreeable, consistent, fair and trustworthy, especially when the chips are down, is to be trusted, loved and sought after as an adviser, comrade and social leader. Mediating conflict in others is a key asset in the quest for a secure social position. There is even honour among thieves, as the saying goes - the key to the Prisoners' Dilemma.. Thus even if we accept a Machiavellian Intelligence hypothesis (Whiten and Byrne R728) including tactical deception, as lying at the root of human complexity, and with it, all of Alexander's arguments about inter-group morality being driven by intra-group competition (p 15), such astute responses as Machiavellian intelligence inspires are likely to embrace genuine indicators of cooperative trust to espouse a win-win, as well as opportunistic covert defection for strategic gain. The filtering by natural selection proposed by Sarah Hrdy, in which maternal ambivalence is attuned to the long term survival of a mother and her descendents applies to all social contracts and to both sexes. We all make a trade off between good character and expedience and we do so trading immediate opportunities for long-term advantages in social standing and the survival of our offspring.

Variance in altruism has been found in a study of 322 twins to have a 42% genetic basis for socially responsible behaviour, with 23% coming from the shared family environment and a further 35% coming from peer group and other non-shared factors Rushton (R588) . Rushton notes: "goodness is somewhat inherent in people. We all join groups and we all want to do the right thing by our group ... there's even honour among thieves." Overall women had higher social responsibility and parents seems to invest more in the social responsibility of their daughters, claiming "boys will be boys". The effect of the family environment is contradicted in some other studies. We thus see both our evolutionary heritage and our culture have strong influences on our human 'goodness'.

Human love is multidimensional. We start by falling in love and continue from sexual infatuation to a close emotional partnership and for many of us, the fulfillment of sexual love in reproduction, leading to a long-term or lifetime adventure of coexistence:

Stay me with apples, for I am sick with love.

These sentiments elaborate down and across the generations in love between parent and child, filial familial love and propensity for good character. Sexual love is more than just reproduction. It is the most powerful force of social bonding in humans, not just a programmed instinct in the reproductive cycle. Sexuality and socalization intermingle psychosexually. Society revolves around the power of sexual love, in song and human drama, from comedy through passion to tragedy. It is also the object of patriarchal religious edict, and violent oppression, because of the very untameable nature of the force it is.

The sexual act itself is a physical and not necessarily loving act, as rape and prostitution confirm, but in sexual love the sexual act becomes the complete expression of the complementation of two beings in the immortal continuity of life. However filial love is a virtue also contained in the natural mammalian endowment of the limbic system. Although not all people are moved to tears, many are, when faced with emotional situations of life, death separation and reconciliation which betray a deep will to love dwelling in the human psyche. Joseph wept in secret when his brothers came even as he sorely tested them. Jesus wept. People literally weep for love! People are also moved to compassion witnessing the plight of others and some live to serve the greater good as their fulfillment in life. Although the psyche can show great egotism, when the barriers of love come down, we finally become one. Through an unswerving faith to one another, borne of ice and fire, out of free choice in the transaction of love, we all gain our place in the completion of existence. This is filial love at its highest - love for all humanity and for life in all its forms.

Love drives even deeper to a deep soul love for all beings simply for the mortal tragedy of ours and their existence as birds of fire on the all-too-brief journey of incarnation. This is also the love of the mystic. The heights of epiphany or samadhi are incomplete without the exaltation of divine love pouring as a cataract of light, as a flame of joy, through our very being, convulsed by the power, gentility, grace and peace of the divine condition and the utter compassion showed by the universe to all incarnate beings. This is also a journey of infinite sadness for all mortal beings, but is also a reconciliation and reunion in atonement for all of us - the homecoming. The mystery of mysteries is that we have evolved into this condition. Key to this is a cosmic change of perspective. The only living strategy with any real future is to participate in the flowering of evolutionary culture. We are then fully part of the fabric, coming to terms with our cosmic responsibility for our actions, as co-creators of the living planet's genetic evolutionary and intentional conscious future.

Mating Minds and Flowering Cultures

Geoffrey Miller's "The Mating Mind" (R464) provides a potent, and prophetically in his own words, "Dionysian" and "chaotic" release unveiling the origins of virtue, and human complexity in culture, specifically through sexual selection. This is an antidote to both the Judeo-Christian foundations of Western conservatism and capitalist greed. It has immense implications for all creative aspects of humanity, from art and music to science, and for the future of our institutions, human society and culture. The core of this idea is that our social structures and our emotional and intellectual life originate from irresolvable paradoxes of reproductive interdependence, through sexual selection. Sexual 'intercourse', the source of our immortality, is now discovered to be also the source of our generosity. All other pretensions of society and intellect are ephemeral, except in so far as they serve this reproductive end for ourselves, or spread to other reproducing beings through literature and culture.

Darwin, in pondering the peacock's tail, recognized that sexual selection is a key complement to natural selection - a chaotic runaway phenomenon, while natural selection is largely conservative. Human evolution has occurred in a context where our principal competitors are other members of our own species and sexual selection is likely to have been the principal force in the evolution of a universal species with an absence of clear predators or specific species on which we depend, being omnivorous gatherers and hunters.

If we are thinking of social institutions, or future utopian world orders, we need to consider that all ape societies are delicate dynamical systems based on a complementation of two disparate social groupings. Firstly the females, distributed across the environment in relation to the occurrence of rich plant foods. In turn the males, either individually or in troops, distribute themselves in different patterns to induce the females into reproductive liaisons. Any attempts we make to design utopian world orders have to take into account evolutionary equilibrium if they are going to be sustainable and not merely imposed structures giving rise to unstable societies which destroy themselves or one another through coercive structures and institutions which fail to recognize evolutionary realities. Our own society is just emerging from several thousand years of frank sexual dominion of man over woman which has resulted in highly artificial institutions and a perception that law can be imposed in contradiction to our own best evolutionary interests. That boom and bust exploitation is a viable strategy, although it is destroying our planet's future fecundity.

Darwin also noted that mutual mate choice could give rise to effective evolutionary selection if mates were able to combine through mutual mate choice to form couplings according to fitness, noting species which had symmetrical characteristics in the light of this, so our dominant motif of overt serial monogamy is an evolutionarily stable strategy. However as we have seen, monogamy always occurs in a fertile covert ground-swell of clandestine affairs which contribute an additional fifth of our offspring, chosen principally through male genetic fitness rather than resources, which ensure a wider mixing of the gene pool than strict monogamy would allow, so strict monogamy is not. Polygyny, and the wandering male as well as female affairs add to our genetic diversity through sexual selection.

Human mate choice is not entirely mutual, but strongly skewed by the natural tendency of males to try to reproduce with many females and to compete and show off to achieve that end. Males in most species display indicators of genetic fitness since they bear no offspring themselves are dependent on females to reproduce, offering only their genes in their sperm. By contrast the human female can get pregnant by any male and will always give birth to her own offspring. Females are thus choosy and males showy. This can give rise to rapid runaway selection, as exemplified by the peacock's tail. To be a genuine indicator of fitness, a display must be costly and hard to fake. Sexual selection also requires the females to be able to be as choosy as the males can manage to display. In the context of intellectual displays, this requires females to be as discerning judges as the males can be performers, requiring both to keep ahead in the red queen race for increasing intellect.

Miller attributes all the creative developments of culture, art, the humanities, intellect and the virtues of compassion and agreeableness to mate choice, partly mutual, but skewed towards female reproductive choice. Darwin who also perceived this possibility, made a serous error in his estimation of this situation: "man [could] have become as superior in mental endowment to woman, as the peacock is in ornamental plumage to the peahen" (Jolly R338 361). Miller correctly points out here that this evolution of woman in the coat tails of man theory does not stack up. It is the demanding nature of the peahen's visual apparatus and her ever-escalating choosiness about display which has driven the poor peacock to a Prisoners' Dilemma of frank, through resplendent disability. If we are considering cultural evolution, the choosiness of the female is always a step ahead of the male and discerning appreciation of eloquent fable and fine art requires as refined an intellect as the performer or the performance can be a faked and shallow affair.

Since the advent of the selfish gene, and the eclipse of group and species selection, evolutionary theorists have pondered how altruism can come to exist. As accounted in Matt Ridley's "Origins of Virtue" (R565), Hamilton firstly introduced the concept of kin altruism - caring for the survival of your relatives because they share some of our own genes, and Trivers complemented this with reciprocal altruism between possibly unrelated individuals. However reciprocation requires a keen episodic memory and is rare in nature. Neither do either of these explain the obvious capacity of humans to be altruistic beyond these horizons in situations where no reciprocation is possible. Compassionate love knows no bounds and asks no specific favours in return.

Miller's answer to this dilemma is that social selection (which is catalytic on sexual opportunity, but in its controlling aspects against defection, is often negative - thou shalt not commit adultery even though 70% of us do it) is too indirect an effect in relation to the immense power of direct reproductive selection, to be the prime mover. The 'true' picture is probably an overlapping mixture with sex the driving force. Miller presents convincing reasons why generosity and compassionate love are the necessarily costly tokens of genuine fitness, that it is sex which has produced not only lust and passionate love, but compassion, agreeableness and generosity to boot. "Sympathy, agreeableness, leadership, fidelity, good parenting, charitable generosity" in Miller's words all derive from sex. It is thus sex which makes us good ethical beings, not social or moral control alone or even principally. This is reflected strongly in the key priorities people have in choosing a partner recorded by David Buss: "love or mutual attraction, dependable character, emotional stability, maturity, pleasing disposition, kind, healthy, smart, educated, sociable, interested in home and family." It is clear these attributes would select for good, amicable, relatively faithful, home builders, particularly among the males, who through astute female reproductive choice, would become innovatively good artists and musicians, entertaining story tellers, affectionate lovers, and humorous companions, while remaining, stealthy hunters, good protectors and astute diplomats. In Matt Ridley's words "domestic bliss". This kind of selection is possible only while females have the conditions and power to apply female reproductive choice. Patriarchal dominion leads rather to women who will produce many sons who can achieve power through status or the force of arms. Furthermore risk-taking male bravado, which makes little Darwinian sense, doesn't impress females, who prefer cautious men (Farthing R200) although they also prefer dominant males (Pelligrini and Long R522). Bravado may rather function to raise male status by impressing other males, only indirectly enhancing mate choice. In speed-dating experiments, although people cite similar social status and background - as the basis of their choices, they act largely on biological indicators - female nubility and male physical attractiveness (Douglas R171), leaving the ideal soul mate for posterity, in the artificially accelerated rush to courtship.

Of course, we are generous because we experience the full spectrum of the mammalian emotional repertoire from hate to love, a huge step of evolution towards a paradigm that goes far beyond individual genetic instincts. However these emotions survive not just because they are 'good', but because they abet survival and pivotally the reproduction of those possessing genes giving rise to such 'empathic' emotions. Rather than strict reciprocation, we have evolved two independent and yet keenly opposed emotional senses, both molded by sexual selection, firstly the capacity for compassionate and generous love and the second to be acutely sensitive to cheating and prepared to punish defection.

Roughgarden (R580), citing the examples of animal 'homosexuality' (Bagemihl R33), and the biology of sex-changing species (p 340), has proposed that social selection, including same-sex bonding (p 384), acts as a major filter to reproductive opportunity. Roughgarden takes issue with the primacy of sexual selection and even goes as far as saying 'sexual selection should be tossed out completely' on the basis of sex changes and the occasional incidence of same sex 'relations' in the natural world:

There are two glaring flaws in Darwin's thinking. In 1871 he wrote, 'Females choose mates' who are 'more attractive ... vigorous and well-armed' just as 'man can give beauty ...to his male poultry' by selective breeding. Hence the peacock's tail, Darwin's frequent example , is supposed to reflect peahen taste in male fashion, and antlers a preference for strong warrior stags. 'Males of almost all animals have stronger passions than females,' he wrote, and, 'The female ...

with the rarest of exceptions is less eager than the male... she is coy.' In Darwin's view, males and females almost universally conform to their preordained roles of horny handsome warriors and discreetly discerning damsels. But the real world is far more diverse than that. In many species, including ours, females are not necessarily less eager than males, nor do females all yearn for Arnold Schwarzenegger. Females often solicit males, and males often decline. Moreover, in many species the supposed sex roles reverse. Even Darwin acknowledged species of birds, like the jacana, in which the females are highly ornamented and the males dull and drab, reversing the peafowl story.

In highly social animals with pronounced sexual activity, such as bonobos (p 66), female reproductive opportunity is influenced by social selection. Participating in same-sex favours which strengthen female coalitions is a key step in social integration for a young exogamous female joining a new troop. Bonobo female-female sexual bonding is strongly linked to the conflict of reproductive interests between female and male in a unique society in which female exogamy combines with female 'dominance' through female coalitions, tipping the sexual dominance from males as in chimps (p 63) to females.

Female Spotted Hyena female with pseudo-penis (Scientific American Jan 94 102)

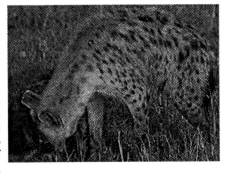

However many species have only a short estrus mating season, and engage in social grooming and amatory behaviors which are not explicitly sexual. This applies to the spotted hyena *Crocuta crocuta*, another species noted for its gender bending, whose dominant aggressive females are 10-20% larger than the males. The hyena is at an extreme of a pattern of female dominance and masculinization common to several mammalian species. One-quarter of mammalian families contain species in which females are larger than males, and there are other female mammals with genitals that are masculinized to some degree, including the spider monkey and European mole. Spotted hyenas have an elongated penis-like vagina, complete with a false scrotum which makes them almost indistinguishable from a male (Gould R248). Consequently their angular birth canal, makes birth a perilous process, with infant mortality up to 40% in first births (Hrdy R323 51). The pseudopenis is unable to accommodate the first birth and the end is inevitably torn open during the first delivery. It is erectile and functions as a 'tool' of social appeasement and familiarization. Subdominant males and females expose their genitals in a paradoxical sign in which erection signals submission, rather than desire, risking serious reproductive injury if the dominant female fails to acknowledge the submission.

However estrus is brief and these encounters are not sexual, but social processes to appease aggression in a mammal so uniquely violent that newborn twins tear at one another, leaving bleeding puncture wounds that frequently result in one or other starving from fear (Meadows R454). Up to a quarter of all young die in this way. The masculinization of the female begins in utero with the conversion of the androstenedione steroid synthesis pathway in the placenta from estrogen to testosterone. However treatments that reduce penis size in other species - prenatal exposure to compounds that inhibit androgens, and castration before puberty - have little effect on genital size in either sex in spotted hyenas, suggesting other genetic mechanisms are also involved. The explanation that hyenas are aggressive group feeders whose high-ranking females enforce strict dominance is also common to several mammal species which do not display these traits. Although a successfully aggressive species, moving from scavenging to predation of animals as large as wildebeast, many of the spotted hyena's characteristics are a direct consequence of adapting to the genetic and hormonal sequellae of female masculinization, whose high costs in many respects are offset by their predatory niche, rather than a manifestation of an evolutionary gender rainbow.

The intriguing examples of sex change in reef fish (p 340), while allowing social factors to influence non-chromosomal sex determination, still hold true to the principles of the Prisoners' Dilemma of sexual selection. Hermaphroditism and socially-driven sex change are adaptions to ensure heterosexual reproductive sex is facilitated under situations of social stratification, which limit opportunities for mating, and are antipodally opposite to same-sex socio-sexual bonding. Neither the natural incidence of hermaphroditism, widespread in plants, as well as animal species such as snails and worms, nor socially driven sex change undermines the power and directness of sexual selection. Nor does it establish that the peacock's tail is to impress other male peacocks, rather than the untamably choosy retinas of peahens seeking sensitive indicators of fitness. Nor does an incidence of frequent socio-sexual bonding, including same-sex couplings, in a few social species such as bonobo, mean that social selection takes primacy, to the exclusion of sexual selection, nor that sexuality is primarily for social bonding rather than reproductive fitness and the survival of successive generations. Only in so far as these two come together, with sexual selection in full play, does the whole process make evolutionary sense.

In human society, despite mild polygynous tendencies, reproductive fitness is measured principally through heterosexual partnering and parenting, particularly mothering. Outside artificial insemination and politically proactive forms of IVF, same-sex bonding is non-reproductive. Nor is it integral to the parenting aspect of reproduction, since the social support required for reproductive success is largely dependent on familial and coalitional relationships of mutual trust in one's community which are manifestly asexual. It is far from clear that same-sex socio-sexual encounters, or the concept of social 'gender' rainbow (Roughgarden R580), mediate human reproductive success in any significant way.

Miller goes on to describe human intellectual, and artistic evolution as a fitness indicator to demonstrate abundant, entertaining, exciting creations, myths, stories and themes which, although not necessarily essential for survival, do indicate a genuine resourceful capacity to fend for a family and to bring skills into play which will, in their application, dramatically improve the survival chances of offspring, partly through the reproductive benefits they will also endow. Mutual mate selection is significantly slewed by the obvious degree to which males display sexually in displays of creativity and power, so in complementary measure by female reproductive choice. This explains why men spend a disproportionate amount of time insinuating themselves into positions of power and striving to become virtuoso geniuses and why consequently more innovation seems to be made by men. This is again consistent with moderate polygyny, rather than strict monogamy.

The adage that men like to be good jokers and that women are discerning appreciators of humour is supported by brain studies (p 390). This lends support to the notion that humour is exists socially as an indicator of male mating fitness. Miller notes: "It's a very powerful and reliable way to show creativity and intelligence". A woman choosing a funny man as a partner would be more likely to have genetically healthy children who will survive and reproduce themselves. Such sexual selection may favour women who like humorous men, and men who like women with an appreciation for humour, as has been evidenced in extensive studies by Bressler and co-workers (R74 with a follow-up in the same journal).

Confirmation of the central thesis in Miller's work - that art, poetry, story-telling and musical and other forms of creativity are indicators of reproductive fitness, giving strategic advantage to the bearer in terms of sexual favours - has received confirmation in the form of research by David Nettle of the University of Newcastle upon Tyne (*Get creative for a varied sex life Steve Connor NZ Herald 3 Dec 2005*). The researchers interviewed 425 men and women about their sexual partners, and found the average number of partners for professional artists and poets (regardless of their fame or otherwise) to be between 4 and 10 compared with just 3 for non-creative people.

Modern humans do display significant sexual differences in cognitive and intellectual expertise (p 388), which are consistent with reproductive realities and the gatherer-hunter complementation of life-styles between the sexes. Men are better as map readers, good at mechanical cognitive tasks and relaxed in situations of working in parallel, as well as tight knit planning, all consistent with good hunting. Women are more proficient at language and at familiarizing themselves a large number of varied objects in the environment, and at networking, consistent with gathering. Consistent with gender complementarities in repro-

58

ductive needs, men tend to hunger for young fertile looking women, while women seek older men with good status and resources. Men are naturally attuned to competing to form hierarchical coalitions while women are broadly better at egalitarian emotional networking. Both sexes however display competition and cooperation, hierarchies and coalitions, depending on the circumstances, and individual human variation is anyway greater than that between the sexes as a whole. The central nature of the sexual relationship in generating loving good-nature, raises a root question of whether external social control imposed by law and punishment, or even by positive filtering of socio-sexual bonding as Roughgarden suggests (p 55) is how society redeems itself, or whether the lubricious, animal, slime of reproductive sex is our royal route to the consummation of love. This requires a revaluation of society as a product of human personal interaction rather than a collective structure imposed upon us.

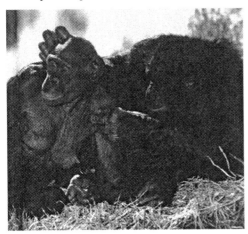

Bonobo affection (de Waal and Lanting R162). As of 2003 projections, all Chimp and Gorilla species may become extinct in the wild within 20 years as a result of the bushmeat industry, habitat damage and ebola.

Part of the evolutionary endowment of human nature is to be sensitively astute at detecting cheating and betrayal and to show personal judgement in balancing real or implied retribution for perceived wrongs, sufficient to avoid exploitation, but tempered with forgiveness and bonding. Defection is as natural a complement to cooperation as chaos is to order, essential to complexity itself. Defection can be creative in a healthy society, where it is outright dangerous in an alienated one subject to inequity and violent repression. Art and music in one society can be perceived as subversion in another.

The source nature of sexual selection in goodness raises serious questions about the concept of original sin. Our society has been dominated for the last 4000 years by themes of male dominion expressed towards woman and nature, in the Eden myth, and in laws and social and religious institutions, from the code of Hammurabi, which prescribes death by drowning for adultery, on down. Our social institutions reflect most closely the hierarchies of dominant male troops. The fight between God and the devil is a male combat myth. Wars and genocide are committed predominantly by men. The competitive nature of capitalism and its boom and bust winner-take-all exploitation are precisely the male reproductive strategy without the balance of female long-term investment which is spread among offspring and over time in a more sustainable way. The rule of law and the imposition of social control are also central characteristics of the alpha male hierarchy.

Beyond sexual differences in the brain is a development, connecting the emotional areas giving peak ecstatic significance in the limbic emotional and memory systems on the one hand and the closely adjacent ultimate centres of meaning and significance in the temporal lobes on the other. These areas, when excited by psychedelic hallucinogens, meditation, prayer, incantation or privation give rise to the peak spiritual experience. They are also intimately involved in expressions of deep religious significance experienced by people in temporal lobe epilepsy. One reading of this 'god spot' is that it is a confluence of higher evolution, leading to societies which can express reverence and ecstatic union in ways which promote social harmony. These do not necessarily have to involve the moral imperatives of conservative religious edict to induce a world order, but emotional and perceptual experience. To be effective they need to be naturally and autonomously expressed and in a way which reflects the dynamics of both sexes, not the coercion of *religio* 'binding again'.

Spiritual experience is also claimed to have a strong genetic basis. Dean Hamer (R276) asked volunteers 226 questions in order to determine how spiritually connected they felt to the universe. The higher their score, the greater a person's ability to believe in a greater spiritual force and the more likely they were to share the gene, VMAT2. Studies on twins showed that those with this gene, a vesicular monoamine transporter that regulates the flow of mood-altering chemicals in the brain, were more likely to develop a spiritual belief. Growing up in a religious environment was said to have little effect on belief. Hamer laconically remarks: "Religious believers can point to the existence of god genes as one more sign of the creator's ingenuity - a clever way to help humans acknowledge and embrace a divine presence". Neurotransmitter differences have also been associated with subjects' readiness to perceive 'synchronistic' unseen influences between events.

An idea of how the God spot might function to produce ordered social structures is gleaned from closely watching chimp societies and the hierarchies topped by an alpha male. Helen Fisher (R208) notes: "The ruler has an important job - sheriff. He steps into a brawl and pulls the adversaries from one another. And he is expected to be a non-partisan referee. When this alpha male keeps fights at a minimum his chimp underlings respect him, support him, even pay him homage. They bow to him, plunging their heads and upper bodies repeatedly. They kiss his hands, feet and neck and chest. They lower themselves to make sure they are beneath him. And they follow him in an entourage. But if the leader fails to maintain harmony, his inferiors shift their allegiance ... subordinates create the chief." The leader of the hierarchy has an investment in keeping the peace, diffusing quarrels and reducing intra-group violence. These spontaneous expressions of reverence are precisely those we display in bowing down to God in expressing a deep inner reverence for a mystery which we believe brings a more harmonious and meaningful order to our lives. We can also see in the Draconian invoking of order by many religions under pain of diabolical punishment in the name of God a runaway example of ape society invoking the strong sheriff who keeps keeping the peace by threat of retribution of the high and mighty upon the weak. The compensating factor in ape society is egalitarian instability - that the alpha male can be deposed by a male coalition (p 63), or in bonobos by an alliance of females in support of a ranking son (p 66).

It is notable here that the females bear allegiance to this 'world order' only in so far as it is consistent with their reproductive choices. Fisher somewhat idealistically describes female chimps by contrast as good networkers: "Female chimps do not establish this kind of status ladder. They form cliques instead - laterally connected subgroups of individuals who care for one another's infants and protect and nurture one another in times of social chaos. Females are less aggressive, less dominance oriented and this network can remain stable - and relatively egalitarian for years. Moreover the most dominant female generally acquires this position by sheer personality, charisma if you will, as well as by age rather than by intimidation." While female bonobos do form large loose coalitions, female chimps spend much more time alone than the sociable males, foraging in their local terrains, or mothering. They do also have a hierarchical ranking although less precisely defined and will drive off outside females who come on to their feeding domains.

The Breakdown of Sexual Paradox and Patriarchal Dominion

Power is the ultimate aphrodisiac
Henry Kissinger - NY Times Jan 19 1971

In 1967 Johnson astounded several top aides and Interior Secretary Stewart Udall by launching into a tirade about his war. Who the hell was Ho Chi Min to think 'He could push America around'? Then he showed in the most unmistakable manner imaginable just what the war meant to him - and it was literally what Carlin insists the war was all about: 'the bigger dick foreign policy theory'. ... The president unzipped his pants, pulled out the member he had named 'ol' Jumbo' and proclaimed 'Has Ho Chi Min got anything like that'? (McElvaine R446 311).

Running throughout this whole account is the unspoken green-eyed monster of jealousy and betrayal, which has always been a universal aspect of the prisoners dilemma of cooperation and defection, despite all attempts to banish or destroy defection by force of violent punishment. In a society of faithful wives, one scarlet woman can command a king's fortune. In a society of faithless harlots one faithful wife can expect the Earth. Neither can be eliminated because the very attempt to do so makes the rarer the more precious.

One can however taboo certain actions by threat or exercise of violent retribution. While not eliminating them entirely, this will at least serve to drive them into the covert undergrowth. This is certainly the case with patriarchal dominion. Once large urban societies developed, the rule of law and the patriarchal imperative passed the ascendancy to the male through social and military instruments of power. Male jealously resulted in adoption of mores which ensured powerful men could secure their own descendents from doubts about paternity which plague the male but are incontestable for the female:

"Momma's baby, Poppa's maybe."

Variation in paternity certainty - the probability that a man is his 'child's' father - can evoke differing forms of society, based either on uncles rearing offspring of their sisters, as with Laban in Genesis, or men rearing the children of their partners, as Jacob chose to do in the patriarchal paradigm. At the critical value of 1/3 the following are equal:

1. You are related to your 'own' children (by your sexual partner) by $(1/2)(1/3) = (1/6)$.
2. Your relatedness to your "full" sister is at least 1/4 (representing your common mother) plus 1/4 (your putative common father) times the paternity certainty of 1/3, totaling $1/4 + (1/4)(1/3) = 1/3$. Since you thus share 1/3 of your genes with your sister and she provides 1/2 the genes of her children, you are related to her children by $(1/2)(1/3) = 1/6$.

In this situation, sociobiology predicts you will invest equally in both your sister's children and your own, all things being equal, since you are related to both sets of children by 1/6. In societies in which paternity certainty falls under 1/3, you should invest more heavily in your sister's children than your own; if paternity certainty is more than 1/3, you should favor your wife's children (Thompson R675 57). It is here also that the balance between allo-parenting by kin and partnership has its basic divide. One also has to take into account that all apes are female exogamous, so the matrilineal human model is exceptional and may constitute only a phase of human cultural development associated with early agricultural cultures such as Catal Huyuk (p 176), though ancient 'venus figurines' (p 92) may suggest an earlier origin.

Genetic testing (Baker and Bellis R37) suggests that 10 - 20% of offspring of an ostensible father are sired by another man - a fundamental expression of covert female reproductive choice so central to evolution and to the greater female reproductive investment. If we turn for a moment to the chimpanzee, we will discover that up to half the offspring are sired in secret trysts outside the immediate male group. This happens despite a consistent presence of a dominant alpha male hierarchy seeking to secure reproductive certainty by a variety of strategies from mate guarding to infanticide. The human statistic represents a moderate swing in favour of human male paternity certainty, well above the level that would equally favour men acting as uncles for their sisters children, however it is still enough to cause extreme violence on the part of males who find out they have been cheated and quite sufficient to provoke a sexist backlash against female reproductive choice.

The principal aim of the patriarchy has been to split the female strategy into clearly-separated faithful wives and whores, thus providing procreation and pleasure. The darker the shade, the more women participating. Upper right triangles are for a 'partnership society', lower left show the female strategy largely bifurcated (divided) by moral edict.

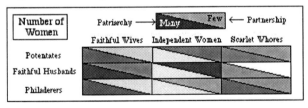

The game diagram (p 60) illustrates three strategies each for woman and men. In a population of faithful wives a rare scarlet woman can have all she asks for. Conversely, a faithful wife is a prized asset in a society of loose women. This rareness factor prevents the annihilation of either strategy and is a common feature of the Prisoners' Dilemma, exemplified in polyphenic species (p 33). A high ranking male may gather a harem, or he may attract an additional concubine, or 'kept woman'. A lower ranking male may choose to be 'dad' declaring as a faithful husband to retain the fidelity of his wife. Others will adopt the 'cad' strategy of loving 'em and leaving 'em.

As we have seen, males specializing in both declared enticement and sneak mate capture occur in many species, from crickets to salmon. In some species these strategies can become entrenched in polyphenism where individuals of a given mating type sport distinct physiologies (p 33). Male orangs have two physiologies, a macho dominant male and a sub-dominant sneak rapist (Hrdy R323 76). Women likewise can adopt several strategies between being 'fast and loose' attracting a temporary mate for immediate gain or a longer term strategy of ostensible monogamy seeking a longer-term resource-bearing partner. Somewhere in between, particularly in matrilineal societies, a woman may decide to retain her own independent status of reproductive choice. As a result of sexual privacy, covert affairs may occur in any of these situations.Such a game theoretic model is supported at a deeper genetic level. It has been found in a study of 3200 women - all identical or non-identical twins, by Tim Spector (Twin Research 2004) that there is a genetic basis for female infidelity, contributing 40% of the variance discovered. There is not a single infidelity gene, but 50 to 100 genes are important, although the researchers managed to pinpoint some of the traits to 3 of the 23 pairs of human chromosomes. The study suggests that a genetic predisposition towards female infidelity may have evolved because it was important in allowing women married to 'low-status' men surreptitiously to become pregnant by 'high-status' men. Spector notes: "Work in the UK has shown that human females generally have affairs with men of higher status than their husbands, perhaps illustrating an effort to mate with a genetically superior partner," consistent with hypergamy (p 31). Slightly more than 20 per cent admitted to being unfaithful in a stable relationship. Some reported no extra-marital affairs or no sexual partners but others said they had had more than 100 sex partners, the average number being between 4 and 5.

> If female infidelity and number of sexual partners are under considerable genetic influence, as this study demonstrates, the logical conclusion is that these behaviours persist because they have been evolutionary advantageous for women.

In an intriguing reflection of the 'dads' and 'cads' male strategy it has been reported that daughters growing up without fathers present reach menarche earlier, suggesting that they may be primed by their early experiences to adopt a more opportunistic 'loose' reproductive strategy based on short term gains in mates, becoming sexually active earlier and with more different partners. This is the opposite of most primates where 'low-ranking' females under stress delay puberty, presumably because of their more perilous reproductive prospects. This has caused some to question whether the effect is simply a maternally-inherited short term investment strategy (R323 189). Noting that precocious sexual maturity can make a girl popular with boys and rejected by other girls in discussing female competition, Anne Campbell (R102 193) comments "early maturing girls have a distinct advantage in terms of mate selection. They garner a disproportionate amount of male interest and by entering the mate market earlier, have a wider choice of prospective men."

The key issue of significance in human culture historically is the imposition of stark divisions on the female sex in the rise of patriarchal dominance. With the emergence of the early urban cultures, male power became enforced by militarization and a simultaneous application of religious and legal edicts under pain of violence and death. The patriarchal imperative seeks to reinforce paternity certainty by rejecting the cultural predicates of matriarchal succession, driving a wedge into the female population to clearly separate women between two exclusive archetypes of the faithful wife for reproduction and the scarlet whore for sexual pleasure, with no ambiguities in between; removing male vulnerability, by threat of death against loss of the tokens of virginity and adultery, in which the female is particularly vulnerable, given stipulations, such as not having cried out. The 'whoring' mixed fertility rites of the goddess and her consort by their many and various names are outlawed by degrees. Imposition of patriarchal dominance would appear to remove the mortal dread men have that their children are not really theirs, but it abets forms of male power which gives some men a disproportionate share of the reproductive resources, as well. The patriarchal imperative does not stop simply with the issue of resolving paternity uncertainty. As power passes to the dominant males, themes of male competition lead to religious and social ideas based on exclusive male domination, the combat between light and dark, jealousy and violence, arms races, expansionist wars, exploitation of resources, and the establishment of hierarchical means of control by the threat and use of force. Mutual grooming and friendship gives way to aggression, abuse and enslavement.

Coupled with the patriarchal imperative are a nexus of effects, all associated with the breakdown of mutual sexual paradox into paradigms of domination - dominion over woman and nature alike. These have been expressed in social power structures, religion, and the rule of law. Patriarchal societies no longer invest cooperatively in abundance, but seek to conquer in unrestrained growth, through militarization, exhortations to population growth, attitudes towards girl children which give males who can be used in combat higher status. They abet attitudes of winner-take-all exploitation, boom and bust, rape of the planet and ultimately that cosmic high noon of male combat myth the apocalypse of arma-geddon and the final day of judgement, the 'rapture' and discarding of the entire natural realm as a husk of the germ of God's will. The result is a frankly unsustainable paradigm of the rule of order in which complexity and diversity atrophy in a war of attrition whose results are scarcity, inequity and further competition or perhaps the final darkness of extinction. The myth of man the hunter thus has its final nemesis, in man the grim reaper of his own misfortune. The Prisoners' Dilemma teaches us that the only sustainable respite from such mutual nemesis is to restore sexual paradox to its condition of climax diversity.

The example of the bonobo (p 66)shows us that social sexuality can act powerfully enough on reproductive choice (and hence reproductive sexuality) to shape it sufficiently to cause a runaway inverse peacock's tail in the form of their enlarged clitorises and ecstatic female-female sexual *hoka-hoka* . However here social sexuality is integrated with the reproductive sexuality of the bonobo matriarchs and is thus not acting against it. Rather the two sexes, caught in a Prisoners' Dilemma game by virtue of their reproductive inter-dependence, each try to shape social sexuality to their own advantage. In the bonobo's case, the females have gained a relative advantage of female social sexual bonding aiding strategic support in dealing with the opposite sex. In some ways the classical Greek male sexual infatuation with the intrinsic superiority of the male sex (p 202) is a cultural equiv-alent of the bonobo female strategy, however the human clitoris, far from being a spandrel as some suggest (p 86), has also had a heady influence on human social sexuality and romantic and family bonding that is key to sexual paradox in our cultural emergence.

The fabric of sexual relations and all the phenomena and styles of relationship, from monogamous devotion, through polygamy, serial monogamy (leading to polygyny in another form), promiscuity (newly packaged in the swingers' lifestyle) and bisexuality (as an extension of sexual openness) are ultimately manifestations of the ongoing reproduc-tive prisoners' dilemma game between the sexes, extended into its social themes of trust and betrayal in relationship, love and security, as well as adventure, conquest and ulti-mately Tantric fusion. Polyamory intriguingly tries to invert the game and its contradic-tions by redefining betrayal as cooperation in an atmosphere of heightened trust, adding profoundly to the fluidity and instability of an already chaotic untameable force of life.

In humans, social sexuality has become a Machivellian and often violent field of contest and conflict over its influence on the reproductive life of the sexes through the bon ding and allegiances it invokes. The Old Testament patriarchal invections by God against Laban's matrilocal traditions (p 189), the whoring ways of the fertility Goddess (p 214) and the associated homosexuality around the temple, are all part of a central Prisoners' Dilemma game, in which the world's major religions, and cultures and empires have risen and fallen by their reactions to social sexuality in their attempts to control the reproductive choice of women and male access to their reproductive capacity. This contest leads to the very precipice of apocalypse, in an inevitable Rape of the Planet, and the mortal male combat of Mutually-assured Destruction and the War on Terror.

Humanity's Evolutionary Heritage

The Contradictory Diversity of Anthropoid Societies

Evolutionary equilibrium means that a strategy has to be optimal to any changes either sex might inflict, or any defection from the game theoretic equilibrium the situation might present. In the context of sex this means that societies need to reflect the complementary interplay between the vastly differing reproductive investments females and males make, the one massive and forthright, and the other opportunistic and competitive.

Diverse ape societies derive their complexity and viability through responding to this sexual interplay, without the extensive capacity humans have for imposing 'artificial' cultural structures upon it. The relative clumping or diffuse nature of plant foods, determine, through the female foraging distribution, and the opportunities it provides males, whether ape species are monogamous (very dispersed females), form harems (clumping sufficient for one male to guard several females - e.g. gorillas) or promiscuous (intermediate distributions requiring free movement of individuals, as in the case of our closest relatives, the chimpanzee. *Pan troglodite*, and the bonobo or pygmy chimpanzee, *Pan paniscus*. In turn these reproductive patterns determine the shifting hierarchies and coalitions of social structure.

The most promiscuous ape societies are the most complex and versatile. Monogamous gibbons lead a solitary and relatively sterile existence in widely spaced territories with little social interaction. For Gorillas there is a little more dynamic movement. Largely affairs are dominated by a silver back who retains dominance over his harem while struggling endlessly against being toppled and his females robbed by a more powerful male. But females will also mate with a younger male if he is present in the group. However only in chimp and bonobo societies do social complexities and subtleties really come to the fore.

Pan troglodyte: Chimpanzee

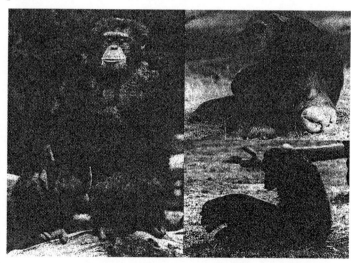

Chimps have a narrow muscular penis inviting intentional displays rather than the fat hydrodynamic penis of the human. Females have a large sexual swelling in estrus, usually mate from behind and females grunt at climax in a way suggestive of 'orgasm' (Pusey R548).

Chimp societies are complex, dynamically changing 'fission-fusion' societies with shifting sexual relationships between females and males, however here the emphasis is on male hierarchies and coalitions. In de Waal's perceptive words (R161 62) "Male chimpanzees hunt together, engage in fights over territory, and enjoy a half-amicable, half-competitive camaraderie. Their cooperative action-packed existence resembles that of a human male, who in modern society teams up with other males in corporations that compete with other corporations." While males display rituals of dominance, amid blustering aggression and reconciliation, females exert significant reproductive choice by subtlety and charisma, with up to half the offspring coming from secret liaisons outside the troop on safari trysts (Fisher R208, Jolly R338). Females seem to be more concerned with establishing and keeping a set of solid relationships with a small selective circle of friends and a few more clearly defined enemies. De Waal notes: "Over the years. I've gained the impression that each female in the Arnhem colony has one or two absolute enemies with whom reconciliation is absolutely out of the question'. Instances which would have been previously attributed to male aggression on closer examination reveal the action was instigated by a female with a long-standing grudge of her own" (Watson R721 117).

When females have sexual swellings indicating fertility, they are extremely gregarious and range over large areas. Otherwise females usually feed alone or are accompanied only by their dependent offspring in core areas of about 2 square kilometers. In the wild they spend about half their time in each mode. In contrast the adult males are more sociable, spending less than a fifth of their time alone and ranging over an area of 8-15 square kilometers, seeking females and protecting and expanding their range against other males. Female distribution in relation to food resources is only a partial explanation for this arrangement because females are also monopolized into seeking the protection of male ranges to avoid aggression against themselves and their infants (Pusey R548 15-17).

Apes, unlike most monkey species, are female exogamous, with half to 90% of chimp females moving to other troops (Hrdy R323 51, Pusey (R548 20), while the males remain with the existing group, which thus consists of males related to varying degrees who have a kin altruistic basis for reproductive cooperation. However males only show significant relatedness in some chimp troops (Taï, but not Gombe) (25). Mitochondrial mtDNA testing of hair suggests that mitochondrial genes are shared between chimps several hundred kilometers apart, indicating wide-ranging exogamy (22). Analyzing DNA found in the hair follicles collected from chimpanzee nests has become a method to test chimp paternity in the wild. At Gombe Julie Constable has found about 20% of conceptions come from low-ranking males with a majority from mating inside the group, particularly with males that were alpha at some time. All three mothers with more than one offspring fathered them by different males, emphasizing both female choice and the shifting nature of male hierarchies. (Pusey R548). In the Taï National Forest on the Ivory Coast, Pascal Gagneaux found only 6 out of 13 cases of paternity could be traced to male residents in the community the females frequented (Strier R660, Pusey R548), linking most to secret liaisons outside.

Incest avoidance and female exogamy in chimps are linked in a way which suggests it is females and not males in humans which should naturally be driving the incest taboo by their exogamy rather than being regarded as mediums of exchange by males, since they have to bear the full reproductive burden of inbreeding. Females coming into adolescence initially mate with most of the males in their own community. However females with older brothers or close relatives cease to travel with them and rarely mate with them. Even if the male shows interest in the female, she will scream and avoid him, presumably as a result of histocompatibility (MHC) odor similarity (p 354) and familiarity during immaturity. Females become fearful of older males in their own community but when they wander with sexual swellings they eagerly meet and mate with males from new communities, either joining the new community permanently or returning pregnant (Pusey R548 19). Sperm competition in utero may allow for selection of sperm with greater viability and genetic fitness. Promiscuity may also aid fertility by promoting histo-complementarity relative to the female's own MHC and immunity type, again through odour (Birkhead R62 204). Mate guarding by an alpha male at the peak of fertility towards the end of the estrus (which ironically means 'gadfly') may also serve to give her access to generally fitter genes, despite her promiscuity.

This pattern of female reproductive choice, despite male mate guarding, is shared among many primate species. Despite living in harems dominated by a 'silver back' male, female gorillas sometimes mate with subordinate younger 'black backs' when they are present (Hrdy R322 147). Recently a mature captive female has been seen teaching her daughter how to bring up a child after she abandoned her first one, suggesting some matrilineal adaption (Leahy R391). A female savannah baboon in estrus will frequently mate with many different males, despite focusing her favours on a few dominant males who can secure her attentions when in peak. These strategies are all consistent with females applying genetic choice and manipulating such services of protection and resourcing as males have to offer.

Both chimps and bonobos share an overt reproductive cycle, and a frankly promiscuous reproductive life, in which the females assume almost all the responsibility for child-rearing. On average a chimpanzee will make love 100 times as often as a gorilla. Rather than a larger body size, the chimp has large testicles which can sustain frequent 'flooding' ejaculates to compete in a promiscuous environment. Copulating with as many males as possible in the vicinity within her immediate troop while she is in overt estrus and can pass without harassment, may serve to reduce a variety of risks of infanticide, although females on the periphery of an established group remain vulnerable to attack both from the existing troop and from outside males, particularly of their male offspring (Hrdy R323 86). The threat of infanticide, of alien offspring and of direct attacks on non-receptive females by male chimps drives females to seek the relative security of a range well within that of her male troop.

At least four female mating modes are in play, mating with the dominant alpha male, openly mating promiscuously with all the males in the troop (to protect against infanticide), going 'on safari' in temporary 'monogamous' relationship with a male with whom a female shares an affectionate bond out of sight of other animals, and 'mate guarding' by a small coalition of males (Jolly R338 78). A female on safari will copulate 5 to 10 times a day, but an estrus female travelling with a group of males may copulate 30 to 50 times in a day (Hrdy R322 148). A high ranking chimp female may stay with the troop giving her offspring added survival support of a central position. The onset of menarche in an adolescent female may occur at about the age of eight but it is several years before her sexual swellings are full sized and grown males pay attention and begin mating in earnest. Even then a female may copulate on the order of 3,600 times during successive subfertile cycles before she conceives the first time, around age 14 and gives birth. Hrdy (R323 185) comments "an adolescent's sexual swellings are especially conspicuous. Like bonobos, young females use them as 'diplomatic passports' that permit safe passage through hostile territories. This way a female can check out competitors and local resources in foreign communities while she decides where to settle and breed." Once she becomes fertile she will be more fecund than older females. A female wandering with such a passport may not be attacked by patrolling males but may not so easily be accepted by resident females in unfamiliar territory (R323 85). Female chimps from dominant ranks are known to commit infanticide against lower ranking females (R323 52). A fertile female who conceives will have made love more than 100 times with as many as a dozen or more males during her ovulatory period. Such motivated sex is lustful and in De Waal's (R163 53) careful words involves 'orgasm-like experiences'. Along with bonobo sexual ecstasy this provides an evolutionary basis for human female orgasm in our common ape ancestors. Once she delivers her baby she does not return to the group but takes it alone and feeds in a small core range to protect it form attack.

Male chimps often form flexible coalitions to collectively depose a dominant male or to attack other groups. They share food as tokens of cooperation. As noted (p 59), successful alpha males often display skills of group mediation and conflict resolution as well as aggression to maintain their position. Coalitions of male chimps also stage raiding parties on neighbouring troops, killing or injuring other males and killing infants. Male monkeys and apes tend to commit infanticide on any offspring not sired by themselves (R323 34) sufficiently frequently to cause female chimps strategic reproductive problems. Infanticide both serves to eliminate genetic rivals before they become active adversaries and is a natural extension of interspecies competition. Males play no part in infant care but may form casual affectionate bonds and be followed by adoring young males.

Chimp societies display many features shared with human gatherer-hunter societies. including a division of labour between meat and plant foods, predominant female exogamy (2/3 of gatherer-hunter societies are male philopatric and less than 1/5 female philopatric), male cooperation in coalitions, reconciliation of aggression within groups, the presence of inter-group violence between males, raiding parties against individuals in other groups, and a similar group size of about 150 to gatherer-hunter bands (Pusey R548).

Chimpanzees use tools for more purposes than any other non-human species (McGrew). Recent investigation indicates young female chimps learn earlier and faster by watching their mothers than males, who are more involved in wrestling play (Lonsdorf et. al. R413). Females learn earlier and ultimately better how to 'fish' for termites and mirror their mother's techniques in a way which males don't. These patterns suggest sex differences in human learning go back six million years. Chimps in captivity also show cultural preferences for conformity with their peers even when they know an alternative tool using strategy is more effective (Nature doi:10.1038/050815-12).

Pan paniscus: Bonobo

The bonobo or 'pygmy chimpanzee' was first discovered only in 1927 from a skull and shortly after recognized as a separate species. It is slightly smaller, darker and more gracile and childlike than the average chimp. This neotonous feature is shared by humans. In 1933 Harold Coolidge (de Waal R163 42) who gave them species status considers them to be anatomically more generalized than chimps and "may approach more closely to the common ancestor of chimpanzees and man than does any living chimpanzee". Adrienne Zihlman has found them to be the closest ape to Australopithecus by several quantitative measures. They are often observed to walk bipedally, especially when carrying food. Like humans, bonobos are receptive sexually for most of their ovarian cycle. They regularly make love face to face as humans do, which chimps do only rarely.

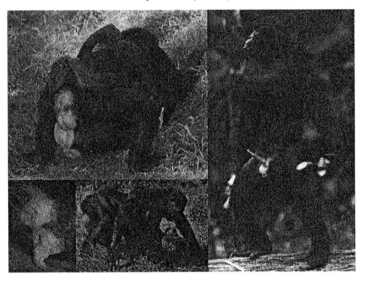

Bonobos mating face to face often stare deeply into one another's eyes and French kiss. Here and below centre two females 'mate' in *hoka-hoka* with the aid of their large clitoris (below left). Right bonobo male giving a penis display (De Waal and Lanting R162, Hrdy R323 ex Amy Parish).

Bonobo societies have become renowned in Franz de Waal's "Good Natured" (R161) as hyper-sexed, promiscuous societies, which use pan-sexuality as a universal social panacea to invite reconciliation for aggression and even at any sight of food, when both males and females will invite sex in a free-for-all. They engage frequent and repetitious apparently orgasmic sex, as much between females (with their especially enlarged clitorises) as between male and female. Males also rub their scrotal areas together in reconciling aggression and occasionally hang upside down in trees rubbing their erect penises together called penis fencing (de Waal R163 54). There are also sexual liaisons between adults and juveniles of both sexes. Frequent sexual encounter has become a contributory phenomenon which generates sufficient cohesion among female coalitions to keep dominant males respectfully deferring to their wishes, trading sex for food in favourable, or indulgent terms, with little molestation of the females. In fact females bond more strongly to one another than to the males and follow them around seven times more. Females use sex to solicit food from males. De Waal notes this wryly as "sex as a weapon." They will also claim food possessed by males if necessary by force. Males tend to follow their mothers. By contrast with chimps, male alliances are little developed and ranking males derive key support from their mothers and the alliance between the females. Females are thus regarded as being dominant.

Robert Jay Russel called the bonobos' propensity for males trading food for sex the 'lemur's legacy', as one of our most remote cousins also share the trait (Taylor R670 81). Timothy Taylor demurs that it is simply the males being courteous and offering the females both food and sex. While this is a nice idea, it negates the subtlety of Machiavellian interplay the whole transaction expresses. Neither does it, as he suggests, imply the female sex drive is less, and we know female bonobos have a great deal of sex themselves. He also observes:

"Most shockingly to human eyes, adults and children have a lot of sex. In fact infants are often initiated by their mothers - the only observed taboo on sex is between mothers and any sons over six years of age." (R670 81).

De Waal (R161 55) proposes that they avoid incest both by a combination of female exogamy and close familial associations and similar body odours inhibiting sexual attraction, driven principally by females avoiding kin. When a young female reaches adolescence at about seven, she stops having sex with her troop and begins to have her first small swellings. This is a major crisis time for a young female. The swellings act as a passport of 'implied fertility' so she can wander freely from group to group and have sex with strange males in the forest without fear of attack, looking for a group with individuals she can bond with and be safe. She invites sex from the other females. Once accepted, her sexuality flowers. She rapidly gains almost continuous sexual swellings which grow in volume with every cycle till they reach full size at about ten. She can expect her first offspring at about thirteen or fourteen. This gives the females ample time to find a home troop and become fully integrated into the community before pregnancy ensues. Unlike chimps where females wander alone with small offspring to protect the young from the risk of infanticide, bonobos return to the troop immediately and infanticide is unknown.

Characteristic of both chimps and bonobos is reconciliation. This is a clear sign of mediation of aggression and implies, despite the relatively peaceful nature of the bonobo that competition, hierarchies and feelings of aggression are still present. In chimps it is the 'underdog' who usually initiates reconciliation, whereas in bonobos it is the 'aggressor', however reconciliation is so beneficial to a group of chimps that if neither of the warring individuals will initiate it, a third party may step in to broker a deal(Dugatkin R175). Reconciliation in chimps is by kissing and cuddling but in bonobos it is mediated through sex. Sex at the sight of food is an immediate mediation of feelings of competition to get enough of a share. Similarly if a male chases another away from a female the males reunite and have a scrotal rub, or if a female hits a juvenile and the mother lunges back they both have sex. Unusually, these types of engagement also occur between troops (de Waal R161 51). The females will groom one another while the males remain tense. Males compete fiercely for rank which is influenced by the rank of mothers, but the female hierarchy, based on age and residency is fairly loose. It is possible the bonobo has been able to engage this strategy because it has access to larger fruiting trees and selects types of abundant terrestrial herbaceous vegetation which can support large groups without conflict. Richard Wrangham has also suggested that the absence of the gorilla in their range opened an evolutionary niche for a less male-dominated social structure. However, missing from both chimp and bonobo societies is any form of pair-bonding or long-term relationship between males and females.

Deaner et. al. (R155) have found that even rhesus macaques are highly strategically sensitive to socio-sexual images. They found that a male would choose a significant cut in a cherry juice offering to look at 'pornographic' images the perineum of a female, or powerful males' faces, both of which are strategically important for reproduction, casting both gossip magazines and human pornographic imagery in a very ancient light.

Australopithecus: Evolutionary Divergence of the Hominid Line

Our closest evolutionary cousins are the chimpanzee and the bonobo, from which we diverged some 5 to 6 million years ago. The divergence of our common ancestor from gorillas, orangutans and old world monkeys occurred at successively earlier dates. This

68

has led to the idea that we are a species in the same genus as Pan. About 5 million years ago, primate evolution split along two tracks: one leading towards humans, the other towards chimpanzees. A million years later, our ancestors adopted an upright gait, and 2 million years after that their bodies and brains began to grow and they started making primitive stone tools. The first modern-looking humans appear in the fossil record about 130,000 years ago. By 50,000 years ago, there is evidence for humans who appear to have distinctly modern bodies and life-styles. They created complex tools and jewelry, built shelters, buried their dead in graves and probably had similar language skills to us.

Sellén-Tullberg and Møller researching the family tree of living primate species by mating type, come to conclusions consistent with the idea that monogamy is a latecomer to the human line (Diamond R165). They suggest that monogamy has not been a trait of our primate evolutionary history, but rather promiscuity in lower primates followed by a common harem-building ancestor, as the gorilla is today. Since recent evolutionary trees place chimps closer to humans than gorillas, the ancestor probably then passed through a promiscuous phase. This missing link probably had the slight evidence of ovulation we find in both primitive primates and gorillas and evolved in opposite directions in humans and chimps, the chimp and bonobo forms of promiscuity emphasizing overt ovulation accompanied by estrus behavior and human monogamy with moderate polygyny favouring concealed ovulation. The overt estrus seen in chimps and baboons is rare in primates and constitutes a specific adaption (Hrdy R323 217).

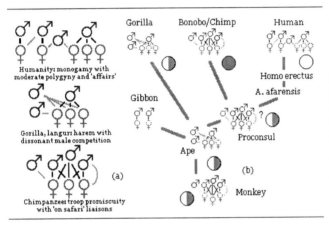

Primate mating patterns and concealed or advertised ovulation. Pink and white discs indicate overt and covert ovulation, half-shaded slight signs (Diamond R165).

Sexual dimorphism varies by different measures from little or none in monogamous gibbons. Slight to moderate differences in bonobos and chimps (various measures range from 6-30% (Reno et. al. R560, Pusey R548 35 Wrangham R751 35). Pair-bonding but moderately polygynous human populations vary from 6 to 23% with an average around through 15%. Harem-forming gorillas, and orangutans and baboons, have a difference of 100% characteristic of species where sexual choice is strongly related to male competition. Matt Ridley (R567 19) comments "Better to be only a little larger than a female and use cunning as well as strength to rise to the top of the hierarchy".

Sexual mating patterns can evolve rapidly (Larsen R389). They can vary as a result of changing environmental and social factors much more rapidly than genotype or phenotype. Savannah and hamadryas baboons have indistinguishable bone morphology, although the latter is a little smaller, and can interbreed where they overlap in eastern Ethiopia, having been previously separated for only about 300,000 years, probably by the latter becoming an offshoot of the former. However they have very different patterns of sexual association. It is thus possible that mating patterns have gone through substantial changes during the time our brain size swelled from the 500cc of *Australopithecus* to the 1400cc of modern *Homo*. Recently a group of savannah baboons was seen to change its social profile from aggressive dominant males to more socially peaceable behavior and grooming, when bovine TB wiped out the aggressive alpha males, and has continued for two decades (Sapolski and Share R598). Savannah baboons live in stable groups, with no exclusive pair bonds, with intra-group relations strongly influenced by alliances among adult females. A troop may contain several competing matrilines and so high social rank of the females is important and markedly enhances daughter's reproductive prospects in infant survival. However high ranking females become more stressed and have more infertility problems as a result (Low R416 60). The social role of males is predominantly to protect against predators such as leopards.

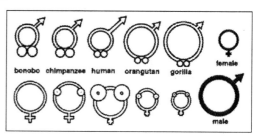

Relative body, penis and testicle size viewed by an ape female and relative body, breast and ovulation signals as viewed by an ape male (redrawn from Jolly R338 180). Humans have intermediate testicles size between promiscuous chimps and lone harem-forming male gorillas, indicating sperm competition and moderate polygyny.

By contrast with savannah baboons, hamadryas are female exogamous. They live in fission-fusion groups, within which exclusive mating units interact with one another through alliances of adult males, leaving females largely powerless (Wrangham R751). Females are abducted as juveniles and taught firm rules of obedience neccesary for survival in their harsher environment, supported by biting on the scruff of the neck if they protest. Despite the paternalism, the sexes are coevolved. The investment of the male is substantial over time, chastising, educating, helping feed, and even carrying his much smaller charges. They will rescue neonates at risk during delivery. Within each large herd, males do not so much as look at females in another alpha male's harem (Hrdy R322 75, 101).

When Raymond Dart in 1925 announced the discovery of *Australopithecus africanus*, he speculated on flimsy evidence that it had been a bloodthirsty carnivore. With it we inherited a pessimistic 'killer-ape' notion consistent with 'man the hunter' (R715, R475), based on the connection between hunting and warfare that aggressiveness drives cultural progress. Konrad Lorenz (R415) in "On Aggression" amplified this claiming our species had not had enough evolutionary time to develop the inhibitions against our own kind, as do full carnivores. With the discovery of violent aggression, murder and raiding parties among wild chimps (Wrangham and Peterson R750) our common origin "suggests that chimpanzee-like violence preceded and paved the way for human war, making modern humans dazed survivors of a continuous 5-million year habit of lethal aggression." However this position has again been modified with the discovery of the more peaceful bonobo and the idea that aggression is an option, depending on environmental correlates and not a fixed drive. Many authors have drawn conclusions about general trends in evolution from apes to humans based on the greater size differences between males and females believed to have existed in early Australopithecines of about 100% compared with modern human differences of only 5-16% across cultures. These conclusions have applied both to Australopthecus, which might be assumed to have been a harem-forming species on this basis, and changes presumed to have accompanied the reduction of these differences later in Homo erectus, for example the rise of pair-bonding. If the sexual dimorphism of Australopithecus is less overall it is as likely to indicate a promiscuous origin.

Work by Owen Lovejoy's group (Reno et. al. R560, Larsen R389) contradicts previous findings of extreme size dimorphism in *Australopithecus afarensis*, our 500cc brained ancestor of some three and a half million years ago. They suggest a sexual dimorphism less than that of humans, consistent with pair-bonding monogamy or promiscuity rather than harems with strong male competition like gorillas as previous studies implied. Canine dimorphism is greater in chimps, leading them to further suggest a monogamous phase. Alison Jolly (R338 362) in reviewing Lovejoy's previous work quotes his central motivating theme - that the reproductive nature of humanity sets us apart from other apes: "the unique sexual and reproductive behavior of [wo]man may be the *sine qua non* of human origin ... he saw the gift that led to bipedalism as monogamy".

However skeletal research suggests bipedalism evolved six-million years ago long before we can expect social patterns characteristic of humanity (Galik et. al. R230). Lovejoy's argument implies monogamy even before we came out of the trees, explaining bipedalism in terms of bringing roots back to a monogamous partner, males' wider ranging avoiding direct competition with closer ranging females based on the claim that human child rearing must have changed very early on to increase survival and shorten birth intervals, given a more slowly maturing infant and the five to eight year interval between births of apes. Jolly laconically notes "meanwhile the females progressively concealed her ovulation so as not to inflame all available males ... but ready to mate with her own man whenever he came home. Both female and male acquired permanent attractiveness, big breasts, big penis which continually advertised both sexiness displays and reassurance to the mate, as in mated birds that engage 'triumph displays'. Feminists were outraged. The idea of hulking polygynous males was horrid, but this kind of monogamy seemed even worse. ... on behavioral grounds, I would opt for big males, small females and a medium level of promiscuity, rather than Lovejoy's monogamy. " Adrienne Zihlman (R766) also has bipedalism evolving from gathering but males learning from their mothers to gather and share with the immediate group in a polygamous rather than monogamous environment.

There is no evidence for Lovejoy's notion of monogamy ever having evolved in a species-wide sense among humans but rather some form of polygamy in a majority of individual societies worldwide. There is a major problem here with the definition of monogamy as an intentional cultural trait defining relationships as one on one in the sense of marriage, with all its trappings of punishments for infidelity. Human societies clearly show they have a large majority of woman-man partnerships with a minority equilibrium of polygynous extended families as male resources permit. This is a complex and flexible form of social system which can provide optimal resourcing to females despite the tensions between co-wives. The idea that archaic humans would have defined a narrow prohibitive monogamous marriage code is contradicted by almost all societies outside Christianity.

Neither do the relative lack of male canines indicate monogamy since even early hominids before the archaeological advent of tool use could have come to depend more on stones than teeth is dominance displays, as noted in Chris Knüsel's theory of bipedalisim in which throwing was the key advantage gained (Taylor R670 36). Agruments in which human emergence is driven by tool use have palled with the discovery that wild gorillas use tools (Public Library of Science Biology Oct 2005) as well as chimps (p 66). Sarah Hrdy (R322 175) also notes that the reduced canines is a weak point in the argument since it does not seem necessary that early man used his teeth in fighting as other primates do. Richard Wrangham (R751) also find the arguments unconvincing: "The anatomist Owen Lovejoy once suggested that bipedalism evolved in order to allow males to bring food to their mates but his much publicized idea of monogamy among the woodland apes now seems farfetched. One of several difficulties is the question of sexual dimorphism in body size. ... Other obstacles to Lovejoy's scheme include scepticism that a male who left his mate to find food for her could guard her from rival males. The absence of any evidence of home bases, the matter of why females became bipedal and evidence that Australopiths life histories resemble those of apes, not of humans as Lovejoy's scheme implied they should. In addition, no living non-human primates exhibit monogamy within social communities. Part of the explanation is that any female who mates exclusively with a low-ranking male within a social group can expect to find her offspring the target of infanticide attempts by more dominant males." The difficulty with arguments based on changes in infant care in Australopithicines is the chicken and egg problem of brain size and what caused it. Australopithecus has a small brain and major child-rearing changes requiring additional partner resourcing are naturally responses to pressures created by delayed development caused by increasing brain size and the need for birth to take place before the brain puts on its spurt of growth. It is thus difficult to place such child-rearing changes before our large brain evolved. When we move to Homo erectus with an increasing brain size, we still find sexual dimorphisms suggested to be a little larger than humans in the range of 20% larger in males, consistent with Jolly's position and with social monogamy emerging later.

Timothy Taylor suggests that breasts and genital hair of the human female are an evolutionary response to bipedal walking:

Stated in brief, I believe that upright walking hid females' engorgable estrus skin between their legs; walking itself both required buttock muscles and hid the female genital opening - an important focus of sexual signaling in primates; the new buttock area became denuded of hair to compensate for the lost sexual signal; and the bare buttocks were mimicked around the front, in the form of bare breasts, [and a pubic triangle of hair against a bare background]. That is, nakedness developed as a form of sexual signaling to compensate for the disappearance of estrus skin, which had formerly performed that function. The emergence of nakedness was thus not a question of losing hair but of extending areas of sexual skin. This process culminated through sexual selection within a cultural environment-clothes and cosmetics enhanced and selectively covered the areas from which hair was lost, and encouraged it to be lost over yet wider areas. In my view, therefore, we have never been truly naked apes (R670 34).

Although acknowledging fatness and fecundity as a genuine indicator of reproductive fitness to carry a baby to term under fluctuating fortunes, and inviting the reader into a sensual notion of nakedness through sexual selection, Taylor cites a simple deterministic environmental sequence the loss of overt estrus signals, for what is a creative product of sexual choice. The critical flaw in such 'external factor' theories is that they attempt to explain the genesis of the most complex system we know of - human culture - in terms of the external advent of a single, generally simplistic, causal factor. The same applies to theories of human emergence based on bipedalism, tool use, hunting, monogamy and even language, each of which is a product of complexification, rather than the cause, although each can facilitate a qualitative leap forward. What is centrally at stake is the complexity of human sexual selection and how it has carried us forward into culture at the edge of chaos (p 506). Central to this idea is understanding how the sociobiology of sex becomes the cultural phenomena which surround us today, not just the social varieties of sexuality itself but all the creative and coercive phenomena of culture, which like our hairlessness and language appear to have been driven by sexual rather than natural selection. To this end Taylor does acknowledge the advent of clothing invites 'gender' - the cultural interpretation of social sex roles.

A similar argument for the human penis holds marginally better, i.e. that a large penis signals an attractive sexual feature, but this is far short of the heady race between the penis and clitoris for insatiable sexual satisfaction Geoffrey Miller conjures up. Timothy Taylor also acknowledges that penis envy is as much a phenomenon of the locker room (R670 24) and male pride among one's comrades as it is to impress the highly elastic vaginas of the girls, just as has been found for risk-taking games like Chicken (p 24). The idea that a bigger penis has direct advantages in fertilization also looks shaky, particularly given that promiscuous chimps have a small penis but large testicles.

Nevertheless, the link between concealed estrus, female reproductive choice, sexual privacy, clothing and the evolution of sensual skin contact raises interesting questions. Ernestine Freidl, studying the ethnographic literature claimed "hidden coitus may safely be declared a near universal", however the same literature has been biased by Judeo-Christian repression of days of sexual license among people like the Huron before anthropologists had the chance to study them. The Yequana of Amazonia consider presence of infants during coitus, an 'important psychobiological link' with their parents (Liedloff). Also it is debatable that early humans living in warms climates concealed much of their anatomy at all. Much of the incidence of clothing in so-called primitive peoples is a recent result of missionary zeal.

Desmond Morris's 'Naked Ape' speculates that the origin of hairlessness in humans arose in males by providing cooling for the peak of the hunt for which humans now required tools and dexterity as well as supreme effort. The fallacy of this argument (R670 27) is that if the selection for hairlessness applied to the males, the females, the females would still be hairier. Women are less hairy than men, so the principal selection has to have occurred in women, implying that it is male sexual selection for females that has driven these major changes defining the human divergence from the apes. Taylor proposes a 'sensual skin' theory that, with the advent of some forms of clothing such as hides, sexual selection for sensual intimate naked skin, (coupled with the other sensuous aspects of female sexual curvature), caused women (and to a lesser extent men) to become the 'hairless ape'. In turn one can see sexual selection shaping male differences in beard hair, and baldness in differing human populations.

Darwin also thought that hairlessness was caused by sexual selection applied to women, which had happened early on in human evolution (R670 35):"No one supposes that the nakedness of the skin is any direct advantage to man; his body cannot have been divested of hair through natural selection". In 'The Decent of Man and Selection in Relation to Sex', he concludes that women lost their hair, because men found hairlessness attractive, not because it was burdensome; women's loss of hair led to a concomitant but less marked loss in men.

As an affectionate father of an infant daughter gently rocked in a baby sling, Taylor cites another single cause theory that the baby sling was the single most crucial step in the evolution towards larger brains (R670 44). The argument is that to get through the pelvis, given the constraints which now make human childbirth difficult and require the rotation of the head during delivery required a slowing of brain development until after birth (human give birth at 29% of adult brain size rather than the 47-8% of chimps) and hence a less developed newborn. The sweeping claim is that the baby sling was the turning point which made possible, not only the 'development of the human brain but human sexual culture and the very idea of gender - the extension of human categories into the realm of objects and ideas ... sex ceased to be necessarily short and sharp and became an act of potentially ecstatic contemplation'. While the baby sling is a major invention of women, central to both the gathering way of life and the capacity to demand feed and hence keep a balance between the number and quality of offspring (p 107) this is another single external factor theory, when it is the inventiveness of sexual selection at play in generating innovations, from the sling through the wheel, to fine music, and the arts of love, rather than the artefacts driving evolution, although they may irreversibly change the social milieu.

Hrdy (R323 264-6) ponders how humans could have evolved at all given our current forces of patriarchal domination so endemic in ape societies as well. "How could females so clearly at risk of reproductive exploitation be selected to produce such a large-brained, slow maturing offspring?" Based on her studies of langurs and other cooperatively breeding primates she proposes that "the earliest representatives of the genus Homo were cooperative breeders" suggesting that a variety of 'allo-mothers' including grandmothers, daughters, siblings, relatives, female friends and incidentally parental partners may all have been involved. This has the virtue of allowing for a flexible interplay of reproductive behavior incorporating both matrilineal and partner-based dynamics. However chimp females our nearest relative are very protective of their young and don't even hand them over to older siblings (Hrdy R323 502). Furthermore in addition to the manifest incidence of pair-bonding across all human societies, mate guarding is an almost universal feature of male mammals and so, even though men may not spend anywhere near as long in infant care as mothers, they are likely to have applied enough selective pressures throughout human emergence for partnership to have played a significant reproductive role. Since mate guarding is a better predictor of monogamy than paternal parental effort, monogamy would be expected to evolve based mutual competition between females for sexual territory. Human females do express preferences for monogamy and resist to a fair degree being co-wives, but moderate polygyny and affairs are common, consistent with a complex and varying social pattern of sexually antagonistic coevolution, poised in a state of paradox between the sexes.

What then of the relationship between our concealed ovulation and monogamy? While 10 out of 11 monogamous species have concealed ovulation, the reverse is not true. Monogamy occurs in only 10 out of 32 primates with concealed ovulation, the majority consisting of promiscuous and harem-forming species. Paradoxically the logic works in reverse for overt ovulation. While most boldly-advertising species are promiscuous (multi-male), 20 out of 34 promiscuous primates have concealed ovulation. Harem-forming species fall right across the spectrum. These confirm that concealed ovulation is a fundamentally successful strategy which can thrive in all mating systems, because it abets female choice, and that overt ovulation tends to be a specialized adaption. Many switches of mating type are believed to have occurred when tree analysis is taken into account. Overall it appears that social monogamy has evolved 7 times in different branches of the primates including humans, gibbons and 5 groups of monkeys, and harems 8 times (Diamond R165 103).

All these societies have frank characteristics of the "sexually-antagonistic coevolution" noted by William Rice (p 16). Male infanticide in all these social systems is in evolutionary conflict with female choice. Concealed ovulation creates a paradox between overt polygyny and the covert polyandry of many 'possible fathers' (Hrdy R324). In promiscuous chimp society by some accounts we have some half the offspring being sired discreetly 'on safari' despite overt ovulation, so the paternity uncertainty is both an overt one shared between genetically related males from the same troop and a covert one of secret unions of more uncertain parenthood. Human societies go further than simple infanticide and stone women for adultery, showing this sexual antagonism to be central to religious imperatives.

Desmond Morris (R475) and others (see Hrdy R322 141) assumed that concealed ovulation and continuous sexual receptivity, rather than the cyclical or seasonal reproductive patterns characteristic of other primates emerged on the basis of 'copulation as a female service' (Symons R665) on a 'man the hunter' basis to give men competing for hunting intelligence more sexual rights to maintain male cooperation in the hunt and enticements for pair-bonding. Taylor also debunks the 'man the hunter' view, as sexist, despite noting that Linda Hurcombe has pointed out that calling the division of labour between gathering and hunting sexist ignores the facts of life ... that a mother holding a young child cannot be a stealthy and fleet of foot hunter (R670 26).

Certainly overt ovulation runs counter to pair-bonding, as noted by Lancaster (R388). However Hrdy (R322 135-144) notes a poor correlation between pair-bonds and high levels of sexual activity in primates (except marmosets). Gibbons, the only monogamous ape for example make love only twice a day during an estrus which lasts a few months every 2 to 3 years with no sexual activity in between. Moreover constant sexual activity is not a good evolutionary basis to select for paternal behavior and could compete with reproductive imperatives. The occurrence of both 'assertive solicitations of males by non-ovulating females among primates which are not pair-bonded and female 'orgasm' in other primates also scotches ideas of its role being unique to humans, for example in making it 'easier for the female to be satisfied by one male'. Non-reproductive female-initiated sexual activity is likely to be selected for to impute paternity and avoid male infanticide in many species. At another extreme Nancy Burley (R93) suggested that concealed ovulation serves to prevent the human female opting out of evolution because of the pain and stresses of childbirth. However this denies women have any sense of their own ovulation which they often do, and ignores women's capacity to resist sex altogether as a means to the same end.

Alexander and Noonan (R7) argue that concealed ovulation, and the breast as a permanent signal of receptivity, enabled a female to hold on to a mate by reducing paternity certainty at the same time as inviting sexual receptivity, making it difficult for a male to know when she is on heat and thus having to stick around. Receptivity is then both an invitation and 'sex as a weapon' to enforce male resourcing compliance. Jared Diamond (R165) calls this the 'daddy-at-home theory'. Diamond argues that a woman had to conceal her ovulation; otherwise her husband would only stay with her when she was exhibiting signs that she was fertile. The rest of the time, he would be out trying to find other women, who were exhibiting signs that they were sexually ready His absence would be detrimental to his children, and by concealing her ovulation, a woman convinced a man to stay by her side and make love to her throughout the month, so that he could be sure he was fathering the children she bore. However Shlain (R625) notes that several flaws and inconsistencies, weaken the argument that promotes sex as the glue holding human relationships together. If sex served the purpose of ensuring the durability of the human parenting commitment, then parents should become more ardent in their lovemaking following the birth of a baby. Instead, the opposite occurs. Both parents routinely report a sharp fall in their respective libidos. Barbara Smuts adds the ironical twist of females tolerating male mates to protect against coercion by other males, thus forcing males to accept these bonds even when they involved lower-ranking males (Pusey R548). Wrangham (R751) has even speculated that pair bonds may relate to food guarding, with the establishment of cooking.

According to the ape family tree (p 68), and the relative success of concealed ovulation across many mating habits, concealed ovulation evolved not to keep dad at home in an already monogamous family unit, but to promote the central reproductive issue for females in ape societies - reproductive choice - immediately equatable with paternity uncertainty of 'polyandrous motherhood' or 'possible fathers' (Hrdy R324). In some primate species such as Barbary macaques, which like chimps are promiscuous multi-male troops and where the attention of several males seems essential for offspring survival, paternity uncertainty may actually aid total paternal investment (Hrdy R322 157). A similar situation prevails in human societies which believe in 'partible paternity' (p 166) the idea that many inseminations are required to form an embryo (Hrdy R323 246). Birkhead (R62 204) notes that extra-pair couplings in socially monogamous birds, aid fertility, reducing the number of eggs which fail to hatch through histo-incompatibility. Human parents with the same HLA leukocyte haplotype also have miscarriage of very early embryos. Prairie dogs also improve their fertility during their afternoon of estrus by copulating with more than one partner.

In the human context sexual privacy along with concealed ovulation acts to optimize covert and particularly female infidelity. According to Geoffrey Miller (R464), such 'reproductive inscrutability' may have catalyzed language, art, science and cultural complexity. Human gossip and judgement of personality tend to focus on detecting deceit from honesty in love and betrayal. The village grape vine round camp fires at night are a prime source of gossip and sexual intrigue. Good art and astute skill in hunting are in turn genuine indicators of fitness giving the entire process of cultural evolution a valid drive in terms of sexual selection. But female 'infidelity' also invites female competition. Several studies in birds confirm the fact that competition between females is a substantial factor inhibiting polygyny, which could, in its absence, be as successful at rearing young as the monogamous state. Ridley (R564) notes that in humans, just like sparrows, "adultery is common. It is commonest between high-ranking males and females of all ranks. To prevent it males try to guard their wives, are extremely violent towards their wives' lovers and copulate with their wives frequently, not just while they are fertile."

Bobbi Low (R416 67) in her own research also confirms that, in human cultures, one of the strongest indicators of polygyny is parasite stress. High pathogen stress accounts for 28 percent of the variation alone and with rainfall seasonality, irrigation and hunting adds to a total of 46 percent of the observed variation in polygyny. High parasite loads favour more careful investment in exogamy, involving on the males' parts wife capturing and seeking wife diversity by choosing partners at a genetic and/or physical distance and promoting genetic diversity in the offspring. Sororal polygyny is avoided. On the woman's side it is better to be the second wife of a healthy man than the sole wife of a parasite-ridden man.

Chris Knight (R373) is scathing of the evolutionary weakness of monogamy because of its sterility and lack of adaptive and social novelty in ape and other animal societies. He notes: "Among non-human primates, monogamy produces not advanced forms of sociability but a very elementary, simple and sparse social life, with little variety or political complexity to select for novel forms of self-awareness or intelligence. Compared with other primates, those which are monogamous appear to eat lower quality diets, have inferior ability to perceive social relationships, and have minimal levels of role differentiation. Moreover monogamous primates are known to be behaviorally more conservative and ecologically more restricted than their non-monogamous counterparts. ... Among non-human primates, in fact, a monogamous mating system appears to have been the least long-term adaptive value and it has been argued that this may apply to humans too." Kinzey (R367) elaborates "The lack of social networks is the major disadvantage of monogamy per se. Promiscuity does not normally occur in any human society but polygyny and polyandry taken together are much more frequent than monogamy. They encompass a greater extension of social networks than monogamy they have greater long-term adaptability and consequently they are more common. Probably the majority of cultures in the world practice some form of extended family in which the living group contains more than a single pair and their children."

In considering human emergence, Carel van Shaik and Robin Dunbar (R163 62) have suggested a radically different basis for pair-bonding as a form of mate guarding to prevent infanticide. Gibbons are socially monogamous, partly because the females distribute themselves too widely for a male to form a harem or a fission-fusion society to form. Consistent with female territory rather than paternal care being a predictor of monogamy, the male does little in infant care although he is remarkable tolerant of juveniles. Their conclusion is that he guards his mate to prevent another male committing infanticide.

Helen Fisher in "An Anatomy of Love" (R208), advances a more flexible version of the monogamy-child care theory, which is not located so specifically early in time as Lovejoy's monogamy theory and is consistent with a later emergence with Homo erectus. She sees in the development of human sexual receptivity and reproductive inscrutability a human origin in which pair bonding had become strong enough that the frank promiscuity of our closest ape cousins had given way to a form of 'serial monogamy' important for successfully rearing increasingly dependent more slowly maturing human infants, lasting for around the four years required for the first offspring to become independent, weaned and able to join a peer play group. If a couple were incompatible or did not have further children, these bonds would frequently dissolve. Unlike people like Desmond Morris (R475) who see female receptivity directed as a monogamous service to males, she notes that monogamy does not imply fidelity and that, on the evolutionary evidence, women pursued a variety of covert affairs as an integral part of their reproductive strategy. This makes much more sense. As Ridley (R564) notes: "The use of veils, chaperones, purdah, female circumcision and chastity belts all bear witness to a widespread male fear of being cuckolded and a widespread suspicion that wives, as well as their potential lovers, are the ones to distrust (why else circumcise them?)" Given an established paradigm of concealed ovulation, monogamy could thus emerge on a 'daddy-at-home' basis, as a late comer, from greater needs for the 'father' to share resourcing, because of the delayed maturation of the human offspring.

Socio-sexual interaction has been proposed to be the prime generator of social diversity because it is the reproductive feedback process through which all other generators of culture such as toolmaking and language are utilized. Sexual paradox thus drives the resulting evolution of the human brain all the way to the Homo level because sexual paradox perpetuates all the way up the tree of increasing social and intellectual diversity (Miller R464). Robin Dunbar (R178) has demonstrated a consistent correlation between social group size and neocortex to brain ratio, across wide groups of primates consistent with brain evolution being primarily related to social complexity. Socio-sexual complexity is also reflected in the dolphin brain's equivalent complexity to the human organ.

Geoffrey Miller notes (R564): "The neocortex is largely a courtship device to attract and retain sexual mates: its specific evolutionary function is to stimulate and entertain other people, and to assess the stimulation attempts of others. ... Just as the peahen is satisfied with nothing less than a visually-brilliant display of peacock plumage, I postulate that hominid males and females became satisfied with nothing less than psychologically brilliant, fascinating, articulate, entertaining companions" - the cultural equivalent of runaway sexual selection - no one can afford to select for anything else and survive.

We can surmise that in the evolution to Homo, females with a less pronounced cycle became more easily able to secure a 'monogamous' partner 'on safari' without attracting the attentions of the dominant alpha male. Covert ovulation gave the females more control over their choice of sexual partners, and provided steadier mates, because it required consistent sexual attention by a male to have any real chance of fertilization. This also favoured sub-dominant attentive males, who gained much greater chances for survival of their offspring. Menstrual synchrony (p 354), would also make it hard for an alpha male to corral all the simultaneously fertile females in a group. We have seen concealed ovulation operates successfully in many mating patterns, so we can't attribute its occurrence in humans to monogamy. Hrdy (R322 158) has this to say of the transition: "A highly assertive female sexuality marked by a potential to shift from cyclical to situation-dependent receptivity constituted the physiological heritage that prehominid females brought to this evolutionary experiment."

The human menstrual period is coupled to the lunar cycle in a way which is different from those of our close relatives. Chimps have a cycle of 36 days and bonobos a doubled cycle of 60 days (de Waal R160). The Barbary macaque's menstrual cycle is 31 and the Japanese macaque's is 28 days in duration (Shlain R625 177). Human cycles average very closely to the 29.53 days of the lunar cycle. About 28% of reproductively mature women show a 29.5 ± 1 day cycle length (Cutler et. al. R141). Vollman et al. (R703-R705) as well as Treloar et al. (R683, R684), have shown that women whose cycles approach the 29.5 day span have the highest likelihood of fertile cycles, while women whose cycles become longer or shorter have a proportionately diminishing incidence of fertile cycles.

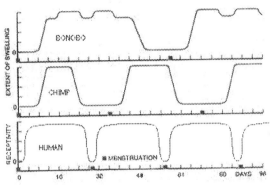

Female receptivity for sex, manifested by swollen genitals, occupies a much larger proportion of the estrus cycle of bonobos and humans than of chimpanzees. The receptivity of bonobos continues through lactation. (In chimpanzees, it disappears.) This circumstance allows sex to play a large part in the social relations of bonobos. (Dahl, de Waal R160, King). Chimps have periods longer than the lunar-related human cycle (p 351), although the bonobo half-cycle is very close.

This differs from the 28 day cycle frequently ascribed to the human female and with it the 28 day menses composed of 4 weeks of seven days, 13 of which comprise a 364 day 'year'. However it is known from deep cave studies that the human circadian rhythm is about 25 hours, not 24, and yet the action of the melatonin cycle keeps it primed to the sun, so many of these primate cycles, including a slightly shorter or longer human cycle could still be held in lunar synchronization by a melatonin-induced non-linear pacemaker effect from the lunar nightly illumination cycle, provided there is exposure to natural moonlight fluctuations, as has been the case until recent times for humans. Coordinated phase relationships between reproductive rhythms and lunar rhythms are documented in the old-world monkey genus Cercopithecus, which includes vervets (Reiter R559).

There are a number of studies that both confirm and dispute the correlation of the moon's cycle and a woman's. The majority of them, however, confirm a statistically significant relationship. The largest, conducted by Walter and Abraham Menaker (R457), collected data on over 250,000 menstrual cycles in over 2,700 women. Their findings revealed that the average length was 29.5 days. Virtually all the studies have been conducted after the invention of artificial light, a fact that could influence each study's outcome. Sung Ping Law (R390) studied women in rural China, a group minimally affected by artificial light. Her published data strongly suggest that the link between the moon and menses was statistically significant. While Law finds menstruation occurring around the ideas of the new moon, Cutler et. al. (R141) working with US university students in a more urban situation claim that menstruation in the lighter part of the month close to the full moon. Criss and Marcum (1981) document that births vary systematically over lunar cycles with a peak fertility at 3rd quarter.

Chris Knight (R373) has proposed that a critical development in human evolution running right through to the cultural phase has been an association between a sex-for-meat exchange between women and men, the moon and menstrual synchrony. In a frankly socialist interpretation of human origins, he suggests that menstrual synchrony, coupled to the lunar cycle enabled the females to exert a form of 'sex strike' in which the males were forced by the women to go 'hunting' in return for sexual favours. Given the human variation in cycle length and the mild and ambiguous coupling with the lunar cycle, the idea of a monolithically consistent sex strike strategy remains speculative, however it may have played a formative role in cultural motifs and had a major influence over the relationship between hunting, sharing and sexual favours in a social ebb and flow from celebration in the moonlight to the stark nights before the new moon. While menstrual synchrony does depend on a relatively non-competitive relationship between the females (unlike savannah baboons), Taylor's idea of it being a survival adaption to enable stressed acyclic women to prime themselves on more fecund womens' cycles (R670 103) is an evolutionarily unstable strategy. Neither does Desmond Morris's critique (R477 159) of sex strike that many of the women would be non-menstruating due to pregnancy and prolonged lactation compromise the validity of the reproductive argument.

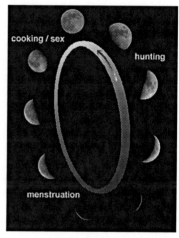

The lunar cycle and sex strike: Menstruation is associated with the dark moon, and the lightening moon gives good evening hunting. Sexual withdrawal is followed by the hunt, capped by the full moon, meat feast and sexual favours.

It is also consistent with Catherine Key's (R349) prisoners' dilemma analysis of human sexual relations (p 34), as reproductive investments shifted to increase the differential between smaller male and larger female reproductive effort with increasing head size, and slowed growth and development, and the ensuing need for females to cooperate to ensure adequate investment from the males through sexual control. Here males become non-reciprocal altruists partly in the hope of securing later matings. One of the strengths of the sex-strike sexual faking theory is that it addresses the question of why symbolic culture evolved, rather than simply how it did so, according to Robin Dunbar (Douglas R170).

Key notes that the presence of estrus females is the best predictor of hunting behaviour in male chimps, just as bonobo males give food for sex and subordinate baboons (*Papio anubis*) court favoured females in a harem in expectation of future matings. Key's Prisoner Dilemma simulations displayed complex system behavior with many strategies needing to be followed by players to survive the reproductive round. Females cooperated with females more than males and under reduced male reproductive effort. However when their reproductive effort was higher females could adopt a strategy of alternate defection tolerating only non-reciprocal altruist males who offered consistent cooperation. Key notes also that women defect when playing the prisoners' dilemma more frequently than men.

In a key way menstruation is a 'no' signal replacing the 'yes' signal of overt estrus, but still implies fecundity overall. Camilla Power (R538) extends Knight's ideas directly into the use of ochre (p 94) as a symbolic substitute extending menstrual 'cheating' into the explosion of the cultural phase through the symbolization of the reproductive strategy.

The significance of menstruation and the moon are coupled in !Kung San (p 113) , Hadza (p 131), and Sandawe rites (p 118). In the San eland dance during menarche, the girl plays the part of a bull, sending out a 'wrong sex, wrong species' signal. Meanwhile, the women of the camp dance around her as if mating with the bull, taunting the local men with their complete lack of interest in them. Power says: "The message to the males is absolutely clear - you go off, you hunt some eland, and then we'll see. It's a sex strike in all but name." The Hadza have a similar ritual called 'epeme', linked to symbolic menstruation and the new moon, associated with a mythical heroine who hunts down male zebra and wears their penises. The Sandawe have a corresponding fertility rite by the light of the full moon in which the women expose their buttocks invitingly to the men in the moonlight.

Leonard Shlain (R625) has extended the significance of menstruation in cultural emergence to development of awareness of 'deep time' over months and the idea of gaining control of one's destiny through women discovering the coupling of their reproductive cycle to the moon and its relationship with birth nine lunar cycles later - a gaining of reproductive power over men which was only later usurped by male control over female fertility and the natural productivity of the planet. However responsiveness to seasonal cycles in the brain is evidenced in the migrations of many species. Nevertheless intriguingly close links among the words for moon, menses, and time are present in every language. The English *menses*,- month, moon and measurement have their roots in the Latin words *mens* 'mind' and *mensis* 'menses' and the Greek word *menos* 'menses'. So, too, do 'mental'. 'meter', 'metric', 'mentor', 'diameter', 'commensurate', 'immensity', 'parameter', 'perimeter' and 'dimension'. Shlain associates this transition with difficulties in childbirth associated with an increase in head size and a transfer from overt ovulation to concealed ovulation with advertised menstruation as a timekeeper. As a laparoscopic gynecologist, he is aware of the increasingly heavy demand on women to replace the iron lost by menstruation (at least in some women) and speculates that this became a burden of this evolutionary adaption which placed women hostage to a degree to the need for a meat component of their diet supplied by the men.

In an interesting twist to the origin of bipedalism associated with the loss of forest and the spreading of savannah around the rift valley is the idea that there may have been large areas of swamp land created during the same epoch. Chimpanzees are much more prepared to walk bipedally when partially immersed and need to do so to breathe. Such a scenario is not inconsistent with the 'aquatic ape' hypothesis (Morgan R471), explaining our hairlessness and other gracile features including a dependency of 98% of the population on eicosanoic acid (a 20 carbon oil) found in fish on the basis of an association with margins of water.

However Elaine Morgan's aquatic ape theory is based on a constellation of unverified assumptions, which don't stand up to closer scrutiny, including 'creative' use of a whole nexus of advantages, from the 'aquatic' hairlessness itself, through the curious vestigal webbing between our digits not seen in apes, to fatty breasts doubling as swimming floats for the kids, long hair to grab mum by in the water, the perceived advantages of 'water birth', rounded buttocks to breast feed on the gravelly shoreline, and subcutaneous fat. According to Taylor (R670 40), despite a suggestive gap in the fossil record, the only evidence for aquatic hominids comes from pre-homo skulls mauled by crocodiles and human subcutaneous fat, which unlike that of marine mammals, fails to insulate us so we rapidly succumb to hypothermia in water. Neither do seals lack fur. Nevertheless it is true that chimps walk upright much more readily when buoyed by water, while foraging in swampland.

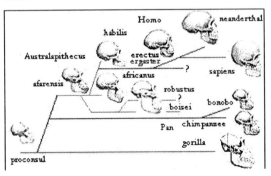

One hypothetical evolutionary tree for humans and related apes. There is much debate about the actual form of such a tree.

Erectus: The Emergence of Homo

Although we may look for historical evidence of evolutionary emergence of Homo in an 'environment of evolutionary adaptedness' in the Pleistocene (Hrdy R323 97), modern humans are an overlapping of many evolutionary processes on vastly different time scales. The molecule prolactin central to human maternal behavior and mammalian lactation generally has an evolutionary history running back to controlling water balance in fresh water fish and metamorphosis in amphibians (R323 130). By contrast changes in allele frequency as a result of sexual selection occur extremely rapidly and could change from a 2% incidence to 98% within 10,000 years (R323 106). Thus although humans have been molded by characteristics emerging over four million or so years, some are much longer and some are subject to extremely rapid selection and variation in modern human societies.

At some point from around the time we began to become bipedal to when the increasing human head size began to cause delivery problems, requiring births of helpless babies, needing more support to survive, this promiscuous ape pattern evolved towards one which gave more emphasis to longer-term semi-monogamous bonds between partners. There are many slightly different renditions of this story, some emphasizing shared child-rearing by female kin and friends rather than male partners. Others vary from emphasizing female reproductive choice to the repressive impact of male coalitions on female reproductive covertness.

Evolutionary conditions now began to favour a stronger pair bond between partners, which would aid offspring survival, at least for the first few years until an infant could join a peer group and fend for itself. Into this picture, we find the development of a form of serial monogamy, extremely rare in mammals, only about 3% of which are overtly monogamous, but much more common in birds where it takes two and a next to incubate and feed the young. The estrus became permanently suppressed, instead of the overt ape form found in chimps, and the female became perpetually sexually receptive, promoting strong psycho-sexual partnership bond formation, developing as well erotic tokens of fecundity in curvaceous fatty, sensitive breasts, only a small minority of whose tissue is involved in lactation, with buttocks and an hour-glass torso indicating ripe fertility.

Some writers, such as Sarah Hrdy (R323), question how much fathers have ever been involved in parenting, citing modern, 'primitive' and ape societies, and others consider that male coalitions may have had a significant influence towards female reproductive covertness rather than female choice, or partners alone. These are all features of a complex evolutionary dynamic whose centre is and has to be the reproductive relationship in a context of a ramifying linguistic grape vine, much of whose gossip, beyond sexual displays and emotional networking, has to have revolved around issues of fidelity and intimations of deceit.

We have noted (p 33), that mutual parenting needs are not a good predictor of monogamy in mammals, but rather the spatial distribution females to form exclusive domains, forcing males to guard a single female (Komers and Brotherton). A consistent and more complex interpretation might thus be that women evolved to have private sex within closely cooperative human social groups in which, like tamarins and marmosets, the females kept other females out of their own private sexual sphere, (Miller R464 185, Hrdy R323 180) by expecting fidelity of commitment from male partners, thus creating small exclusive sexual ranges, keeping track of the consistency of their lovers through gossip with other women during gathering forays, at the same time embracing the prowess of good hunters. The relative difficulty for males of crossing between partners without friction would then bias the natural male tendency towards polygyny towards overt monogamy with secretive affairs unless a male could openly supply resources sufficient to protect and support two partners. Human pregnancy is about as much of a maternal crisis as a twin birth would be for a tamarin. Maternal ambivalence would thus seem to be inevitable, and like other mammals to fall both on a male partner and on other kin in the kind of cooperative breeding arrangement Hrdy has associated with allo-mothering.

The crucible for such evolution, rather than the small-brained *Australopithicenes*, with a cranial volume of some 450 cc similar to other apes, appears to be the major push made by *Homo erectus* and his alter-ego *Homo ergaster* who is consigned by some to an African rather than adispersed Asian locale (Dennell and Roebroeks R156), from a 750cc brain to 1250cc close to our own average size of around 1400cc. This expansion occurring between 1.6 million and 500,000 years ago achieved even in 75,000 generations, has to have been driven by a high degree of selection unlike any selection we see today in the relatively static brain size of modern humans. It is somewhere in this process, we can expect the human head size and retarded development to have played an increasingly significant role. There is little evidence of changes of tool-making during this time, with the handaxe playing an almost unchanging role, as continuing stereotype , but by 790,000 years ago, there is already evidence of control of fire, associated with flints and wood of six species including olive, wild barley and wild grape (Goren-Inbar et. al. R247).

There is some evidence that colonization of cooler climates may have been consistent with the use of skins or other forms of clothing. Analysis of erectus skulls and the discovery of a hyoid bone involved in speech vocalization is also consistent with an increasing use of language in erectus (Broadfield et. al. R78). On the other hand 1.6 million year old Nariokotome *Homo ergaster* skeleton, which does have some evidence of Broca's area (Taylor R670 41) has been claimed to have too narrow a spinal cord at the neck to have enabled the chest control for speech and some later examples have a high ape-like larynx that might be incompatible with speech (Ridley R567 219). Evidence for development of auditory areas associated with language goes back much further. Early work by Tobias (R680) and others suggest that the beginning of brain asymmetry in early Australopithecus exists. There are current studies on chimpanzees that suggest that there are certain very specific lateralized brain functions having to do with language which are present in chimpanzee brains. In particular is the 'planum temporale' which is a specialized area in the auditory association cortex which receives sounds, and attaches meaning to them. In most of the chimp brains tested, this area was larger on the left side hemisphere than in the right one, which is also the human pattern (Begley, 199R51 9). This evidence is also supported by Kanzi, a bonobo who has been in a language learning environment for nearly 20 years and has a very good level of comprehension of spoken English. He was tested on 660 novel English sentences and responded to the correctly on 72% of the trials, which was an equivalent response rate to that of a two year old human child tested on the same problems. (Savage-Rumbaugh et al. R600). Tobias (R680) had suggested that Homo habilis might have a Broca's area and Falk (1992) feels that by specialized measuring techniques she has confirmed its presence. A team of researchers has also established that Homo heidelbergensis thought to lead to Neanderthal had a hearing profile consistent with attention to speech rather than the high and low alert frequencies of chimps (DOI: 10.1073/pnas.0403595101).

The shape of the Neanderthal larynx and tongue was not positioned in the same way as ours for language (Comrie et. al.) and the skull shapes are significantly different (Harvati et. al.).

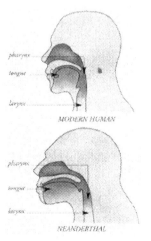

MODERN HUMAN

NEANDERTHAL

On the other hand the Neanderthal throat is believed to have been less suited to verbal vocalization. Recent research, both from mitochondrial DNA (Krings et. al. R384), and from careful skull measurements (Harvati et. al. R290), suggests Neanderthal diverged from the line of Homo some 465,000 years ago and are a distinct species. Ridley (R567 214) has also drawn attention to the FoxP2 transcription factor gene on chromosome 7 whose mutations can give rise to severe selective language impairment and appears to be associated with fine motor coordination of the larynx. Mutations in this gene are rare. There have only been two functional mutations detected, one in the ancestors of mice and one in those of orangutans. But there has been a double mutation in this gene and the paucity of 'silent' neutral mutations which don't change the protein suggests it is a very recent change, later than 200,000 years ago, which has swept through the population by conferring a major selective advantage. However there is evidence for Neanderthal bone flutes (Gray et. al. R259) similar to those found all the way to Dolni Vestonice (p 173).

There are hints that these differences in Neanderthal are linked to social differences in sex roles. Lewis Binford speculates that the pattern of bones and tools in the French cave of Combe-Grenal reveals two separate but contemporaneous kinds of living area, one suggesting a life lived very locally, the other showing the comings and goings of more mobile folk. Binford calls the first type "the nest", and believes its occupants were females and their dependent children, foraging in the immediate vicinity. The second kind – smaller, more peripheral to the cave itself, he calls "scraper sites," suggesting these sites were produced by males. There is a connection between the two types, but a small one. Binford sees some provisioning of the young on the part of the males, but only in a haphazard sort of way. This dual pattern occurs through the 75,000 Mousterian years in Combe-Grenal, unlike the way modern men and women live together and divide the labor of food procurement and preparation between them. The Neanderthal sexes may thus have lived more apart with independent food preparation, different land-use patterns, different uses of technology, suggesting sexually mature males and females were not bound together by the long-term, reasonably stable sexual and economic relationships that exist between the sexes in all known human communities today (Shreeve R628 331). Dental evidence also suggests Neanderthals had a more rapid growth, becoming fully mature at 15, consistent with a higher mortality rate (Rozzi and de Castro R583) in contrast to delayed human development, although this is contested (R197). However at Shandar there is evidence of burial and caring for the disabled (Taylor R670 108).

We propose the driving force for human brain growth was the complexification of the entire world of Homo brought about by the involution of semantic language into consciousness (and thus society) as an outgrowth of gesture and emotional vocalization and that it has been driven principally by social complexity, expressed in mate selection and social standing. Mirror neurons have been cited in this regard (p 379). In this description, the evolution of language is a crisis of social interaction generated by genetic systems through the dynamic capacity to encapsulate language as 'memes' rather than hard-wired genetic determinism.

Orthodox ideas of language evolution emphasize how natural selection shaped our ancestors to improve their talent for complex communication. Noam Chomsky (R117) famously pointed out that infants learn language quickly and reliably from sparse and chaotic input. For him and many linguists, this 'poverty of the stimulus', is evidence that much of our language ability is innate, directly encoded in our genome, and takes the form of a neurologically hard-wired universal grammar. Steven Pinker (R531) argues that the ability to communicate effectively would have given early humans a 'fitness advantage'. Natural selection favoured genetic mutations that improved our language faculty, so they spread through the hominid gene pool. The legacy is that we all have brains adapted for speech. However the development of the human brain, unlike that of song birds, doesn't simply consist of an enlarged language centre but an entire enlarged and complexified cerebral cortex, indicating evolution has been in the direction of adapting to a universal increase in complexity of the social environment.

Right: Homo erectus hand axe - almost unchanging over long epochs. Sculpture from Berekhat Ram, Israel dating from strata c 233,000-470,000 BP hints at an early origin of primitive art in Homo erectus. Inset: 'Neanderthal' flute 45,000 BP Divje babe I Slovenia.

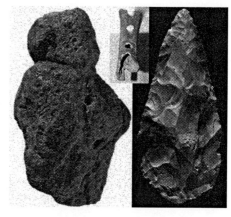

A theory of language as an evolutionary 'parasites' reaching towards internal efficiency has recently been advanced. Darwin, the founder of the evolutionary approach speculated that language was potentially an invention (R148 60): "Man not only uses inarticulate cries, gestures and expressions, but has invented articulate language, if indeed the word *invented* can be applied to a process completed by innumerable steps half consciously made". Morten Christiansen (Christiansen and Kirby R120) questions the need to invoke a Chomskian generative grammar. Instead, he argues, language has adapted to utilize more general cognitive processing capacities that were already part of our ancestors' brains before language came along.

Among these, he focuses on 'sequential learning' - the ability to encode and represent the order of the discrete elements in a sequence. This ability is not unique to humans: mountain gorillas, for example, use it in the complicated preparation of certain spiky plant foods, where a sequence of tasks is required to remove the edible part. Language, he says, is a 'non-obligate mutualistic endosymbiont' - a kind of evolutionary structure like a 'symbolic virus'. Kirby suggests our brains are not so specifically designed for language and that we appear to be biologically adapted to language because language which evolves much faster than biology has culturally adapted to us, gaining semantic power and representational efficiency as it evolves. Languages as different as Danish and Hindi have evolved in less than 5000 years from a common Proto-Indo-European ancestor. Yet it took up to 200,000 years for modern humans to evolve from archaic *Homo sapiens*. The latest estimates of the oldest skulls discovered, from the Omo river by Richard Leakey are 196,000 years (McDougall et. al. R434). Pinker (R533) notes steps of this type in the experiments of Martin Nowak's group (R496, R497) in establishing both sequential symbols such as vowels and consonants to form a word and positional syntax in which words describing single events give way to active characterization of a type of event. Both are adaptive responses to informational crisis as a large number of symbols each associated with a single context or event involves too many similar symbols to adequately discriminate one from another. The emergence of such structures could in turn have enabled the semantic enfolding of the rational mind. Reading written language is clearly such and adaption of visual pattern recognition and other skills

Ape communication is a fluid mix of gesture, body, hand and facial movements, and vocalizations, all of which play a role in expressing meaning in emotional terms. Yawning is catching in chimps suggesting self-awareness (DOI 10/1098/rsbl.2004.0224). Karen McComb (R444) tested an idea of Robin Dunbar's that language arises from mutual or reciprocal grooming as ape societies become lager and more complex. In a study of 42 primate species she found that call repertoire and time spent grooming increases with group size.

Corballis (R132) suggests language arose from a selective convergence of these diverse attributes to give rise to semantic language, possibly also accompanied by a convergence of other faculties such as mental perspectives of others, consistent with an early common origin of click sounds (p 106). Gestures like the shrug are also ancient responses, while smiles, and snarls with all their dimensions from appeasement to tooth threatening exposure go all the way back through our primate relatives. Laughter is an example of a central chaotic and explosive emotional response to contradiction, or surprise, which is suggestive of an ancient origin, earlier than language as we know it, in sharing emotional reactions, which also appears to have a basis in sexual courtship and family bonding:

> "Women laugh most in the presence of men they find attractive.
> Men are the leading laugh getters, women are the leading laughers"
> Robert Provine University of Maryland (R371)

The advent of semantic exchange would place a huge new evolutionary burden on all areas of the cortex by exploding time, space and society into an historical process in which more and more contexts, individuals and situations came to be named and hence distinguishable from one another. Such a language involution would then place a burden of selection on larger brains which could handle the new and diverse complexities of a world imbued with historical and semantic meaning requiring slowed fetal development and a new awareness of social and sexual relationships and their implications. We can see the germ of this complexity in ape societies, such as grazing gelada baboons where there are a host of cries indicating all manner of interactions, from courtship, through male competition, to emotional 'social contracts' of mutuality, reciprocation, aggression and reconciliation, as well as group warnings about predators. Among these, sexual courtship and competition are both very strong and also very subtle fleeting yet highly focused influences, as a glance at a female macaque inciting an extra-alpha 'safari' coupling behind the alpha males' backs indicates. This supports a general role for Machiavellian social interactions, with a core emphasis on reproduction and sexual selection driving the burgeoning complexity of semantic language, consistent with both Geoffrey Miller's sexual selection ideas and honesty and deceit in wider social contracts. Consistent with this view is the fact that the sneakiest monkeys have the largest brains (DOI: 10.1098/rspb.2004.2780)). Dunbar (R177) suggests that, as neocortical size increases, more subtle social and political strategies, such as tactical deception come into play. As a result, lower-ranking individuals are able to find loopholes in the social dominance hierarchy. Their special cognitive capacity makes them able to improve their reproductive success, in spite of lower rank - in line with the Machiavellian Intelligence hypothesis (Whiten and Byrne R728, R729). Boehm (R67 182) comments that the political invention of egalitarian society during this process enabled such individuals to forgo or invoke strategies of social deception, suggesting that lower ranking coalitions bluffed or forced their way, as male coalitions of chimps can do, to form large, stable and purposeful coalitions which are at the root of our social egalitarianism, politics and morality.

Erectus is conceived as a gatherer-hunter species, so one can envisage a leading edge of such evolution applying to coalitions of gathering females consistent with sexual differences in human language acquisition in humans today. This in turn could have driven increased opportunities for female reproductive choice and the growth of a capacity to define long-term relationships and forms of serial monogamy within an existing social grouping not found in ape societies, where monogamy occurs only outside immediate social groupings, which are either harems, or promiscuous troops. We can envisage a continuing trend of sexual selection, increasing long-term partnership, female cooperation in gathering and social cohesion, the avoidance of male-driven infanticide and strong sexual selection for males with a good social capacity for fathering, entertainment, protective prowess and partnership.

A new human-like species *Homo floriensis* - a dwarfed relative who lived just 18,000 years ago in the company of pygmy elephants and giant lizards - has been discovered in Indonesia, which may be a remnant of *Homo erectus* stock adapted for small size (R81, R479).

Sapientia: Adolescent Adam and the Unbearable Beauty of Eve.

The emergence of modern *Homo sapiens*, is accompanied by a slight decrease in brain size from an average of about 1500cc to 1400. Although this is well within the range of human variation between 1100 and 2000cc, it does suggest that some form of compactification has taken place. One view of this is that the development of culture and language has actually made it cognitively easier for the brain to assimilate the world around us. Another suggested by Matt Ridley (R567 34) is that a reduction of aggression may be accompanied by a neotonic (tending towards embryonic form) reduction of the limbic brain areas associated with aggression, which appear to be among the latest to mature. A similar argument has been made about the evolution of the bonobo by comparison with chimps. More extreme such reductions in brain size have been seen in breeding domesticated animals from the wild

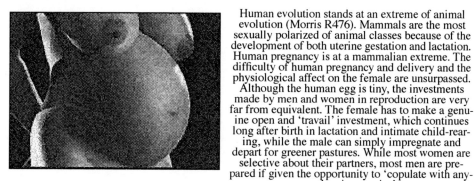

Human evolution stands at an extreme of animal evolution (Morris R476). Mammals are the most sexually polarized of animal classes because of the development of both uterine gestation and lactation. Human pregnancy is at a mammalian extreme. The difficulty of human pregnancy and delivery and the physiological affect on the female are unsurpassed. Although the human egg is tiny, the investments made by men and women in reproduction are very far from equivalent. The female has to make a genuine open and 'travail' investment, which continues long after birth in lactation and intimate child-rearing, while the male can simply impregnate and depart for greener pastures. While most women are selective about their partners, most men are prepared if given the opportunity to 'copulate with anyone bearing ovaries'..

The sexual evolution of the female human has become unique in many diverse ways.

Female humans have evolved physically to become perpetually attractive to males, through continual receptiveness, able to make love 'in continuum', over prolonged periods, resulting in an intense sustained form of social bonding unparalleled in other socially monogamous species. These evolutionary characteristics involve the whole female body in such a way as to advertise ripe fecundity - fat-engorged breasts, hour-glass torso, larger buttocks. Despite Hrdy's demurring at Buss's 'patriarchal' emphasis on feminine beauty in sexual selection (R95), this uncontrollable beauty of the feminine form, which has obsessed artists, scholars, lovers and fearful religious patriarchs alike is an aspect of human sexual evolution which, like the female's choosy preference for 'declared' monogamy to a resourceful partner, rings true throughout our evolutionary and cultural emergence.

This is complemented by a sensual sensitivity capped by a profound female orgasm which is tuned for reproductive selection of highly desired partners, whether long-term, or a secret love tryst. Ovulation is cryptic mid way between menstrual periods, making it difficult for any male to be sure whether or not he has succeeded in the fertility quest without sticking around. The sexual act is pursued largely in privacy which makes it as hard as possible for others to trace the intimate details of who was present and what went on. Sexual relationship is intense and long-lasting and has the capacity to become an abundant and fulfilling life transaction which has a major role in establishing a primary child-rearing resource in long-term partnership with a male, as well as the thrill of the chase in a strange affair.

There is also a great variety of sexual development among individual women. By comparison with the peacock's tail as a powerful indicator of alpha male genetic prowess and little else, human females appear to have evolved sexual diversity as a signal to accomplished and desirable males that they are uniquely different, alien, alluring, exotic and erotic in the extreme, thus responding to the innate philandering polygyny of the male and the high variance in male resources, by evolving sexual variety as an irresistible enticement.

Human pregnancy is at an extreme of living species, leaving the female vulnerable and travail in her final months, with birth a major compromise to fit the human head through the birth canal, and lactation and child rearing expanded into a fully fledged cultural discovery process which takes more care and effort than any other species. This is complemented by a human male who can excel as 'dad' but can also betray as a 'cad', who may oppress as a 'despot', or come to the rescue as a temporary hero. This perpetuates a situation of sexual paradox in which neither gender has ultimate control of their own reproductive destiny.

Into this mix enters an evolutionary race between the clitoris and the penis, the clitoris becoming ever more demanding and the penis more satisfying - the principal instruments of emotional lust, love and togetherness, a glue cementing the human family, from which all our notions of passion, romantic and compassionate love emerge. The human penis is the thickest, and most hydraulic of ape penises, by comparison with the thin pencils of muscle and bone sported by other apes. Jared Diamond laconically complained of the great failure of modern science to come up with an adequate theory of penis length, suggesting it might relate to aggression displays with other males (Blum R65 31). This is matched by the time and energy involved. Humans make love for periods of ten minutes to half an hour or so. Gorillas barely manage one minute. With bonobos its over in fifteen seconds and excitable chimps barely make seven seconds. The entire species is founded on premature ejaculation.

The answer to the enigma of the penis according to Geoffrey Miller (R464) lies in its mysterious sister-spouse the clitoris. The apparently vestigial, but astonishingly powerful clitoris, despite its small size, has twice as many sensitive nerve endings as the penis. The clitoris and its hidden complement, the G-spot, now came into play in an evolutionary 'amatory race' with the penis, aptly described by Geoffrey Miller: "The penis evolved to deliver more and more stimulation, while the clitoris evolved to demand more and more." Both of these, according to Miller, were driven by female reproductive choice, the clitoris, which is not prominently displayed to male view and hence choice, unlike the estrus, swollen buttocks and reflex pheromones of apes, as a discriminator of sexual love, and the penis as an indicator to, and satisfier of, women's mate choices. In fact female orgasm dwarfs that of the male in its capacity for extremes of ecstasy, body-wracked convulsions and multiple, or even continual orgasm, undiminished by the 'downfall' and refractory 'impotence' following male ejaculation. It is also, unlike the physical necessity of male orgasm for insemination, an ephemeral discriminator, of male ardour, never dependable but coquettish and precocious, depending on the mood of the moment, which does not serve the routine life of monogamous pair bonding so much as it acts as a sense organ of novelty and excitement - an evolutionary discriminator which separates the man who can really give the lady "all she desires" from the boys who shoot once and think they are king of the road. A central part of male sexual denial in the desire to sexually dominate is a vain attempt to deny the full flood of female ecstasy and its implications.

Shlain (R625) describes three theories of female orgasm which sexologists and interested anthropologists have whimsically given the names Pole Ax, Upsuck, and Cuddles. Pole Ax is the idea that laying a women out with a powerful orgasm will cause her to lie down and keep the sperm in place ensuring fertilization in a bipedal upright species with a downward pointing vagina. Baker and Bellis (R37) have suggested that female orgasm, particularly the stronger variety which may accompany a passionate affair, may provide and 'upsuck' which selectively improves the chances of conception with the partner of choice. This in association with the tendency of women to be more prone to sexual activity during ovulation, with both their existing partners and others, could provide another partial explanation for its role in reproductive terms, which so far remains unproven. The third theory Cuddles, postulates that Mother Nature bestowed on '*Gyna sapiens*' a multisynaptic orgasm to help a couple more thoroughly bond with each other through mutual great sex. However this is again a little naive in terms of their differing strategies and ignores the fact that natural selection has not seen fit to take this route in other socially monogamous species.

Mary Sherfey (R624) in "The Evolution of Female Sexuality" noted that "to all intents and purposes, the human female is sexually insatiable in the presence of the highest degree of sexual satiation". Despite being based on the now believed to be false notion of a primal matriarchy and having no clear evolutionarily rationale, Sherfey's view coincides with that of pre-Victorian Europe where female sexual precociousness was recognized in an "exuberant and inexhaustible appetite for all variety of sexual pleasure", (just as it is feared in the Old Testament and Amazonian societies). Kim Phillips in "Medieval Maidens" (R527) has noted that in old Europe mutual orgasm was deemed necessary for conception.

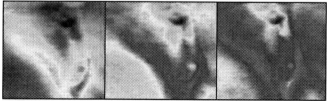

Infrared imaging: Female sexual arousal is accompanied by blood flow to the labia and clitoris just as it is to the penis. This is central to the nature of human courtship and bonding between the sexes (p 361) but does it also function to confuse or even diminish paternity certainty?

By contrast, the Victorian era ushered in the notion that "the majority of women (happily for them) are not much troubled by sexual feelings of any kind" - a form of psychic female circumcision partly in concordance with the Darwinian awareness of greater reproductive variation and sexual competition in males. In response to Sherfey, Donald Symons (R665) comments "It is difficult to see how expending time and energy pursuing the will-o'-the-wisp of sexual satiation, endlessly and fruitlessly attempting to make a bottomless cup run over could conceivably contribute to a female's reproductive success" noting it would both interfere with food gathering and child care and even subvert female choice. This case is based on females having little variation in reproductive success and that copulating with many males cannot improve their reproductive success.

This has led to the notion that both female orgasm and the clitoris are 'spandrels' like the appendix and male nipples as Stephen Jay Gould specualted - evolutionary relics, or results of underlying sexual homology. Some support for the idea comes from twin studies in which there is a 32-45% genetic factor involved in the wide variation in orgasmic ability of women from 14% who always succeed, through 32% who only do some quater of the time to 14% who cannot reach orgasm either by sex or masturbation (Spector et. al. R642). ElizabethLloyd (R410) takes this case further, that like stump-tailed macaques and bonobos, female orgasm is more for female-female social bonding than reproductive advantage - a spandrel for pleasure, riding on the coat-tails of male evolution, extending this to questionable claims based on FGM (p 285). However the 'choosiness' of the clitoris, in coitus does not imply no reproductive advantage but high discrimination in reproductive choice.

Sarah Hrdy's (R322 - R324) view, offers an ironic twist, which has formidable undertones. She proposes that females evolved an interest in promiscuous sex so that many males would 'presume' that they could have 'fathered' a female's child. Multiple male care for, or at least lack of harm to, her offspring would result, thus enhancing her fitness and offspring survival. Hrdy and others have also seen the human female's loss of physical signs of ovulation in this light: Concealed ovulation was naturally selected since it helped to *decrease* paternity certainty. Hrdy, despite extolling a life of monogamy herself, argues that paternity uncertainty was an advantage for evolving hominid women, but that, as human society developed, males devised ways to increase paternity certainty (through seclusion of women, chastity belts, and so on), women lost their autonomy, otherwise at a high level among primate females, as a result of male success in increasing paternity certainty.

One should note that although human ovulation is concealed, males still find a woman more attractive during ovulation and can tell that the vaginal mucosae, rich with fern-like polymers to aid sperm transit are unusually slippery and attractive. Kuukasjärvi et. al. (R386) note that female body odours are more attractive to men during mid-cycle.

Her experience with primates (R322 160-180) has led her to realize that there are a variety of reasons why females may elicit sex with more than one male, both in the relative frenzy of estrus and outside it. These actions are both an expression of graduated female sexual choice, focusing on prime genetic partners towards the peak of estrus, from a wider range she entices beforehand and they serve her reproductive efficacy in claiming many 'fathers' thus helping to give her offspring the relative protection of the males in her vicinity and reducing risks of injury or infanticide - specifically by reducing paternity certainty! Notably human step fathers are 65 times more likely to kill infants (p 49). Noting the behavior of macaques and experiments on the stimulation of female rhesus monkeys, she has even gone so far as to suggest that the unique features we experience in female orgasm serve this promiscuous end, continuing after a male has completed his all-to-transient act of insemination and thus inviting the implied attention of more ardent suitors:

"What we know about primates suggests that prehominid females embarking upon the human enterprise were possessed of an aggressive readiness to engage in both reproductive and non-reproductive liaisons with multiple, but selected, males. What happened next is, and probably will always remain, shrouded in mystery. We can only document the attitudes prevalent in human cultures during historical times. There can be no doubt from such evidence that the *expectation* of female 'promiscuity' has had a profound effect on human cultural institutions."

This explanation is frightening, with dark undertones, explaining in one step why female sexuality is repressed cauterized and incised by a fearful patriarchy, perceiving that it *reduces* paternity certainty. Eighteen years later Hrdy (R323 222-3) plays devil's advocate to her own radical position, in the light of our excoriating patriarchal history.

"Female libido and sexual assertiveness are dangerous predispositions in such contexts, more likely to get a woman beaten disfigured or killed than to increase her reproductive success ... Knowing how risky extra-pair sex can often be for females in my own species has led me to wonder if female orgasms may be a once adaptive retention, now no longer selected for, like the grasp of a just-born baby for maternal fur that no longer exists, a reflex gradually fading out of the human repertoire".

Jared Diamond (R165) compares Alexander and Noonan's "daddy-at-home" theory with

Sarah Hrdy's "many fathers" theory. Hrdy contrasts langurs, which have concealed ovulation with chimps which have overt ovulation, noting that overt ovulation is a rare (only 27 out of 175 primate species) evolutionary response to full-developed promiscuity, in which females mate with as many males in the troop as possible to avoid any of them having a reason to commit infanticide. Effectively this advertises to all "come and get me" for a gang bang while dealing with the matter effectively and quickly. By contrast, langurs have a single male in a harem and the females have concealed ovulation, again as a hedge against infanticide, because this makes it possible for the females to mate with a stray male outside the extended family without either her 'husband' or the 'gigolo' knowing whether she has gotten pregnant, or by whom. In more sinister terms it helps protect the female from infanticide when stray gangs of males take over the harem and displace the protecting male. Sperling (R643) has claimed that, although Hrdy's vision of primates may be more acceptable to feminists, it is still based on unwarranted assumptions interpreting primate behaviors as end points, in evolutionary adaptations which are also more complex, varied, and context-dependent than sociobiological theory suggests. However this looks more of a case of denial of the disquieting roots of human culture which religious conservatives and gender feminists alike would seek to avoid, lest they throw their preconceived defences into disarray. Evolutionary ecologists maintain that social behavior, including that in humans, is influenced in subtle but fundamental ways by natural selection, fitness and sexual selection without the hard-line genetic determinism of earlier sociobiologists.

None of this complex picture of polyamory amidst social monogamy in humans implies that fidelity reigned, even if emerging Homo was predominantly patrilocal like other apes and pair-bonding was a strong feature associated with the needs of slowly-developing infants. Human males have medium sized testicles and killer sperm consistent with moderate sperm competition, but less than those of the larger ejaculates of promiscuous chimps. As a proportion of body size human testicles are five times the size of gorillas and one third the size of chimpanzees (Ridley R567 21). In the Cosmopolitan survey of 1980 half of married women under 35 had been unfaithful and 70% of those over. Likewise for men sewing wild oats is accepted as natural. Human males are about 10% larger than females consistent with moderate polygynous competition, but not the large harems of gorillas. Men are more aroused by images of males competing for a female than readily available females and produce better sperm after watching such images (.Biology Letters doi:10.1098/rsbl.2005.0324).

Into this arena falls the highly contentious question of whether human male acts of sexual coercion also have a biological basis, or are a cultural expression of male power and patriarchal dominance (p 47). While some authors such as Thornhill and Palmer (R677) argue for a sociobiological basis, others in reaction (Travis R682) see the question of 'rape' as at the very least a multi-disciplinary issue. This is clear from our studies of slavery and concubinage (p 195), where forms of effective male coercion have become institutional, however one can also argue that these are obvious expressions of sexual sociobiology. Moreover rape is rare in our primate cousins with one notable exception. In one study almost half the copulations in an orangutan troop happened after fierce female resistance had been overcome by the males (Sparks R641 153). Immature male orangs, which have a distinct phenotype (p 33), use sexual coercion as their main mating strategy. Baboon males also engage in aggressive sex which appears reluctant on the part of the female (R641 156). Jolly (R338 80) comments that real rape is very rare in primates besides ourselves and orangutans but that it *is* natural in humans, although whether it is inevitable or right is a separate question.

Human females have a more heavy reproductive commitment than almost any other species, with massive pregnancy, difficult childbirth, and a period of vulnerability after lactating, with a small infant on the hip. To spread their massive out-front investment it is essential for virtually every species for the female to be able to exert genuine female reproductive choice. When reproduction depends also to some degree on the partnership and resourcing of a male, this involves a dissonance between the resources of the partner and the best genes available. Both humans and colonial monogamous birds solve this dilemma by investing about 80% in their overt partner's genes and up to 20% in those from covert affairs. The best genes may also be a relative issue. As noted in terms of the histocompatibility preferences (p 354) and the incidence of potential mate infertility in both monogamous birds and humans (Birkhead R62 204) this may also serve to secure partners who, relative to the given female, have high fitness in immunological and histological terms and possibly higher than their resourcing partner. Men are renowned for spreading their wild oats, but women are subject to dire punishments for infidelity because of the fear males have of the 'pollution' of their reproductive chances and the life dilemma of bringing up another man's child. Consequently females have sought not only concealed estrus but privacy in sexual intercourse to protect them from real risk of ostracism, desertion, infanticide, injury and death. The veil, stoning, burning, and drowning , disfiguring, female genital mutilation, chastity belts and chaperones all attest to the deep and powerful nature of male jealousy and fear of female infidelity in major traditional societies. But this is not infidelity, so much as the prisoners' dilemma and the differing genetic strategies of each sex speaking.

Barash and Lipton (R40 154) note the irony of how universal jealousy is in males, even more so in those whose beliefs are towards promiscuity: She notes that Wilhelm Reich the imprisoned founder of 'orgone' sexual energy therapy insisted in his work and his writings that monogamy was an unhealthy state for human beings, undermining their sexual health and stunting their emotional lives. Yet his wife reports that Reich was often insanely jealous:

"Always, in times of stress, one of Reich's very human failings came to the foreground, and that was his violent jealousy. He would always emphatically deny that he was jealous, but there is no getting away from the fact that he would accuse me of infidelity with any man who came to his mind as a possible rival, whether colleague, friend, local shopkeeper, or casual acquaintance."

Polygyny is practised in the 85% of human societies which permit it pretty much to the extent which differing male resources allow. Distribution of wealth occurs in a rough inverse cube law, so one in eight men has the resources of twice the average male and can support two wives. Although there is often jealousy and dissension in polygynous partnerships, some women decide that it is better to be a second wife of a well-appointed male than dependent on a poor, or a genetically, physically, or intellectually disadvantaged man with few, or no resources. Although the fertility of a polygynous wife may be on average lower than a monogamous one, the principal wife is likely to gain a higher fertility (Hrdy R322 133). By contrast overt polyandry is almost unknown, occurring only in 0.5% of societies, and then only to retain family land ownership. In addition, genetic testing confirms 4-30% of ostensible children of a given father in human societies (p 92), and 10-20% in monogamous colonial birds are the offspring of a secret affair, confirming that monogamy is 'social', as biologists state. There is a peak in human divorces around the time a single child would become able to fend for itself in a social grouping when they can run and talk (Fisher R208). Humans are thus serially monogamous for a time phased to carry out our basic reproductive function, in this way producing a majority of our offspring.

Many writers gloss the question of monogamy and its alternatives with their own orientation. Male researchers tend to stress the 'seeking wild oats in young buxom fertile women' scenario while female writers veer towards a plea for monogamy, or serial monogamy, on a resourcing basis. Geoffrey Miller (R464) espouses the role of a resourceful lovable male who extols mutual mate selection while espousing sexual selection and its inevitable reproductive choice (and hence infidelity), as central to our cultural flowering. In being so affectionate to monogamy he looks ever more like a lekking grouse strutting ever-so-astutely on the human stage of sexual charisma. From her side Helen Fisher conveniently champions a short four-to-five year serial monogamy and separates monogamy from fidelity, thus bringing into swing all sorts of strange affairs characteristic of unfettered female choice, keeping the field wide open for female reproductive 'inscrutability'.

Sarah Hrdy (R323) quite rightly homes in on the parental aspects of reproductive process as equally essential to reproductive efficacy, as is sexual choice, in espousing the need to emphasize infant survival and its flip-side - infanticide in social relationships. She also advances a role for allo-parenting - the extended family help of daughters, grandmothers etc. with child support , rather than a dependence on 'monogamous' male partnership in human evolution. It is important to take this into account as it occurs in various forms among mammals and primates and is a human cultural motif which is prevalent or even predominant in some cultures. It extends to the historical epoch in *beena* marriages of biblical times typified by Jacob's sojourn with Laban. It also reflects the very significantly lower paternal investment made by men in many cultures, although many of the founding cultures we know of from Africa do have affectionate fathers (p 109), (p 124).

Hrdy's evidence for obligate allo-parenting (R323 90), where its role is critical to infant survival comes only from "many species of birds, and about 10 percent of mammals, including a tiny fraction of primates (humans and a few species of monkeys and prosimians that bear multiple young)". However she notes (R322 97) that in many primate species, including squirrel monkeys, howlers, vervets and colubines, mothers readily give up their newborns to the attention of others. A newborn langur may spend half their first day with other females. On the other hand baboons and rhesus monkeys refuse to give up their infants for some weeks. This sharing offers advantages of unencumbered foraging and additional protection and even, in an emergency, adoption. It also gives young females, who have not given birth, a chance to learn infant care. However it also involves negatives. In macaques and baboons where there are several competing matrilines, high ranking females may take infants of low-ranking females and injure them or refuse to give them back, causing them to starve (R323 52). Young females may not be fully competent and drop their charges. The recurrent observations of abuse suggest not all females who borrow infants are doing so merely to care for them. Most allo-mothers are also exploiting their charges in some way, using them as pawns in social interactions or as props to practice maternal skills (Hrdy R322 98, Low R416 187).

Allo-mothering does not occur in apes, and so cannot fairly be advanced as an evolutionary strategy in the transition from apes to Homo, except as a human innovation. Chimp females do not release their offspring to the care of others even older siblings (Hrdy R323 161, 502), and have a 5 to 8 year gap between pregnancies (Jolly R338 362) (5 to 6 years for bonobos) so do not have the repeated reproductive pressures of many cooperate parenting species such as tamarins who have multiple births. Chimp mothers only resume estrus after lactation stops at three to four years, although this is not true for bonobos (de Waal R163). While chimp mothers often wander alone with infants, a strategy of defence against infanticide, bonobo mothers with coalitions which make infanticide an unknown rejoin their group immediately after having given birth and copulate within months. The closest we come to such activities in apes may be male games with infants in bonobos (Enomoto, R193). Like reciprocal altruism, allo-parenting is not just an issue of mutualism but of trusting interdependence. On the other hand there is good evidence in human society for a relatively high degree of mutual help with child care among families, particularly in matrilocal and or matrilineal societies, but also in patrilocal societies where there is adequate access and contact between maternal kin, and where there is respect for the bond between a first time mother and her maternal grandmother as in the !Kung.

One explanation for human menopause is that a slowly maturing, long-lived species may gain an evolutionary advantage from a 'biological clock' which causes a female who has reached the age where her children have offspring to enter menopause and to invest in the welfare of her children's offspring rather than her own. Chimps, unlike Humans remain fertile until too old to bear pregnancy (p 348). Kristen Hawkes (R296, Blurton Jones, Hawkes, et. al. R66) has put forward evidence from groups such as the !Kung and Hadza. A study (Lahdenpera et. al. R387) of 2,800 18th and 19th century women has confirmed that they had two extra grandchildren for each decade they lived after 50, confirming a selective advantage for grandparenting resulting from the help and experience received.

Judith Rich Harris (R287) also stresses the importance of horizontal peer groups in human development as opposed to the manifest vertical importance human societies pay to kinship and family parenting. Although these horizontal and vertical influences are largely complementary in any society, as we have noted in the prisoners dilemma, peer groups form an extension of the allo-parenting concept, as children mature. Human families and extended families are well positioned to gain help from existing daughters, as well as siblings, uncles and aunts. Humans also engage in more complex reciprocal and mutual relationships than any other species and social networking, even in the face of patriarchal dominance appears to be a central aspect of how human females maintain a state of relative autonomy, even under repressive conditions. Given the relatively low level of paternal investment in infant care in most patriarchal societies, such factors are certainly no less important.

Ironically, Hrdy gained this perspective in a climate of anxiety about her own absences and the allo-parenting of her own offspring (which she fittingly (62) calls "the day care factor") by a paid care-giver, while she was engaged in field studies, and her husband was occupied in a medical practice, placing her in a privileged position, not dissimilar to a tamarin mother. The allo-mothering issue is thus close to home and by no means entirely objective, although it is a dilemma of maternal ambivalence shared by many women in attempting to resolve the Hamiltonian prisoners' dilemma of the mother-child relationship:

"One angle to the story had to do with women who combined motherhood with demanding careers, a reasonable line of inquiry since my daughter had just been born ... No doubt Trivers spoke straight from the heart when he told the reporter 'My own view is that Sarah ought to devote more time and study and thought to raising a healthy daughter That way misery won't keep travelling down the generations'. Needless to say these off the cuff remarks, which cut straight to the heart of feminist wariness of evolutionists were prominently published. Here was not just a reference to inter-generational transmission of bad mothering ... this was a reference to the ghosts in my nursery. Was I offended? After all my daughter's father was an infectious disease specialist working long hours and Professor Trivers, also a father was just as consumed by his work as I was in mine. Clearly in addition to the assumption about what infants need, there was an assumption being made about precisely who should meet those needs. Progenitors of one sex only had to realign their priorities to prevent 'misery' passing down the generations. At the time though, the unfairness of this logic was far less riveting than my own nagging anxiety lest Trivers was right"... vocation or reproduction. Twenty years later I still return to this topic with trepidation (Hrdy R323 490).

Anne Campbell (R102 250), perhaps as a result of dealing with female competition and girl gangs, give a more prosaic gloss:

Polygyny is a system that has been and is practised in many societies but it is one that most women have resisted (it generates strong conflicts of interest between co-wives) and while men may have envied polygynists, democracy has meant that their envy has ultimately overthrown the system. Monogamy seems to have won for now.

It is not democracy, but Christian anti-sexual morality that has outlawed polygynous marriage in the Western world. She then goes on to cite the experiment by Holland and Rice (p 16),which forced monogamy on normally promiscuous house flies. This demonstrated that their usual arms race of semi-toxic male semen and female immunity resistance waned, leaving the females defenseless to the toxicity of natural males and the males unable to compete. It also showed that the monogamously sequestered flies had more successful offspring under these artificial conditions. This is placing monogamy in double jeopardy - it is not an evolutionarily stable strategy in house flies and enforcing it is causing the loss of adaptive characteristics. Should we all seek stricter morals to increase the human population at risk of losing our own adaptability and creative ingenuity?

Bobbi Low's (R416) extensive study in "Why Sex Matters" considers human marriage patterns best fit a form of serial monogamy, but classifies humans as 'slightly polygamous', based on the manifest differences in variance of reproductive potential between men and women, noting (55): "Most societies with a one-spouse-at-a-time rules would be called polygynous in a biological definition." Deborah Blum (R65 110) admits Low's evidence: "In the United States though, she suggests we maintain a kind of informal polygamy. The overall pattern in America is that more divorced men than divorced women remarry and when they do remarry, more of the divorced men begin new families ... it turns out that we in the United States look more like polygamists in general, than serial monogamists". However she then envisions hopefully (109-125) that we are 'travelling toward monogamy' - going so far as to identify monogamy with 'equal parenting partnership': "If we want to define ourselves as a monogamous species, then we need to accept all the biological implications" - namely equal parenting family values in which both partners 'bring resources, love and affection to all aspects of marriage' - this said from a position of a career marriage in journalism where a 'traditional' set of sex roles is *sine qua non* 'inappropriate'.

Sexual double-think in Western society. Left the typical pattern of serial monogamy: adventure, betrayal and divorce is really a cover for male polygynous desires, covertly expressed in the lone polygamous carousing alpha male underwear among a 'harem' of bras and panties (right).

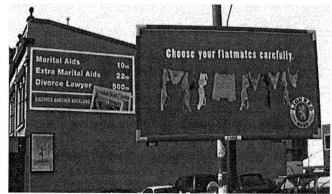

Barash and Lipton (R40 153) in "The Myth of Monogamy" sum up this complex situation:

"Having looked, although briefly, at the diversity of human mateships, what can we conclude? For one thing, it seems undeniable that human beings have evolved as mildly polygynous creatures whose "natural" mating system probably involved one man mated, when possible, to more than one woman. It is also clear than even in societies that institutionalized some form of polygyny, monogamy was nonetheless frequent, although, for men at least, this typically meant making the best of a bad situation. (Worse yet was bachelorhood.) There is also great diversity, however, in the patterns of monogamy, ranging from frequent extramarital sexuality, condoned and sometimes even encouraged by the social code, to occasional affairs, frowned upon but not taken very seriously, to rigid monogamy, jealously and violently enforced ... although even here it seems likely that the rules of absolute sexual fidelity are often violated, in secret. Certainly there is no evidence, either from biology, primatology, or anthropology, that monogamy is somehow 'natural' or 'normal' for human beings. There is, by contrast, abundant evidence that people have long been prone to have multiple sexual partners. In a sense, however, even if human beings were more rigidly controlled by their biology, it would be absurd to claim that monogamy is unnatural or abnormal, especially since it was doubtless the way most people lived, most of the time ... even while men strived for polygyny and women (as well as men) engaged in EPCS (extra pair couplings). This is clearest for men, if only because polygyny has often been institutionalized-and, thus, proudly displayed by the male 'winners' - whereas EPCs among Homo sapiens, as among most living things, have been much more covert, because of the costs of disclosure. Nonetheless, male philandering would never have become part of our biological heritage if women did not permit some men, at least on occasion, to succeed in their quest for EPC. Which is to say that, whether officially polygynous or monogamous, women-perhaps no less than men-have long sought extramarital lovers. What makes human beings unusual among other mammals is not our penchant for polygyny but the fact that most people practice at least some form of monogamy."

Barbara Smuts' (R638) ideas of the evolutionary origins of patriarchy, or male dominance begin with the same assumptions, that nonhuman and human primates seek to maximize their fitness and that males and females have different reproductive strategies. In short, males go for 'mate quantity' whereas females pursue 'mate quality'. Smuts is quite explicit about not seeing human behavior as 'genetically programmed' and argues that "natural selection has favored in humans the potential to develop and express any one of a wide range of reproductive strategies, depending on environmental conditions". Smuts focuses her attention on male aggression against females and female resistance to this aggression - that males are aggressive against females in order to mate with them, to pursue 'mate quantity'; but females, following their own reproductive interests, can and do resist. At the same time, there is variation in the extent to which females can successfully resist male aggression. Consideration of the numerous factors that may be involved concerns females' ability to resist male aggression by forming alliances with other females against males. Among the many primate species in which females bond together, this strategy works quite well. Among others, such as the common chimpanzees, females disperse at maturity to join new groups where they do not have female relatives to protect them. Among the bonobos, females disperse out but are also able to form alliances with unrelated females in the new groups. Thus, among common chimpanzees we see relatively high levels of male aggression against females, whereas among bonobos male aggression is successfully resisted and males do not sexually coerce females. Applying the same logic to human evolution, she proposes that the prevalence of patrilocal residence in human societies means that women are often deprived of the support of female kin and allies, leaving them more vulnerable to male aggression "In pursuing their material and reproductive interests, women often engage in behaviors that promote male resource control and male control over female sexuality. Thus women, as well as men, contribute to the perpetuation of patriarchy". Here Smuts suggests that in some circumstances women can facilitate their own reproductive success not so much by allying with other females as by allying with mates who command more resources and by complying with customs that increase paternity certainty, promoting patriarchy. Smuts is correct in that cultural developments appear to have developed strategies of reproduction which have acted to enforce male domination to the detriment of sexual paradox. Human society is integrally complex and responds both to evolutionarily acquired traits and cultural interaction in choosing complex forms of social adaption (Stone).

Gatherer-hunter societies with ancient roots, as well as most current societies show a spectrum of relationship patterns in which monogamy predominates, adultery is frequent and in addition to sewing wild oats, outside the Christian sphere, up to 15% of men who have the resources to support two families are in polygynous marriages. Serial monogamy accentuates this polygynous tendency. The possible sperm retention of female orgasm, occurring simultaneously or subsequent to male ejaculation and the fact that women having affairs frequently mate close to ovulation and have a predominance of powerful retentive orgasms all attest to an evolutionary basis for 'infidelity'. Even if an 'unfaithful' woman has sex more often with her husband, she is still more likely to conceive by her lover. On the male side, sperm competition supports the same conclusion. Men also make larger ejaculates when they are away from their wives during the day, again indicating sperm competition.

The evidence of genetic testing suggests up to 30% of offspring of ostensible fathers (with a possible average figure around 4%) are sired covertly by another man confirms female reproductive 'inscrutability' is likewise operating at a steady level (Bellis et. al. R55).

Steatopygous fat buttocks are shared by some !Kung genotypes (Low R416, Hrdy R323) and the paleolithic 'Venus' figurines such as Lespugue (right). Among the !Kung (then called Hottentot), Darwin's informant reported, a truly sexy woman was one who was unable to rise from level ground because of the weight of fat on her buttocks (Low 81). Unlike apes, human babies are usually born with a healthy store of fat. Mothers also accumulate reserves of fat on the breasts and buttocks to provide for, and indicate fecundity (Hrdy R323 126).

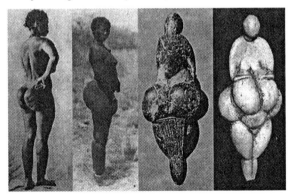

Concealed ovulation empowers the potential mother, both in long-term relationship, by keeping the daddy around, and the strange affair, by enabling covert infidelity and encouraging other men to consider themselves possible fathers, as long as this doesn't result in public accusations of 'loose promiscuity'. It thus entices toward monogamy, while promoting female reproductive choice. Given menopause and the much higher female fertility in the years after menarche, the higher mortality rate of young males and the male desire for fertile partners, rather than the resourcing and protection women seek, older men tend to seek young nubile partners they believe can produce the offspring they themselves are unable to. It is thus easy to see how female beauty becomes a biological indicator of fitness, with all the evolutionary manifestations of fecundity, in breasts, buttocks, hour-glass waist-hip ratio and the accessory features, including bodily symmetry which epitomize female beauty and which a variety of evidence shows is a genuine indicator of genetic fitness and a key indicator of reproductive potential.

Female concern for physical beauty as a reproductive asset is attested to throughout archeological history from the ochre and beads in Blombos cave (p 94), ancient venus figures and jewelry at Dolni Vestonice to the mirrors and jewelry at Catal Hüyük. While male Paleolithic art focuses on the prowess of the hunt, female representations are of fecund anatomy as in the lunar Venus of Lauselle (p 174).

The significance in Homo sapiens of the unique features of female sexual evolution is enshrined in many of our founding archetypal myths including the Fall from the paradise in Genesis, where it is Eve's natural beauty which is tragically linked to her earthy temptation:

> *Eve was said to be so beautiful that no one could look upon her.*
> *For her the sun and clouds would arc into a rainbow*
> *the flowers would bloom where she walked*
> *and the birds burst into spring song (Kabbala).*

The relatively smaller reproductive investment of the human male in each offspring than the female favors polygyny, various of forms of which are common from hunter-gatherer bands through the Jews of Old Testament times to many modern cultures, including the Islamic world. A male will tend to seek to fertilize several females to broaden his reproductive potential, simply because he lacks the power for autonomous reproduction and must invest in mating strategy and less-direct child support. An astute female may in turn seek covert adultery to be fertilized by a highly-regarded, manifestly fit or histocompatibly exotic male who is not her immediate 'domestic husband' to seek the 'best of both worlds' - genetic and resource-bearing. Women prefer men with complementary histocompatibility (giving off a exotic pheromones) when ovulating, but revert to preferring familial antigens when on the pill (mimicking data on mice during pregnancy). The newly recognized VNO organ of smell appears to be specific in sensing for such physical nuances. The pattern is in this sense 'cooperative' between the genders as a reproductive strategy shared by humans and monogamous birds, in the prisoners' dilemma of sexual paradox, except when it is repressed, e.g. by draconian male suppression of female infidelity. Such 'moderate infidelity' is indicated by the existence of 'kamikaze' blocking sperm in humans, the intermediate physiology of human testes between the promiscuous chimp and polygynous but non-promiscuous gorilla, the sperm-retentive nature of female orgasm and the concealed estrus itself, which is clearly a form of 'evolutionary female empowerment' consistent with it evolving in a context in which female sexual choice has been an ongoing reality, putting the female in Matt Ridley's words 'one step ahead of the male'. It is also consistent with the privacy of sexual relations which make it difficult or impossible to detect covert infidelity.

In hunter-gatherer societies, the male opportunist streak would have been far more easily satisfied by adultery than by polygamy. In most gatherer-hunter societies it is uncommon to find a man with more than one wife and very rare to find a man with more than two, but wherever adultery has been looked for, it is common. By analogy with monogamous, colonial birds, therefore, one would expect to find human beings practising either mate guarding, or frequent copulation. Richard Wrangham has speculated that human beings practise mate guarding in absentia. Men keep an eye on their wives by proxy. If the husband is away hunting all day in the forest, he can ask his mother, or his neighbour, whether his wife got up to anything during the day. In the African Pygmies Wrangham studied, gossip was rife and a husband's best chance of deterring his wife's affairs was to let her know that he kept abreast of the gossip. Wrangham goes on to observe that this is impossible without language. So he speculates that the sexual division of labour, the institution of child-rearing marriages and the invention of language - three of the most fundamental human characteristics that we share with no other ape - all depended on each other (Ridley R564 220).

On a counterpoised tack, Chris Knight (R373) and Camilla Power (R538), (p 77) have suggested that the lunar and menstrual cycles became locked into the strategic relationship between the sexes in terms of a meat for sex exchange in a real, or imputed 'sex strike' by the women, associated with inducing the men into resourceful hunting and with maintaining female reproductive choice over the men around 500,000 years ago, when brain size started expanding rapidly in the form of a phase of sexual withdrawal . This is in line with Catherine Key's Prisoners' Dilemma analysis (p 34) of the shifting reproductive investments towards greater female commitment, given both increased risks and difficulty of delivery and longer child-rearing with a slowed neotonous infant growth pattern as part of an adaption to the larger brain size within the constraints of cervical delivery. Camilla Power (R538 310) proposes that women extended any patterns of lunar menstrual synchronization by faking the signs. She suggests that menstruating women would have become a threat to other females by attracting much-needed male attention, particularly when menstruating women were rarer as a result of pregnancy and anovulatory demand breast feeding (p 107). So women who were nursing and pregnant took control of the situation by feigning menstruation. What began as impromptu borrowing of one another's blood or using animal blood became ritualized culturally in the use of red ochre. She points out that the word 'cosmetics' comes from Greek, *cosmos*, or order. "In traditional cultures cosmetics are not mere frippery. They define who belongs to which group, who can touch who, and who can mate with who. The regularized use of cosmetics as a sexual signal could even have been the thing that marked off modern humans." So perhaps lipstick is not just the key to culture, but also to the origin of our species. Ian Watts' study of 74 sites in southern Africa dating from more than 20,000 years ago, including Blombos, reveals an explosion in the use of red ochre and other red pigments between about 100,000 and 120,000 years ago (Douglas R170). Findings in Zambia and the re-dating of Border Cave in South Africa may push the date of the earliest use back to 170,000 years ago in Zambia. Some have yet to be convinced about the symbolic purpose of ochre and say the use is rather to do with preserving animal hides. Chris Henshilwood suggests the shells were jewelry or for accounting and associated with peoples such as the San. Independently from the suggested link between ochre, menstruation and sexual control, the early appearance of cultural forms in cosmetic and jewelry suggests females had a formative role in the emergence of culture. Timothy Taylor (R670) questions why ancient cosmetics should apply to women rather than men, since men like peacocks are the more competitive sex, but a simple argument based only on male reproductive competition ignores the manifest complexity of human sexual selection by both sexes.

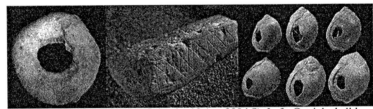

Ancient beads and marked ochre (New Scientist 10 Apr 2004 8). Left: Ostrich shell beads Yoilangalani river Serengeti National Park (c 40,000 - 110,000) Centre: Scored ochre block. Blombos (c 77,000). Right: Pea-sized *Nassarius kraussianus* shells pierced and showing wear from leather thongs.
Blombos cave (c 75,000) (Henshilwood R302, Holden R316).

Briffault (R75v3 572) sees the relationship between woman as danger, menstruation, and the moon as universal to our cultural origins:

"The maleficent, or more properly speaking, the dangerous and dreaded character which is ascribed to women extends ... to that celestial body which is everywhere intimately associated with women, namely the Moon. The tabu with which the menstruating woman is invested attaches to the cause of menstruation also." (583) The Moon is the regulator and according to primitive ideas the cause of the periodical functions of women. Menstruation is caused by the Moon; it is a lunar function , and is commonly spoken of as the 'moon'. It is frequently regarded as being the result of actual sexual intercourse between the Moon and women. ... The Maori expressly affirm that 'the moon is the husband of all women', and that their mortal husband is only as it were a subsidiary co-husband. The 'heitiki' which represents a foetus ... was said to have been given to the women by the Moon. The situation is similar with Soma the Moon God. In Persia the moon is keeper of the seed of the bull as the Moon and its crescent shape is associated with the bull's horns. Sin the Moon God is also a bull who sought to renew the seed of royalty eternally. The Moon is in this role primally male preceding its association with the Moon Goddess (592) .

The social pattern of overt monogamy and covert adultery is common to all socially-monogamous animals which gather together in close communities and have a degree of resource dependence on a male to assist in child rearing. Adultery is thus a biologically important contributor to the genetic diversity and genetic fitness of humanity. (Fisher R208, Ridley R564, Watson R721). It should thus not be suppressed or exposed to genetic testing to the point where female reproductive choice becomes unraveled.

The two sexual hormones are also intimately interwoven (p 347). Women also have circulating testosterone and have been found to become resilient to stress when given small traces of testosterone analogues and to respond to pornographic enticement with a testosterone burst of 80% over background, compared with a similar male burst of 100%. Complementing this, males require estrogen to be fertile (p 349). Progesterone is likewise present in both sexes and has a pronounced daily fluctuation in men peaking in the evening when love-making is common (Scientific American Jan 94 103). Men also respond to female ovulation, with increased testosterone levels, although it is largely concealed, and the men may not consciously recognize they are doing this. It may even be that they are responding to the women's tendency to engage sex more often and passionately around ovulation. There are also indications that women prefer men with marginally more female characteristics, suggesting a Dionysian direction of human evolution, consistent with the more evolved (neotonous or child-like) female physique. The ironic exception is when they are in mid ovulation, when they prefer the strong features of a fit high testosterone male.

As noted, Smuts (R638) has suggested that females may have by evolutionary reliance on male resources, inadvertently promoted patriarchal control of the female. In patriarchally dominant societies women who give birth to more male offspring may have a better chance of reproducing their genes through high-born sons who have greater reproductive opportunities. Sex ratios in highly fed animals can reach 1.4 males to each female. Sexual bias in animals may be partly a result of a process of selective abortion, even sometimes of whole high-female litters. However, it turned out to be more the mothers rank in the social group which influenced the sex of their offspring. Valerie Grant discovered that mothers who subsequently had daughters rated 1.35 on a psychological dominance scale, but those who later had sons rated 2.26 - a highly significant difference, possibly mediated by testosterone levels. In studies of some feudal societies Laura Betzig and Sarah Hrdy have noted bias towards more males among elite class groups, while the peasantry have a compensating slight bias towards more daughters. This is reflected in patterns of marrying up in the Indian dowry (p 288). The requirement for a 50:50 ratio of sons and daughters stemming from the collectively equal reproductive potential of each sex as a whole will lead to such compensation. Since the male inherits his rank, the female has a chance to marry up, but because she moves, she cannot carry her rank and family connections, with implications about the dowry in its varying forms (Ridley R564). There are also differential effects on a mothers life-span, with sons reducing life-span by 34 weeks, possibly because of testosterone immune reduction and the impact of a larger baby, and daughters extending it by 23 weeks. This is consistent with boys being favoured when mothers have better resources (Science 296, 1085).

A 2004 study by the US National Bureau of Economic Research, based on data from 86,436 births established that 51.5% of babies born to couples living together at the time of conception were boys, compared to 49.9% among parents who were not. Studying brothers and sisters, the study found that couples who were living together before conception were 14% more likely to have a male child than when they were not. There are reports dating back to the 19th Century of a lower percentage of boys being born to women who were not married. Studies in modern Kenya have found a similar trait among polygynously married women. Male embryos are less robust than their female counterparts, and so require a greater degree of nurturing through pregnancy if they are to survive to full term.

It may be that a woman who is in a stable relationship may be in a better position to provide this care. Karen Norberg R493 notes "There are several possible mechanisms that could explain the effect. Factors operating at conception could include the mother's or father's hormone status, or the timing or frequency of intercourse; factors operating later in pregnancy could result in sex biases in risk of miscarriage." The natural bias of the sex ratio of about 106 boys to 100 girls may compensate for sex-linked diseases such as muscular dystrophy, which affect males through their single X-chromosome.

Sarah Johns (R334) asked 609 first-time mothers, who had already given birth, to guess when they thought they would die. By subtracting the mother's age, she then calculated the number of years each woman thought she had left to live. As the number of perceived years left rose, so too did the chance that they had had a son. Every extra year on the clock increased the odds of producing a male by 1%. The finding backs up a 30-year-old hypothesis that suggests women can bias the sex of their unborn babies, to enhance the chances of their genes being passed on to future generations. Boys need more looking after than girls, the theory says. So when food is scarce and resources are low, females preferentially give birth to girls because they are more likely to live through the hard times. But boys are able to produce more offspring, so when resources are plentiful, mothers should be more likely to give birth to boys, to maximize the number of potential grandchildren. The research accords with other human and animal studies. Mhairi Gibson showed that rural Ethiopian women with low levels of nutrition are more likely to give birth to girls. As we have noted, this is consistent with the Trivers-Willard hypothesis of women biasing the sex of their offspring biologically to suit their reproductive prospects (p 30). However there is no evidence that genes can cause some mothers to conceive embryos exclusively of one sex or the other. Researchers at the ART Reproductive center Beverly Hills found that couples seeking pre-implantation genetic diagnosis (p 400) to correct a run of one sex, produced embryos equally of both sexes (Independent).

Evolutionary adaptions, based on female choice are likely to have been central to human intellectual and cultural development, through the expanding social fluency required to adapt to gender paradox, despite the severe repression of 'deceitful' and 'polluting' behavior in females by virtually all patriarchal societies. Brain asymmetries usually associated only with human language have now been discovered in chimps, suggesting the adaptions leading to language go all the way back to the great ape ancestor. Language and tool-making are becoming less-likely candidates for distinguishing human evolution from the great apes. However maintaining a resourceful social and reproductive position in the face of covert sexual deceit requires astute judgement, sensitive 'intelligence', poetic eloquence, skilled craft, astute affection and all the diverse resourcefulness that language and tool-making can bring. All the trappings of culture and intellect come down ultimately to one genetic reality - reproduction - and acceptance, or affirmative choice, by the opposite sex.

Continuing reproductive asymmetry in human society is supported by the near uniformity of the human Y-chromosome in Africa. This is significant in the context of the putative origins of human diversity in Africa as evidenced by the African root of the 'mitochondrial Eve' - the earliest common female ancestor of modern humanity (p 103). The male need to seek as many sexual partners as possible also explains why male mammals don't lactate and feed their young (Diamond R165). This process is enhanced by full internal fertilization and particularly uterine live birth, which breaks sexual symmetry completely at the outset. Male child-rearing occurs primarily in externally fertilizing species such as fish and amphibians, and in warm blooded nesting birds where two partners are required to ensure survival of the offspring, however it is essential for men to father their children in a world which is both culturally complex requiring all the astuteness both parents can muster to succeed and where maternal ambivalence is a necessary part of female choice given that we are a species in which the female has a higher risk and more massive investment than almost any other.

A feel for the difference between the reproductive strategies of the genders can be gleaned by comparing the Eves and Adams (the first common ancestor) of a given group with well-established genealogies. Generally the Y-chromosome Adam is only about half as many generations back, because the much greater diversity of reproductive frequency among males quickly floods the population with a few successful genotypes. The mitochondrial Eve, the mitochondrial ancestor of all humans currently alive, has been traced to Africa some 140,000 years ago, with 80% of human diversity still present in African people. The Y-chromosome Adam has been found to be much younger. This challenged by the regional development hypothesis which itself postulates sexual exchange as the formative influence on the co-evolution of human genotypes across vast regions of the planet. The Y-chromosome in Africa is of particularly low variation, although the putative Y-chromosome ancestor has also recently been linked to Africa (p 105). Part of the problem here is that the Y chromosome is suffering genetic minimization (p 343).

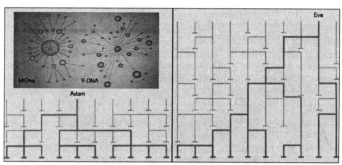

Substantial differences between the age of the primal Adam and Eve in modern genealogical trees demonstrates a greater diversity of reproductive potential in males than females (Jones). Inset: Differing evolutionary trees of mitochondrial and Y-chromosome DNA illustrated (Sykes R664)

Human sexuality is a complex, fluid and culturally-responsive mix of overt and covert strategies - of professed monogamy and concealed or expressed infidelity. While women, no matter the degree of repression, endeavour to exercise reproductive choice, men with the resources do so, practise polygyny, either by loving em' and leaving em', having kept women, parlor maids or, outside Christian influence, overtly polygynous marriages. Long-term partnership, serial monogamy, polygyny, sewing wild oats and covert affairs are central continuing motifs of human reproductive strategies in the complex prisoners' dilemma game of advertised monogamy to secure long term resourcing and concealed or expressed reproductive opportunity on the part of both sexes. Rather than perceiving monogamy, and fidelity to be righteous in conflict with unholy polygamy, strange affairs, amid deceit, we need to respect the subtlety and maturity of human reproductive choice as at the heart of the creative complexifying power of sexual paradox. Looking back towards our cultural emergence, the lessons if any are that imposing moral rules by force has if anything undermined a natural state of creative paradox evident in our founding tribal societies, replacing it with an often violent male dominance.

Evidence on Human Evolution from Chimp and Human Genomes

The biology chapter (p 328) contains background information on many of these ideas.

Goodman (R245) compared sequences in 97 genes from both human and ape species. When non-synonymous DNA regions are compared, where there are strong selection constraints for unique function we have 99.4% identity to chimps and bonobos. When synonymous sequences are compared we are 98.4% identity. Figures are around 98.7% when general point mutations are considered (Ebersberger et. al. R179) and significantly lower at 94.6% when changes from insertions and deletions are taken into account (Britten R77). These appear to be important for regulatory changes in existing genes. When differences in gene expression, particularly in the brain are taken into account chimps and humans have a 10% difference of expression of such genes according to Svante Paabo.

A detailed study of comparable chromosomes, human 21 and chimp 22, (R719, R490) has exposed a complex evolutionary process during and since human-chimp speciation, with transposable elements playing a significant and possibly crucial role in the divergence between the species. The 1.44% divergence in single base substitutions is consistent with previous studies, but these changes are widely dispersed across genes, so that 83% of the 231 coding sequences, including functionally important genes, show differences at the amino acid sequence level. In addition there are 68,000 insertions and deletions causing significant changes to 20% of the proteins. The insertions are driven primarily by insertion of Alu and LINE L1 elements (p 331), occurring more commonly in the human line, as well as LTR (long terminal repeat) and endogenous retroviral elements (p 332). Random deletion events also occurred, resulting in net chromosomal shrinkage. Neither do conserved regions correspond to transcribed functional genes. The most strongly conserved corresponds to a 'genetic desert' containing no coding sequences for proteins, consistent with the regulatory role of other human ultra-conserved regions (Bejerano et. al. R52).

Gene regulation is also significantly different between the species, with 20% of the genes showing significant differences in their pattern of activity. 15% of 'CpG-islands', associated with gene regulation, also differ between the species (Ebersberger R179). Two genes, the human versions of which contain large sections that are missing in the chimp, NCAM2 and GRIK1, are both known to be involved in neural function. The effects of such changes can be seen predominantly in the regulation of brain genes particularly those to do with further cycles of cell division during development. Starting with a set of about 12,000 genes, Cáceres et. al. (R96) found 91 that differed significantly in human and chimp brains. In 83 of these cases, the human brain had higher gene activity. In contrast, where genetic activity differed in heart and liver, human genes had decreased activity just as often as they had increased activity. However even subtle changes in a single key gene can have major effects. Ridley (R567 36) notes that ASPM (p 103), a large 10,434 'letter' gene contains 28 functional exon regions, of which numbers 16 to 25 contain isoleucine-glutamine repeats which seem to determine how many cell generations occur in brain development in the vesicles about two weeks after conception. Humans have 74, mice 61 and fruit flies 24, in proportion to the number of neurons in the adult brain of each. Significant divergences have also been discovered in microglial cell sialic acid receptor genes (R327).

A detailed map of human evolution is emerging from comparison between the results fo the human and chimp genome projects (R116). The discoveries so far are summarized below.

The single nucleotide divergence between chimp and human is only 1.23% (35 million base pairs) if which 1.06% corresponds to fixed fixed divergence between the species once 14-20% of intra-speces polymorphisms are taken into account. The correspondingly higher divergence of the Y of 1.9% Y and lower of the X of 0.94% indicates the male mutation rate is 3-6 times the female rate. This mutational discrepancy between the sexes supports the necessity of female reproductive choice in all hominids, including humans.

CpG (cytosine-guanine) bases are prone to deamination to TpG and constitute the dominant form of chemical damage, causing 25.2% of mutations but only occurring in 2.1% of bases. Mutation rate variations between sexes are not CpG correlated because chemical damage is time related as opposed to replication errors from the 5-6 fold higher number of cell divisions in spermatogenesis.

Mutation rates also vary with location with 15% more near the ends of chromosomes, with higher local recombination rate, high gene density and high GC content. This effects the shorter chromosomes more significantly. Dark bands which are gene poor have a 10% higher mutation rate. Telomere regions have a higher rate rate in hominids than in murids, suggesting less selective pressure.

Insertions and deletions are rarer individually than point mutations but are larger, so 1.5% of the euchromatic differences are species specific, a larger difference than point mutations. Overall indel divergence is about ~45 Mb in each species or about 3% of the gemone dwarfing the single nucleotide divergence. Most are very small, but the total contribution is 73% from larger >80bp indels. Over a third of these come from repetitious micro-satellite and satellite sequences, a quarter are caused by transposable elements, with a residue coming from deletions in the other species. 8.3 Mb of these in humans contain 34 exon regions indicative of new genes.

The history of transposable elements (p 332) differs significantly between the species. Endogenous retroviruses have died out in humans except for HERV-K with 73 human insertions (of which 66 have only the long terminal repeat remaining, indicating old insertions) This occurs also in chimps 45 insertions (44 LTR only) but chimps have other active ERVs. PtERV1 has over 200 copies over half of which are full length indicating active insertion. SINEs in particular Alu has been 3 times more active in humans (7000/2300 lineage specific insertions) mostly due to two new subfamilies (Ya5 Ya8), but baboons are 1.6 times higher still. Old Alu elements lie in GC rich gene-rich regions but newer ones are in AT rich gene-poor regions where LINEs also accumulate, consistent with L1-based retrotranscription. There is similar L1 activity in both species (~2000 insertions), as well as 200 human and 300 chimp processed LINE-related retrogenes (pseudogenes). SVA an Alu repeat with a CpG island and potential transcription factor binding sites occurs (~1000) in both species. 3 human genes show SVA insertions resulting in species differential transcriptions. There are also 612 human and 914 chimp Alu-Alu deletions, 26 and 48 L1 deletions and 8, and 22 LTR deletions, none involving exons of human genes in chimp.

There are also larger scale inversions and fusions. Chimp chromosomes 12,13 now called 2A,2B fused to make human chromosme 2. There have also been pericentric inversions.

Orthologous proteins are very similar between the species, with 29% identical. Recombination is limited by a low cross-over rate with 1kb only having only ~1 crossover every 100,000 generations, or 2 million years.

Estimates of the effects of natural selection, neutral evolution and other factors can be gleaned by examining KA the amino acid substituting mutations, KS the synonymous mutations and KI the non-coding mutations. KA is 37% higher in the most distal 10 Mb than in proximal regions so careful averaging across the genome is needed. Both KA/KS and KA/KI are around 0.23 << 1 indicating significant purifying selection. This value is 35% greater than for murids (rodents) indicating either greater positive adaption or fewer evolutionary constraints. There is also weak purifying selection on silent sites in exons compared with introns In terms of gene evolution a KA/KS of 0.23 indicates 77% of amino acid substitutions are sufficiently deleterious to be eliminated by natural selection. 4.5% of human-chimp orthologues (585/13,454) have KA/KL>1 indicating strong selection, however because of the low divergence between the species, about half could occur by chance variation among genes. The high KA/KS for these genes also shows that 25% of amino acid substitutions contribute to the current human genetic load. The KA/KS for human polymorphisms of 0.20-0.23 is very similar to that for human chimp divergence, indicating little positive selection across the genome driving evolutionary divergence, because positive selection would cause many selective sweeps and reduce polymorphisms, indicating fewer evolutionary constraints in the hominid lines than in murids. X has KA/KL = 0.32 skewed high and low with higher selection on testis-related genes. The median is similar to autosomes indicating a skewed subset with vry high evolutionary selection. Many low values indicate greater purifying selection consistent with being genes expressed in the hemizygous single X state in males, and high values could also result from positive selection from adaptive hemizygosity of the X in males, particularly if a substantial proportion of these genes are recessive.

Genes involving disease resistance, reproduction and reproduction (seminal protamines and seminogelins), and nocioception (awareness of pain and toxic substances) stand out as rapidly evolving. Gene evolution is faster on rearranged chromosomes 1, 2, 5, 9, 12, 15, 16, 17, 18. Rapidly evolving gene clusters are associated with immunity, host defense, chemosensation and inflammation. Hominid lines show increased divergence of genes associated with ion transport, neruotransmission, sound perception and reproduction by comparison with murids. Large gene families such as those involved in immunity and olfactory are harder to test but are also subject to accelerated divergence.

Six regions of low diversity have been noted, consistent with linked genes hitchhiking on strong selective sweeps in recent human history. In addition one region containing several high diversity-divergence scores contains genes noted for selective mutations, FOXP2 (involved in speech), as well as CFTR (connected with asthma resistance). Other selective sweeps have also been discovered in recent human evolution associated with brain size determining genes microcephalin and ASPM.

Many brain genes are more strongly conserved than other genes, although brain evolution may be affected by new alternative splicing arrangements in a small subset of genes, and strong selective sweeps made by new highly selective genes. Gene conversion with a pseudogene for example in the human linehas altered sialic acid expression in brain tissue so that only human microglia express sialic acid.

Human Nature, Gender Roles, Sexual Plasticity and Cultural Liberation

Anthony Giddens (R236) has made the point that modern sex is characterized by the emergence of 'plastic sexuality' (R670 266) - the detachment of sexual life from any biological or reproductive imperative (p 396). We have already examined (p 39) whether there is such a thing as human nature in the debate between the proponents of sociobiology in its various forms and those who 'espouse' the ultimate supremacy of culture. This debate has pitted an early wave of male-oriented sociobiologists with a genetically deterministic overview, against cultural feminists and defenders of the 'post-modern' sociological idea that culture takes us unilaterally beyond the confines of nature. The pendulum has again shifted with a more resourceful and flexible view of our evolutionary heritage as a set of genetic potentialities which are able to respond to changing circumstances in a dynamic society, just as the genetic basis of our brain is able to generate an organ capable of responding to all the diversity and contradictions that culture and nature bring forth.

Sigmund Freud once claimed "anatomy is destiny" (R670 7). In writing "The Prehistory of Sex" (R670) Timothy Taylor's retort is that "culture is freedom" and he has set out to refute the sociobiological thesis specifically to affirm the liberating effect culture has on sexuality. However the main emphasis of his idea of cultural freedom is the tacit acceptance of the 'sexual rainbow' of whatever social gender role a person cares to define for themselves in the pursuit of the pleasures of love - in particular the perceived liberations of homosexuality, transvesticism and sex-reversal.

This begs the question of the how the human species will continue to survive if we choose to define sexuality purely in social terms as 'gender roles' between consenting adults and neglect the integrating factor of reproduction and its manifestations in the complementary roles of woman and man, parenthood, family life and the extension of genealogy into relatedness generally, as a fabric of society, which carries us from generation to generation. It is this sense of ongoing relatedness that has given sex its meaning in all societies, and in turn given all human societies the ultimate resources in love and kinship which have sustained each as a living people with a sense of cultural identity and life direction.

The idea that culture is freedom ignores both the very coercive cultural restrictions many major world cultures have placed on sexuality and gender roles in defiance of nature to our detriment, and the blinding stereotypy of many forms of modern sexual variety, from hardcore porn to the kings and queens of drag, despite the healing effect of more liberal attitudes to sexual relationship and sensual pleasure, the exploration of exotic arts of love, from the Karma Sutra to the Scented Garden, and the capacity of us to see and feel the other gender in ourselves, rather than being starkly confined to iconic masculinity or femininity.

Young people will continue fall in love innately, as they have done since time immemorial, and will do so as biological beings, regardless of the enticements, or repressions, which cultures seek to impose. The power of falling in love and the intoxication of the love quest becomes ever more a light into which the moth will fly for life itself, even when faced with punishments as dire as death by stoning for adultery for any form of transgression. This is the emotional ground swell that sociobiology seeks to uncover so that we can better understand who and what we are as sexual beings. Our evolutionary heritage is our best defence and most trustworthy resource in the face of rapid social and cultural change. We are not cultural blank slates who can define ourselves and our sexual identities ad hoc without losing our relationship with nature and life itself.

We shall now investigate the cultural phase and show that in founding human societies, rather than clear motifs of sexual domination, a state of strategic paradox occurs, reflecting both the manifest complementarity between the sexes and the division of labour and it is this state of strategic paradox that has led to the explosion of social complexity we associate with the emergence of culture. The key to cultural emergence is a complex form of mutual sexual selection, in which the choices made by each sex upon the other are dynamically responsive to the social environment in which they are taking place, in a way which has facilitated all the stunning differences between us and the higher apes, from the sensual beauty of the female form to the mesmerizing enchantments of good music, art, myth, resourceful technical innovation and last, but not least, the sensual arts of love. Sex HAS become manifestly social, not just a reproductive process, and capable of a great deal of cultural diversity, but it is in the continued passage of the generations and the continuing dance of reproductive sexual choice between woman and man that all the characteristics of the 'sexual rainbow' find their genetic, social and cultural meaning and acceptance. The lesson, if any, from looking at our evolutionary heritage is that cultures will survive and succeed best when they resonate with the best in human nature and express it meaningfully in the span of life as a whole. We shall see in succeeding chapters that cultures have risen and fallen by either repressing sexuality and sexual diversity with dire punishments, or indulging every form of gratification the mind can hunger for without any limit to perversity. Seeking to discard human nature altogether in a cultural glasshouse is likewise a cul-de-sac.

Culture Out of Africa

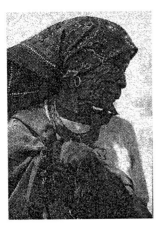

Nisa - (redrawn from Shostak R627)

When the gods gave people sex, they gave us a wonderful thing.
Sex is food: just as people cannot survive without eating,
hunger for sex can cause people to die.
!Kung saying - Nisa.

Sexual Paradox in Human Origins

A consistent and powerful hypothesis about human emergence is that the complementary reproductive strategies of
females and males led to evolutionary gender paradox in
early human societies and hence cultural complexity based
on sexual relationships driven to a considerable extent by
female reproductive choice. The males, to achieve reproductive success needed to compromise their competition to
fit with the cooperative nature of the human group, centered
on the family and gathering and social relationships with
the females. Selection among males reinforces not just the
traditional hunting prowess and toughness ('he-man') but
diverse social skills ('domestic bliss') - "a mosaic of qualities that reflect the necessities of
compromise ... good with the children, relaxed, eloquent, knowledgeable". Women in turn
are the immediate progenitors of offspring, nurturing an articulate and cooperative group
culture as well as being societal family-builders and resourceful gatherers of diverse plant
species. In this way human culture evolved in a social setting where male reproductive
success was mediated through the social awareness of the female gatherers, upon whom
the child rearing and basic food resource of the society depended.

Our early human record speaks of a 100,000 year period of gatherer-hunter emergence in
which women and men enjoyed a degree of reproductive autonomy and choice regained
by our own societies only in part in the last century. Homo sapiens has spent the vast
majority of this time leaving only flaked tools with only minor changes of design, the
social aspects of culture, which are not so easily left in artifacts may have become highly
attuned to complex and subtle interactions. Although so-called "primitive" cultures are
diverse and parallels, between modern gatherer-hunters and our ancestral origins remain
speculative, among the few primitive hunter-gatherers still existent, egalitarian societies
such as the !Kung-san 'bushmen' of the Kalahari, the Sandawe and Hadzabe of Tanzania
and the Biaka and Mbuti 'pygmies' of the Congo Basin have much to teach us both genetically and culturally.

Genetic Emergence of Modern Humans

Chromosomes contain a variety of markers that can be used to compare diverse populations and infer an evolutionary relationship between them. These include the slowly varying protein polymorphisms of coding regions which are useful for long-term trends, single
nucleotide polymorphisms, and non-coding region changes (mutation rates about 2.5×10^{-8} per base pair per generation and useful for reconstructing evolutionary history only over
millions of years) insertion and deletion events (about 8% of polymorphisms, extending
from one to millions of nucleotides), particularly those driven by transposable elements
such as the LINEs and even more frequent SINEs (p 332), non-coding micro-satellites
(mutation rate 10^{-5} - 10^{-2} due to repeat slippage) and mini-satellite regions of repeating
DNA (mutation rates as high as 2×10^{-1} due to meiotic recombination in sperm) that both
evolve rapidly and are not subject to the strong selection of coding regions which can differentiate changes over the much shorter time scales of modern human migration.

The insertions and deletions of the million or so Alu elements in the human genome (p
332) are particularly useful, as the most active sub-population of about 1000 Alu is
actively transcribing and undergoing rapid change. A subpopulation of Alu are capable of
generating new coding regions (exons), when inserted into non-coding introns between

spliced sections of a translated mRNA, because one base-pair change within Alu leads to formation of a new exon reading into the surrounding DNA. This is not necessarily deleterious because alternative splicing still allows the original protein to be made as well. We have the highest number of introns per gene of any organism, and thus have to have gained an advantage from this costly error-prone process. Alus may have given rise, through alternative splicing, to new proteins that drove primates' divergence from other mammals. Recent studies have shown that the nearly identical genes of humans and chimps produce essentially the same proteins in most tissues, except in parts of the brain, where certain human genes are more active and others generate significantly different proteins through alternative splicing of gene transcripts. Our divergence from other primates may thus be due in part to alternative splicing.

If we consider the likely effects of the out of Africa hypothesis, we would expect that founding African populations not subject to active expansion and migration would have greater genetic diversity and that the genetic makeup of other world populations would come from a subset of the African diversity, consisting of those subgroups who migrated.

In the case of mitochondrial mtDNA (mutation rate about 2.5×10^{-7}) and its hyper-variable D-loop (mutations rates as high as 4×10^{-3}), which is transmitted only down the maternal line (see Tishkoff and Verrelli R679 for caveat) and the non-recombining majority of the Y-chromosome which is transmitted only down the paternal line, each with no recombination, we would expect greater diversity going deeper into the historical tree of divergence, with certain existing groups who have retained the founding patterns of survival and have not undergone rapid population expansions to retain an increasingly diverse source variation. All these features are broadly observed in the genetic data to date.

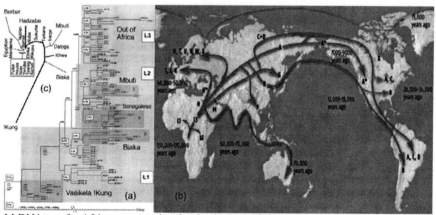

(a) MtDNA tree for African groups showing haplotypes of !Kung, Mbuti and Biaka as well as the line coming out of Africa (Chen et. al. R115). (b) Diagram of world migration and regional differentiation of successive mtDNA haplotypes (Gilbert R237). (c) mtDNA distances between founding African groups including Hadza (clicks) Khwe is from (Knight et. al R372). Recent mtDNA evidence suggests a first wave of migration down the coast of Asia all the way to Australia (Forster et. al. R216).

Most studies of non-coding regions of autosomal, X-chromosome, and mitochondrial mtDNA genetic variation (which are desirable markers because they are not so subject to selection and thus have relatively neutral drift) show higher levels of genetic variation in African populations compared to non-African populations, using many types of markers. Although some studies of Y-chromosome variation have observed higher heterozygosity levels in non-African populations, the African populations have higher levels of pairwise sequence differences, consistent with these populations being ancestral. High levels of diversity in African populations alone do not prove that African populations are ancestral. A recent bottleneck event and/or colonization and extinction events among non-African populations, or a more recent onset of population growth in non-Africans, could also cause a decrease in genetic diversity (Tishkoff and Verrelli R679). In fact the complete inter-fertility of all human populations and the relative lack of genetic divergence by comparison with the few remaining chimp colonies in the wild (Hrdy R323 183) does indicate a significant bottleneck. The genetic data is consistent with a human emergence from a population of only 10,000 around 100,000 years ago. This is also consistent with the delayed maturation, long birth spacings as a result of prolonged lactation and high infant mortality seen in gather-hunter populations such as the !Kung. At such low growth rates a population of 100 would take 50,000 years to reach 10,000 (ibid).

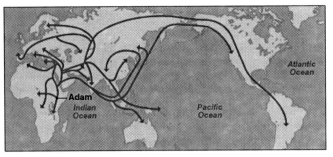

Patterns of male migration. The Genographic Project - a partnership between National Geographic and IBM - will collect DNA samples from over 100,000 people worldwide to provide a high-resolution genetic map of human migration.

However studies of protein polymorphisms as well as mtDNA haplotypes, X-chromosome and Y-chromosome haplotypes, autosomal microsatellites and minisatellites, Alu elements, and autosomal haplotypes indicate that the roots of the population trees constructed from these data are composed of African populations and/or that Africans have the most divergent lineages, as expected under a recent African origin rather than a multi-regional emergence model. Additionally, studies of autosomal, X-chromosomal haplotype and mtDNA variation indicate that Africans have the largest number of population-specific alleles and that non-African populations harbor a subset of the genetic diversity that is present in Africa, as expected if there was a genetic bottleneck when modern humans migrated out of Africa. Analysis of genetic variation among ethnically diverse human populations indicates that populations cluster by geographic region (i.e., Africa, Europe/Middle East, Asia, Oceania, New World) and that African populations are highly divergent. The mtDNA studies hypothesize a primal female ancestor - the African Eve - around 150,000 years ago (Chen et. al. R115) while the Y-chromosome Adam is more recent, at around 90,000 years ago (Underhill et. al. R698) consistent with the greater reproductive variance of males than females. Differences between the Y- and mtDNA distributions (p 143) indicate how migration, intermarriage and female exogamy have affected the gene pool. The genetic patterns of both these and autosomal microsatellites (Zhivotovsky et. al. R764) are consistent with founding African diversity with migratory radiations to form other world populations, with deep founding radiations to the forest people such as the Biaka and Mbuti, Khoisan click-language speaking !Kung-san bushmen of Botswana and the Sandawe of Tanzania, and possibly the Hadzabe, as well as the forest people such as the Mbuti and Biaka 'pygmies' who have adopted the Bantu languages of the farming neighbours with which they now share semi-symbiotic relationships. Along with some Ethiopian and Sudanese sub-populations, these groups may represent some of the oldest and deeply diversified branches of modern humans.

Such recent genetic evidence has laid bare the relationships between some of the founding human groups spread across Africa from the 'Cushite' horn of Ethiopia to the southern Kalahari. Mitochondrial DNA studies have highlighted the ancient origin of the !Kung San and of pygmy peoples of the Congo Basin such as the Mbuti and the Biaka.

Y-chromosome studies have shown the !Kung share a most ancient haplotype with subpopulations from Ethiopia and the Sudan. According to an overall survey of genetic research by Sarah Tishkoff of the University of Maryland, the most deeply ancestral known human DNA lineages may be those of East Africans, such as the Sandawe, who share many phenotypic features and a click language with the !Kung. This suggests southern Khoisan-speaking peoples originated in East Africa. The most ancient populations are now believed to also include the Sandawe, Burunge, Gorowaa and Datog people of Tanzania. The Burunge and Gorowaa migrated to Tanzania from Ethiopia within the last 5,000 years consistent with an ancient founding population in this area. Echoes of the earliest language spoken by ancient humans tens of thousands of years ago may have been preserved in the distinctive clicking sounds still spoken by some existing African tribes.

Highlighting unique features of human genetic evolution, two key genes whose mutations cause microcephaly are involved in brain development, consistent with increased brain size, whose rapid spread through the human population coincide with spurts in human culture. Microcephalin (R197) appeared ~37,000 years ago coinciding with the birth of culture and ASPM (p 68) spread from the Near East around 5000 years ago (R455). These are consistent with an overall examination of linkage disequilibrium in single nucleotide polymorphisms (Moyzis et. al. R482) which indicate that about 7% of our genes have been subject to selection in the last 50,000 years, a figure similar to domestication of maize, including genes for protein metabolism, disease resistance and brain function.

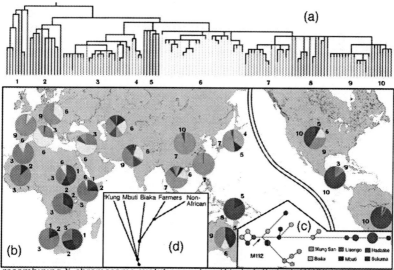

(a) Non-recombining Y-chromosome evolutionary tree (Underhill et. al. R698) (b) Geographical distribution showing the ancient haplotype shared by the San and Ethiopian and Sudanese sub-populations. (c) Genetic distances between Khoisan and forest peoples sharing M112 a Y-chromosome allele common only in these groups showing great genetic distance between Hadzabe and San peoples (Knight et. al. 2003) . (d) Autosome satellite analysis confirming ancient divergence of San and forest peoples leading to migration from Africa (Zhivotovsky et. al. R764).

In a counterpoint to these studies, Rohde and coworkers (R577, R299) estimate that the repeated spreading of family trees by sexually recombining mobile populations and differences in reproductive rates leads to an estimate of the most recent common ancestor of our global populations existing just 3,500 years ago, excepting these most isolated groups.

The clicks made by the San people of southern Africa and the Hadzabe of East Africa may thus be the linguistic equivalent of living fossils, preserved from a much older and more primitive tongue. A study by geneticists and linguists has found that people who use click sounds as part of their vocabulary have almost certainly inherited them from a common ancestor who spoke one of the earliest proto-languages. The investigation, led by Joanna Mountain and Alec Knight of Stanford University in California (R372), centered on the genetic relationship between the Hadzabe of north-central Tanzania and the Ju'hoansi San (!Kung) who live on the Namibia-Botswana border. Although separated by thousands of miles, both groups use the same sort of click sounds and accompanying consonants to communicate, yet their DNA shows they are only very distantly related and must have been geographically separated for at least 40,000 years.

Distribution of African populations 8000 BC (R127).

Key Click Language Consonants:

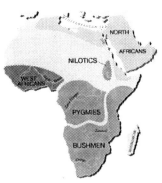

/ Dental click in which the tip of the tongue is placed on the hard ridge behind the upper incisors. When the tongue is pulled away, a short, gentle sound is produced similar to the Englishman's "tsk tsk" when expressing disapproval.

! In this click, the tip of the tongue is pressed against the alveolar ridge (where the hard palate begins to curve up to the soft palate) to produce, when sharply released, a loud, popping sound.

≠ The front part of the tongue is pressed against the alveolar ridge. On release a sharp, flat snap is produced.

// Lateral click, the front part of the tongue remains on the hard palate while air vibrates at the sides.

There is continuing historical and mythological evidence that these peoples were widespread across the African continent before the Bantu expansion about 2000 years ago. Kikuyu myths tells of the 'ground people' or Athi, from whom they 'bought' their land. The Egyptians referred to the Mbuti as 'the people of the trees' renowned for their singing and dancing. Pharaoh Phiops II (about 2300 B.C.) mentions a Pygmy dancer brought back from an expedition to the forest, while Homer, Herodotus, and Aristotle are but a few others to mention Pygmies or small African people, often called Aka a name still used today for the Biaka. The earliest humans in Gabon were believed to be the Babinga, or 'Pygmies', dating back to 7000 B.C. The Bantu name 'Twa' for the pygmies is the same word the Zulus use for the Khoisan click-language speakers they found in their early migrations into what is now Natal province of South Africa. One San tribe there today is still called Twa.

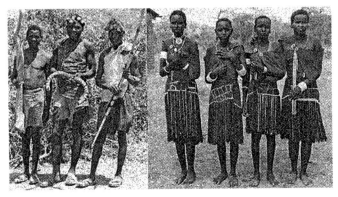

Hadzabe men and Datog women two diverse groups with ancient genetic and cultural roots (Tishkoff).

There is continuing debate between anthropologists, sociobiologists and evolutionary psychologists about whether any group can be regarded as more 'primal' than another in cultural terms or used to infer any universal foundations for emergent human nature (Marks R429 169). Although in a sense all humans alive today are 'equally evolved', the !Kung, Sandawe, Mbuti, Biaka and related groups share both a 'founding' genetic 'footprint' at the base of modern human diversity, indicating long periods of conserved population, and cultural practices which reflect long periods of time in which they have had a low-impact, low-change pattern of survival, despite some contact with other groups and changes in their habitat and life-style, for example imposed by other migrating peoples. These cultural and genetic reasons combine to give validity to their capacity to teach us about human origins.

!Kung San: Egalitarian Gatherer-Hunters

The !Kung San of the Kalahari provide a unique perspective on our possible hunter-gatherer origins. As we have noted, they stand close to the root of both the mitochondrial Eve tree and the Y-chromosome Adam tree. There is more variation in the mitochondrial DNA of such ancient groups than between diverse world peoples, because their population has been relatively stable over long periods, so the original pool of diversity has increased over time without one woman's genes growing to swamp the others in number of offspring.

The !Kung San camp in groups of perhaps 20 to 40 people, always ready to move on - within the constraints of access to water holes - when the food supply looks better elsewhere. Group composition changes as the more stable units that are nuclear families come and go somewhat independently of one another, banding together with one set of relatives for awhile, perhaps, and then with another.

In a !Kung San population studied by Nancy Howell of the University of Toronto, women experience their first menstruation at an average age of 16.6 years, and it is at about that age that they first marry (Daly and Wilson R143 40). The husband is likely to be at least 5 years older than his wife, and may not be the man she would have chosen for herself. Adolescent fertility is low, and the first child is born at an average maternal age of 19.5 Nursing commonly continues until age 4 and exceptionally until age 6. The child is typically weaned only when the mother discovers that she is again pregnant and informs her disgruntled toddler that her milk and energy are henceforth required by a younger sibling-to-be. Well-nourished but thin, !Kung San women seldom conceive within the first couple of years of nursing due to the frequency of suckling on demand.

!Kung San mothers carry their babies in slings, allowing them to suckle essentially at will throughout the day and night. Timothy Taylor has suggested (R670 44) this is a key cultural invention of women leading to culture. The baby nurses for a couple of minutes about once every quarter hour throughout the daylight hours. This demanding nursing schedule does not seem to vary much for at least the first 2-3 years of the baby's life. Such frequent suckling day and night has hormonal consequences for the mother that tend to inhibit ovulation and hence delay her next conception.

In the rare event that a baby is born before the mother feels she can safely wean its older sibling, or it has a birth defect, then she may feel compelled to abandon the newborn. Howell reported 6 infanticides in 500 live births, but there is probably some under-reporting, since !Kung San women, consider infanticide a major personal tragedy and would sooner not dwell on such painful memories. By custom, a !Kung mother goes into the bush alone to give birth. If she comes back with the baby, it is recognized and protected as a group member. However if she abandons the baby before returning, she is not regarded as someone who has killed a person (Hrdy R323 468).

Although neither contraception nor abortion was evidently practiced, a healthy fertile !Kung San woman - if she had the good fortune to survive until menopause - was likely to produce only about five children. Despite her best efforts, one of these five, on average, would die before its fifth birthday, of malaria, perhaps, or some other disease. Even more heartbreaking would be the deaths of two older children, nurtured through several years only to succumb to disease or accident or violence while still unmarried and childless. A girl who lived to reproduce - and only 48% of female babies did so - could expect to raise successfully one son and one daughter who would marry and produce children of their own (Daly and Wilson R143 40). The eloquent !Kung San 'autobiographer' Nisa, for example, lost all of her children, at various ages and in various ways, and thus suffered the grief of a middle age without descendants (Shostak, R626). Other women were luckier. All available evidence suggests that the general features of a !Kung San woman's reproductive career as described above - the wide birth spacing, the prolonged demand nursing, low fertility, high childhood mortality, and the other demographic details-are indeed representative of hunter-gatherers, and of the life history that has characterized Homo for thousands of millennia . Raising 2 or 3 children to competent maturity-the life's work of a successful woman-has typically required hard decisions about priorities, attentive management of social relations, ingenuity, luck, and decades of hard labor.

Children always accompany their mothers so they don't get lost in the wilderness. The carrying sling represents a major technological invention which makes it possible for woman gatherers to both look after their children and also bring back enough food for the groups to survive well without a regular kill. Carrying young children can become back-breaking when food is gathered miles away and has to be carried back as well. The !Kung have a proverb 'Women who have one birth after another like an animal have a permanent backache!' and the back-load hypothesis has been advanced as an explanation of birth spacing. (Hrdy R323 197). !Kung mothers may be thus balancing the optimum survival of the children they do have partly by the mother's endocrine system making sure the mothers also replace their reserves. By contrast with a !Kung mother who may carry an infant nearly 5,000 miles overall by the age of 4, Hadza women who travel shorter distances to forage and can thus also more often leave a child in camp have a shorter inter-birth span.

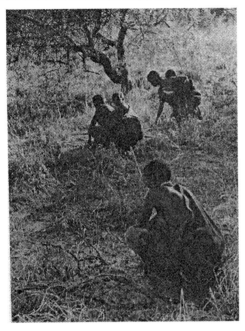

!Kung women gathering together with children in slings (Shostak 1981)

In such societies the gathering of the females provides up to 85% of the diet and the meat of hunting only 15%. One estimate of time spent is 12 hours a week, on about two days, gathering and 21 hours hunting (Ruether R585 160) leaving substantial leisure time for intense social life: trance dancing, story telling, exchange of gifts, rites of passage. As a social activity done largely independently from the men, gathering provides a social concourse and opportunity for reproductive freedom lying largely beyond male control. Hunting's intermittent spectacular success, is symbolic of sexual prowess and is often engaged in a spirit of social altruism through sharing the proceeds, by contrast with gathering, which is performed for the benefit of immediate families. Boasting is discouraged among hunters and may result in jeering insults about one's genitals. Male hunters often prefer to seek large prey, which in turn encourages a pattern of sharing both because the bounty is great and because success is intermittent. There is evidence that at least some Bushmen may have also previously learned to herd cattle (Robbins et al R575).

Kristen Hawkes' 'show off' hypothesis suggests that the prime motive of hunting is not the food resource itself, but the social status among neighbours (Hawkes et. al. R295), and sexual favours it elicits from the women (Hawkes R294). Large game like the eland represent 'prowess' rather than protein which could be gained more easily from hunting small game. That "women like meat" was the standard explanation for why a poor hunter remains a celibate bachelor. (ibid). Helen Fisher (R207) gave expression to this idea in 'The Sex Contract', which Chris Knight (R373) extended to the idea of a fully fledged sex strike in 'Blood Relations', involving lunar-menstrual synchrony (p 354). Polly Wiessner has a more Machiavellian version of this theory from studying the !Kung and foragers of New Guinea, in which "the hunters are sharing meat in order to influence the political composition of the group, since kin and others helpful for rearing their offspring tend to gather around successful hunters" (Hrdy R323). This is a natural counterpoint in which parenting and sexual choice are complementary facets of the reproductive imperative. Both contrast markedly with the earlier "man the hunter" theories of De Vore and Washburn (R715), in which the driver for cultural diversity is male prowess in hunting and toolmaking to provide for their very dependent offspring and 'captive' one-man wives.

Marjorie Shostak (R626) notes: "Here in a society of ancient traditions, men and women live together in a non-exploitative manner, displaying a striking equality between the sexes. Other contemporary gathering and hunting societies have a similar high level of equality - higher at least than that of most agricultural or herding societies. This observation has led to the suggestion that the relations between the sexes that prevailed during the majority of human prehistory were comparable to those seen in the !Kung today." The !Kung are likewise described by Patricia Draper (R173, Sanday R596 124-5), as sexually egalitarian. Draper says that !Kung females are autonomous and participate in group decisions because they do not need the assistance of men at any stage in the production of gathered foods. Nor do they need the permission of men to use any natural resources entering into this production. !Kung men and women live in a public world, sleeping and eating in a small circular clearing, within which all activities are visible. Lorna Marshall (R433) notes: "There is no privacy in a !Kung encampment, and the vast veld is not a cover. The very life of these people depends on their being trained from childhood to look sharply at things ... They register every person's footprints in their minds ... and read in the sand who walked there and how long ago. There are inherited positions, such as the 'headman', but these are said to be essentially empty of behavioral content" (Sanday R596 125). There are many similar examples of self-sufficiency and autonomy of women in foraging societies.

Even when fathers are obviously devoted to their offspring, fatherly love is rarely translated into direct care of infants. Hrdy (R323 211) states that during the first six months of his daughter's life, this doting !Kung San father will hold her less than 2 percent of the time, although this may neglect night times spent sleeping together.

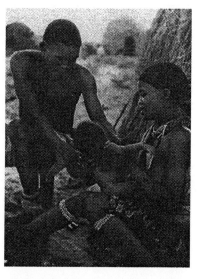

!Kung fathers are affectionate, indulgent and devoted and form intense mutual attachments with their children. Although they do not spend as much time with their children as the mothers and often hand them back for the less pleasant task of child care, fathers, like mothers are not viewed as figures of awesome authority and their relationships with their children are intimate, nurturant and physically close (Shostak R626 45-6).

Bushmen fit into the Kalahari ecosystem at more than one level; they compete with all the animals for water, share the prey of the smaller carnivores, rival the lions and other big predators for the larger game and contest the claims of the scavengers to fresh carrion. Their hunting is not so intensive as to disturb the natural balance. Because they are few and their subsistence comes from so many different points in the food-web, no single animal species is endangered. They kill only to consume, and their usual method of hunting using poisoned arrows and waiting for the animal to fall, they create less disturbance than a lion or leopard, and do not frighten the animals from the hunting grounds. When Bushmen still inhabited the more hospitable parts of the subcontinent, they often trapped the hippopotamus and other large animals by digging holes, disguised with branches, in busy game paths, with upward pointed stakes coated with poison. Early travellers walked in constant danger of a fatal accident, because there were so many of these cunningly concealed pitfalls.

In the central Kalahari, the Big Rains reunite the small groups of Bushmen who dispersed during the dry season (Johnson et al R336, R701). Everywhere they usher in a time of plenty for the Bushmen. Game becomes more numerous and, within a few weeks of the first rains, the ripening of the ochna and grewia berries heralds the richest season. In this season, men and women are continually on the look-out for hives. As the sun sets they may pause to see in which direction a bee flies, because they know that at this time they fly straight back to their hives. When Bushmen find a hive they smoke out the bees and remove the honey, but if the hive is not yet ready for opening, the finder will mark it and return later for the honey. This is truly a case of 'finders keepers' for if another comes and removes the honey from a marked hive his crime is regarded as being worthy of death. Long after the Bushmen had disappeared from the southern areas, the sharpened hardwood pegs they had driven into the faces of precipices to reach the hives and the small heaps of stones with which they had sealed their ownership remained as evidence that this land had once been theirs.

Draper, who accompanied foraging !Kung women of the Kalahari on gathering expeditions, notes that the male hunters depend on the information women bring back about the "state of the bush." If on a gathering expedition women discover fresh tracks, they send an older child to deliver the report to the men in camp. Since women are skilled in reading the signs of the bush, upon their return to camp, men query them about evidence of game movements, the age of animal tracks they may have encountered, and the location of water.

Although all !Kung agree that meat is the most desirable and prestigious food, the hunters cannot always provide it, and the vegetable food gathered by women is the staple, contributing about three quarters of the daily food intake by weight. Draper challenges the view that gathering is a monotonous routine requiring no particular intelligence. Successful gathering among the !Kung involves the ability to discriminate among hundreds of edible, inedible, medicinal and toxic species of plants at various stages of growth. This kind of intelligence is fully as important to !Kung survival as the physical strength, dexterity, and endurance required for success in hunting. It also appears to be an evolutionary trait which still displays itself in studies of the sexual brain in Western subjects.

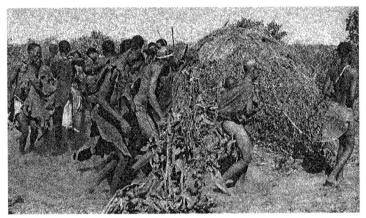

!Kung eland ceremony for the menarche (redrawn from R701).

In !Kung society, all manner of sexual liaisons occur, from partnership and serial monogamy, through open polygyny, to a variety of affairs pursued with passion by some members of both sexes, although extramarital sex is 'forbidden' by the male elders unless to entertain an age mate of the husband. There is at least begrudging respect for a woman's determination to love whom she will, with some intermittent male violence, often mediated by the group. Wife sharing has also been reported. The infrequent custom of /kamberi allows men to exchanges wives for a while if the women agree. 'If you want to sleep with another man's wife first let him sleep with yours'(R82 335). However a husband may be enraged if he finds his wife has been unfaithful and may kill one or both with poison arrows (R82 275).

Although adult !Kung disapprove of child sex games, they only discourage something if they see it mildly saying "Go play nicer games!". Child sex games are common. Boys solicit sex games with the girls and girls also play sex games together (R627). Nisa had a complex love life involving husbands she loved and others who tried to possess her as well as many secret and not-so-secret affairs, proceeding from diffident childhood sex games with both sexes (R627 31) to the passionate enjoyment of sexual love (p 102):

> [Nisa] began telling me about her own childhood; her [childhood] homosexual loves, her initial refusal to have sex with boys [for fear of the sexual act], the boyfriend she loved, who taught her to play "house" and her eventual enjoyment of sex.

Trial marriages are common, especially when they involve young girls. A father or mother may take their daughter back if she is not treated adequately. Nisa had several trial marriages before having to begin making love in marriage before her first menstruation. On her first trial wedding night she had to endure her first trial husband sleeping with another man's wife who was there to chaperone to ally her fears of being a child bride. She also had to endure adult married sexual relationship before she had had begun to menstruate. !Kung are modest and cover their genitals and a woman's buttocks, but breasts are left bare for nursing.

Shostak (R626 267) notes that infidelity is frequent in !Kung oral history and myth and it was acknowledged and talked about in the 1950s ... it is therefore not likely to be of recent origin. From Nisa's dialogue she says:

"The best insurance against complications arising from love affairs is not to be found out. Great care must be taken to arrange meetings at safe times and places, away from the eyes of others. ... . Those who tell what they know may become central figures in fights that ensue or even be held responsible for the outcome. ... To succeed at and to benefit from extra-marital affairs, one must accept that one's feeling for one's husband 'the important one from inside the hut' and one's lover 'the little one from the bush' are necessarily different. One is rich, warm and secure. The other is passionate and exciting, though often fleeting and undependable. Since such affairs are not openly condoned, it is most important that a lover have 'sense' that he be discrete and play by the rules. He should also show his affection - by arranging rendezvous, by being faithful and by giving gifts. I have told you about my lovers, but I haven't finished telling you about all of them, because they are as many as my fingers and toes."

Commenting on Shostak's work Hrdy (R323 230) notes:

"Nisa's biography provides a !Kung San forager's perspective on the tensions underlying human pair-bonds. Nisa marries four times, always monogamously. When her first husband, Tashay, brings home a second wife, Nisa recalls, "I chased her away and she went back to her parents." Several of Nisa's marriages dissolved under the strain of infidelities, either her husband's or her own. In addition to her four husbands, eight lovers pass in and out of her life. Nisa is quite obviously in love with several of them. 'Pair-bonds' were formed, but the relationships did not last. Two of Nisa's pregnancies probably derive from affairs with men other than her husband at the time. As Nisa's daughter Twi grows up to look more and more like her husband's brother, with whom Nisa was having an affair when the child was conceived, her husband reminds her that his younger brother is the likely progenitor and therefore "will help take care of her." Whenever Nisa finds herself between husbands, when she is widowed or divorced, she sets out across the Kalahari to find her brother and live with him" .

"Hunter-gatherer societies like the !Kung San are as egalitarian as traditional societies ever get. Nisa's husbands were physically stronger than she, able to dominate her, but if she was unhappy enough, Nisa could always vote with her feet and leave. Even when Nisa was caught by her husband in flagrante delicto with a lover and beaten and threatened with murder, others stood up for her, and life went on. In more patriarchal societies, her perpetual adulteries would have been lethal. Since none of Nisa's children survived to adulthood, the life of this spunky woman can scarcely be said to typify success in evolutionary terms. Yet the tensions that characterized her marriages are the same ones that Nisa's mother mentions. Again and again, her predicaments crop up in women's life stories. Nisa cherished her freedom of movement, her freedom to choose mates, and, if her husband did not provide sufficient food, her freedom to negotiate with lovers. Each husband, on the other hand, wanted multiple wives for himself but also to maintain exclusive sexual access to Nisa. There is a dynamic tug-of-war in these relationships that is at odds with conventional pipe dreams about humans having an innate tendency to form long-lasting pair-bonds, unions in which both sexes have a powerful commitment from within to adhere. Such cases make it hard to sustain the illusion that lifelong monogamous families are the natural human condition. Monogamy in Nisa's case is more nearly a compromise than a species-typical universal. Monogamy is the most harmonious common ground she and her husband of the moment can arrive at. And when it works, children benefit. Monogamy reduces inherent conflicts of interest between the sexes. Her reproductive success becomes his, and vice versa, promoting harmonious relations between genetically distinct individuals striving toward common goals. Sociobiology is not a field known for the encouraging news it offers either sex".

Although initial marriages are often arranged by families, subsequent partnerships and their dissolution can come at the initiative of either sex. Women such as Nisa speak of a woman having lovers as a blessing - she can on her travels gain many tributes of food, affection, bonding and possessions that make life good. Domestic disputes which could become violent are often settled by protestations of concern from neighbouring families in their close-knit shelters. When a man does not help his partner she may scold and curse him publicly until the grumbling of the other forces him to take responsibility. When a major dispute threatens to burst into violence, it is confronted by the entire band in frank and forthright discussion, which leaves the offender in no doubt about the consensus of opinion concerning his behaviour and where it is likely to lead him. When their leisure is not beset with pressing problems, they exchange banter and merriment by the firelight, often talking about their relationship long into the night.

Bushmen and Forest Peoples show remarkable balance between the sexes and reverence for women, particularly for the menarche, as a sacred force, which rather than being a defilement, is regarded as a time of psychic power, having vast influence on hunting and the existential flow. Although the !Kung name offspring down the paternal line, they recognize that a husband should first live with the wife's family to aid in hunting. Sarah Hrdy (R323 192) points out that this measure is also a key to the success of !Kung motherhood through grandmotherly allo-parenting of the daughter through her first offspring, providing the key know-how to give the child the best chance of survival and the mother first-hand experience to benefit future children.

The !Kung myth of the striped mouse contains a specific warning that rampant patriarchy nearly led to the destruction of society and recounts how mutuality between the sexes was rescued. An attractive young beetle woman was imprisoned by her father, the lizard, in a house in the earth. The lizard is an image of awareness bound too closely to the earth and its rocks to be good for the future. Hence the beetle woman, its future self, though also intimately of the earth, was winged, capable and desirous of taking to that other great opposite of creation, the sky. But the father, as so many fathers throughout the masculine-dominated past and present, denies the daughter, the soul in him, the right to raise life towards the heavens and so fulfil the end to which it had been born. At this point the Praying Mantis, who has appeared on Bushman earth as the instrument of ultimate meaning, has a dream and sees how life itself would be denied and arrested if the tyranny of the lizard were allowed to continue. He, therefore, sends the long-nosed mouse into battle against the lizard. We already know the reason for a mouse, but why a long-nosed mouse? Because the nose which informs life of things not seen in the night or hidden by distance and other forms of concealment, is one of the earliest of our many images of intuition. But like all intuition, wise and sensitive as it may be, it lacks the cunning of the serpent which is necessary to overcome the lizard. Inevitably the long-nosed mouse is killed by the lizard and, though followed by countless gallant long-nosed kinsmen, all are killed and the lizard remains an adamant and triumphant impediment to becoming' a new being. Happily, Mantis is informed of the disaster in a dream and decides to send the striped mouse into battle instead. The striped mouse, of course, has a sensitive nose but it is not too long, there is no hubris of intuition, and its stripes are of even greater significance. They are the outward signs that it is a more differentiated form of being and consciousness. He kills the lizard, calling out as he does so, 'I am killing by myself to save friends', and hastens to free the beetle woman, the feminine in life. All the dead forces of intuition, the long-nosed mice, are resurrected and this army of tiny visionary creatures are led back to the palace of the Praying Mantis. Jubilant they follow the striped mouse and the beetle woman marching at his side, feeling herself 'to be utterly his woman'. As they march, they wave high above their heads like flags the fly whisks which the Bushmen of the great plains of the south alone had made out of animal tails (van der Post R701 148).

Under the harsh conditions of the desert it will be several years after puberty before a girl reaches menarche (Hrdy R323 187). A girl's first menstruation is a reverent occasion, danced over for several days and nights by women, old men watched by young male onlookers - it is spoken of in awe by the !Kung in the same terms as a young warrior shooting his first big game animal - 'she shot an eland!' The first menstruation is believed to give the girl supernatural potency (nlum), powerful enough to disturb the fate of the village in the hunt, if a man sets eyes on the girl during the 'period'. Consistent with the 'wrong sex, wrong speices' signal (p 77) is the fact that the women expose their buttocks to the girl and whoever may be playing the bull (Power and Watts R538 323). This reverance, accompanied by 'awe' and 'silence' on the part of the girl lasts through to the second menstrual period.

This is in stark contrast to the negative connotations of menstruation as 'unclean' in many cultures and religions. The most ancient of all !Kung music is the 'eland music' that is sung only by women and only when the dance the eland dance in celebration of a young girl's first menstruation (Johnson et. al. R336). Although not matrilineal, they are 'matrifo-cal' in respect for menarche and mothering (Ruether R585 160).

Chris Knight (R373) sees these rites as founding human motifs in a 'sex-for-meat' exchange phased with the lunar cycle which Camilla Power has highlighted as a 'wrong sex, wrong species' signal (p 77). Evidence of the ancient use of ochre (p 94) and its use among San groups to adorn the 'new maiden' and/or the women of the band and to protect adolescent boys in the hunt is consistent with this interpretation. Consistent with the idea of a sex strike is the nineteenth century anecdote from Smith's notebook (R538 322):

The Bushmen when they will not go out to steal cattle, are by the women deprived of intercourse sexual by them and from this mode of proceeding the men are often driven to steal in oppoosition to their better inclination. When they have possessed themselves by thieving a quantity of cattle, the women as long as they exist appear perfectly naked without the kind of covering they at other times employ.

Also consistent with the sex strike concept is the 'normative belief associating menstrual with lunar periodicities' among San peoples. The /Xam, !Xu, G/wi and/or G//ana would not release a girl from seclusion until the appearance of the new moon. Shostak (R626 68) also notes belief in menstrrual synchrony among !Kung women. Also consistent is the fact that the most productive hunting by many San groups and the Hadza consists of night-stand hunts over game trail leading to water holes, optimally during the second quarter of the waxing moon and thereafter. The use of spears rather than poisoned arrows in this con-text attests to its ancient roots, extending back to the last interglacial (Power and Watts R538 321).

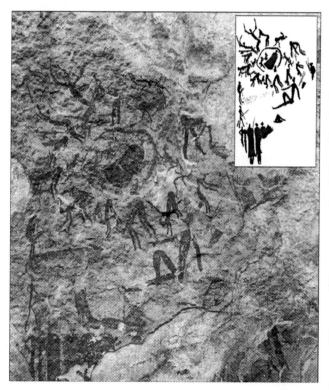

Fulton cave drawing (R701) 1000 BC (BBC 'New light shed on SA cave art' 7 -2-03) cele-brating the first menstrual rite, Drakensberg Mountains, Natal (van der Post). The central fig-ure is a young enrobed woman undergoing her first menstrua-tion ceremony in a special shel-ter. Circling her are clapping women, female dancers and (in the outer ring) men with their hunting equipment. Two figures hold sticks; the women bend over and display 'tails' as they imitate the mating behaviour of elands. Among living San, such rituals are intimately con-nected with success in hunting. Each male figure has a bar across his penis. This may be the artist marking the marital abstinence associated with menstruation and valued as a condition of hunting luck. The other figures may represent the few men who join in the dance, some holding sticks. The sur-rounding figures, are all bend-ing over, their buttocks playfully thrust in the direction of the menstruating girl. These details match those of hunt-linked menstrual rituals still practised by San and related groups in recent times (Knight R373, Lewis-Williams R401).

Peggy Reeves Sanday (R596) perceives the evolution of abhorrence of menstruation as a counterpoint between the blood of life and the blood of death wrought by the male hunter, explaining the subsequent fear and 'taboo' associated with the period in terms of avoidance of sex, restrictions on dress, movement and contact with food, ritual equipment, rivers and being secluded in huts, both as a reflection of the male fear of the danger of the female as life-giver, and the life and death counterpoint blood implies. The !Kung no longer practice male circumcision as initiation to adulthood. Female circumcision is not practiced.

The San have been immortalized by anthropologists as 'the gentle people', and indeed they have fought no wars that anyone can still recall, but this does not mean that retaliatory violence is alien to them (Wilson and Daly R143 224). Richard Lee collected the accounts of 22 homicides which had taken place among the traditional foraging !Kung San during a 50-year period, or about 29.3 homicides per million persons per annum, a figure common to large Western cities. Bearing in mind that the men are lethally armed with poisoned arrows, and there is no central authority, this is hardly surprising. Although the Bushmen are profoundly less homicidal than the Yanomamo, they have one thing in common: Each has a societally acknowledged right ultimately to use lethal force to resolve disputes between them. Anyone can literally 'take the law into his own hands' because in such societies that is where justice and judgment ultimately reside. There is no 'government' to keep men in awe, no impersonal authority to decide who is right and who is wrong. As one of the !Kung men in an argument about a marriage put it to his adversary, their dispute could be quickly settled with an arrow. Just one little arrow (Chagnon R110 212). Like their more warlike counterparts on other continents, they avenged slain kinsmen. If a killing occurred it was more likely than not to be followed by a retaliatory killing; 15 of the 22 homicides were parts of blood feuds. A group of the San had also recently avenged a murder by sneaking into the killer's group and executing every man, woman, and child as they slept (Pinker R532 56). Although !Kung society is by no means completely non-violent, people manage to resolve virtually all their disputes through personal dialogue and remonstration, without recourse to a tribal police or vigilante justice. Neither do male elders have definitive authority, particularly over women, although they strive to impose their decisions in resolving disputes. Close-knit neighbours also mediate domestic violence. There is a noticeable ebb and flow of the incidence of wife beating with less in the dry months when people congregate in extended-families than in the wet season of more nuclear families (Broude R82 313).

Old man in menstrual rite representing the eland (R701)

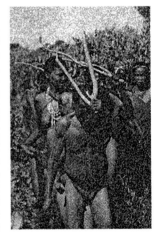

Bushmen believe in the existence of two gods: a greater god manifesting the creative force and a lesser god invoking the malevolent forces of uncertainty and misfortune, each with a shadowy consort (Johnson et al R336,van der Post R701). They have many names, but the !Kung Bushmen most commonly call them ≠Gao!na and //Gauwa, while to the /Gwi they are N!odima and G//awama. The Bushmen do not see these as a good and bad god. When a missionary inquired into a Bushman's ideas of good and bad he was told it was 'good' to sleep with another man's wife, but 'bad' if he slept with yours. Still lamenting the Bushman's ignorance of absolute morality, he later asked the man, whom meanwhile he had discovered 'was in the habit of smoking wild hemp', what he thought was the most wonderful thing he had seen. The reply he was given, that no one thing was more wonderful than any other and that all the animals were the same.

≠Gao!na, the !Kung Great God, using one of his seven divine names, created himself:

"I am Hishe. I am unknown, a stranger.
No one can command me.
I am a bad thing. I follow my own path."

Then he created a Lesser God who lives in the western sky where the sun sets; and after this two wives for himself and for the Lesser God. ≠Gao!na, tallest of the Bushmen, was in his earthly existence a great magician and trickster with supernatural powers, capable of assuming the form of an animal, a stone or anything else he wished, and who changed people into animals and brought the dead back to life. But as the Great God who lives beside a huge tree in the eastern sky, he is the source and custodian of all things. He created the earth with holes in it where water could collect and water, the sky and rain both the gentle 'female' rain and the fierce 'male' rain thunder and lightning, the sun, moon, stars and wind. He created all the plants that grow on the earth. He created the animals and painted their individual colours and markings, and gave them all names. Then came human beings, and he put life into them; and gave to them all the weapons and implements they now have, and he implanted in them the knowledge of how to take all these things for themselves. Thus their hunting and gathering way of life was ordained from the very beginning and ≠Gao!na ordained that when they died they should become spirits, //Gerais, who would live in the sky with him and serve him. He set the pattern of life for all things, each in accordance with its own rules.

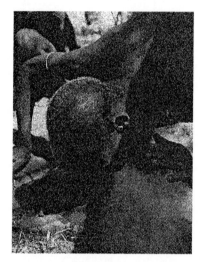

The !Kung include among their herbs traditional use of cannabis as a mind-altering substance. Dagga is consumed in traditional underground water 'pipes' (Johnson et al R336)

The !Kung pray to ≠Gao!na not as a remote being, but as intimately involved with their lives, sometimes calling him father. They pray for rain, for success in hunting, for healing both of physical and social ills. Only a really great medicine man might see ≠Gao!na face to face, but this is said to be very rare; much more frequently ≠Gao!na may appear to anyone in a dream to encourage or advise. ≠Gao!na does not reveal himself to ordinary humans, for so great is his power that, were he to come too close, he would destroy them unintentionally. But he nevertheless retains an interest in them. He is in no way concerned with their, but is aware of them, and if their behaviour offends him he will deal with them appropriately. But he is not truly a god of vengeance. When he deals harshly with someone, it is not an act of retribution but a demonstration of his power. This is the power of the unknown, the 'stranger', which explains why lightning strikes one man dead, and not the other standing beside him. The dead man, it is reasoned, must have offended ≠Gao!na by referring to him by one of his divine names, or perhaps he abused food. But he is not continually on the look-out for offenders. It is only when they happen to come to his attention that he demonstrates his power, and so sometimes people do offensive things and get away with it. Chiefly he acts for the benefit of mankind, for he supplies rain, food, children and poison for the arrows.

//Gauwa, the lesser god, who lives between two great trees in the western sky, also performs deeds that may be either beneficial or harmful to humans, but most are harmful. He is pictured as a very small Bushman, an incompetent who, even when well-intentioned, may bring misfortune by mistake. Although he is supposed to be subservient to ≠Gao!na and to act at his behest, he also sometimes acts on his own initiative while travelling about in a whirlwind, causing sickness and death to those he touches in passing. The people say that at certain times they catch glimpses of //Gauwa among the shadows of the trees.

≠Gao!na is said to live in the sacred Tsodilo Hills whose sexual story is a legendary comment on !Kung sexual relations. A man had two wives, but he loved one wife more than the other, and this caused a big quarrel. The one he didn't love hit him on the head, causing a deep wound. Then she ran off into the desert. But the Great God, ≠Gao!na, decided that because there was no peace among them, he must turn them all into a stone. The man became the largest of the hills; the unloved wife became the smallest hill that stands alone;

and the loved wife, with her children, became the cluster of hills in the middle. But they believe there are supernatural powers in the Hills because ≠Gao!na himself lives there. It was there that he created and kept his cattle, sheep, goats, and all sorts of different animals. The !Kung claim you can see footprints in the rocks. But ≠Gao!na also played ribald tricks on his wives before he ascended into the heavens (Shostak R626 325).

Bushmen of the Orange believed that people and all animals had originated together in a hole in the ground, from which they came speaking the same language. Throughout a day they issued in a continuous stream from this hole between the roots of a giant tree that spread its branches over a vast territory. When the still of evening set in, they all gathered beneath the tree for the night, people and animals together. The Creator warned the people that, no matter how cold it became during the night, they were not to light a fire. But it grew steadily, colder, Until just before dawn, when the people could no longer endure the cold, they lit one. Immediately the animals took fright at the blaze and stampeded, losing, their powers of speech in their panic. And ever, since that time they have fled from man.

The !Kung cosmos is also inhabited by trickster heroes, such as Mantis, who has a key mythic role in the creation process. For the Bushmen of Lesotho, Mantis or, /Kaggen, the first being, made all things by ordering them to appear. He created the Sun, Moon, Stars, wind, mountains and animals. A quarrel began between /Kaggen and his wife over a knife she made blunt by using it to sharpen her digging stick. As a result of his anger, she gives birth to an eland calf in the fields. /Kaggen leaves the calf in the bush while be goes away for three days to obtain arrow poison, his two sons find the calf and kill it for food. /Kaggen accuses his sons of 'spoiling' the eland. He instructs his sons to put the blood of the calf in a pot and churn it with a stick. The blood splatters and becomes snakes. They try again, and the blood that is spilled turns into hartebeest. /Kaggen is still not satisfied. He orders his wife to clean out the pot and to bring fresh blood from the paunch of the little eland. To this he adds fat from the heart, and when the blood spatters this time, each drop becomes an eland bull, and all the bulls surround /Kaggen and his sons and menace them with their horns. 'See how you have spoilt the elands,' says /Kaggen, and he chases them away. The next time the blood is churned it produces eland cows, in such numbers that the earth is covered with them. 'Now go and hunt them and try to kill one', says /Kaggen. 'That is now your work, for it was you who spoilt them.' But they fail, and so /Kaggen himself goes out and spears three bulls. Thereafter, with his blessing, his sons are also successful. Some myths speak of regeneration. The mythical Mantis, in his human person as one of the 'early race', finds that his grandson has been killed by baboons, who are playing a ball game with the child's eye. Mantis joins in the game and, gaining possession of the eye, places it in a pond, where it once more becomes the complete child, the grandson whom the baboons had killed.

The Bushmen of the Cape directed some of their prayers to the Moon, which they believed controlled the rain. And Rain they considered to be a supernatural personage, who sometimes appeared as a black bull. In terms of their conception of nature, Rain was to be shown respect, because he came armed with thunderbolts to chastise those who offend him, and girls were the objects of his special attention. Thus women did not walk about in the rain, lest the lightning seek out their scent. If a shower caught them in the open, they took care whenever the lightning flashed to look immediately at the place where it had struck, believing that in this way they were able to turn back the thunderbolts aimed at them and that Rain would then pass them harmlessly by. It is said that girls killed by lightning were taken away to become stars, or be the wives of Water as the flowers that grow in pools.

Natural and supernatural forces also have a power of their own (Johnson et al R336, van der Post R701). Trance dancing leads the participants to a place where they experience the mystery beyond directly for themselves in personal vigil, not indirectly through intercession of a priest. What Westerners would call 'supernatural' forces are so active in the natural world of the Bushmen that the distinction between them is blurred. In so far as a duality does exist, it is transcended frequently by 'medicine men'. But the state of transcendence is not the exclusive preserve of the 'medicine men', although they are more accomplished at attaining it. It is achieved by everyone who goes into a trance during the 'healing dance'. Someone who achieves this state is said by the !Kung to !kia. This is a condition which is experienced rather than conceptualized, and it seems to correspond to the transcendental experiences of mystics. Among the Bushmen, the medium is the dance, but the description they give of the inner physical process that produces the !kia state is strikingly similar to the way in which the kundalini form of yoga practised in India is said to operate. The !Kung say that !kia occurs when a subtle energy, called nlum, is heated in the lower stomach region by the dance and rises up the spine as a vapor until it touches the base of the skull, at which point the energy is diffused throughout the body, like an electric current, causing the flesh to tingle and all conscious thought to cease.

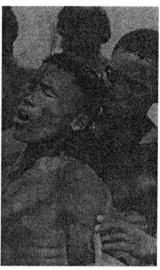

Entering trance (Shostak R626)

People in this state are able to cross into the province of the supernatural and engage the spirits of the dead in battle on their own ground A person charged with nlum repulses the spirits and is cured of his physical and metaphysical ailments, actual and potential. Those who attain it use it to cure other members of the community who fall victim to the arrows of misfortune. It would be a misuse of this power to keep its benefits for themselves. Nlum energy is the universal 'medicine' that was given originally to man by ≠Gao!na and has been passed on from man to man ever since. All who can !kia are thus in this sense 'medicine men' and participate in the religious experience. But some 'medicine men' are more accomplished than others. Those who have absorbed a lot of nlum leave their bodies during the trance and ascend the invisible thread to visit //Gauwa in the western sky, and the greatest of the 'medicine men' sometimes even catch glimpses of ≠Gao!na himself.

Many Bushman groups today tell a story concerning the origin of death which is essentially the same as the account given by the Cape Bushmen in historical times. According to this tale, man may blame his mortality on an ancient argument between the moon and the hare. It is said that, in the days when the earth was inhabited by the 'early race', Moon declared that, just as he was dying and being reborn repeatedly in the cycle of his phases, so too would people die and be reborn. But Hare, who was mourning the death of his mother, denied this, saying that his mother was truly dead and would not return. They argued for some time about this, but Hare insisted that when someone died he remained dead. Eventually, Moon offered to demonstrate his own cycle of death and rebirth, but Hare refused to watch. This so enraged Moon that he struck Hare in the face and split his lip. Hare retaliated by scratching Moon's face, leaving permanent scars. Losing his patience, Moon withdrew the offer of immortality and decreed that Hare was no longer a person but an animal, to be hunted, savaged and eaten by wild dogs. Henceforth, said Moon, all men would die and not return. From that time the hare has been an animal with a split lip, and men have been mortal.

The spirits of people who have died in old age are not so much feared, because death is natural for the aged and they have had time to come to terms with it gradually. In fact, old people accept that in times of great thirst and famine, when their band is perpetually on the move in search of food, it may become necessary for the other members of the band to leave them behind, with no more than a fire to warm them and a circle of dry thorn bush to protect them from the hyenas during what will probably be their last hours. But it is not as if they were abandoned utterly to their fate. Whether they stay behind or continue with the band, the choice is unlikely to alter their fate, except that, if they continue, their presence could be the cause of the whole band having to share it. If the others find food and water before it is too late to save them, some of the men return with supplies to fetch them. If not, the old people know how their end will come. The others, knowing it too, never return to that spot, and neither will their descendants, until its deathly associations have been expunged from collective memory.

All places associated with death are left strictly alone. A body is buried in a squatting posture facing the Great God's home in the eastern sky, and all the personal possessions of the deceased are broken over the grave, so that people passing that way will recognize it as a grave and keep away from it. The campsite is then abandoned, and the band moves to another place and does not camp there again for at least two generations.

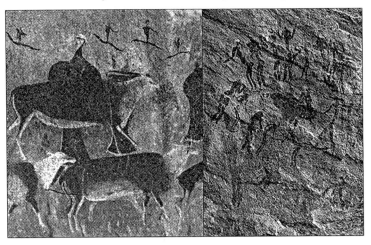

Left: Hunting eland Kamberg (Mohen R467) Right: San painting of the healing or trance dance Lonyana Rock Kwazulu-Natal. Figures dance around a seated figure apparently healing another reclining person enveloped in a kaross, a short skin-cloak. (Rock Art Res. Inst., Univ. of the Witwatersrand, SA)

The !Kung believe in an afterlife, in which their spirits become //gauwasi, who live in the eastern sky as servants of ≠Gao!na. Life dies in the body and does not leave it, but the spirit survives, and the //gauwasi come to fetch it when someone dies, removing it through the head of the corpse and taking it to ≠Gao!na, together with the heart and blood of the deceased. These he hangs on a branch over a fire, and in the smoke, the heart, blood and spirit are reconstituted. As //gauwasi, they have eternal life. They age, but do not die, because //Gauwa renews them with a special medicine before they become too old. They have bodies, as they had on earth, and they have their own supplies of the same types of food they ate formerly. They also retain their former spouses, but eternity is a long time for even the best of marriages to endure, and so if any of them tires of a partner, he or she may cause a mortal woman or man to die in order to provide a replacement in the spirit world. This explains why a beautiful woman or eligible hunter sometimes dies without apparent cause.

The !Kung have elaborate processes to deal with nature carefully which serve to ensure the land can still provide wildlife and plants. These help ensure nature is respected and the fragile ecosystems they depend on to eke a living are not compromised for their future offspring. A wide range of edible roots, bulbs, berries, fruits, melons, nuts and wild leaf vegetables are available, but as several are usually in season at the same time, some may be eaten only occasionally. The Bushmen naturally indulge their preferences when they can and concentrate on the more appetizing of the plant foods that may be gathered in any given season.

Sadly the San peoples are being driven off the Kalahari in Botswana to make a wildlife reserve, so the most valuable ancient gatherer-hunter archetype of human survival over evolutionary time is to be traded for a tourist spot on the very land which they have preserved for millennia, a way of life which has now all but become lost as they forsake the gatherer-hunter way, losing for us all our most robust strategy for planetary survival.

Sandawe: Even More Ancient Roots

The Sandawe people are a small group living in north central Tanzania. They are a remnant of the earlier inhabitants of the area, thought to have once covered all of eastern and southern Africa. Southern Cushites then Eastern Cushites were followed by the Highland Nilotes (Kalenjin Cluster), then the early Bantu. Oral traditions of the Kikuyu of Kenya refer to the Athi (the ground people), whom the Kikuyu paid for the right to move into their land. The Athi are thought to be the original San people of the area.

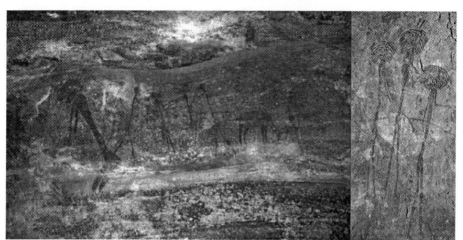

Kolo Rock painting Tanzania Believed to have been painted by ancestors of the Sandawe 4000 BP. Left: May be a healing ceremony. Originally thought by Mary Leakey to represent an abduction..

The Sandawe are racially different from the surrounding tribes. Whereas most of the tribes in Tanzania are Bantu people, the Sandawe are San. They have lighter skin and are smaller, with knotty hair like that of the Bushmen, commonly referred to as peppercorn hair. They have the epicanthic fold of the eyelid (like East Asian peoples) common to the Bushmen.

Much of Sandawe life focuses on a series of fertility rites known as phekumo. The dances of phekumo are held after sunset, the only illumination allowed being the benign, 'cool' light of the moon. Linking the phekumo with the eland-bull dance of girls' puberty rites among the north-western Bushmen is the native claim that such dances were organized in the past by men who had daughters who had begun to menstruate (Ten Raa R672 36). Menstruation as such is associated with the darkness of new moon; but the nocturnal dances get under way only as the moon approaches fullness at around the beginning of the moon's second quarter.

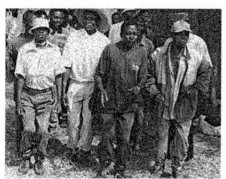

The Sandawe are today no longer gatherer hunters (Tishkoff).

The dance is begun by the women, who go round in circles:

They carry their arms high in a stance which is said to represent the horns of the moon, and at the same time also the horns of game animals and cattle. The women select their partners from among the opposing row of men by dancing in front of them with suggestive motions. The selected partners then come forward and begin to dance in the same manner as the women do, facing them all the time (Ten Raa R672 38). As the dance warms up, the movements become more and more erotic; some of the women turn round and gather up their garments to expose their buttocks to the men (rather than to the newly menstruating girl as in the !Kung): Finally the men embrace the women while emitting hoarse grunts which sound like those of animals on heat. The men and women lift one another up in turn, embracing tightly and mimicking the act of fertilization; those who are not dancing shout encouragements at them ... What the women are in fact doing, writes Ten Raa (ibid), is to re-enact the role of the moon in the basic creation myth, according to which the moon entices the sun into the sky for the first celestial copulation. The women are the moon; the men, the sun. The whole rite is held under the aegis of the moon, and has the explicit purpose of 'making the country fertile'.

Mbuti: Father, Mother, Lover, Friend

The Mbuti Forest People share significant ancient characteristics with the bushmen and form the largest single group of pygmy hunters and gatherers in Africa (Sanday R596 93). Around 2500 BC the Egyptians referred to the Mbuti as 'the people of the trees' renowned for their singing and dancing. These records support the Mbuti remaining stably in this habitat for 4000 years. Because of fission into small isolated groups they have lost their original language and adopt those of neighbouring Bantu tribes with whom they share a semi-symbiotic relationship and more features than the !Kung.

Like the !Kung, the Mbuti have a minimal differentiation of sex roles. Mary Douglas says of the Mbuti (R172) 'Neither sex, age nor kinship order their behavior in strictly ordained categories'. They have no concept of pollution 'of death nor of birth nor of menstruation'. Forced marriages and divorces are very rare. Eligible men and women are free to chose their spouses, but the approval of both sets of parents is usually sought. As a gesture of appreciation to the family of the women, the man usually offers an antelope to the father of the bride. *Arobo*, or free love, is practiced by youth. The Mbuti consider youth to be a period of experimentation and exploration and adolescents are free to satisfy their sexual curiosities. Despite their premarital permissiveness, children outside of marriage are rare. Ther eis no social prohibtion on married men having affairs but they are discrete to avoid angering their wives (R82 276). A Mbuti girl is ritually deflowered by her boyfriend. The girl remains in a hut surrounded by armed women and the boy must fight the whips and missiles aimed at him to get in. If he succeeds he pays an axe as price and spends the night with her (R82 64). There are no prohibitions on sex during menstruation among the Mbuti (R82 226).

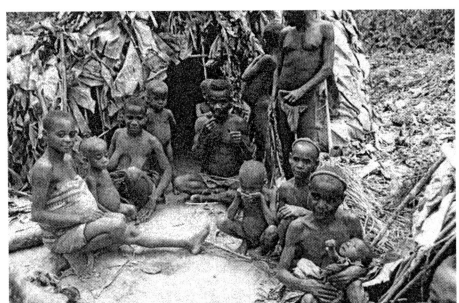

A Mbuti camp (daryl@nevadasurveyor.com). Pygmy representatives have asked the United Nations to set up a court to try government and rebel fighters from DR Congo for acts of cannibalism against their people. Sinafasi Makelo, a representative of Mbuti pygmies, told the UN's Indigenous People's Forum that during the civil war his people had been hunted down and eaten. 'In living memory, we have seen cruelty, massacres, and genocide, but we have never seen human beings hunted down as though they were game animals,' he said. 'People have been eaten. This is nothing more, nothing less, than a crime against humanity.' More than 600,000 pygmies are believed to live in the DR

Congo's forests. Both sides in the war regard them as 'subhuman'. Some say their flesh can confer magical powers (BBC). The Biaka are also threatened by logging, which damages the forest, drives cris-crossing roads into their territory and frightens away the game as well as poaching of the game animals they hunt.

Their habitat and their heaven is the Ituri Forest. The forest is their godhead, and different individuals address it as 'father', 'mother', 'lover', and/or 'friend'. They say that the forest is everything: the provider of food, shelter, warmth, clothing, and affection. Each person and animal is endowed with a spiritual power that "derives from a single source of power whose physical manifestation is the forest itself". Disembodied spirits deriving from this same source are also considered to be independent manifestations of the forest. The forest lives for the Mbuti. It is both natural and supernatural, something that is depended upon, respected, trusted, obeyed, and loved. The forest is a good provider. At all times of the year men and women can gather an abundant supply of mushrooms, roots, berries, nuts, herbs, fruits, and leafy vegetables. The forest also provides animal food.

There is little sexual division of labor. The hunt is frequently a joint effort. A man is not ashamed to pick mushrooms and nuts if he finds them, or to wash and clean a baby. In general, leadership is minimal and there is no attempt to control or dominate either the geographical, or human environment. Decision making is by common consent: Men and women have equal say because hunting and gathering are both important to the economy. The forest is the ultimate authority. It expresses its feelings through storms, falling trees, poor hunting all of which are taken as signs of its displeasure. But often the forest remains silent, and this is when the people must sound out its feelings through discussion. Diversity of opinion may be expressed, but prolonged disagreement is considered to be 'noise' and offensive to the forest. Certain individuals may be recognized as having the right and the ability to interpret the pleasure of the forest. In this sense there is individual authority, which simply means effective participation in discussions. The three major areas for discussion are economic, ritual, and legal matters having to do with dispute settlement. Participation in discussions is evenly divided between the sexes and among all adult age levels. The avoidance of differentiation between the sexes is consistent with the principle of egalitarianism that rules Mbuti life in the forest.

Mbuti (www.nevadasurveyor.com)

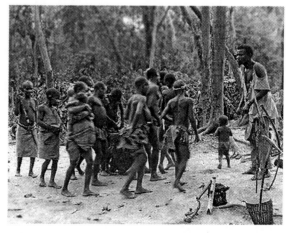

Some sexual differentiation, occurs in the emotional connotations associated with mother and father and is acted out in one of the most important Mbuti ceremonies. Motherhood is associated with food and love, and fatherhood with authority, although fathers physically nurture their children. The mother is regarded as the source of food; all food that is collected or hunted is cooked and distributed by women. Hungry children look to their mothers for food, not to their fathers. Sexual differentiation is acted out in the molimo ceremony, which is held irregularly, when someone dies or when conditions of life are generally poor. Its goal is to awaken and 'to rejoice the forest.' The festival symbolizes the triumph of life over death. The central ceremonial symbols are the molimo fire and the molimo trumpets. Both are associated with life, regeneration, and fertility. Both are believed to have been once owned by women and stolen from them by the men. The trumpet is sometimes referred to as an animal of the forest: It is symbolically fed, it is passed through the fire, and during a dance it is used by a young man to imitate the male and female parts in the sexual act. The trumpet is the only sign of the presence of a supernatural power during the molimo festival.

The trumpet is supposed to sing and to pass on the song of the Mbuti into the forest. It is kept out of the sight of women and children, who are supposedly forbidden to see it. The Mbuti do not consider the trumpet to be sacred in itself - it is simply a vehicle for transferring power between the Mbuti and the forest. The molimo festival includes two rituals that separate male from female. Both focus on an old woman who symbolically kills and scatters the molimo fire (the symbol of life) and later ties all the men together with a roll of twine. The old woman dances the fire dance led by a chorus of women singing molimo songs (supposedly known only by men). The men follow in obedient chorus. The high point of the dance comes when the old woman jumps into the flames, whirls around, and scatters the molimo fire in all directions within the circle of men surrounding her. The men, still singing, gather the scattered embers, throw them back onto the coals, and dance while the flames begin to rise again as if they had brought the fire back to life. The old woman repeats her dance, each time seeming to stamp the fire out of existence, after which the dance of the men gives it new life. Finally the old woman and the women leave the scene. A little later the old woman comes back alone. The men continue singing while she ties them all together, looping a roll of twine around their necks. Once all are tied they stop singing. The men then admit to having been bound and to the necessity of giving the woman something as a token of their defeat, so that she'll let them go. After a certain quantity of food has been agreed upon, the old woman unties each man. No one attempts to untie himself, but as each man is untied he begins to sing once more. This signifies that the molimo is free. The old woman receives her gifts, and before leaving several weeks later, she goes to every man, giving him her hand to touch as though it were some kind of blessing.

Colin Turnbull (R694, R695), the major ethnographer of the Mbuti, suggests that in the fire dance women assert their prior claim to the fire of life and their ability to destroy and extinguish life. However, he asks, was the old woman really destroying the fire? Perhaps when she kicked the fire in all directions among the men she was giving it to them, to gather, rebuild, and revitalize the fire with the dance of life. In discussing these ceremonies, Turnbull suggested to me the possibility that they symbolized the transference of power from women to men. As he put it, "Women have the power which they give to men for them to control" (personal communication). If this is indeed the case, and it is difficult to be sure, then whereas in some societies men take power from women, Mbuti women give power to men (Sanday R596 23).

Explaining to Colin Turnbull the reason for the molimo ceremonies, held when the Mbuti feel that all is not well between themselves and the forest, upon which they depend for everything, an old Mbuti man said: "The forest is a father and mother to us and like a father or mother it gives us everything we need food, clothing, shelter, warmth . . . and affection". Normally everything goes well because the forest is good to its children, but when things go wrong there must be a reason. Things go wrong, the old man said, at night when the people are asleep, when no one is awake to protect humans from harm. At night army ants may invade the camp or leopards may come in and steal a hunting dog or even a child. The old man said that such things would not happen when people are awake. Thus, he reasoned, "When something big goes wrong, like illness or bad hunting or death, it must be because the forest is sleeping and not looking after its children." Because things go wrong when the forest is 'asleep,' the forest must be 'awakened' so that it looks after the interests of the people. The old man said: "We wake it up by singing to it, and we do this because we want it to awaken happy. Then everything will be well and good again. So when our world is going well then also we sing to the forest because we want to share our happiness. One way the Mbuti 'awaken' the forest is to sound the molimo trumpets. These trumpets are referred to as 'the animal of the forest' and are kept from the sight of women, who are supposed to believe that the sound of the trumpet is made by an animal and that to see the trumpet would bring death. It is also believed that the women used to possess the molimo trumpets and that they were stolen from them by the men. This is the main reason why the women must be barred from viewing the trumpets. Were they to have access to the trumpets, it is thought, the women might try to seize them from the men (Sanday R596 187).

A ceremony called the 'lesser' molimo is held when hunting is bad. This ceremony involves men alone. After supper the women and children are bundled away safely in the huts and the men prepare for a night of eating and singing to the forest. When the men sing in the camp, the sound of the trumpets echoes the men's song from the depths of the forest. Sometimes the sound of the trumpet is that of an angry animal who will endanger the lives of women and children. Other times the trumpet's sound is mournful and pleads with the forest and men for food. The trumpets are fed food and water and passed through the flames of the molimo fire in an act that signifies the male role in copulation . These acts suggest that men are responsible for the well-being and fertility of animals. The 'lesser' molimo ceremony is one of the few times when men and women are separated and men imitate a dominant role. This ceremony signifies the responsibility of men in connection with animals and the hunt. Women and children are bundled off into the huts in order to protect them from the dangerous forces emanating from the forest world during the night. The animal nature of men is expressed in the association of the trumpets with masculinity and animality. The manipulation of the trumpets during the ceremony, however, indicates also that with the aid of their forest, men are meant to control animal nature for the good of the community.

The idea that the trumpets were stolen from women suggests that it was from women men believe they found the means to control the destructive forces that stalk the forest at night and that it was from women they received their animal nature. Stealing the trumpets implies also that masculinity must be aggressively separated from femininity, that men in order to be powerful and to have control must take these rights from women by force.

The whole community participates in the 'greater' molimo, a ceremony held when hunting is bad, someone has died, there is widespread sickness, and death seems to rule life. In this ceremony the Mbuti conception of male and female is thrown into sharp relief. While the 'lesser' molimo is spoken of as 'waking' the forest, the 'greater' molimo ideally is a festival of joy. The purpose of this ceremony, Turnbull says, is to symbolically establish the triumph of life over death. The focal role in this ceremony is played by an old woman This woman, together with the nubile girl with whom she dances, symbolizes the forces of life and of death. The old woman is referred to as 'mother,' the same term used to address the forest in its capacity as giver of life and death. In her ceremonial acts the old woman symbolizes these two forces. When she stamps out the fire, the symbol of life, she enacts the meaning of death. When she scatters the embers and allows the fire to be revitalized and rebuilt by the men, she enacts the transference to men of the role they are to play in connection with life. The men revitalize and rebuild the fire with a dance that simulates copulation. Turnbull says that fire is primarily connected with women; the hearth is often referred to as the vagina. When the men rebuild the fire and sing to the forest, they are serving as agents for restoring order. Women, on the other hand, appear to be placed in the role of either giving or taking life. They do not, at least within the framework of the molimo ceremonies, act as mediators between positive and negative forces. The symbolism of the old woman tying the men with a roll of twine suggests that in their role as life takers women have ultimate control but that this control is inimical to the survival of the group. When the old woman ties the men, they stop singing, which means that the male capacity to rejuvenate the forest has been bound. The men say: "This woman has tied us up. She has bound the men, bound the hunt, and bound the molimo. We can do nothing." By untying the men the old woman gives them control once again. But in order to be freed the men must admit that they have been bound and they must give the woman something as a token of their defeat. Once she has been given an agreed-upon quantity of food and cigarettes, the old woman unties each man. As each is untied, each begins to sing again. Once more the molimo is free.

Turnbull says that the molimo festival serves as an integrating factor in Mbuti life. It also expresses the latent antagonisms that exist between the sexes while uniting the band in a common expression of their dependence upon the forest. The molimo forces "an acknowledgment of the most basic dependency of all, that of life and death". The molimo is also an enactment of the interdependence between male and female. The latent antagonism between the sexes to which Turnbull refers could be viewed as an expression of the basic antithesis between forces meant to give as well as take life (associated with females) and forces meant to regenerate the forces of life from those of death (associated with males). The molimo expresses the double nature of women as well as of men. Men and women stand for life and death in different ways, women more directly than men. Men regenerate life in the 'greater' molimo and enact the role of destructive animality in the 'lesser' molimo. Though the old woman's superior position is assured by the deferential behavior of the men, it is the ceremonial give-and-take between male and female and between men and the forest that controls and harmonizes opposing forces in the Mbuti forest world.

Blood symbolizes both life and death. As noted previously, menstrual blood in particular symbolizes life. The blood that comes for the first time to the young girl comes as a gift, received with gratitude and rejoicing, because she is now a potential mother and can proudly take a husband. The girl enters seclusion, taking with her all of her friends. Here they celebrate the happy event and are taught the arts and crafts of motherhood by an old and respected relative. They learn to live like adults and to sing the songs of adult women. Pygmies from all around come to pay their respects, because for them this occasion is one of the happiest, most joyful occasions in their lives.

Chris Knight (R373 388) notes:

"The onset of a girl's first flow is marked by a joyful ritual known as the elima, this word denoting in the first instance a large hut in which one or more pubescent girls are joined by female relatives for a period of singing and celebration. During this, the girls are taught to be proud of their bodies both sexually and in terms of reproductive potential (Turnbull 1976: 167-81). The elima forges strong bonds of solidarity between girls who together 'have seen the blood'; it simultaneously achieves 'at least a temporary obliteration of the bonds of the nuclear family' (Turnbull 1966: 136). A girl who has begun to menstruate for the first time is said to be 'blessed by the moon' and becomes the focus of rejoicing as everyone is told the good news: 'The girl enters seclusion, but not the seclusion of the village girl. She takes with her all her young friends, those who have not yet reached maturity, and some older ones.' They enter a single communal 'women's house' (the elima) where the girls celebrate the happy event collectively. During the ethnographer Colin Turnbull's fieldwork visit, two young women experienced their first menstruation at the same time, and entered the house together, along with their female friends. Turnbull's (1976: 169) description is enough to refute the view that such 'seclusion' must always and everywhere be a degrading experience: Together they are taught the arts and crafts of motherhood by an old and respected relative. They learn not only how to live like adults, but how to sing the songs of adult women. Day after day, night after night, the elima house resounds with the throaty contralto of the older women and the high, piping voices of the youngest. It is a time of gladness, Turnbull continues, not for the women alone but for the whole community. People from all around come to pay their respects, the young men standing or sitting about outside the elima house in the hopes of a glimpse of the young beauties inside. And there are special elima songs which they sing to each other, the girls singing a light, cascading melody in intricate harmony, the men replying with a rich, vital chorus. For the pygmies the elima is one of the happiest, most joyful occasions in their lives.

Mbuti boys sometimes sleep together in one hut and, during these occasions, are likely to be in close physical contact, with legs entwined, or thrown around one another's waist or hips. But no homosexual activity occurs, and the idea of something of the sort horrifies the Mbuti, who only refer to homosexuality when they are extremely provoked and wish to level an enormous insult at a man (Broude R82 298).

Male circumcision represents a 'pass through age' ritual, and for them makes a difference not only between boys and men, but between the Village and the jungle. When a group of boys reaches the age of 8 to 12 years take place the 'encoumby' (the name given by this people to the ceremony). Each boy is prepared by their own mother and aunts. Their body and face are painted with white and black colors. The body is dressed with some kind of skirt made with fibers from palm tree. The group is taken to the center of village and begins a dance, meanwhile women and girls leave the village announcing the beginning of the party. The origin of the custom is explained by the following legend: "The tradition of circumcision was made an institution by a woman ('amiana'), come from west, and her husband ('tocool'). They saw the monkeys making a circumcision and adopted the practice. The season for the ceremony is announced by a bird, who flies high and which cry is very recognizable. 'Monkey' may the nickname given by them for other human groups). The high flying bird is to distract the subject so the cut can be made "See the birdie!"

Biaka: The Forest's Family Care-givers

The earliest humans in Gabon were believed to be the Babinga, or Pygmies, dating back to 7000 B.C., who were later followed by Bantu groups from southern and eastern Africa.

Like the Mbuti, the Biaka, Ba'Aka, or Aka Forest Pygmies of the Central African Republic and Gabon do not have formally defined sex roles. The sexual division of tasks is never rigid and compulsory. Biaka life is characterized by gatherer-hunting with an emphasis on hunting in a semi-symbiotic relationship with neighbouring farming villagers. Sexual relations are extremely egalitarian and cooperative. Violence by men against women is extremely rare. Women share autonomous power although men hold symbolic roles and men play an exceptional role in infant care.

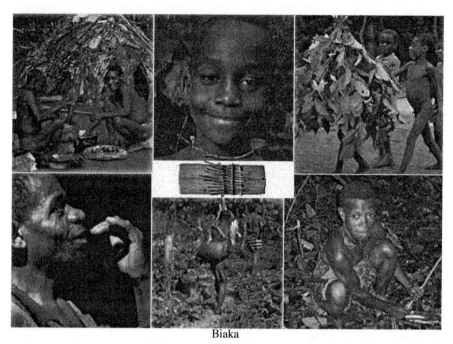
Biaka

Unlike the Mbuti Pygmies in the Ituri who speak the same language as their village neighbors, the Biaka speak their own language (diaka), as well as the language of their neighbors

All women get married, generally by age sixteen to seventeen years of age. Men first marry two to four years later than women. Aka prefer to marry far away, and clan exogamy is practiced. About 17 percent of Aka men have more than one wife, and about one of four marriages ends in divorce. Most of the divorces come at an early age before children are born. Most of the early divorces are initiated by women, whereas most divorces after age thirty-five (when women have completed fertility) are initiated by men.

Fertility is high and infertility infrequent. Female infertility is rare among the Aka; only one women was reported infertile. Birth intervals are about 3.6 years shorter than the 4.0 year interval found among the !Kung San , but substantially higher than the 2.9 year interval estimated for the Yanomamo. The completed fertility of Aka females is about 5.6 lying between the 4.7 live births found with !Kung San females and the 7.9 live births found with Yanomamo women (Hewlett R305).

The camp generally consists of groups of three to four adult males (about half the males) from the same patriclan (usually brothers or first cousins), their wives and children, an elderly mother of some of the adult males, an older divorced sister of the patriclan and her children, a daughter of one of the adult males and her spouse who is performing bride service (about a fifth of the males), and one or two visiting families (about two fifths of the males).

The Aka are patrilineal, having shallow patriclans (dikanda), and are generally patrilocal except for a few years after marriage when the male provides bride service in the camp of his wife's family. While the core of the camp usually consists of about thirty five people consisting of adult males belonging to the same patriclan (dikanda) -that is, individuals tracing their ancestry patrilineally to a mythical plant or animal. Clan identity is weak. Few Aka know the mythology associated with their clan and Aka rarely invoke clan obligations if family members do not help out in subsistence activities. Aka adults can seldom remember patrilineal links back more than two generations and matrilineal relatives are visited frequently. Female lines are also recognized by the term *mobila*. This term refers to the lines of mother, mother's mother, father's mother, and father's mother's mother.

Two to four clans gather together for net hunting which is pursued in the dry season. Aka tend to travel in a 50 km radius area from their place of birth, and get to know about 700 Aka in this area. Aka males generally have a greater exploration range than females. The 'exploration range' is where subsistence activities take place, a spouse is encountered, and other aspects of geographical as well as social knowledge are acquired and transmitted.

Aka know hundreds of forest plants and animals, but subsist primarily on 63 plant species, 20 insect species, honey from 8 species of bees, and 28 species of game. The Aka collect roots from 6 species of plants, leaves from 11 species, nuts from 17 species, and fruits from 17 species. They collect 12 species of mushrooms, 4 types of termites, crickets, 3 types of grubs, and 12 species of caterpillars. The Aka hunt for 7 species of large game with the spear (primarily hog and elephant), 6 species of duiker with the net (primarily the blue duiker), 8 species of monkeys with the crossbow, and 7 species of rat, mongoose, and porcupine with a variety of small snare and net traps. The Aka clearly identify forest zones rich in particular plant or animal species.

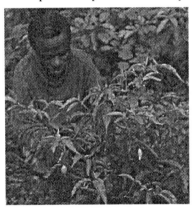

Tamassi, head of a pygmy family with eboka. Myths tell of the discovery of the hallucinogen iboga (p 477). The wife of a pygmy finds the plant and uses it to communicate with the spirits of the dea in the form of her husband who has become scattered as the plant. Suggesting discovery of the sacrament by women (D. Lieberman dan@iafrica.com).

Zame last of the creator gods gave us Eboka. One day he saw the pygmy Bitamu high in the Atanga tree gathering fruit He made him fall. He died and Zame brought his spirit. He took the fingers and the little toes and planted them in various parts of the forest. They grew into the Eboka bush (Furst 245).

During the year the Aka spend about 56% of their time in hunting, 27% of their time in gathering, and 17% of their time in village work for the Ngandu. The Aka spend up to 90 percent of their time net hunting in the drier season (January to May), while during part of the rainy season (August to September) 60% of their time is spent collecting food, especially caterpillars. Much of the vegetable food in the Aka diet is obtained by trading meat to farmers for manioc and other cultigens. Researchers suggest the forest does not yield enough carbohydrates (specifically, wild yams) for people there to live independently. They hypothesize that Pygmies originally lived on the margins of the forest exploiting both forest and savannah habitats and did not move into the forest until forest farmers moved in with them. The forest is sanctuary to the Aka while the village is a place of doubt and suspicion. In the forest, Aka sing, dance, play, and are very active and conversant. In the village, their demeanor changes dramatically - they walk slowly, say little, seldom smile, and try to avoid eye contact with others. Although both men and women collect leaves, fruits, nuts, mushrooms, and termites, women do the majority of the collecting. They may do this as a conjugal unit or individually. Men do the majority of the honey collecting, especially if it involves climbing a tree large in diameter. Both men and women net hunt, usually together, but sometimes individually, and men and women both use small traps to hunt, often together, but again, sometimes individually. Only men use the spear and crossbow to hunt.

As with the Mbuti, most camp members - male and female, young and old - participate in the net hunt . Unusual for the sexual division of hunting generally, women net-hunt more frequently than men. From the time Aka leave the village and return to the forest (February-March) until caterpillar season (July-August), they often net hunt six days a week, four to nine hours per day. Net hunts decrease in frequency during the caterpillar season and the major rainy season (August-October); individual and small group foraging techniques (e.g., spears, crossbows, traps) are utilized more frequently during these seasons. There is no stalking of game, once the nets are set the object of the "beaters" is to make as much noise as possible in order to wake up the nocturnal duikers, the primary targets of the net hunt. It is one of the few hunting techniques where ears are just as important as eyes and where women carrying infants and older children can contribute to the success of the hunt.

There are few Aka status positions. There is no chief in the sense of a person commanding ultimate authority, yet there is the kombeti, who is generally more influential in subsistence and camp movement discussions. The *nganga* is the traditional healer and provides a wide range of services to the community--such as divination on hunts, curing of witchcraft, and herbal healing. Most Aka camps have an nganga. Ngangas can cure all forms of illness (e.g., malaria, worms, bad luck, attack by witchcraft), see into the future to help one make decisions about travel, marriage or friendships, and can see game animals deep in the forest while on the net hunt. Women are also skilled in plant healing as traditional doctors. Specific remedies include those to help a girl find a husband, or for a woman who is having problems desiring her husband. Witches or sorcerers (the Aka make no distinction) practice secretly and are unknown to the general population, although ngangas are highly suspect. The *tuma* is the great hunter who has often killed several elephants on his own. He leads spear hunts and important hunting and seasonal rituals, and organizes the training of young boys in the men's secret society. The status positions are usually held by males.

Aka who believe in bembe, the creator of all living things, believe also that bembe retired soon after creation. The most consistently mentioned divinity or spirit is that of dzengi, a forest spirit. All Aka adolescent boys are taken on an elephant hunt by a tuma to learn how to hunt elephant as well as to learn about the secret lore of dzengi. While women are kept peripheral to powers and secrets of *dzengi*, most women I spoke to about dzengi were not mystified or fearful of dzengi or the mens' secrets, and in fact, sometimes laughed and said it was just a way the men tried to keep knowledge and power from them.

The Aka are fiercely egalitarian and independent. No individual has the right to coerce or order another individual to perform an activity against his/her will. Even when parents give instructions to their children to collect water or firewood, there are no sanctions if they do not do so. Aka have a number of informal non-institutional methods for maintaining their egalitarianism. First, they practice prestige avoidance; one does not draw attention to his or her activities. There are certainly exceptional hunters, dancers and drummers, but individuals do not brag to others about their abilities. Second, they practice the rough joking described among the !Kung San. For instance, if a man is boasts about the amount of honey he collected, others will joke about the size and shape of his genitals. And third, they practice demand sharing. This simply means that whatever one has will be given up if requested.

Sharing, cooperation, and autonomy are but a few other of the Aka core values. The community cooperates daily in the net hunt, food hunted is shared with members of the camp, and decision- making is the reserved prerogative of the individual; if one is not content with living conditions, for instance, one moves to another camp. As a result, camp composition changes daily.

Aka infant mortality at 20 percent is indistinguishable from the infant mortality rates of the !Kung (20.2 percent) and the Yanomamo (21.8 percent). The Aka are more peaceful than many other hunter-gatherers and horticulturists. Accidental and violent deaths were relatively infrequent especially in comparison with the Yanomamo and !Kung San. The causes of death study also indicated that males at every age were at greater risk of death than were females. Young adult males (18-25 years) were at especially high risk relative to female risk of death at the same age. This pattern is consistent with that found among the Yanomamo and !Kung San. Aka infancy has the following characteristics: constant holding and skin-to-skin contact, high father involvement, multiple care giving, indulgent care, lack of negation, early training for autonomy and subsistence skills, parents as primary transmitters of culture, and precocious motor and cognitive development. Infants are held almost constantly, and have skin-to-skin contact most of the day as Aka seldom wear shirts or blouses. They are nursed on demand and attended to immediately if they fuss or cry. Aka parents interact with and stimulate their infants throughout the day.

Aka fathers do more infant care giving than fathers in any known culture. There are various aspects of Aka infancy that contribute to and reflect the intimate nature of the father's role.   Aka fathers hold or are within an arms reach of their infant about half of a twenty four hour period and perform 22 percent of the care giving of 4-month-old infants in the camp. They are the second most active care givers after the mother and their style of care-taking is characterized by its intimate, affectionate, and helping-out nature, rather than by its playfulness. Numerous others help out with infant care. While in the camp setting, Aka one-to-four month-old infants are held by mothers less than 40 percent of the time, are transferred to other care givers an average of 7.3 times per hour, and have seven different care givers on average that hold the infant during the day. The multiple care giving decreases as the group moves out of camp to travel or go net hunting. Like the !Kung, Aka infants are carried vertically most of the day. Infants will sleep for hours in their side sling as parents set up nets and chase after game. The increased vestibular stimulation may con-tribute to the Aka infants' precocious motor and cognitive development.

Generally, it is difficult for parents to get their older children to do much for them. The parents may yell at their children, but more often than not, they just go and get what they need by themselves. Children are independent and autonomous at an early age. Infants are allowed to crawl or walk to wherever they want in camp, and allowed to use knives, machetes, digging sticks, and clay pots. By three or four years of age children can cook themselves a meal on the fire, and by ten years of age Aka children know enough subsis-tence skills to live in forest alone if need be. Respect for an individual's autonomy is a core value among the Aka, and it is demonstrated and encouraged in their patterns of infant care. The great respect for autonomy is consistent with another Aka value - inter-genera-tional equality. This is a positive description of what villagers would call lack of respect for elders. Violence or corporal punishment for an infant that misbehaves seldom occurs. In fact, if one parent hits an infant, this is reason enough for the other parent to ask for a divorce.

While fathers are very active in infant care, they do not usually participate in the birth of their infants. Unlike some other forest people the mother is first to suckle her newborn. Usually only women and young children attend births. If a father attended and helped in the delivery of his infant because his wife gave birth while they were walking together in the forest he is not teased or stigmatized for his participation. Both mother and father observe food taboos during the pregnancy and until the infant can walk well. There is also a postpartum sex taboo until the child can walk very well. Most Aka know about the post-partum sex taboo, but limited interview data and impressions indicate it is not observed. Even if one does break the rule there are indigenous medications to remedy of the trans-gression.

Aka male-female relations are extremely egalitarian by cross-cultural standards. What is especially remarkable about the Aka is the amount of time husband and wife spend in cooperative subsistence activity. Husband and wife are together on a regular basis to net hunt, collect caterpillars, termites, honey, fruit, and sometimes fish. On net hunting days husband and wife are within view of each other 47 percent of the time. They are not only in association with each other, but actively cooperating in subsistence activity. On days when there is no net hunt, it is not unusual to see a husband and wife going out together to collect plants or honey. Wives are less likely to participate in cross-bow hunting for mon-keys and trap-line hunting for medium size game, and never participate in spear hunts for wild pig and elephants. Aka husbands and wives are together often and cooperate in a wide variety of subsistence tasks throughout the year; they clearly care for one another, but it is also clear that Aka men and women like to be with members of the same sex at least as much as being with their spouses.

Men contribute slightly more to the diet while in the forest camps because in addition to the net hunting, men hunt for monkeys, pigs, elephants, and most of the honey. In the village camps females are the primary providers, contributing at least 70 percent of the calories. Women not only contribute substantially to the diet, but have considerable control over the distribution and exchange of food. Both women and men butcher and distribute game captured on the net hunt, and if it has been a reasonably good hunt women will prepare pots of food for other camp households. Women also distribute gathered food--mushrooms, fruit, nuts, tubers. Besides having a central role in the distribution of food, women are primarily responsible for exchange with villagers.

The political power and social prestige of Aka women is pronounced, but is not as structurally salient as that of Aka men. Aka men hold all the named positions of status - kombeti, tuma , and nganga--but as mentioned already, these men hold no absolute power. They influence people through their hospitality, persuasiveness, humor, and knowledge, not by their position. Aka women challenge men's authority on a regular basis and are influential actors in all kinds of decision-making. There is something of a queendom in many camps as the mother of the men who form the core of the camp is often the eldest patriclan member. Since men marry younger women, Aka women usually outlive their husbands by many years. These grandmothers eventually move back to the camp of their patriclan. Women in this position are vivacious characters and become respected patriclan spokespersons. The men in the named status positions are usually her sons.

Husbands and wives cooperate in a wide range of activities, but there is respect for each other's feelings and peculiarities. Husbands cannot force their wives to come on the hunt, and the wives cannot force their husbands to look for honey. Spouses can and do ridicule each other with rather crude joking (e.g., uncomplimentary remarks about the size and shape of their partner's genitals), but for the most part the partner does not pay much attention to the ridicule. If the couple does not get along, divorce is a matter of one partner simply moving out of the house.

Physical violence in general is infrequent and violence against women is especially rare. The lack of violence enhances female autonomy and encourages husband-wife cooperation and trust. Husband-wife conflicts do of course occur but they are usually resolved through talking, rough joking , leaving camp for awhile, or mediated assistance from other camp members. Female violence can occur against men, such as cutting their husband's face with a knife or hitting their husbands with logs from the fire for sleeping with other women. Women, however, are more likely to show their anger and displeasure with their husband by tearing down the family house. Aka women make the houses, and Aka men are not very good at it (they usually make lean-tos). Female autonomy and the lack of violence against women is also demonstrated by the frequent travel of women, alone or in small groups, throughout the forest.

Husband and wife are together often, know each other exceptionally well, and cooperate on a regular basis in a diversity of tasks. Men and women have distinct tasks, but there are few underlying beliefs that one sex is naturally inclined to perform certain tasks. Aka men are similar to men cross-culturally in that men predominate in the named status positions, only men hunt large game, and polygyny is relatively common. Aka male-female relations have commonalties with male-female relations cross-culturally, but the Aka are probably as egalitarian as human societies get.

Hadzabe: Emerging Sexual Tensions

Like the San and Mbuti, the Hadza are gatherers and hunters. They hunt game, gather edible plants and honey, and move from place to place whenever the weather changes, or the wild herds migrate, or they just feel like moving. In small groups of about eighteen adults and their children, they pitch camps among the rocks and trees of the dry savanna.

It takes less than two hours for Hadza women to build a new camp. They make huts by bending and weaving branches into round structures about six feet high, then covering them with thick clumps of long, golden grass. Or, if the weather is very wet, the women may skip the hut building and choose a dry cave to set up a camp that includes a hearth, cooking vessels, sleeping mats made of animal skins, and tools for sharpening stones and scraping skins. Some rock caves have been used intermittently over thousands of years and are decorated with ancient rock paintings.

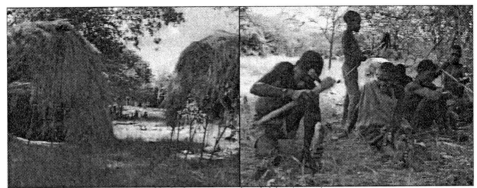

Hadzabe camp and activities (www)

Men and boys hunt with bows and arrows, almost always alone. Women and girls do not hunt. By the age of 10, an Eastern Hadza boy will have made himself a sturdy bow and a set of arrows to kill hyrax, rabbits, squirrels and birds. Men tend to make long bows, about six feet in length, which are exceptionally powerful and heavy to pull. Hadza hunt from very close range to shoot impala, zebra, eland or giraffe. Some Hadza also eat predators, including lion, leopard, and other wild cats, or perhaps scavengers like jackal, hyena and vulture, but they draw the line at reptiles like monitors, snakes and lizards. Like the !Kung, they use poisoned arrow tips to hunt large animals. Once a beast has been wounded, the hunter waits a few hours for the poison to act and then tracks the wounded animal until it dies.

Most meat is eaten where it falls. Hunters take each day as it comes and generally hunt alone to feed themselves, however they occasionally go out at night, encircle a troop of baboons, and kill them. They take meat back to camp only if there is a surplus and they feel like making the effort. Most men content themselves with vegetable foods and small animals. The men frequently gamble their few possessions in a game of chance throwing wooden discs until one matches the large one. Far from resenting these non-hunters, the few big-game hunters readily share meat with them as well as with women and children. A good hunter will be favored by women and will tend to be welcome, perhaps even pampered, when he joins a camp. Like the !Kung, the interactions of Hadza people are relatively free of jealousy, resentment, elitism, tyranny, or any concept of private property.

Hadzabe woman and man (www)

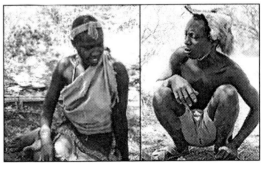

Gathering begins early in Hadza childhood, when babes help their mothers, big brothers and sisters pick berries, dig edible roots, and gather seeds and pulp from baobab trees. Like the San this food supplies 80 percent of the normal diet by weight. Hadza people obtain the remaining 20 percent of their food from meat brought back to camp and wild bee honey taken from hives in the bush.

Hadza women make skirts from the skins of female impala, sometimes decorated with beads, shells and bells. A second garment, made of cloth and beads for a married woman, or strings and beads for an unmarried woman, hangs in front. The upper garment, also made from impala hide, can be used for warmth or to carry berries, babies, firewood or meat. Men and boys of the Hadza tribe wear the skin of a small animal as a loincloth, its tail hanging down between their legs. They wear sandals to protect them from the thorns on the savanna.

Hadza people generally come and go as they like. They may travel alone, join a camp, move to a different camp, or gravitate to a small area and live there with any group that happens to come along. The major exception is demonstrated by married couples, who may stay together for twenty years and tend to live with the wife's mother. If husband and wife live apart for two weeks or more, they are likely to be considered unmarried. Spouses of either gender may abandon the marriage and seek a new partner by reverting to the dress of unmarried members of the tribe.

In the rock-strewn hillsides of Tanzania, Hadza foragers collect all the tubers and baobab pods they need without having to travel more than two miles from camp. Mothers are rarely gone longer than an hour. Infants are left behind at around two rather than the four characteristic among the !Kung, often with subadult caretakers. Because they have the option to leave babies with an allo-mother, Hadza mothers can produce infants after shorter intervals than !Kung mothers without compromising survival. As a consequence, the Hadza population is growing by 1% a year rather than holding steady (Hrdy R323 197).

A camp has no organized leadership and no sense of itself as a permanent group. They are far more likely to move on than create conflict. Dissidents are more likely to leave a camp than face a conflict. Conflict is often concealed behind ecological excuses, such as an claiming the berries are better or the game more plentiful somewhere else.

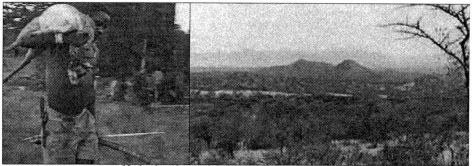

Hadza hunting and their traditional lands (www)

Hadza women depend on their female kin to act as buffers against a husband's violence. The mother of a beaten woman may threaten to take her daughter back, and a wooman's relative may band together to beat the husband with their digging sticks if his abuse of his wife becomes too severe (Broude R82 313). Hazda men who have a grudge against another camp may attack, or rape, the women without repercussions (R82 252). On the other hand if a Hadza man leaves his family for more than a few weeks they say "his house has died". Marriage last only as long as the two live together on a regular basis. The man no longer has rights over the woman and any children they share and it is up to the woman whether to take him back or not if he returns (R82 76).

"In the Hadza matriarchy myth of *Mambedaka*, the original owner of the sacred *epeme* meat is an old woman who dresses as a man, hunts zebra and wears a zebra penis which she uses to have sex with her 'wives'. She demands that men bring the epeme meat to her cooking pot which she distributes to the 'wives'. Men have no share in the sacred meat until the violent overthrow of *Mambedaka's* rule" (Power and Watts R538 323). This is again a depiction of the logic of women procuring fatty meat from men by signalling 'wrong sex, wrong species (p 77). This interpretation, like many others in more patriarchal societies speaks of an overthrow of female power over sexuality by the men. Consistent with this trend, among the Hadza there is an extraordinarily intense consciousness of sexual difference, which divides the sexes into "two hostile classes, each of which is capable of organizing itself for defense or virulent attack against the other" (Sanday 1981):

This opposition between the Hadza sexes is more pronounced during the dry season, when camps are bigger and large animals and humans congregate near the few available sources of water. During the wet season, however, food becomes both abundant and evenly dispersed, and the sexes live together relatively harmoniously in small, widely scattered camps, subsisting on roots and small game. In these small wet-season camps, men and women are not segregated greatly. Only the large camps of the dry season seem to stimulate sexual segregation and mutual hostility between the sexes. It is common for the relationship between the sexes among the same group of foragers to change, depending on seasonal activities or a switch from nomadic to sedentary life. In foraging societies, when food is abundant and dispersed, small family groups wander with relative ease in their environment and the sexes are integrated in most activities.

This ease disappears during the dry season, when the food supply fluctuates, or is concentrated in certain areas, bringing animals and people into competition for the same water resources. Hadza men hunt large game, which implies danger, and they gamble in camp, which conveys a concern with chance. In the concentrated settlements of the dry season, the Hadza believe that contact with menstrual blood is dangerous. This is the wedge that drives the sexes apart - as is the case in most societies in which sexual separation is rigid. When a Hadza women menstruates, she avoids certain activities, which would be polluted by her contact. In addition, her husband of the moment, whoever he may be, must abstain from his ordinary activities lest he endanger the rest of the camp's chance of success in hunting. Just as the !Kung say a menstruating girl at menarche has 'shot her first eland' the Hadza say 'she has shot her first zebra', consistent with the link between menstruation and hunting.

For the Hadza, the dry season marks the phase of social aggregation when their most sacred rituals are held - The épeme dances held on each night of the dark moon for the duration of the aggregation. All camp fires are extinguished and the women call upon each man in turn to dance, referring to him exlusively in consanguineal kinship terms [therefore, as borthers and sisters rather than lovers]. In Hadza belief women synchronize their menstruation with the dark moon, hence at the time of epeme rites. The dance emphasizes gender segregation cross-cut by kinship solidarity. As well as being a healing dance, it is believed to ensure success in forthcoming hunts, when portions of the fattiest meat will be offered in birdeservice. A coherent pattern emerges: First, men should not hunt nor have sex while their wives are bleeding; second, the most successful hunting in the dry season occurs around full moon; and third, menstruation normatively occurs at dark moon, at the same time as the most sacred ritual. (Power and Watts 322).

The most important Hadza ritual, the Epeme Dance, is a solemn affair carried out in total darkness on moonless nights. The men become sacred beings and dance, one by one, communicating with the women, who sing sacred accompaniment in a special whistling language reserved for this context. The men are secretive about what is going on and sit apart from the women and children. Despite this, the ritual emphasizes the shared interests of men and women, especially as parents of children. This ritual is considered indispensable for Hadza well-being. It may be interpreted as a recurring ceremonial reconciliation of men and women, and indeed all Hadza. Attendance is obligatory for all the camp's dwellers (Lee and Daly R394).

Adding to sexual tensions, the Hadza also appear to have partially adopted both male and female circumcision from neighbouring tribes on their periphery although this is disputed:

Bagshawe (1925) said the old men and women circumcised boys and girls but no ritual was involved and he felt the practice had only recently been adopted from neighboring tribes. Based on my interviews, I suspect he was right. Linguist Dorothea Bleek (1931) visited the Hadza in 1930 and said that unlike other tribes, circumcision was unknown to the Hadza. Hadza men are not circumcised today and only a certain unknown fraction of women are. Given all these differences, it appears there may have been more influence from Isanzu then than now, at least along the margins of Hadza country. (Marlowe R430)

Hadza men and women are differentiated in religious contexts. Men are initiated into an egalitarian community of men which has privileged rights over certain portions of the best meat or most game animals. Initiated men meet on their own and have secrets from women and children. Men are liable to respond violently to perceived encroachment on their secret activities. Women too have secrets from men. Female circumcision, in which the men have little interest, is organized by the women alone, and is seen as a matter entirely for women. After the operation, the newly circumcised young women chase after and violently attack the men, especially their potential husbands, with specially deco- rated staves. There are at present some indications that Hadza women may, on their own initiative, soon decide to give up circumcision (R394).

Peggy Reeves Sanday (R596) notes the sexual tension involved:

"The sexual segregation and taboos restricting the activities of Hadza men and women during the dry season may well be the means by which the Hadza handle their perception that the odds are stacked against them, that their lives are at the mercy of random blows inflicted by nature. We can only speculate why people handle their fear at such times by separating the sexes and deeming menstrual blood powerful and dangerous. To many peoples, blood means the source of life and the signal of death. A people's experience with blood must be more negative than positive when their lives are threatened by starvation, thirst, or by the hungry animals they hunt. Little information exists on the mortality rate of hunters. If, as in warfare, hunters risk death, then they must be extraordinarily cautious. A hunter who has had recent contact with a menstruating woman possibly carries the smell with him, warning the animals of his presence. Unfortunately, we have little information on how hunted animals are affected by the smell of menstrual blood. Restrictions separating the sexes are more elaborate in concentrated settlements. When humans congregate in larger settlements, the smell of menstrual blood must be more obvious. It is a frightening smell because it is reminiscent of death. Being a fluid that flows from the body, menstrual blood is like the fluid that drains from the newly dead. Both types of fluids represent the loss of a vital essence. The more people experience death in nature, the more likely they are to view menstrual blood as dangerous. Such a response to menstrual blood is illogical, because blood in women signals their readiness to bear life, whereas the blood drawn by hunters signals death. However, by killing animals, men also bring life in the form of animal protein - a food with a high prestige value wherever men hunt. If the blood that flows from women can only be equated with life, then why is it so often equated with danger? Perhaps the answer lies in a rather simple proposition. If blood is associated with life and death in the experience of males, a balance is achieved by associating female blood with life and danger. If humans do strive to achieve such a balance, we would expect, to the extent that men have more experience with blood and death, that the blood of women would be endowed with corresponding connotations."

Ashanti: Sexually-balanced Separation

Ashanti carved box (www).

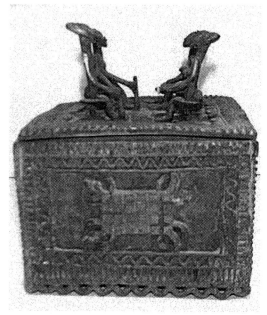

*Mawu, the female principle, is fertility,
motherhood, gentleness, forgiveness;
while Lisa is power,
war-like or otherwise,
strength and toughness.
Moreover, they assure the rhythm
of day and night.
Mawu is the night, the moon,
freshness, rest, joy;
Lisa is the day, the sun,
heat, labour, all hard things.
By presenting their two natures
alternately to men,
the divine pair impress on man
the rhythm of life and the two series
of complementary elements
of which its fabric is woven.
The notion of twin beings . . .
expresses the equilibrium
between opposites,
which is the very nature of the world.
Dahomean Mawu-Lisa cult.*

In many societies male leadership is balanced by female authority. Among the Ashanti, Iroquois, and Dahomeans, though women were not as visible as men in external public affairs, their right to veto male actions formed checks and balances in which neither sex would dominate the other. We thus have defined sex roles and separate spheres of influence and power, but these do not automatically result in male dominance.

The Ashanti, one of the great West African Kingdoms, convey the essential outlines of the segregated-but-equal sex-role plan (Sanday R596 27). The Ashanti were polygynous, matrilineal and avunclocal or virilocal, that is daughters move in with their husbands family, but this actually means the family of the husband's maternal uncle, because sons are expected to live in the household of their mother's brother. This is a common pattern in matrilineal societies, as it brings the adult male members of a matrilineage into a single residential unit. Both men and women could own land but a women could inherit only from a woman and a man from a man (Low R416 203). Ashanti wives occupied separate quarters.

Ashanti society was divided into a number of chiefdoms composed of eight dispersed matriclans, recognizing a remote common ancestress. At the apex is the king, the *Asantehene*, with his court. Clustered around are a group of Ashanti chiefdoms, each a largely autonomous unit that, in major outline, reproduced the higher jurisdiction of the king but owed allegiance to the unity of the state. Each chief had a council of hereditary advisers or elders, and succession to chiefly office (like succession to the title of king) was inherited through the female line. The unity of the new empire was symbolized in the Golden Stool which, being without past, was regarded as having descended from the sky and contains the soul of the Ashanti nation, the people's power, health, bravery, and welfare (Sanday R596 28).

Everyday life was organized around the group of related men and women lining in village or township wards. These groups, called localized lineages, trace their descent through females. Each has a male head, who is often one of the chiefs councillors. He is chosen by the consensus of the older men and women and with their assistance is responsible for the welfare of the entire group. In lineage affairs there is a "high degree of equality between male and female members." The lineage head is assisted by a senior woman informally chosen by him and his elders. This is extended to the kingdom as a whole and to each chiefdom. The senior woman of the royal lineage is the Queen Mother. She has her own stool, which is senior to the chief's stool. Traditionally, the Queen Mother has had the most to say in selecting a new chief or king. No one can be put upon the stool who is vetoed by the queen and her veto cannot be overruled. After the chief or king is 'enstooled,' he sits down on the right of Queen Mother to receive the homage and oaths of allegiance of the assembled subchiefs or chiefs. As long as he is in power, Queen Mother's place is on his left hand. Pre-menopausal women were barred from war, but Ashanti queens might accompany an army to war if they were post-menopausal (Sanday). Others assumed responsibility for civil government in the absence of the king on a military campaign. Each queen mother had the right to choose the king's senior wife, or replace her if she died. The queen mother thus had direct political power, and influence over coalition formation. The classic study of the Ashanti states the recognized seniority of the woman's stool is no empty courtesy title. But for two causes, [the physical inferiority of women, menstruation and ritual avoidance] the stool occupied by the male night not be in existence at all" (Low R416 203).

Today, in addition to her power to select a king when the stool is vacant, the senior Queen Mother controls all the Queen Mothers of Asante. The Ashanti regard for women comes from their idea that the lineage - and the clan that incorporates several lineages - is synonymous with blood, and that only women can transmit blood to descendants. A man cannot transmit blood, and so no Ashanti can have a drop of the male parent's blood in his or her veins. Males transmit *ntoro*, meaning soul or spirit. The Ashanti trace blood through the female line alone, because of the blood observed at menstruation and child-birth. It is agreed that a male has blood in his body, but he does not transmit it to his offspring. People say that if a male transmitted his blood through his penis he could not beget a child. The word ntoro is sometimes used to mean semen.

Ashanti women are definite about their own importance. They say: "I am the mother of the man ... I alone can transmit the blood to a king ... If my sex die in the clan then that very clan becomes extinct, for be there one, or one thousand male members left, not one can transmit the blood, and the life of the clan becomes measured on this earth by the span of a man's life". As the Queen put it: "We in Ashanti here have a law which decrees that it is the daughters of a Queen who alone can transmit royal blood, and that the children of a king cannot be heirs to that stool. This law has given us women a power in this land so that we have a saying which runs: 'It is the woman who bears the man' (i.e., the king)".

The importance of women is also seen in Ashanti religion and ritual. Priestesses partici-pate with priests in all major rituals. Sky and Earth are the two great deities. The Ashanti creation story emphasizes the complementarity of male and female and of sky and earth: It is said that a very long time ago one man and one woman came down from the sky and one man and one woman came up from the earth. From the sky also came a python who made its home in a river. The first men and women did not bear children, they had no desire, and conception and birth were not known at that time. The python, on learning that the couples had no offspring, bade them to stand face to face and plunging into the river he rose up and sprayed water on their bellies and then ordered them to return home and lie together. The women then conceived and brought forth the first children into the world. These children took the spirit of the river where the Python lived as their clan spirit. Members of that clan hold the python as taboo; they must never kill it, and if they find a python that has died or been killed by someone else, they put white clay on it and bury it human fashion.

Asase Ya, the name of the Earth Goddess, means 'the soil, the earth', but not what grows or stands on it. People say: 'We got everything from Asase Ya, food, water; we rest upon her when we die . . . every one must pass into the earth's wallet'. Just as the sky is believed to be the source of the Golden Stool, the symbol of the Ashanti confederacy, the earth is believed to have been the source of the aristocracy of the Ashanti clans. On Thursdays, the day set aside for the observance of 'Old Mother Earth', the Ashanti farmer will not break soil. In the past, infringement of this rule was punishable by death (Sanday R596 31).

Female power among the Ashanti, as among the Iroquois, is associated with a ritual orien-tation to plants, the earth, and fertility. Like the !Kung, the Ashanti also equate menstrua-tion and childbirth with hunting and warfare, emphasizing the complementarity of female reproductive functions and male activities considered vital to social survival. This kind of orientation, together with the belief that the child is formed from the mother's blood, gives Ashanti women power and authority in everyday affairs. Like the !Kung, it is said that some Ashanti originated from the earth. The earth is believed to be filled with the spirits of the departed forbearers of the clan. These spirits are thought to be the real landowners, who still continue to take a lively interest in the land from which they had their origin or that they once owned.

The Golden Stool (the male symbol of leadership), which is believed to have originated from the sky, cannot come into direct contact with the earth; it is always placed upon an elephant's skin. The feet of the king of Ashanti can never touch the ground, "lest a great famine should come upon the nation."

There is a sacred grove in a forest that is marked as the most hallowed spot in all Ashanti territory. At this spot, it is said, some clan forbearers belonging to certain ruling clans came forth from the ground, and settling near by, increased and multiplied, learned to use fire and other arts, till eventually, compelled by increasing numbers, they scattered and became the clan or 'blood' from which the rulers of the united nation later chose their kings and queens (Sanday R596 116). This is notably similar to the !Kung myth and it has been suggested that the Ashanti adopted the beliefs of a more ancient people when they migrated into the area which is also littered with ancient remains. Again like the !Kung they specifically equate menstruation with hunting the prize animal - "the Bara state has stricken her. She has killed an elephant." and childbearing with being a warrior. This is an occasion for elaborate ceremonials and exchange of gifts. A mother's first act, upon learn-ing the news from her daughter, is to inform the villagers, the Sky God, the Earth Goddess, and the ancestors. Taking some wine and spilling it on the ground, the mother says:

> *"Supreme Sky God, who is alone great, upon whom men lean and do not fall,*
> *receive this wine and drink.*
> *Earth Goddess, whose day of worship is a Thursday, receive this wine and drink.*
> *Spirit of our ancestors, receive this wine and drink.*
> *This girl child whom God has given to me, to-day the Bara state has come upon her.*

0 mother who dwells in the land of ghosts, do not come and take her away
and do not have permitted her to menstruate only to die" (Sanday 94).

Although the blood denotes the possibility of life, it also reminds people of death. The advent of puberty means that the child of a departed ancestor will soon die in order to be reborn into the world of the living. People say, "A birth in this world is a death in the world of ghosts." Menstrual blood implies power, and there are many taboos in connection with ii. During the puberty ceremonial, a girl is taken to the river, where she is disrobed and immersed three times with the words: "We quench the bara fire at its source". Again like the !Kung menstruation evokes supernatural danger. Menstrual blood is thought to nullify all supernatural powers possessed by persons, spirits, or objects. These powers, if rendered inactive by contact with a menstruating woman, have to be "recharged, as it were, by propitiation, extirpation, and augmentation rites, to placate them and build them up anew."

If a woman dies during childbirth, she is treated like a warrior who has lost an important battle. A ceremony is conducted that only pregnant women attend. The goal of the ceremony seems to be to chastise the woman who has died, and hence has failed in her primary duty, and to prevent other such failures. They feign shooting the evil and holding knives say: "We told you to fight but you could not fight, when our turn comes to fight we swear the oath we shall not pass out." Thus, the Ashanti impose hunter and warrior imagery on female reproductive functions. By phrasing the natural rhythms of life giving and life taking in the same terms, the Ashanti establish a symmetry between male and female.

The Ashanti were considered extreme enemies of Islam. They had a taboo against male and female circumcision, and no one could become elected as a chief if their skin were cut. Divorce was permissable if either party was a thief or insults kin, the husband was impotent or infertile, or the wife was quarrelsome or practised witchcraft, and was frequent, even among established relationships, because of conflicts of loyalty to partners and children (Broude R82 72). Incestuous sexual intimacy between brother and sister is strongly denounced, partly because it undermines the kinship of matrilineal descent through sisters (R82 149). They did however negotiate promissory marriages and had symbolically dire penalties for anyone caught in adultery with the chiefs wives (Low R416 49):

"the culprit through whose cheeks a sepow knife has already been thrust is taken ... the nasal septum is now pierced and through the aperture is threaded a thorny creeper ... by which he is led about . For other sepow knives are now thrust through various parts of his body, care being taken not to press them so deeply as to wound any vital spot. He is no led by the rope creeper ... to Akyermade where the chief of that stool would scrape his leg , facetiously remarking as he did so ... 'I am scraping perfume for my wives' next to the house of the Chief of Asafo where his left ear is cut off thence to Bantama where the Ashanti generalissimo scrapes bare the right bone. ... then he was made to dance all day after dark his arms were cut off at the elbows and his legs at the knee he was ordered to continue dancing but since he couldn't his buttock flesh was cut off and he was set on a pile of gunpowder which was then set alight Eventually the chief gave permission to cut off the offender's head".

Dogon: Male Dominion by Primal Violence

The Dogon of Mali illustrate how sexual identities become antagonistic when the sexual spheres become separated and patriarchal dominance is exerted in violence against the female in the name of social order. Their cosmology more than any other explains how control of the female and violence to her to maintain paternity certainty are the prime 'thrust' of patriarchal dominion.

The Dogon are a society of millet and onion farmers who reside in a system of stone canyons and plateaus on the southern edges of the Sahara, where temperatures are high and food, water, animals and plants are scarce. On their small fields they cultivate their staple diet stored in high quadrangular granaries around which they build their house. They possess an unusually complex and advanced cosmology, with intimate knowledge of the stars and planets, a numerical system, extensive physiological and anatomical knowledge, genetics and a systematic pharmacopoeia. (Griaule and Dieterlen R263 57). They believe that the star Sirius is a binary system, with a smaller counterpart, invisible to the naked eye, orbiting it. This was recorded in 1931, 40 years before the existence of Sirius B was confirmed with telescopic photography for the first time, and 6 years before the first Christian missionaries made contact with them. Their mythology includes Saturn's rings, and Jupiter's four major moons and a knowledge that planets orbit the sun.

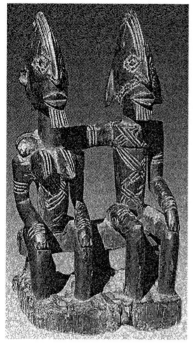

Dogon primordial couple (www)

The Dogon claim they were part of the ancient Mandingo empire of Keita, (10th - 13th cent.) which dominated a greater part of West Africa. They emigrated from the west bank of the Niger River to northern Burkino Faso, where local histories describe them as *kibsi*. Around 1490, they fled a region now known as the northern Mossi kingdom of Yatenga when it was invaded by Mossi Islamic authority calvary. They ended up in the Bandiagara cliffs region, safe from the approaching horsemen. Carbon-14 dating techniques used on excavated remains found in the cliffs suggest that there were inhabitants in the region before the arrival in the Dogon, dating back to the 10th century. They slowly absorbed this Tellem culture who became part of their mythology.

Although unusual for Africa, a continent with many matrilineal societies, their classically patriarchal family system, endorsing polygyny, with patrilocal residence, patrilineal inheritance, and male-biased institutions, including preferential inheritance of property by sons has many parallels with societies in Asia and, to a lesser extent, the Western world.

Sarah Hrdy (R323 254) and Meredith Small (R634) describe various aspects of Beverly Strassmann's discoveries (R657 - R659):

Polygyny among the Dogon—as in other patriarchal societies—occurs hand in hand with various means of monitoring female sexuality. Countering millions of years of evolution, the Dogon have become a culture where ovulation cannot be concealed. Each woman's menstrual cycle is open to public scrutiny. By custom, as soon as she detects bleeding, a woman must relocate to a special hut, as documented in about 2 percent of tribal societies.

The menstrual huts are situated outside the walled compounds of the village, but in full view of the men's thatched-roof shelters. As the men relax under their shelters, they can readily see who leaves the huts in the morning and returns to them in the evening. And as non-menstruating women pass the huts on their way to and from the fields or to other compounds, they too can see who is spending the night there. Failure to comply with the rules, especially cheating (pretending to menstruate when a woman is actually pregnant), brings social reprisals in the real world, and the prospect of worse punishments in the supernatural one. In this way, a man can be confident that any woman he marries is not already pregnant by another man. The huts are cramped, dark buildings - hardly places where a woman might go to escape the drudgery of work or to avoid an argument with her husband or a co-wife. The huts sometimes become so crowded that some occupants are forced outside - making the women even more conspicuous. Although small children can go with their mothers to the huts, they are not allowed to spend time with the rest of their families. Yet they are still expected to do their usual jobs, such as working in the fields.

The explanation is that a menstruating woman is a threat to the sanctity of religious altars, where men pray and make sacrifices for the protection of their fields, their families and their village. If menstruating women come near the altars, which are situated both indoors and outdoors, the Dogon believe that their aura of pollution will bring calamities upon the village. The belief is so ingrained that the women themselves have internalized it, feeling its burden of responsibility and potential guilt. Violations of the taboo are rare. A menstruating woman who breaks the rules knows that she is personally responsible if calamities occur.

However Beverly Strassmann who investigated their habits proposes the menstrual taboos are actually expressing a carefully defined reproductive protocol. She notes: "There are two important pieces of information for assessing paternity: timing of intercourse and timing of menstruation. By forcing women to signal menstruation, men are trying to gain equal access to one part of that critical information." Such information is crucial to Dogon men, because descent is marked through the male line; land and the food that comes from the land is passed down from fathers to sons. Information about paternity is thus crucial to a man's lineage. And because each man has as many as four wives, he cannot possibly track them all. So forcing women to signal their menstrual periods, or lack thereof, helps men avoid cuckoldry. When she leaves the hut, she is considered ready to conceive. When she stops going to the hut, she is evidently pregnant or menopausal. And women of prime reproductive age who visit the hut on a regular basis are clearly infertile.

The Dogon do use that information to make paternity decisions. In several cases a man was forced to marry a pregnant woman, simply because everyone knew that the man had been the woman's first sexual partner after her last visit to the menstrual hut. Strassmann followed one case in which a child was being brought up by a man because he was the mother's first sexual partner after a hut visit, even though the woman soon married a different man.

In addition to menstrual monitoring, ancient female incentives for confusing paternity are countered by removing each girl's clitoris. The Dogon take it for granted that after clitoridectomy a woman will find sexual intercourse outside marriage less tantalizing, not worth the risks. In this way, older men with several young wives can be as certain of paternity as any primates in the world—Dogon certain.

Dogon women mostly play by the rules. In 86% of the hormonally detected menstruations, women went to the hut. Moreover, none of the tested women went to the hut when they were not menstruating. In the remaining 14% of the tested menstruations, women stayed home from the hut, in violation of the taboo, but some were near menopause and so not at high risk for pregnancy. None of the women who violated the taboo did it twice in a row. Even they were largely willing to comply. In general, women are cooperative players in the game because without a man, a woman has no way to support herself or her children. But women follow the taboo reluctantly. They complain about going to the hut. And if their husbands convert from the traditional religion of the Dogon to one that does not impose menstrual taboos, such as Islam or Christianity, the women quickly cease visiting the hut.

Like the !Kung a woman in a natural-fertility population such as the Dogon has only about 110 menstrual periods in her lifetime. The rest of the time she will be pre-pubescent, pregnant, lactating or menopausal. Women in industrialized cultures, by contrast, have more than three times as many cycles: 350 to 400, on average, in a lifetime. Women spend most of their reproductive years in lactation amenorrhea, suppressing ovulation from nursing each child on demand. . Dogon women bear eight to nine children on average.

Does certainty of paternity ensure that Dogon men invest more in their children? Not necessarily, especially not if they have several wives and many sons. As in most patriarchal societies, a man's attention tends to be focused on gaining and maintaining prestige, with its corollary of more wives and more children.

Typical for this area, child mortality among the Dogon is very high. 46% will die before age five. What is more noteworthy, though, is that the chances of a child dying are 7 to 11 times higher if the mother is in a polygynous family, working together with and sharing meals with cowives, than if she is married monogamously. In a monogamous union, a mother's loss is equally the father's. But in the case of a man married to three wives, the polygynist comes out ahead reproductively even if more than half his children die.

Unlike a mother's goal, which is generally "quality," well-spaced, healthy offspring, each one well provided for, the Dogon's father's goal is "quantity"—as many children as he can have, even if many die. Among the Dogon, this is particularly unfortunate, because land is increasingly in short supply, and men can bequeath a homestead only to one select son, or to a couple of sons. Yet men have little incentive to take fewer wives. For women work hard. Owning them confers prestige, a higher standard of living, and reproductive success.

Dogon mothers claim that their sons are being poisoned by co-wives. Strassmann was invited to attend rituals at which masked dancers intimidate women to deter wives from such nefarious pursuits. Indeed, wild-sounding accusations about children poisoned by cowives can be extensively documented in Malian court records. Occasionally women actually confess to poisoning a rival's child. But why primarily sons? Because daughters leave home when they marry, and it is sons who are favored, and who remain at home to compete with their father's other sons for inheritances of scarce land.

Why don't wives married to the same man manage to cooperate more? In some societies, they do, especially if the husband marries sisters. Among Australian Aborigines, wise men often seek to marry wives who are related to each other precisely because such women are known to get along better. But among the Dogon, the benefits of reduced strife do not outweigh the benefits to the patriarch of discouraging his wives from forming alliances. The patriarch's strategy is to "divide and conquer." Strassmann notes that sisters and other related women are specifically prohibited from marrying into the same patriline. Such strictures make it hard to sustain the functionalist argument that these polygynous families are set up for the common good, with eugenic intent to promote the well-being of all concerned. In a world where the optimal number of fathers per child is pretty obviously at least one, not some fraction of one, most Dogon men still aspire to be polygynists.

In 'Conversations with Ogotemmeli' Marcel Griaule (R262) recounts a cosmological tale of sexual origins from the creator God and Mother Earth in which sexual antagonism leads to an order reinforced by male and particularly female circumcision at every stage. Despite being a type of joint creation including an androgynous primal couple, the entire cosmology is both sexual and confrontational. We can see frankly enshrined a root collision between male and female sexual and orgasmic capacity, and its 'cutting' out of the female to 'feminize' her in the (negative) image of man. At every stage this creation myth re-emphasizes the dominance and invincibility of the male in setting out the 'world order'.

Dogon mythology describes the creation of the universe in terms of contrasting motions. In his initial act of creation, the one God Amma, threw out the seed of the world, which radiated out in four directions forming the surface of the earth. The stars came from pellets of earth he flung out into space. He had created the sun and the moon by a more complicated process: the art of pottery.

The God Amma took a lump of clay, squeezed it in his hand and flung it from him, as he had done with the stars. The clay spread and fell on the north, which is the top, and from there stretched out to the south, which is the bottom, of the world. It extends east and west with separate members like a fetus in the womb. This body, lying flat, face upwards is feminine. Its sexual organ is an anthill, and its clitoris a termite hill. Amma, being lonely and desirous of intercourse with this creature, approached it. That was the occasion of the first breach of the order of the universe.

At God's approach the termite hill rose up, barring the passage and displaying its masculinity. It was as strong as the organ of the stranger, and intercourse could not take place. But God is all-powerful. In the primal act of female circumcision, he cut down the termite hill, and had intercourse with the excised earth. But the original incident was destined to affect the course of things for ever; from this defective union there was born, instead of the intended twins, a single being, the pale fox, or jackal, symbol of the difficulties of God.

God had further intercourse with his earth-wife, and this time without mishaps, the excision of the offending member having removed the cause of the disorder. Water, which is the divine seed, was thus able to enter the womb of the earth and the normal reproductive cycle resulted in the birth of twins. Two beings were thus formed. God created them like water. They were green in colour, half human beings and half serpents. From the head to the loins they were human: below that they were serpents. Their red eyes were wide open like human eyes, and their tongues were forked like the tongues of reptiles. Their arms were flexible and without joints. Their bodies were green and sleek all over, shining like the surface of water, and covered with short green hairs, a presage of vegetation and germination.

These spirits, called Nummo, were of divine essence like himself, and developed normally in the womb of the earth. They are androgynous couples who each embody the proper balance of the sexes. Their destiny took them to Heaven, where they received the instructions of their father. They were of the essence of God, made of his seed, which is at once the form, and substance of the life-force of the world, from which derives the motion and the persistence of created being. This force is water, and the Pair are present in all water: the water of the seas, of coasts, of torrents, of storms, and of the spoonfuls we drink.

The Nummo, looking down from Heaven, saw their mother, the earth, naked and speechless, as a consequence of the original incident in her relations with the God Amma. It was necessary to put an end to this state of disorder. The Nummo accordingly came down to earth, bringing with them fibres pulled from plants already created in the heavenly regions. The purpose of this garment was not merely modesty. It manifested on earth the first act in the ordering of the universe and the revelation of the helicoid sign in the form of an undulating broken line, for the fibres fell in coils, symbol of tornadoes, of the windings of torrents, of eddies and whirlwinds, of the undulating movement of reptiles. In these fibres full of water and words, placed over his mother's genitalia, Nummo is thus always present.

Thus clothed, the earth had a language. It was good; nevertheless from the start it let loose disorder. This was because the jackal, the deluded and deceitful son of God, an unnatural and socially disruptive creature born without placenta and thus robbed at birth of his female counterpart desired to possess speech, and laid hands on the fibres in which language was embodied, that is to say, on his mother's skirt. His mother, the earth, resisted this incestuous action. She buried herself in her own womb, that is to say, in the anthill, disguised as an ant. But the jackal followed her. There was, it should be explained, no other woman in the world whom he could desire. The hole which the earth made in the anthill was never deep enough, and in the end she had to admit defeat. The myths of the pale fox demonstrate the chaos resulting from this imbalance of male and female qualities. This prefigured the even-handed struggles between men and women, which, however, always end in the victory of the male.

The incestuous act was of great consequence. In the first place it endowed the jackal pale fox with the gift of speech so that ever afterwards he was able to reveal to diviners the designs of God. It was also the cause of the flow of menstrual blood, which stained the fibres. The resulting defilement of the earth was incompatible with the reign of God. God rejected that spouse, and decided to create living beings directly. Modeling a womb in damp clay, he placed it on the earth and covered it with a pellet flung out into space from heaven. He made a male organ in the same way and having put it on the ground, he flung out a sphere which stuck to it. The two lumps forthwith took organic shape; their life began to develop. Members separated from the central core, bodies appeared, and a human pair arose out of the lumps of earth.

At this point the Nummo Pair reappeared. The Spirit drew two outlines on the ground, one on top of the other, one male and the other female. The man stretched himself out on these two shadows of himself, and took both of them for his own. The same thing was done for the woman. Thus it came about that each human being from the first was endowed with two souls of different sex, or rather with two principles corresponding to two distinct persons. In the man the female soul was located in the prepuce; in the woman the male soul was in the clitoris. Man's life was not capable of supporting both beings: each person would have to merge himself in the sex for which he appeared to be best fitted. The Nummo accordingly circumcised the man, thus removing from him all the femininity of his prepuce. The prepuce, however, changed itself into an animal which is "neither- a serpent nor an insect, but is classed with serpents." This animal symbolized the pain of circumcision and the need for the man to suffer in his sex as the woman does.

The man then had intercourse with the woman, who later bore the first two children of a series of eight, who were to become the ancestors of the Dogon people. In the moment of birth the pain of parturition was concentrated in the woman's clitoris, which was excised by an invisible hand, detached itself and left her, and was changed into the form of a scorpion. The pouch and the sting symbolized the organ: the venom was the water and the blood of the pain. Dual souls were implanted in a new-born child by holding it by the thighs above the place of the drawings with its hands and feet touching the ground. Later the superfluous soul was eliminated by circumcision, and humanity limped towards its obscure destiny.

As if this surgical excision of the female identity were not enough the creation process continues with the complete take-over of Mother Earth by male identity. The divine thirst for perfection was not extinguished, and the Nummo Pair, who were gradually taking the place of God their father, had in mind projects of redemption. But, in order to improve human conditions, reforms and instruction had to be carried out on the human level. The Nummo were afraid of the terrifying effect of contact between creatures of flesh and blood on the one hand and purely spiritual beings on the other. There had to be actions that could be understood, taking place within the ambit of the beneficiaries and in their own environment. Men after regeneration must be drawn towards the ideal as a peasant is drawn to rich farmland. The Nummo accordingly came down to earth, and entered the anthill, that is to say, the sexual part of which they were themselves the issue.

In the fullness of time an obscure instinct led the eldest of the offspring of the primal pair towards the anthill which had been occupied by the Nummo. He wore on his head as headdress and to protect him from the sun, the wooden bowl he used for his food. He put his two feet into the opening of the anthill, that is of the earth's womb, and sank in slowly. The whole of him thus entered into the earth, and his head itself disappeared. But he left on the ground, as evidence of his passage into that world, the bowl which had caught on the edges of the opening. All that remained on the anthill was the round wooden bowl, still bearing traces of the food and the fingerprints of its vanished owner, symbol of his body and of his human nature, as, in the animal world, is the skin which a reptile has shed.

Liberated form his earthly condition, the ancestor was taken in charge by the regenerating Pair. The male Nummo led him into the depths of the earth, where, in the waters of the womb of his partner he curled himself up like a fetus and shrank to germinal form, and acquired the quality of water, the seed of god and the essence of the two Spirits. And all this process was the work of the Word. The male with his voice accompanied the female Nummo who was speaking to herself and to her own sex. The spoken Word entered into her and wound itself round her womb in a spiral of eight turns. Just as the helical band of copper round the sun gives to it its daily movement, so the spiral of the Word gave to the womb its regenerative movement. Thus perfected by water and words, the new Spirit was expelled and went up to Heaven.

All the eight ancestors in succession had to undergo this process of transformation; but, when the turn of the seventh ancestor came, the change was the occasion of a notable occurrence. The seventh in a series, it must be remembered, represents perfection. Though equal in quality with the others, he is the sum of the feminine element, which is four, and the masculine element, which is three. He is thus the completion of the perfect series, symbol of the total union of male and female, that is to say of unity. And to this homogeneous whole belongs especially the mastery of words, this is, of language; and the appearance on earth of such a one was bound to be the prelude to revolutionary developments of a beneficent character. What the seventh ancestor had received was the perfect knowledge of a Word-the second Word to be heard on earth, clearer than the first, destined for all mankind. Thus he was able to achieve progress for the world. In particular, he enabled mankind to take precedence over God's wicked son, the jackal. In the future order of things he was to be merely a laggard in the process of revelation.

The potent second Word developed the powers of its new possessor. Gradually he came to regard his regeneration in the womb of the earth as equivalent to its capture and occupation, and little by little he took possession of the whole organism, making such use of it as suited him for the purpose of his activities. His lips began to merge with the edges of the anthill, which widened and became a mouth. Pointed teeth made their appearance, seven for each lip, then ten, the number of the fingers, later forty, and finally eighty, ten for each ancestor in a kind of vagina dentata of genealogy.

These numbers indicated the future rates of increase of the families; the appearance of the teeth was a sign that the time for new instruction was drawing near. But here again the scruples of the Spirits made themselves felt. It was not directly to men, but to the ant, avatar of the earth and native to the locality, that the seventh ancestor imparted instruction. At sunrise on the appointed day the seventh ancestor Spirit spat out eighty threads of cotton; these he distributed between his upper teeth which acted as the teeth of a weaver's reed. In this way he made the uneven threads of a warp. He did the same with the lower teeth to make the even threads. By opening and shutting his jaws the Spirit caused the threads of the warp to make the movements required in weaving. His whole face took part in the work, his nose studs serving as the block, while the stud in his lower lip was the shuttle. As the threads crossed and uncrossed, the two tips of the Spirit's forked tongue pushed the thread of the weft to and fro, and the web took shape from his mouth in the breath of the second revealed Word. By so doing he showed the identity of material actions and spiritual forces, or rather the need for their co-operation.

Consistent with this stark division between the sexes, the Dogon divide their community into two opposed categories: living or pure man, and impure or dead man. The Hogon, the most important village chief, is leader of the pure men, while the Olubaru, the highest official of the Awa society, is leader of the impure men. The Awa society assumes control during the ceremonial period, while the Hogon is the leader of the community during the rest of the year and assumes ritual duties at the time of agricultural rites. The impure perform rituals associated with death, such as the preparation and burial of the corpse, the sacrifice and eating of sacrificial animals, and the construction and maintenance of the menstrual huts.

Female Power and Male Dominance

In 'Female Power and Male Dominance' Peggy Reeves Sanday (R596) analyzed over 100 societies seeking the causative or contributory factors leading to male dominance. She examined societies both from their creation mythologies and actual social patterns. She divides societies in three types, 'equal' where women and men shared power and there was little or no aggression or suppression, 'mythically dominant' where there was male aggression in the presence of female economic or political power, and 'unequal' where males were both mythically and practically dominant (R596 164). Dominance was expressed in both exclusion of women from political and economic decision making and male aggression against women in several forms: the ideal that males should be tough, brave and aggressive, the existence of exclusive men's houses or spaces, frequent quarreling fighting or wife beating, institutionalization or regular occurrence of rape and raiding other groups for wives. She cites a variety of anthropological theories for male dominance giving some validity to each of them and then developing a theory of her own which is a form of the prisoner's dilemma polarization.

Marvin Harris has suggested imbalance between protein sources and population density leads to male dominance. This has several suggested manifestations. Female infanticide ensues to produce hunters and warriors to compete for the available protein supplies. This slows population but causes a shortage of marriageable women requiring men to take them from hostile groups. Polygyny, the mark of a successful and powerful hunter and warrior exacerbates the shortage. Male supremacist institutions arise as a by-product of warfare, male monopoly over weapons, and the use of sex to nurture aggressive male personalities. There is some debate about this issue. Sanday (R596 45) claims the Yanomamo have a protein deficiency with 85% of the diet from plant sources, noting they have a specific word for craving meat. However this proportion for gathering is similar to the !Kung diet and although the !Kung hunt with lethal weapons war is unknown. Chagnon (R110 94) has this to say: "The most prominent champion of the protein theory is an anthropologist named Marvin Harris. We disagree a good deal and have 'debated' the protein issue publicly on a number of campuses. The argument began when I cautioned the protein-deficiency advocates that the Yanomamo did not suffer from a protein shortage and that their warfare (and the warfare in any group) was too complex to reduce to a single variable."

Charted results from Sanday (R596) indicate that sexually equal societies are likely to be aboriginal and peaceful while migratory and warlike societies are likely to be mythically or materially male dominant. A constant food supply also favours equality while stress from erratic food supply is associated with male dominance. The form of the society is also reflected in its creation myths with mythical or actually male dominates societies having male creation mythologies unlike sexually equal societies. Joint creations are not necessarily indicative of equal societies. Extremely warlike patriarchal societies such as the Yanomamo and Jivaro use joint creations specifically to portray sexual antagonism.

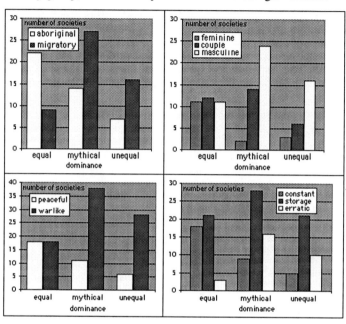

Ernestine Friedl (R223) suggests that men have greater control than women over the extra-domestic distribution and exchange because of the male monopoly on hunting large game. Among shifting agriculturalists this becomes male monopoly on clearing land and its cultivation. Warfare then becomes the domain of males because they are the expendable sex in reproductive terms. There is also some evidence to support this as a contributory factor.

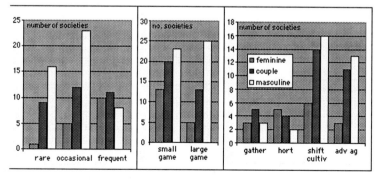

Rare and occasional parental care of young children is associated with male creation myths, hunting especially of large game and shifting cultivation and advanced agriculture are likewise, while gathering and horticulture are associated with balanced or feminine creation myths.

Martin and Voorhies (R436) deduce that paternal descent and residence rules are adaptive where resources are scarce or where populations have been subjugated by patrilineal invaders. Matrilineal and matrilocal patterns are accommodating and integrative while patrilineal ones acquisitive and internally divisive. There is also evidence for this factor both in the social forms equal and unequal of these differing residence and lineage patterns and in the fact that matrilineal and matrilocal societies have become rarer over time, having been displaced by more aggressive patrilineal and patrilocal systems.

Hrdy (R323 252) states: "Such matrilineal arrangements are fragile, and they quickly disappear after contact with patrilineal herders, agriculturalists, or wage economies. A mid-twentieth-century survey revealed 15 percent of the world's cultures were matrilineal, and they were becoming scarcer." Hrdy notes that 70 percent of human societies were living in male philopatric arrangements. About two-thirds of these patrilocal societies have patrilineal descent groups, and most are polygynous and founded on paternity certainty at the expense of female choice. "Elaborate modes of socialization, rituals, and whole mythologies have grown up to endorse male control over the inconvenient sexual legacy that women inherited from their primate predecessors". Low (R416 223) likewise associates the male inter-group violence occurring in 60% of human societies with primate raiding parties (p 148).

However, unlike the matriarchal origins of Bachofen and the hopes of some feminist authors, genetic studies on the Y-chromosome and mitochondrial mtDNA distributions (Seielstad et. al. R620) indicate that human societies have been predominantly patrilocal with moderate polygyny throughout human emergence with an eight times higher rate of female migration overall. Thus while more extreme forms of patriarchal dominion have definitely emerged, human sociobiology over the last 100,000 years appears to have been similar to ape societies rather than like many monkeys and other mammals in which related females reside together.

Matrilocal and matrilineal societies each tend to be more equal then patrilineal and patrilocal societies, which tend strongly to mythical or actual male dominance.

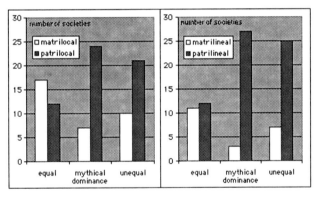

This picture was further refined and a more complicated picture emerged with the work of Giovanni Destro-Bisol and Gabriella Spedini three years later (New Scientist 7 Feb 2004 40-42). In this study gatherer-hunter societies tended to have higher male migration, possibly associated with greater male mobility in the division of labour, and agricultural populations had more female mobility possibly associated with the rise of agricultural patriarchy. Large spreads of male Y-chromosomes were also associated with the Batu migrations although these would have also been accompanied by women. There were clear signs of Y-migration into pygmy populations where we know there has been cultural adaption. Conversely there is an outward flow of female mtDNA from Pygmy to Bantu, reflected in a low bride price and a reputation for high fertility, but higher-class Bantu women did not 'marry down' in the other direction. Western Biaka have 62% of a Bantu Y-mutation called M2 coinciding with the beginning of the Bantu migrations. By contrast a much lower Y-influx has occurred in the !Kung who do not traditionally intermarry with Bantu. The Pygmy Y-inflow may have been caused by affairs with Bantu men, pygmy women returning after divorces, or adopting mixed marriage offspring. Destro-Bisol sees agriculture as being responsible for a traditions from cultures which buffered genetic underpinnings allowing adaption to diverse environments, to "the driving factor for establishment of more complex societies with social inequalities within and between populations".

Sherry Ortner (R506) describes women as associated with nature and life while men's role is driven in compensation to take up the projects of culture. Lacking creative functions man must assert his creativity externally. Simone de Beauvoir notes: "It is not in giving life but in risking life that man is raised above the animal; that is why superiority has been accorded in humanity not to the sex which brings forth but to that which kills." John and Beatrice Whiting take a more psychological point of view in the male need to break a primary identity with powerful women particularly when expressed primarily in the domestic sphere in a way which later can be rejected when a young male finds differing realities in the wider world. Margaret Mead notes the difficulty of striking a balance between the need to reproduce and overpopulaion and that different reactions to population stress involve rejection of powers of fecundity for example in a fixed circut of energy, male only fertilization powers.

These views can be readily combined into a pespective where males are more vulnerable to their feelings of mortality because they do not themselves give birth to new life, they are also fearful and uncertain of their paternity by contrast with the certainty a female has, and they are naturally in sociobiological terms the competitive sex who risks life to reproduce and who throughout the mammalian evolution has sought to jealously guard mates and female resources as a means to secure reproductive advantage.

Peggy Reeves Sanday (R596) takes up Mary Douglas' (R172) idea that patriarchal dominance is part of a people's response to stress. She notes however that adaption to stress does not always involve the subjugation of women. Where there is cooperative immersion in nature and the feminization principle male dominance is unlikely. She thus articulates a two stage process leading from aboriginal cooperative societies to male dominance in which the cultural configuration first enters a divergence of sex-role plans into a dual-sex configuration such as we have seen in the Ashanti, the stage is set for mythical male dominance when competition under stress drives the separate complementary spheres into a symmetry-breaking into dominance. This two-step evolution is really a presentation of the prisoners dilemma and its bifurcation between cooperation as a feminine strategy and competition to the point of violent defection as a masculine strategy.

There are further sociobiological interpretations of this process which are also consistent with the above interpretations but lead to a more historically realistic description of how major societies including our own cultural tradition have entered a major epoch of male dominion. In sexual selection there is always a counterpoint between female reproductive choice and male competition and mate guarding. The exact balance varies from species to species with a degree of genetic conflict from example between hierarchies of male chimps who practice infanticide and raids on other groups and loose female coalitions who in the case of bonobos have managed to achieve a relatively high degree of female power.

It is easy to see that the first migrations of homo sapiens were into niches not previously occupied by modern humans, and only sometimes by relatives such as Neanderthal and so there was initially little need for inter-group competition and stress between modern humans. Populations could also gravitate to regions where the food supply was relatively constant and plentiful. However once modern human populations spread widely, the niche opens for a more predatory type of male-dominating culture to take selective advantage, based on male coalitions, warfare, abduction of females and rapid population growth fuelled by resource exploitation. Such societies would be associated with migration, war, food stress caused by ecological instability, patrilineal inheritance, patrilocal residence, drives for increased population rather than attempts to balance fertility and male domination of females. Viewed in this way the emergence of male dominance is as natural as the emergence of carnivores, but its also raises serious questions of ecological stability of the human species if the population of predatorial societies begins to exceed that of the 'hosts'.

These processes can become profoundly amplified by technological changes such as the transition from gathering to horticulture espoused predominantly by women through to large-scale plow agriculture dominated by men, and a parallel transition from hunting through to shepherding and animal husbandry again male dominated. Major inventions such as metallurgy, the wheel and the domestication of the horse not only transformed society in peace time but gave huge new opportunities for migratory warfare. New types of society evolved in which several of these motifs come together such as the liaison between planter queens and shepherd kings in Sumeria portrayed in the tale of Inanna and Dumuzi (p 180).

Sexual Paradox and Cultural Sustainability

The evidence is that the sexes have complementary evolutionary strategies, the male based on competition, by dominant rank or subterfuge, exploitation of reproductive advantage, even at risk of death, exponentiation of resources to provide unbounded reproductive opportunity, and maximum investment in the current opportunity, without necessarily providing long-term. By contrast the female investment is more out-front, honest and massive over time, seeking to spread the benefits over all offspring in a way which conserves scarce resources in a way which is sustainable over time. By being closer to the immortal flow of life in the cytoplasmic continuity of the birth process the female is also more liable to make a cross-generational investment than the male who does not reproduce directly and lives in mortal fear of cuckolding.

No one who would question the idea that sexual paradox has been the evolutionary driving force for our linguistic articulacy, diverse crafts and skills, abstract reasoning and technology can deny that sexual relationship is the dominant theme in spoken fable, written literature, music and song, now winging the 'air-waves' of radio and television throughout human culture (p 349). Without it, mass media and popular literature, and the trappings we associate with 'culture' would atrophy, if not collapse. This view is central to all social theories of the evolution of intelligence through the dissonance between trustworthiness and deceit, the subtleties of detecting and concealing deceit and the complexity of the social 'grapevine'. Notably gatherer-hunters such as the !Kung spend long evenings discussing their sexual and emotional relationships and the resulting stresses, often through to the dawn.

Acknowledging our sociobiological roots does not mean conceding society and culture are biologically determined, but simply that biology cannot fail to contribute its heritage, subtle or frank, to the form of society and culture. Any culture which ignores, or rejects, its biological foundations will experience dissonance or repression. To ignore such factors will mean that they play out their effects in less constructive ways, despite social taboos. To repress them will result in tyranny and human misery. However in acknowledging and taking advantage of our biological roots, we may not only come to a point of genuine personal and cultural freedom of expression, but also gain the capacity to enjoy a sustainable evolutionary future. Neither does a complementary view of gender divide the sexes, for the feminine is present in both men and women, as the small spots in the yin-yang symbol of the Tao attest.

The evidence from both primate and human gatherer-hunter societies shows that the patrilocal kinship common to apes does not automatically lead to a cultural emergence based on patriarchal dominance, or women being treated as commodities. Male dominance may arise rather through cultural stress and the development of patterns of social predation. At issue in our view of gender and culture is not whether individual women have better innate ecological sustainability than men, because survival of the species depends ultimately on both, but the more subtle question of the survival value of the complete human reproductive strategy, with the feminine playing a full and pivotal part as a complementary contributor to the male, in conceiving and forming whole sustainable societies. Repression of the reproductive protocols of an entire sex in a society could thus have potentially disastrous consequences.

It behooves us to consider whether current ideals of partnership involving a division between the illusion of strict monogamy and images of sexual attraction based on the heroic fantasy of a 'rebel without a cause' serve the creative needs of human cultural evolution. It is not clear the ideal of the delinquent 'he-man' portrayed on the media serves reproductive interests of women, in a society of increasingly single-parent and dysfunctional families. A non-violent society of 'conjugal bliss' follows only from a more open and honest approach to sexuality and our biological roots, in which women are able and encouraged to make good choices which abet the best in male resourceful defence and support of the family, agreeableness, humour, affection, and all the features of artistry and skill the 'good hunter' can provide, as Geoffrey Miller (R464) suggests (p 53). Moreover this needs to happen with some respect, and room for, female reproductive choice to occur, in all its gambits, from established long-term partnership, to more secretive affairs, along with a reasonable degree of ethical compassion on the part of men towards supporting, with love, those offspring who are not their own children, without stripping bare all the devices of sexual selection, through genetic testing and paternity suits.

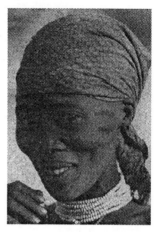

NISA (redrawn from Shostak R626)

We have to lay at Adam's feet, in the spermatogenic evolutionary strategy, responsibility for all the unstable features of competitive and exploitative instability society is displaying. Instability which compromises our future viability and sustainability - an endlessly exponentiating relentless industrializtion, extinction-risking boom and bust economics, winner-take-all exploitation of natural and non-renewable resources, population crisis, environmental impacts which are never addressed until the damage is possibly irreversible, and the devastation of a billion years of evolutionary diversity. The use of controlled violence combined with reproductive competition has led to war, atrocity and genocide as well as the development of industrial civilization and post-modern culture. These features began with the patriarchal dominion of large city states, exacerbated by patriarchal religious leaders who insist on the male right to reproduce as well as man's dominion over nature. They have resulted in war and genocide to the point of final end-game 'solutions' such as sheol and the nuclear madness of mutually assured destruction. For this reason it is necessary to exorcise the doctrine of original sin which has cursed Eve throughout the history of patriarchal monotheism.

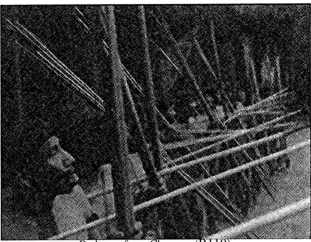
Redrawn from Chagnon (R110)

Sexual Polarization in Warrior Cultures

We now examine a spectrum of societies from the greater Amazon to see sexual relations in dynamic evolution, particularly in the context of warrior conflict and violence, but also in terms of partible paternity and matrilineal sexual relations and parenting. These show interesting features relevant to understanding similar divergences between matriliny and patriliny in the emergence of urban cultures central to human history.

Carol Ember (R189 - R191) has calculated that 90 percent of hunter-gatherer societies are known to engage in warfare, and 64 percent wage war at least once every two years. W. T. Divale (R168), investigated 99 groups of hunter-gatherers from 37 cultures, and found that 68 were at war at the time, 20 had been at war five to twenty-five years before, and all the others reported warfare in the more distant past (Pinker R532 57). Donald Brown (R83) thus includes conflict, rape, revenge, jealousy, dominance, and male coalitional violence as human universals . Most attacks in traditional societies are ambush attacks, often well coordinated to take advantage of the element of surprise, and often with numerical superiority. A description of such attacks would differ little from the description of a male chimpanzee raid (Low R416 223).

Amazonian Indian societies, including the Yanomamo and Jivaro provide an example of the extreme consequences of male domination and its ensuing tendency to conflict and violence. The death rates of Yanomamo men from warfare or homicide for example are 25-40% and Jivaros of 60%. By comparison with these figures !Kung rates of male homicide are as little as 0.3%. Although these societies are very different from modern urban cultures, they provide an insight into how male dominance leads to patterns of violence, polarization, instability and deprivation which have direct relevance to our own futures. .

Yanomamo: The 'Fierce People'

The Yanomamo have been referred to as 'one of the most aggressive, warlike, and male-oriented societies in the world' (Sanday R596 45). They live in southern Venezuela and adjacent portions of northern Brazil in some 125 scattered villages ranging from 40 to 250 inhabitants. In the 1960s they were still actively conducting warfare. Chagnon (R110) called them 'the fierce people' because, he says, "that is how they conceive themselves to be, and that is how they would like others to think of them". Traditionally they were hunters and gatherers. Today 85% of their diet consists of cultivated plants high in calories but low in protein. Hunting and fishing are the only source of protein, and men spend as much time hunting as they do gardening. They are aware of their need for animal protein. They have two words for hunger: One means an empty stomach and the other means a full stomach that craves meat. Game animals are not abundant and an area is rapidly depleted, keeping groups constantly on the move. Hunting often provides barely enough protein but at other times there is an occasional abundance sufficient to fed the whole village (Sanday R596 45).

Chagnon (R110 205) notes: "Among the more significant results of my analysis were the following facts, which put the nature and extent of violence among Kaobawa's people into regional perspective:

1. Approximately 40% of the adult males participated in the killing of another Yanomamo. The majority of them (60%) killed only one person, but some men were repetitively successful warriors and participated in the killing of up to 16 other people.
2. Approximately 25% of all deaths among adult males was due to violence.
3. Approximately two-thirds of all people aged 40 or older had lost, through violence, at least one of the following kinds of very close biological relatives: a parent, a sibling, or a child. Most of them (57%) have lost two or more such close relatives. This helps explain why large numbers of individuals are motivated by revenge.

Because of the emphasis on warfare and hunting, male babies are preferred. Men make it known that their wives had better deliver a son or suffer the consequences. Women will kill a female infant or allow it to starve to avoid disappointing their husbands. The shortage of women produced by infanticide is exacerbated by taboos prohibiting sexual intercourse at certain periods and by the tendency for influential men to have more than one wife. In one village, for example, there were 122 males and 90 females. About 25% of the politically important men in that village had two or more wives. Sexual intercourse is prohibited when a woman is pregnant or nursing. This creates considerable concern within the village over the acquisition and possession of sexually active females. Teenage males frequently have homosexual affairs because the females of their own age are usually married. By the time a young man is 20, however, he is anxious to display his masculinity and becomes an active competitor for the favors of sexually active women. This leads to considerable friction between men within the village.

Percentage of male deaths caused by warfare, Jivaro and Yanomamo (Pinker R532)

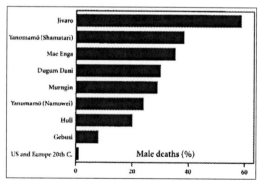

Although boys spend most of their time with their mothers, they quickly learn that there are status differences between males and females. From an early age, boys are treated with considerable indulgence by their fathers. Boys are encouraged to be 'fierce' and are rarely punished for beating girls in the villages, as their fathers beat their wives. Many Yanomamo make statements like 'Men are more valuable than women ...boys more valuable than girls.' Female children assume duties and responsibilities in the household long before their brothers are obliged to participate in comparable useful domestic tasks. Little girls are obliged to tend their younger brothers and sisters, and expected to help their mothers in other chores such as cooking, hauling water, and collecting firewood (Chagnon R110 122).

By the time girls reach puberty they have already learned that their world is decidedly less attractive than that of their brothers. Most have been promised in marriage by that time. Girls have almost no voice in the decisions reached by their elder kin in deciding whom they should marry. They are largely pawns to be disposed of by their kinsmen, and their wishes are given very little consideration. In many cases, the girl has been promised to a man long before she reaches puberty, and in some cases her husband-elect actually raises her for part of her childhood. In a real sense, girls do not participate as equals in the political affairs of the corporate kinship group and seem to inherit most of the duties without enjoying many of the privileges, largely because of age differences at first marriage and the increase in status that being slightly older entails. Marriage does not automatically enhance the status of the girl or change her life much. There is no 'marriage ceremony,' and the public awareness of her marriage begins with hardly more than comments like 'her father has promised her to so-and-so.' She usually does not begin living with her husband until she has had her first menstrual period, although she may be 'married' for several years before then. Her duties as wife require her to continue the difficult and laborious tasks she has already begun doing, such as collecting firewood and fetching water every day.

Firewood collection (redrawn from R110).

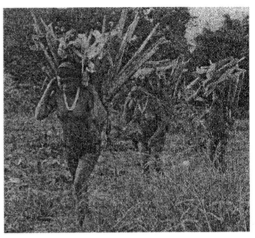

Firewood collecting is particularly difficult, and women spend several hours each day scouring the neighborhood for suitable wood. The women can always be seen leaving the village about 3 or 4 pm and returning at dusk, usually in a procession, bearing enormous loads of wood in their pack baskets. By the time most women are 30 years old they have "lost their shape" because of the children they have borne, the children they have nursed for up to 3 years each, and the years of hard labor; and they seem to be much more often in 'bad moods' than men. They seem, in these moods, to have developed a rather unpleasant attitude toward life in general and toward men in particular.

Many Yanomamo women show the effects of brutal treatment by men: They are covered with scars and bruises from violent encounters with seducers, rapists, and husbands. By displaying their ferocity against women, men show other men that they are capable of violence and had better be treated with respect and caution (Sanday R596 45).

Women must respond quickly to the demands of their husbands and even anticipate their needs. It is interesting to watch the behavior of women when their husbands return from a hunting trip or a visit. The men march dramatically and proudly across the village and retire silently into their hammocks, especially when they bring home desirable food items. The women, no matter what they are doing, hurry home and quietly but rapidly prepare a meal. Should the wife be slow at doing this, some irate husbands scold them or even beat them Chagnon (R110 124).

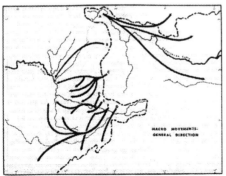

Patterns of migration of Yanomamo settlements including fissioning of villages illustrate impacts of migration of a warlike patriarchal society (Chagnon)

Some men seem to think that it reasonable to beat their wife once in a while as if the objective is 'just to keep her on her toes'. Most physical reprimands meted out take the form of blows with the hand or with a piece of firewood, but a good many husbands are more severe. Some of them chop their wives with the sharp edge of a machete or ax or shoot them with a barbed arrow in some nonvital area, such as the buttocks or leg. Some men are given to punishing their wives by holding the glowing end of a piece of firewood against them, producing painful and serious burns. The punishment is usually, however, more consistent with the perceived seriousness of the wife's shortcomings, more drastic measures being reserved for infidelity or suspicion of infidelity. It is not uncommon for a man to injure his sexually errant wife seriously and some men have even killed wives for infidelity by shooting them with an arrow. Women who are not too severely treated might even measure their husband's concern in terms of the frequency of minor physical reprimands they sustain. I overheard two young women discussing each other's scalp scars. One of them commented that the other's husband must really care for her since he has beaten her on the head so frequently!

A man in one of the villages Chagnon (R110 124) studied shot his wife in the stomach with a barbed arrow. Considerable internal injury resulted when the arrow was removed and the girl nearly died. Another man chopped his wife on the arm with a machete. A fight involving infidelity took place in one of the villages. The male culprit was killed in the club fight, and the recalcitrant wife had both her ears cut off by her enraged husband. A number of other women had their ears badly mutilated by angry husbands. The women wear short pieces of arrowcane in their pierced ear lobes; these are easily grabbed by the husband. A few men jerked these so hard that they tore their wife's ear lobes open.

A woman can usually depend on her brothers for protection. They will defend her against a cruel husband. If a man is too severe to a wife, her brothers may take the woman away from him and give her to another man. It is largely for this reason that women usually abhor the possibility of being married off to men in distant villages; they know that their brothers cannot protect them under these circumstances. Women who have married a male cross-cousin have an easier life, for they are related to their husbands by cognatic ties of kinship as well as by marriage (Chagnon R110).

> The Yanomamo have a concept, *buhi yabrazi*, that I thought, at first, could be translated into our notion 'love.' I asked ... "Do you 'love' so-and-so?" naming their brother or sister. "Yes!" "Do you 'love' so-and-so?" naming their child? "Yes!" "Do you 'love' so-and-so?" naming their wife. A stunned silence followed, then peels of laughter. "You don't 'love' your wife, you idiot!" The divorce rate is about 20% but marriages seldom last till children reach maturity. Few children are still part of an intact nuclear or polygynous family by the time they reach ten years of age. There is a somewhat rare way a woman can escape the tragedy of marriage to an especially cruel or undesirable husband. They have a word for this: shuwahimou. This is applied to women who, on their own initiative, have fled from their village to live in another village and find a new husband there. It is rare because it is dangerous. If her own village is stronger than the one she tees to, they will pursue her and forcibly take her back - and mete out very severe punishment to her for having run away. They may even kill her. Most women who have done this have done it to escape the savage treatment they have received at the hands of a cruel husband (Chagnon).

Where women are captured during fighting, or are simply kidnapped, their feelings may carry little or no weight. All women fear being abducted by raiders and always leave the village with this anxiety at the back of their minds when their village is at war. They take their children with them, particularly younger children, so that if they are abducted, the child's future will not be put in jeopardy because of the separation of the mother. They are therefore concerned with the political behavior of their men and occasionally goad them into taking action against some possible enemy by caustically accusing the men of cowardice.

A woman gains increasing respect as she ages, especially when she is old enough to have adult children who care for her and treat her kindly. Old women also have a unique position in the world of intervillage warfare and politics. They are immune from the incursions of raiders and can go from one village to another with complete disregard for personal danger.

Headmen can be violent warriors who are oppressive despots, or more astute leaders experinced at conflict resolution. Kaobawa as a headman stands at the mild, quietly competent end of the spectrum. He has had six wives - and temporary affairs with as many more, at least one of which resulted in a child that is publicly acknowledged as his. When Chagnon first met him he had two wives, Bahimi and Koamashima. Bahimi had two living children, others had died. She was the older and enduring wife, as much a friend to him as a mate. Their relationship was as close to what we think of as 'love' in our culture as any seen among the Yanomamo. His second wife was a girl of about 20 years, Koamashima. She had a new baby boy when I first met her, her first child. Bahimi was pregnant, but she destroyed the infant when it was born - a boy in this case - explaining tearfully that the new baby would have competed for milk her youngest child, who was still nursing. Kaobawa claims he beats Bahimi only 'once in a while, and only lightly' and she, for her part, never has affairs with other men (Chagnon R110 27).

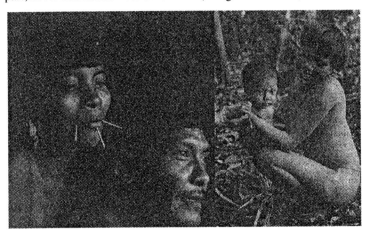

Kaobawa and his wives (redrawn from R110).

We also find patriarchal sexual sharing in Yanomamo families. "There was speculation that Kaobawa was planning to give Koamashima to one of his younger brothers who had no wife; he occasionally allows his younger brother to have sex with Koamashima, but only if he asks in advance. Kaobawa gave another wife to one of his other brothers because she was beshi ('horny'). In fact, the earlier wife had been married to two other men, both of whom discarded her because of her infidelity" (Chagnon R110 27).

Clandestine sexual liaisons often take place at daybreak, having been arranged the previous evening. The lovers leave the village on the pretext of going to the toilet and meet at some predetermined location. They return to the village, separately by opposite routes.

Another form of permitted affair is called hoimou 'to befriend' or 'act like a friend' to a woman. This type of relationship might occur, for example, when the members of a village have to take refuge with an ally. The allies invariably enter in nohimou relationships with the women of the refugees. The refugees are reluctant to give their women as wives to the men of the host village, but they are obliged to permit them to have sexual access to the women. These kinds of affairs also develop within a village between a man and the wife of a friend, or, with single girls. Again, when men go on visits to other villages and bring trade goods, they frequently are permitted to have affairs with the hosts' women, particularly if the men have brought goods that are highly prized by the hosts (Pasternak et. al. R517 173).

Gregor (1995 29) mentions the game of Kanupai ('taking a wife', marrying), and Ukitsapai (being jealous'). The latter game involves the children sneaking off on cross-marital assignations, 'only to be surprised by furious spouses'. Becher (R50 140) notes:

"It is especially popular to play 'mother and child' or 'married couple'. In the latter game sexual activity is already often involved. As long as the children have not yet reached puberty, the adults laugh about it. It is only the mothers of girls who are a little annoyed when they hear about it. They do not regard it as tragic, however, since they themselves were reprimanded about it by their mothers when they were little girls".

"Marriages are arranged by older kin, usually men, who are brothers, uncles, and the father. It is a political process, for girls are promised in marriage while they are young, and the men who do this attempt to create alliances with other men via marriage exchanges. Ideally, all Yanomamo men should marry a cross-cousin. Patrilineal descent, combines with the maintenance of complementary patrilines to make a bilateral cross-cousin marriage ideal. This creates a unique kinship system in which a wife may be both a maternal and paternal cousin of the husband and vice versa, combining the mother's brother's daughter and father's sister's daughter linkages. This also means that women who marry cousins have more kin support among their in-laws. Mother's brother's are conveyors of affection because of the implied link to marriageable cousins.

Population pyramid for remote Yanomamo groups illustrates the effects of female infanticide and young male homicide on particular age groups. There is also a pronounced female mortality a decade after the male which may be due to childbirth. Inset bilateral cousins resulting from reciprocation between kin groups (Chagnon R110).

Most fighting within the village stems from sexual affairs or failure to deliver a promised woman, or out-and-out seizure of a married woman by some other man. This can lead to internal fighting and conflict of such intensity that villages split up and fission, each group then becoming a new village and, often, enemies to each other" (Chagnon R110 7).

The headman has somewhat more responsibility in political dealings with other Yanomamo groups, and very little control over those who live in his group except when the village is being raided by enemies. Most of the time men like Kaobawa are like the North American Indian 'chief' whose authority was characterized in the following fashion: 'One word from the chief, and each man does as he pleases' (Chagnon R110 27). This has led to the Yanomamo being described as egalitarian, however in reproductive matters nothing is further from the truth (Low R416 117).

Chagnon (R110 205) notes the reproductive advantage being a killer: "The most unusual and impressive finding, one that has been subsequently discussed and debated in the press and in academic journals, is the correlation between military success and reproductive success among the Yanomamo. *Unokais* (men who have killed) are more successful at obtaining wives and, as a consequence, have more offspring than men their own age who are not unokais. The most plausible explanation for this correlation seems to be that unokais are socially rewarded and have greater prestige than other men and, for these reasons, are more often able to obtain extra wives by whom they have larger than average numbers of children. Thus, 'cultural success' leads, in this cultural/historical circumstance, to biological success. Unokais had, on average, more than two-and-a-half times as many wives as non-unokais and over three times as many children".

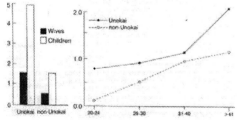

Among the Yanomamo, the reproductive context of men's warfare is clear. Men who participate in revenge raids and ambushes have more wives, and more children than others, and men who avoid warfare suffer reproductively. Because sexual selection can rapidly amplify alleles for male violence, the population becomes dominated by aggressive young males (Low R416 223).

The effects of this sexual selection for mutual competition and warfare are regionally pronounced (Chagnon R110 87):

"The most startling difference is the degree to which violence and warfare-and the consequences of these distinguish highland and lowland groups from each other. Warfare is much more highly developed and chronic in the lowlands. Men in the lowland villages seem 'pushy' and aggressive, but men from the smaller, highland villages seem sedate and gentle. Not unexpectedly, alliance patterns are more elaborate in the lowlands and dramatic, large, regular feasts are characteristic, events in which large groups invite their current allies to feast and trade. Larger numbers of women in lowland villages are either abducted from or 'coerced' from weaker, smaller neighbors, including highland villages. By contrast, highland villages have fewer abducted women, and when they do, they usually come from other small highland groups, not from the more bellicose, larger, and more powerful lowland villages. Fewer of the adult men in the highland villages are unokais, who have participated in the killing of other men. There, the average fraction of adult males who have participated in the killing of another person is over twice as high (44%) but the average number of victims killed per unokai is only slightly higher in the lowland villages, 1.13 compared to 0.96. The percentage of females in the lowland villages who have been abducted is significantly higher: 17% compared to 11.7% in the highland villages".

What of women's costs and benefits in this polygynous society? In some societies, polygyny, despite its likely costs, could have real resource benefits for women-if men vary in wealth. But Yanomamo men do not, so a polygynous Yanomamo woman must share the re- sources of her husband with co-wives, even though he has nothing more than a monogamous man. Furthermore, Yanomamo men have a large say in arranging marriages. Polygynous households tend to have smaller gardens for their family size than monogamous house- holds, but economically, the only difference between polygynous and monogamous households is that polygynous households receive more food from others. A high-status Yanomamo man, therefore, though he does not directly provide wealth, may indirectly create some benefits for his wives (Low R416 117).

Some leaders are mild, quiet, inconspicuous most of the time, but intensely competent. Other men are more tyrannical, despotic, pushy, flamboyant, and unpleasant to all around them. They shout orders frequently, are prone to beat their wives, or pick on weaker men. Some are very violent (Chagnon R110 27). The men of a village are constantly fighting among themselves or going off to raid other villages. An enraged husband who has caught another man with his wife will challenge him to what is called a club duel, in which the two will flail at one another's heads with heavy clubs resembling pool cues, 8 to 10 feet long. When the blood starts to flow from one of the blows, almost all of the men in the village will rip a pole out of the house frame and join in the fight in support of one of the contestants (Sanday R596 47).

Warfare between villages is commonly for abducting women, due to the unbalanced sex ratio created by female infanticide. Yanomamo regard fights over women as the primary cause of their wars. Male supremacy is part of a self-perpetuating cycle of violence. Males are reared to be fierce in order to compete for protein resources, garden plots, and women. To display their fierceness, men beat women, fight other men, and go to war. To defend against counterattacks, more fierce males are needed, and male infants are favored over female infants. Infanticide is necessary in order to achieve a balance between population size and protein resources. The shortage of women causes sexual frustration and jealousy. Having several wives is the insignia of power and influence, which only increases the level of sexual frustration and the motivation for going to war (Sanday R596 45).

The Yanomamo cosmos is comprised of four parallel layers, analogous to historical stages, lying horizontally, each on top of the other. The upper-most layer is at present considered to be 'empty' but long ago some things originated there and then moved down to the other layers. This layer is called the 'tender' plane and is sometimes described as 'an old woman', a phrase used to describe an abandoned garden or a female no longer able to produce offspring. The next layer is called *hedu*, 'the sky'. Its top surface is made of earth and is the eternal home for the souls of the departed. Its inhabitants are spirits of men who garden, make witchcraft, hunt, and eat. Everything that exists on earth supposedly has its counterpart in hedu. Its bottom surface is the visible portion of the sky. Man dwells below the sky on what is called 'this layer' or *hei*. It originated when a piece of hedu broke off and fell to a lower level. It consists of a vast jungle in which the numerous Yanomamo villages are dispersed. Finally, there is another place underneath this layer, which is almost barren. A single village of spirit men, the *Amahiri-teri*, live underneath the earth layer. It was formed after the earth layer when another chunk of hedu fell down and crashed through the earth. It hit earth where the Amahiri-teri lived and carried their village down to the bottom layer. When this happened, only their garden lands were carried to the lower layer; the Amahiri-teri thus have no place in which to hunt for game and must send their spirits up to earth, to capture the souls of living children and eat them (Sanday R596 47).

Yanomamo men take hallucinogenic Anadenanthera snuff *ebene* containing dimethyl tryptamines almost daily (Chagnon R110 54) and spend a great deal of their time in shamanic encounters using the many kinds of colourful spirits or hekura to devour enemies souls or to help their hosts cure sickness in the village. Sexual restraint accompanies the shamanic quest, which is encouraged partly as a way of reducing sexual friction in a polygynous society where women are in short supply. However an experienced shaman in tune with his *hekura* can abandon these restrictions (Schultes and Hofmann R612).

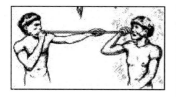

Snuffing pipe (R612).

The present-day Yanomamo are descended from the 'first beings', or 'those who are now dead'. The 'first beings' lived on earth and departed for hedu after a major disaster in which most of them were killed. The chain of events bringing an end to the 'first beings' and resulting finally in the creation of the 'fierce people' is set off by meat hunger, cannibalism, and rape. Cooperation and sharing are conspicuously absent.

A mother who keeps her knowledge of fruit cultivation a secret gives a piece of fruit to a child, who then dies. Hungry for meat, another woman, who is the daughter-in-law of the offending mother, asks if she may eat the child, and her request is granted. Also hungry for meat and out of revenge, the father of the eaten child eats the mother of the child eater. This man is killed by the sons of the mother, who then become afflicted with sex hunger, which may be equated with meat hunger since the Yanomamo use the same verb for eating and copulating. To satisfy their sex hunger, the two sons rape the daughter of another 'first being'. They then change the girl's vagina into a mouth, with teeth that bite off the penis of the next man who seduces her. One of the brother's sons gets very thirsty, and to quench his thirst, the father digs a hole too deep from which water flows endlessly, causing a great flood in which many of the 'first beings' are drowned. Those who escape do so by climbing mountains, which is why the first beings may be said to have ended up in the sky, or hedu. The mother of the girl who had been raped and whose vagina had been changed into a mouth plunges into the lake caused by the flood, and eventually she makes it recede. She still remains there, having been changed into a serpent-like monster by one of the brothers. To this day, the Yanomamo are afraid to cross large rivers, for fear that she will eat them or create large waves (Sanday R596 48).

Among the very few original beings left after the flood was the Spirit of the Moon. He comes down to earth from hedu to eat the soul parts of children. Eventually some earth beings (it is not clear whether these are 'first beings') manage to pierce his flesh with an arrow, causing him to bleed profusely. Where his blood hit the earth, a large population of men (no women) are born. Most of the Yanomamo alive today are descended from the blood of the Spirit of the Moon. Where his blood fell the thickest, wars were so intense that the people in that area exterminated themselves. Where it was thinner, the people were less fierce and did not become extinct. The most docile Yanomamo are thought to have been created from the right leg of one of the blood men, and women from the left leg. Thus, there are three types of Yanomamo - fierce men, docile men, and women (Sanday R596 49).

According to the tale, only men appear to have survived the flood, with the exception of the raped girl's mother. Only men are thought to have been created from the blood of the moon spirit. This, in addition to the idea that there are different types of Yanomamo, suggests the theme of a group of migrating males who, long ago, came from another land and, along the way, killed or incorporated men from other groups to obtain sexual access to women and rights to hunting territory (R596 49). The treatment accorded Yanomamo women certainly appears to perpetuate the relationship between conquerors and the conquered in a harsh environment. The cycle of violence and sexual inequality we observe among the Yanomamo can be viewed as part of an extreme adaptation to extreme circumstances in the struggle for survival. In their origin tale, cannibalism, rape, and murderous revenge are responses to the tensions created by a precarious existence and by the perception that the universe contains powerful and uncontrollable forces that may at any moment destroy all life. These forces are set in motion by the minds of men in their struggle to maintain the upper hand in a losing battle. If the Yanomamo believe that they exterminated themselves once before, they must live with the fear that it will happen again.

Elena Valero, a Brazilian woman was kidnapped by Yanomamo warriors when she was eleven years old at a time when intertribal warfare and raiding for women was still endemic. No sooner was she kidnapped than Elena Valero's captors were themselves attacked by rival Yanomamo. Again she was taken captive and handed over to one of her abductors as a wife. She would spend the next twenty years among the Karawetari, marry twice with different captors and bear three children before finally escaping. She would witness, and hear about, many more raids. But none were so horrifying as the second one: 'They killed so many. I was weeping for fear and for pity but there was nothing I could do. They snatched the children from their mothers to kill them, while the others held the mothers tightly by the arms and wrists as they stood up in a line. All the women wept'. They fled before the raiders, taking their children with them. 'The men began to kill the children; little ones, bigger ones, they killed many of them. They tried to run away, but [the Karawetari raiders] caught them, and threw them to the ground, and stuck them with bows, which went through their bodies and rooted them to the ground. Taking the smallest by the feet, they beat them against the trees and the rocks. The children's eyes trembled. Then the men took the dead bodies and threw them among the rocks, saying, 'Stay there, so that your fathers can find you and eat you.' One woman pleaded, 'It's a little girl, you mustn't kill her.' Another gambled desperately to save the life of a two-year-old snatched from her arms by telling the raider, 'Don't kill him, he's your son. The mother was with you and she ran away when she was already pregnant with this child. He's one of your sons!' The man mulled over this possibility before replying, 'No, he's [another group's] child. It's too long since [that woman was] with us.' The man then took the baby by his feet and bashed him against the rocks. When much later, anthropologist Napoleon Chagnon interviewed different Yanomamo groups, people told him about women being kidnaped, their infants merely left behind to starve. (Hrdy R323 241).

Hrdy (R323 468) notes: that in some Amazonian tribes too much or too little hair on a newborn can be seen as a sign of sexual misconduct. When she gave birth to a 'half-caste' Elena Valero was told by the other women "kill hm at once", but the man who had taken her told them to go away saying "Let her bring him up, even if he has no hair".

Jivaro: People of the Shrunken Heads

The Jivaro are even more extremely violent than the Yanomamo, having a war homicide rate of about 60% of men, although modern changes are leading to social resolution of physical conflicts. They are renowned as the one Amazonian tribe who practised head-shrinking. They refused to be suppressed by the Inca and revolted against the Spanish Empire and thwarted all subsequent attempts by the Spaniards to conquer them. In the year 1599, the Jivaros banded together and killed 25,000 white people in raids on two settlements. The attack was instigated over the natives being taxed in their gold-trade. After uncovering the unscrupulous practices of the visiting governor, molten gold was later poured down his throat until his bowels burst. Following his execution, the remaining Spaniards were killed along with the older women and children. The younger useful women were taken as prisoners to join the clan.

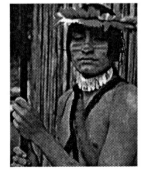

Like the Yanomamo, perpetual animosity existed between the neighboring tribes of the Jivaro. The Shaur and Achuar Jivaros, once deadly enemies have only recently formed a tribal federation. Among the Jivaro, as among the Yanomamo, there is no stratification - but egalitarian warriorship. During times of peace there's no chieftain. When wars erupt, older experienced men who have killed many men and captured many heads are chosen as war chiefs. No Jivaro can be chosen if he has not killed. Bloody feuds, reported as functioning to obtain women, are frequent and follow familial lines (Low 192). A fundamental difference between wars enacted within the same tribe and against neighboring tribes is such that wars between different tribes are in principle wars of genocidal extermination. A significant goal of these wars was geared toward the annihilation of the enemy tribe, including women and children. This was done in order to prevent them from seeking revenge against the victors in the future. There were however, many instances where the women and children were taken as prisoners and forced to become a part of the victors families. A woman who fights, or a woman who refuses to accompany the victorious war-party to their homes and serve a new master, exposes herself to the risk of suffering the same fate as her men-folk. Up de Graff (R700 273) describes a foray with the Jivaro:

> "A Huambiza woman who had fallen in the fight wounded by 3 spears. Little did we imagine what the ultimate issue might prove to be, when we attacked that morning. The woman lay there where she had been borne down by the spear-thrusts. The Agurunas eager to collect her head, went to work while she was still alive, though powerless to protect herself. While one wrenches at her head another held her to the ground, and yet another hacked her neck with his stone-ax. Finally I was called upon to lend my machete, a far better implement for the work in hand. This was truly an act of mercy, to put the poor creature out of her misery as soon as possible. It was truly a hideous spectacle."

On the whole, the Jivaro Indians attributed each death to supernatural causes rather than accepting natural death. Following each death a vicious cycle of retaliation ensues in which someone is always held accountable for the murder of another. This cycle of blood-revenge is perpetuated by religious reasons by which the soul of the victim requires that his relatives should avenge his death. Because witchcraft and sorcery can account for the majority of murders and natural deaths within a tribe, it is not surprising that the medicine men, or shamans, are most susceptible to attack as they are frequently accused of using their powers against others. If the surviving members do not retaliate against he slayer, the anger of the vengeful spirit may in fact turn against themselves. If blood-revenge cannot be directed to the actual slayer, it may be directed toward one of his relations. Once a murder has been avenged, blood-guilt or *tumashi akerkama* is atoned for and the offended family is satisfied. Younger males, often as young as six, listen to fathers describe the various crimes that had been committed against them. A strong sense of family justice is instilled and expectation to avenge previous injustices committed against family members.

The Jivaro believe that "witchcraft is the cause of the vast majority of illnesses and non-violent deaths" (Harner R285 142) in the world and that they are only part of a large spiritual world. The Jivaro believe in a total of three souls for humans. The *Arutam* soul is acquired through a vision quest at the sacred waterfall. Attainment of the Arutam soul is not, however, guaranteed by this quest. This soul is considered vital to the possessor's health and safety. Arutam possession is almost assured protection from death by physical violence, poison or sorcery. Only after obtaining the Arutam soul, can the second soul be obtained. This soul, *Muisak*, is known as the avenging soul. Muisak avenges the death of a person who has died as a result of physical violence or of sorcery. The soul attempts to kill the murderer, but at times misses the target, harming innocent family members. Commonplace accidents, such as drowning or being bit by a snake, are believed to be the result of a Muisak. The concept of the Muisak furnishes the Jivaro the rationale for head taking and shrinking (*tsantsa*). By shrinking their enemies' heads, they prevent attacks from the avenging soul. Because of its seemingly minor role in their day-to-day survival, the Jivaro place less emphasis on the third soul, known as *Nekas Wakani*. This soul enters the body at birth. It leaves the body at death, and is believed to roam the deceased's former home. It is the task of the living to feed the Nekas Wakani soul. If this task is not performed properly, the third soul may take a demon form and cause harm to the living.

The Jivaro have two kinds of shamans that help them control the supernatural forces: bewitching shamans and curing shamans. Each type of shaman is a specialist who uses hallucinogenic drugs to deal with the spirit world including *Yaje, Caapi* or *Ayahuasca*, This is an extremely powerful indole hallucinogen containing an admixture of two plants, Psychotria viridis and Banisteriopsis caapi, the first containing dimethyl tryptamine and the other harmine as a monoamine oxidase inhibitor potentiator. Yage is one of the world's most potent hallucinogens with a folklore of telepathic and remote viewing powers.

The most important spirits are the *tsentsak*, called spirit helpers. Individuals who are not shamans cannot access this spirit world, however, so there is great demand for 'specialists who can cross over into the supernatural world at will to deal with the forces that influence and even determine the events of the waking life'. This means that a great deal of the vision quest is preoccupied with potentially homicidal events in the supernatural world colouring their entire spiritual cosmology with the motifs of male combat and retribution.

Harner noted that 1 out of every 4 men in the village were shamans, and this was especially true for males whose fathers were shamans. However, women were welcome to become shamans as well; all that was required was the acquisition of tsentsak and the ability to use natema. When a curing shaman drinks hallucinogenic brews, she will enter a trance at which point she can see through the patient's body "as though it were glass".

The Jivaro divide work according to the sex of the objects worked with. They believe everything in the world is either male or female. Women should prepare food because fire is female. Women should make and clean pots because clay, being part of Mother Earth, is female. They have declared cotton to be one of the few male plants. The Jivaro men therefore do all the spinning, weaving, and making of clothes. Fiber, the Jivaro believe, is male. So the men make all baskets. Baskets themselves are female, so women tote the heavy loads. On the role of women Jivaro note man (the sloth) is son of Sun and Moon, while woman (wife) comes from the egg of the Chingaso. Thus man is lazy - most of work being done by women!

Anne Christine Taylor in "The Gender of the Prey" (R669) explores relations of matrimony and the web of connections between conjugality and taming, between women and game animals, between seduction and predation. Through an examination of Jivaroan notions about parent-child relations, she shows how the complex of predation, linked to affinity, is articulated to a representation of identity figured by vegetal cloning, a form of reproduction that is both monosexual (purely feminine) and mono-generational, 'mothers' being their own 'daughters' and vice-versa. Thus, the production of 'true persons' depends crucially on the masculine capacity to kill, insofar as homicide is viewed as the principle responsible for the separation between generations, hence the creation of kinship.

The women of the Aguaruna Jivaro of northern Peru kill themselves more frequently than do men in a ratio of from 2:1 to 9:1. In 31 percent of the cases, their relatives say that the motive for death was because the woman was scolded or beaten by either her kinsman or her spouse for failure to perform domestic duties. Women have little control over their marital situation: "men are often reluctant to protect their daughters or sisters from abuse by a brutal husband, except perhaps during the initial trial period of a marriage. This state of affairs changes dramatically when a woman kills herself, for then her kinsmen angrily demand an explanation from her husband - and they also seek compensation or exact retribution through a vengeance killing. Women thus use the implicit or explicit threat of suicide to gain leverage over their husband, as a way of preventing beatings or discouraging the formation of a polygynous household ... in some cases the husband may face actual physical danger if his wife's family holds him responsible for her death" (Brown M R86 7). It seems that female suicide is so common among the Aguaruna that it has lost its effectiveness as a way of influencing male behaviour; men become inured to it. "some men ... were quite fatalistic, arguing that it didn't matter how they treated their wives since women are likely to kill themselves anyway". Because of the demand for women a girl may be promised as a wife when she is as young as five and some are betrothed shortly after birth (Chagnon R82 48).

Although changing times and cultural influences are causing the warrior mentality to be moderated by dialogue many of the founding motifs remain. As with the Yanomamo political power among the Shuar Jivaro, is a quality of individuals. Spiritual power, rather than having been an abstraction of social control, has similarly expressed this individualism, which refers primarily to individuals and not to groups of persons, such as kin-groups castes or classes. The vision quest forms the precondition for the achievement of power: In the course of visionary rites people can integrate the invisible power and endow them with certain abilities in dealing with their natural and social environment .

One of the major preconditions for a 'good life' is successful conflict management. Only those people who can stand their ground in a conflict, lead a good life. On the one hand this means being able to successfully carry out a conflict, and on the other hand it also comprises a talent for peaceful settlements. The victorious warrior, who kills instead of being killed, the charismatic speaker, who succeeds in creating alliances, the woman, whose strong words settle domestic quarrels, they will all gain their influence in the community through their strength in conflicts (Mader R419).

All traditional male 'positions of leadership' are directed to conflict resolution: The warrior distinguishes himself by settling a feud by force; the influence of the 'Great Old Man' endows him with an important vote in deciding about the manner of dealing with conflicts, which reach beyond the local group (for example whether a member of his alliance-group should carry out a blood revenge or not. In contrast to this, female power in this society is connected to a greater extent with the woman's role as the provider of food, although conflict management does constitute an important aspect of a woman's mastering of life and her social actions. In this, women attain a vital function in the solution of domestic quarrels. They also performed important duties in the course of traditional warfare.

Women and shamans are always mentioned in one breath as the main causes for the high potential for conflict in this society. "This is why there were so many wars in the former times ... The issues were not land, or any treasures, or any market, issue was either women or witchcraft." This is again reflected in an origin myth based on antagonism between male and female spirits in which war is instituted to the antagonism remains perpetual (Sanday R596 181). Conflicts in connection with unpermitted sexuality and witchcraft can go from misunderstandings or altercations between husband and wife to strained relations between local groups due to accusations of sorcery, and on to armed conflicts between groups of allies. This again could lead to protracted cycles of blood revenge.

The connection between amoral or deviant behaviour and blood revenge ensues from the conception of shamanic power on the one hand, and the sanctions for adultery on the other hand. In the traditional culture of the Shuar and Achuar adultery represents one of the worst violations of the social order. It endangers the alliances which have been formed through marriage and threatens the stability of the political framework. Fathers and husbands are the authorities who control female sexuality. In the case of an infringement of the rules, it is their duty to impose sanctions. Among other forms of punishment, these can also take the shape of the death of both accessories. Should one of the two perpetrators be killed in a concrete case, the conflict usually expends to a blood revenge feud: 'You can kill a woman out of jealousy, but then this woman's family will declare war on you. Let's suppose a man had a wife. If another one did not respect this fact, he became jealous. He killed and started a war. Thus war came about and this war was endless, until everybody was dead'.

In this culture female attraction and shamanic power are both conceived as forms of power with a great ambivalence: Just like the shaman can use his power not only for healing but also for bringing about illnesses and calamities, a woman can also, apart from making her husband happy, attract suitors and lovers. Female beauty is always subject to a touch of immorality, while the productive qualities of a woman have a very high social rating. As one Jivaro put it:

> "In former times, when you had a lover, this was a matter of outmost secrecy, so it would not be found out. Only the two people concerned were allowed to know, nobody else. No look, no greeting, no smile must betray you. There were experts in this, who could keep their affairs totally secret: They were lovers only when they were alone, but in public nothing was to be seen. My lover can publicly insult me, she can spit in my face, but we both know that we are lovers. But you don't let anything on in front of other people, thus you avoid death. But today, what with the young Shuar, as soon as a young girl grants them a smile, they say: She is my lover! ... The young men talk: She is like this, her body is shaped like that - they make their relationship a public affair and everybody starts commenting on it. These things, this lack of respect, this is what happens today, whereas in former times nobody knew anything."

Tukano: The Mournful Sound of Hidden Trumpets

An elaboration of the nexus of warrior male and the power of female sexuality permeates the mythology and ritual practices of the Tukano, another north Amazon tribe, described here in the contest of the Desana group.

Male initiation is climaxed by an hallucinogenic rite called *Yurupari*. Yurupari dances have been widespread, especially in western Amazonia. They characteristically use sacred bark horns and are taboo to women, who are forbidden to see them and flee to the forest at the first sound. The ritual communicates with male ancestors, propitiates fertility spirits, effecting cures of prevalent illnesses, and improving the male prestige and power over women and is centered on the taking of the hallucinogenic drink *Yaje*, or *Ayahuasca*.

"A deep booming of drums from within the maloca heralded the appearance of the mystic Yurupari horns. With only very slight urging from one of the older men, all females from babes in arms to withered, toothless hags betook themselves to the fringing forest, to hear only from afar the deep, mysterious notes of the trumpets, sight of which is believed to spell certain death for any woman...". Payés and older men are not above aiding the workings of the mystery by the judicious administration of poison to any over-curious female. "Four pairs of horns had been taken from places of concealment, and the players now ranged themselves in a rough semi-circle, producing the first deep, lugubrious notes... Many of the older men had meanwhile opened their boxes of ceremonial feathers and were selecting brilliant feather ruffs, which were bound to the mid-section of the longer horns... Four oldsters, with perfect rhythm and dramatic timing, paraded through the maloca, blowing the newly decorated horns, advancing and retracting with short dancing steps" (Schultes and Hofmann R612 123).

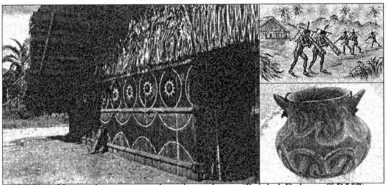

Maloca, Yurupari trumpets and uterine yaje urn (Reichel-Dolmatoff R557)

The initiates are deemed to be menstruating (Jackson R330 190). Both the maloca and the jar are symbolic of the uterus. The shamanistic descent is a return to the uterine state at the beginning of existence.

Younger men were beginning the first of the savage whippings, and the master of ceremonies appeared with the red, curiously shaped clay jar containing the Yaje. The thick, brown, bitter liquid was served in pairs of tiny, round gourds; many drinkers promptly vomited ... Whipping proceeded by pairs. The first lashes were applied to the legs and ankles, the whip flung far back in a deliberately calculated dramatic gesture; the blows resounded like pistol shots. Places were immediately exchanged. Soon the whips were being freely applied, and all the younger men were laced with bloody welts on all parts of the body. ... About a dozen of the older men were outfitting themselves with their finest diadems of resplendent guacamayo feathers, tall, feathery egret plumes, oval pieces of the russet skin of the howler monkey, armadillo-hide disks, prized loops of monkey-hair cord, precious quartzite cylinders, and jaguar-tooth belts. The men formed a swaying, dancing semi-circle, each with his right hand resting on his neighbor's shoulder, all shifting and stamping in slow unison. Leading he group was the ancient payé, blowing Tobacco smoke in benediction on his companions from the huge cigar in its engraved ceremonial fork, while his long, polished rattle-lance vibrated constantly. The dignified ceremonial chant was intoned by the group; their deep voices rose and fell, mingling with the mysterious booming tones of the Yurupari horns (Schultes and Hoffman R612).

The Tukano believe that when, at the time of creation, humans arrived to populate the Vaupés, many extraordinary happenings took place. People had to endure hardship before settling the new regions. Hideous snakes and dangerous fish lived in the rivers; there were spirits with cannibalistic proclivities; and the Tukano received in trepidation the basic elements of their culture. There lived among these early Tukano a woman; the first woman of creation, who 'drowned' men in visions. Tukanoans believe that during coitus, a man 'drowns' - the equivalent of seeing visions.

In the beginning of time, when the Anaconda-Canoe was ascending the rivers to settle mankind all over the land, there appeared the Yaje Woman mother of the Yaje vine:

"The canoe had arrived at the House of the Waters, and the men were sitting in the first maloca when the Yaje Woman arrived. She stood in front of the maloca, and there she gave birth to her child; The Yaje Woman took a plant and cleaned herself and the child. This is a plant the leaves of which are red as blood on the underside and so was the long umbilical cord. It was red and yellow and white, shining brightly"(Halifax R274 224-6).

"Inside the maloca the men were sitting, the ancestors of mankind, the ancestors of all Tukano groups. To each one the yaje vine was to be given, and they had gathered to receive it. Then the woman walked toward the maloca where the men were sitting and entered through the door, with the child in her arms. When the men saw the woman with her child they became benumbed and bewildered. It was as if they were drowning as they watched the woman and her child. She walked to the center of the maloca and, standing there, she asked: 'Who is the father of this child?' The men were sitting, and they felt nauseated and benumbed; they could not think anymore. The monkeys too could not stand the sight either. They began to eat their tails. The tapirs, too, were eating their tails which, at that time, were quite long and the squirrels, too. There was a man sitting in a corner and saliva was dripping from his mouth. He rose and, seizing the child's right leg, he said: 'I am his father!' 'No!' said another man; 'I am his father!' 'No!' said the others; 'We are the child's fathers!' And then all the men turned upon the child and tore it to pieces. They tore off the umbilical cord and the fingers, the arms, and the legs. They tore the child to bits. Each one took a part, the part that corresponds to him, to his people. And ever since each group of men has had its own kind of Yaje. The Yaje woman became pregnant from the old man, the Sun Father; he was the phallus. She looked at him and from his appearance, from the way he looked, the seed was made because he was the Yaje Person. The Sun Father was the Master of Yaje, the master of the sex act. In the House of the Waters, by looking at the Sun Father she became impregnated through the eye."

"The Yaje Woman had come with the men. While the men were preparing cashiri the Yajewoman left the maloca and gave birth to the Yaje vine in the form of a child. It was night. The men were trying to find a way to get drunk. The animals that were eating their tails were cohabiting because they had become intoxicated. The Yaje should have produced only pleasant visions, but some became nauseated and so they rejected it. The woman had walked to the center of the maloca. There was a box of feather headdresses; and there was a hearth. When she walked in, only one of the men had kept a clear head and had not become dizzy. The men were drinking when she had her child, and at once they became dizzy. First they became dizzy; then came the red light and they saw red colors, the blood of childbirth. Then she entered with her child, and when she stepped through the door they all lost their senses. Only one of them resisted and took hold of the first branch of Yaje. It was then that our ancestor acted like a thief; he took off one of his copper earrings and broke it in half, and with the sharp edge he cut the umbilical cord. He cut off a large piece. This is why Yaje comes in the shape of a vine. They all tore off bits and pieces of the child. The other men had already taken their parts of the child's body when at last our ancestor, bmika, took the part corresponding to him. Our ancestor did not know how to take advantage of Yaje; he became too much intoxicated."

There are many themes entwined here. Firstly an admission that the agent of the male vision quest has been stolen from the female horticulturists. The blood of birth is intermingled with the blood of death. The tradition is founded on murder of the child as well as vegetative propagation and this murder comes from male conflicts over paternity. Finally the visionary experience is also sexual merging and has become a representation of coitus and the power of women as mortal danger, which is however at once the goal and final destination of the mystical and supernatural quest.

The impregnation of the Yaje woman is also central in the falling out between the sexes at the cosmic origin. This is another version of the creation myth in which incest and female lust conspire to cause a primal schism associated with menstruation and incest and their taboos. The sun and moon are brothers and the sun first issues three principles, that of order of the day, that of corporeality and bodily health, and centrally that of hallucinogenic powder. But the daughter of the sun scratched is penis and found that powder epena snuff which is thus called 'the semen of the sun' (Reichel-Dolmatoff R556 28):

"The Daughter of the Sun had not yet reached puberty when her father made love to her. The Sun committed incest with her at Wainambi Rapids, and her blood flowed forth; since then, women must lose blood every month in remembrance of the incest of the Sun and so that this great wickedness will not be forgotten. But his daughter liked it and so she lived with her father as if she were his wife. She thought about sex so much that she became thin and ugly and lifeless. Newly married couples become pale and thin because they only think of the sexual act, and this is called gamuri. But when the Daughter of the Sun had her second menstruation, the sex act did harm to her and she did not want to eat anymore. ... When the Sun saw this, he decided to make the invocation that is made when the girls reach puberty. The Sun smoked tobacco and revived her. Thus, the Sun in his remorse established customs and invocations that are still performed when young girls have their first menstruation" and the rules of exogamy.

Relaters of this tale state that the daughter was the instigator of this incest by being too 'frolic-some'."

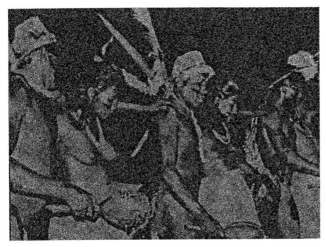

Tukano ayahuasca ritual at which both sexes are present (McKenna R449)

The incest of the Sun and his daughter/wife, who may be identified with Venus, is complemented by the saga of the Moon. In various twists to the tale, the Moon became jealous of the Sun's wife and tried to abduct her. The Sun and Moon danced and the Sun took the Moon's crown leaving only a single silver feather and copper earrings causing him to be diminished (R556 24). It is also said that the Moon cried for three nights and hid when the act of incest took place, and when he shows his full face the spots of blood of the Daughter of the Sun are seen upon it (R556 60). The moon is *nyambi abe* - the nocturnal sun a negative, evil part, associated with illegal love rather than legitimate affection, and since then has continued to be a seducer and nocturnal adulterer - since he showed no remorse when he abducted the Daughter of the Sun. Consequently an eclipse of the Sun by its dark brother is fearful, but an eclipse of the moon is a lucky night for provocative action. He descends in the night to cohabit with (the Tukano word is the same as to 'eat') women in their sleep and in their nightmares to incite them to sexuality and adultery. He is even believed to frequent cemeteries in acts of necrophilia. However he is also associated the dew which is his saliva a seminal fluid which fertilizes nature and beneficially influences the gestation of women who are pregnant. In the nights of the full moon these women will sit talking outside of the maloca, receiving the fecund power that emanates from the lunar rays (R556 72).

The Tukano know that only by a mixture of semen and the woman's secretions can an embryo be created, but they believe the quantity of semen is very small, requiring several copulations to achieve fertilization. It is considered proof of this that children are said to be more like their mothers (R556 73) an example of partible paternity.

The Tukano have ceased warfare for at least fifty years and have resolved the incessant round of male violence by developing ideas of 'closing the circuit of exchange' through exogamic and reciprocity which extends to language group exogamy where husband and wife do not speak the same language. Marriage is achieved by the careful exchange of daughters between groups. This is a close variant of the kinship pattern we have noted in the Yanomamo and indeed cross-cousin marriages are preferred.

Almost all marriages are monogamous and polygamy is reduced to about one percent confined to headmen and regarded as somewhat selfish because it deprives another man of a tradeable wife (Jackson R330 130). The monogamous trend is possibly partly due to the influence of Christian missionaries as we shall note about the Shipibo. Monogamy has the effect of reducing female scarcity and male friction, but finding a wife is a complex inter-social exchange which ideally involves 'pair marriages' by exchanging women preferably sisters of the respective husbands, but it may involve owing another group or trading an under-age girl, because of imbalances in the number of young females. People say pair marriages are more stable because each depends on the stability of the other and sisters may be called back if one of the liaisons breaks down. Possessions cannot be substituted for a deficit in traded females, so the debt has to ultimately be repaid in like kind. Like the

Jivaro, human activities are assigned a sexual nature and are for example forbidden to cook their own food as this is a female activity. On the social plane men are identified as hunters and women horticulturists. Following a classic division Jean Jackson (R330 190), consistent with Sherry Ortner (R506) (p 144), says Tukanoan society defines the men as more 'cultural' and the women more 'natural'. Only men are thought of as true spiritual beings.

Regardless of who is responsible for beginning a flirtation the least disruptive view is that the outsider women are the troublemakers. Male solidarity must be maintained and a rift between brothers is a serious matter. Themes of women being sexually provocative, demanding or even voracious appear and reappear in the myths. To be seductive a woman must make an overture, not just 'look' sexually inviting. Mock abductions still occur in the form of elopements with ritual parrying exchanges between the groups.

Consistent with the pattern of sexual segregation, in public spouses almost never show affection, not even touching one another, except when joking or grooming or administering healing. They play down any highly charged emotional encounters and politeness prevails to keep the collective peace. This can make it easier for newly weds to accustom themselves to their new environment. When problems do surface a new bride finds herself more powerless than she ever will be again. Nevertheless the women do form strong bonds together, sharing the same dilemmas and vulnerabilities - a coalition of exogamous females in the 'affine' patrilineal kinship group.

Male sexual activity is linked to a general loss of male potency and purity. The themes of woman as outsider and polluter are pertinent to this, as is the overall theme of potential danger resulting from excessive contact with women regardless of the activity. There is a story about the Yurupari horns that shows that males view their sexuality as essential to break up the solidarity of the females and to separate and continue the generations:

> "The women who were not as lazy as the men, got up before dawn to bath and being clever obtained the horns and hid them in their bodies, first in the arm bone then the vagina. The women grew very strong and refused to have sexual relations or bear children. The men, realizing the people would cease to exist consulted a shaman, who managed to find a trick to recover the horns. Since then men get up before dawn to bathe and the women cannot see the horns for they would fall sick and die" (Jackson R330 188).

Even when female power is seen as neutral or good, it still must be supervised by men. Even mothers milk must be made safe by the shaman before being fed to babies. Couvade or sympathetic pregnancy likewise instills in the male a compensation for the uninterrupted continuity of conception and birth for the female which is punctuated by the male life-giving semen, 'soul stuff' and names.

The cultural focus of the Desana is the hunt, and as hunters they live in close contact with their natural environment and seek to restrain the tendency to overexploit it. The principle underlying this interdependence is the concept of the great circuit. There is only one Creation, only one potential of energy in which all participate, both men and animals, society and nature. The hunter needs animals to be able to live and to procreate new generations and must, therefore, foster the increase of the species. The game animals, on the other hand, according to the Desana, acknowledge the interest of the hunter in their increase and thus become his dependents. But at the same time they fear that human sexuality, which always diminishes the total potential, may set a limit to their own powers of procreation. The sexual act executed freely leads to multiplication; repressed, it leads to the restriction of the species. Only its selective control, by man, establishes a balance and guarantees survival.

When an animal is killed, the energy of the local fauna is displaced into the field of society. This must eventually be replaced by masculine energy called tulari. Anything perceived as having force, power, and impulse is tulari. Anything that attracts or is a recipient is boga. Hunters represent tulari and animals boga. Hunting is a courtship and a sexual act, which must be prepared for with great care. The verb to hunt translated means 'to make love to the animals.' It is said that 'to kill is to cohabit.' The hunter must make himself sexually attractive to the animals. One of the principle conditions in preparing for the hunt is sexual abstinence because, in the words of a Desana male, 'The animals are jealous.'

The central preoccupation of Desana religious thinking is thus the control of human and animal fertility. It is not sex in its carnal, erotic meaning that preoccupies them but the simple fact of male fertilizing power that acts upon female principle and thus creates a new being. Sexuality is thus the most simple expression of an economic principle.

Over time there has been a growing scarcity of game and an increase in the female sphere of horticulture (to supply other groups). This means to men that male energy is being depleted and causes them to become anxious about their sexual and procreative powers. Sexual repression is one means by which men seek to restore these powers to original levels, as well as excluding women from male ritual equipment and certain ritual activities. By so doing, men ensure that human female energy (boga) will not contaminate male energy (tulari) needed for success in hunting. This causes psychological problems, expressed 'in the high incidence of homosexuality' and 'acts of aggression'. Men order women around, occasionally subject them to sexual assaults, and exclude them from the ritual activities.

The Desana insist that they are hunters but meat furnishes only a small proportion of the total daily food supply They say that many of the plants grown by them were introduced in recent times. They fish, but this activity also seems to be an introduction from other groups. They illustrate cultural and demographic effects of a dependence on hunting in an area where hunting is neither profitable nor easy which causes stress and instability.

The Creation of the Universe was the primordial fertilizing act that established the great model for the continuity of life thus created. But Creation, for the Desana, resulted in essentially two beings, man and animals, the hunter and his prey. Since then, the fertility and fecundity of both have been the great framework within which existence and life are developed. Outside of this framework, there is no possible place for the Desana (Reichel-Dolmatoff R556 97, Sanday R596 191).

However although the relations between the sexes are segregated and opposed, they are still understood as completing between them the potential for the continuity of existence of the people as family and kin, which is the prime motive for all cultural activity.

Mundurucu: Stealing the Women's Trumpets

An explanation for the hiding of the Yurupari trumpets is suggested by the story of he Mundurucu, another tribe in the Eastern Amazon. Women originally found the sacred trumpets, after hearing them by a lake, and catching the fish who were their guardians, using a soporific nut. The women gained ascendancy over the men and the sex roles were reversed, with the exception that women could not hunt. During that time women were the sexual aggressors and men were sexually submissive and did women's work. Women controlled the "sacred trumpets" (symbols of power) and the men's houses. The trumpets contained the spirits of the ancestors. The brother of the women who found the trumpets complained that the ancestors insisted ritual offerings of meat. The men demanded the trumpets. At first the women marched round the village playing the trumpets and insisted the men went into the dwelling houses but the men agreed to go for one night only. The women entered the men's house and forced the men to return with them to make love all night so they became slippery. In the morning the men stole the trumpets. Since women did not hunt and could not make these offerings, men were able to take the trumpets from them.

The trumpets are long, hollow tubes in which the ancestral spirits are believed to dwell, "just as the real cavities of women contain the regenerative potential of the people and the clans." The sacred trumpets have a wide mouth, and on certain ritual occasions a gourd of meat is placed before the mouth of each instrument, a symbolic offering of food to the totemic ancestors who are contained within. In the mouth of the trumpets there are two strips of the wet and pliant root of the paxiuba palm, placed side by side and bound together near each end. Blowing through the mouth causes the halves of the unbound middle section to vibrate, making a deep, rather mournful-sounding note. It is believed that the ancestral spirits are pleased by the playing of the trumpets, as they are by being fed meat after a successful hunt. Feeding the spirits and playing the trumpets is a form of fertilization; it pleases the spirits and the game increases. The pliant, wet opening of the mouth of the trumpets and the internal cavity containing the ancestral spirits suggests vaginal and uterine symbolism. By taking the trumpets, men symbolically seize ownership and control of female generative capacities. The trumpets are secured in special chambers within the men's houses and no woman can see them, under penalty of gang rape (Sanday R596 39, Murphy and Murphy R484).

In order to please the trumpet spirits, men bring back heads of non-Mundurucu they have taken in warfare. Men also seek enemy trophy heads to offer to the spirit mothers of animals, who must continually be propitiated to ensure success in hunting. Trophy heads are believed to charm the spirit mothers into improving the supply and availability of game. Just as men once gained control from women by robbing them of the sacred trumpets, men attempt to gain power over the spirit mothers. This can only be done by shamans, men believed to have special powers to contact the supernatural world. The shaman acquires power over the spirit mothers by killing certain animals when they are pregnant and extracting the fetus. But the spirit mothers also have power over the shaman: If he is not careful to observe certain rituals, they can turn the shaman into an animal (Sanday R596 39).

The men sleep in a men's house and the and the women and children in the village dwellings and men relate to men and women to women in a sexual division. Females are excluded from all formal leadership and religious positions. Fear of women dominates their male dominant myths. The Mundurucu believe that women's vaginas were originally shaped from the creator hero's clay models by bestiality in sexual intercourse with animals. A Mundurucu male who sees a woman sitting with her legs apart will call out that his mouth is open. The armadillo-trickster is said to have smeared rotten Brazil nuts on them to give the vagina its 'bad smell' (Sanday R596, Murphy and Murphy R484).

The Mundurucu are patrilineal but they are matrilocal, so a woman is likely to be living with maternal relatives. This gives the women a great deal more practical autonomy and their own sphere of existence. This means that although the men dominate the women in leadership and myth, much of the life goes on around the homes frequented by women, children and male family relatives. Some men keep an extra hammock in the dwelling house to lounge in during their visits, but they sleep in the house only when ill or they need the care of their wives. The solidarity of the mother-daughter and sister-sister extends to a union of all the women of the household and ultimately the village. Most work is done by the women in companionship, or cooperation with other women.

Talk among the women continues whenever they are together. They gossip about the men and one another. The women exchange notes about the sexual escapades of others, or their laziness. A woman who has loose sexual morals becomes a butt of gossip, partly because she breaches the moral solidarity of the females as a group and invites the intervention of the men who may stage a gang rape which is an assault on the women as a whole, however a woman who engages only in occasional dalliance and protests seduction suffers only female gossip. If a woman even looks at a man directly or sits with her legs apart it is a blatant invitation to sex. Thus women and men do not touch and women keep a contained distance from contact with men folk. They consider a woman who is promiscuous has been the victim of male witchcraft, but if all cures fail, gang rape ensues. Up to twenty men from the village drag her out to the fields and violate her because she has threatened their sexual superiority (Murphy and Murphy). A woman who goes alone out of the village is always considered to be heading for a tryst and even if she is not, any male has the right to accost her and demand that she have intercourse. Women always travel together to avoid being sexually assaulted.

Antagonisms between the sexes are very real and evident, ritualized by the men and verbalized by the women. Women say a man mever comes home except for water and sex. The women dislike gang rapes however rare and the separation of the men in the men's house instead of a family unit. They complain that the men are lazy. The men are regarded as exploitative and dominant but not superior. Men give little help with infants but take a measured interest in children once they can walk. However there are few physical attacks, between men or against women, even in cases of perceived adultery.

Marriage is a simple practical affair generally preceded by a relationship. Its primary evidence is bringing the days hunting kill to the bride. Polygyny is no longer accepted. It is vehemently opposed by the women who refuse to cohabit with another 'wife'. Divorce and death is frequent and most married people have had several previous partners, thus practising a form of serial monogamy. There is a lot of passion and little trust in the early phases of marriage. Some sexual mistrust continues even in established relationships. Women complain that they are kept pregnant at the behest of the men or that they are lazy. The primary loyalty of the women lies with her female house mates and not her husband.

Sex is not restricted to the house and hammock and couples go into the forest to secluded grassy areas to have sex. Intercourse is customarily in the missionary position. Orgasm is sometimes reached by women, but mostly only by the man. There is little foreplay and sexual encounters are brief in consummation. The woman usually derives far less satisfaction, but she knows sex is the means to get and hold onto a husband. Although opportunities are restricted, most men and women occasionally have adulterous relationships, men for variety adventure and sexual gratification, women for complex reasons including revenge for male adultery. Infanticide is infrequent but common enough to affect population size.

Ache: Dimensions of Partible Paternity

A fascinating perspective on the extent and nature of affairs and sexual intrigue in such societies is given by the Ache, who live in eastern Paraguay, in the southwestern part of the Brazilian highlands. As in many tribes, including the Mundurucu and Yanomamo, the Ache believe fetuses are a composite product of several different men with whom the mother had sexual relations - that a baby is sired by more than one man, a biological fiction anthropologists refer to as 'partible paternity.' That is, fetuses are thought to be built up over time, like the luster on pearls, by repeated applications of semen. This both makes affairs less of an immediate threat to the husband who is regularly with his wife and leads to significant ambiguities and multiple paternity.

All Ache groups in recent times have been gatherer-hunters. Apparently, for the last four hundred years they have engaged only in hostile interactions with outsiders and have not traded, visited, or intermarried with the other nearby populations. Only four Ache groups numbering about 600 existed in the nineteen seventies when they made permanent contact with outsiders and became 'civilized'. In their traditional gatherer-hunter mode, they live in small bands of fifteen to seventy individuals, moving throughout the forest. Bands comprise closely related kin and some long-term friends. Large sibling groups of both sexes tend to remain together along with additional kin. Men spend almost fifty hours per week getting food. They hunt peccaries, tapir, deer, pacas, agoutis, armadillos, capuchin monkeys, capybara, and coatis; they collect honey, which accounts for 87 percent of the calories in the Ache diet. Men often hunt in ways that look inefficient from standard optimal foraging perspectives, but in fact such men seem to be pursuing a high-risk, high-gain, show-off strategy that may often fail but can produce big, flashy hunting successes - and, with success, more sexual access to women. Women spend about two hours a day gathering; they collect fruits and insect larvae, as well as extract the fiber from palm trees. Women also carry the family's children, pets, and possessions. Their care of children and possessions constrains their ability to forage. Men may travel with the women's group, but more often they set off in small groups to search for game, spending about seven hours per day hunting. In the late afternoon, families gather and prepare food. Hunters rarely eat from their own kills, and much food is shared, leading early observers to argue that the society was completely egalitarian. While meat is apparently shared evenly under most circumstances, honey and gathered items are not. Further, when a man dies, his young dependent children are far more likely to die than if he had lived. While reciprocal sharing of meat is ordinary, when a man has died reciprocity can no longer be extended, so meat is no longer shared with the widow and children. The Ache are polygynous, and during young adulthood they may switch spouses frequently. This pattern seems to have changed little after contact with Europeans. After marriage, residence is typically matrilocal. Many children have multiple recognized fathers. Reproductive success is difficult to measure under such circumstances, but despite the fact that the Ache have little in the way of heritable wealth (which in so many societies correlates with reproductive success for men), status matters: the best hunters have the greatest reproductive success (Low R416 223).

An Ache woman rests during early stages of labor (Hrdy R323 248).

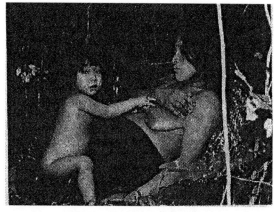

Ache men would donate any spare meat they had to women they wanted to have sex with. They were not doing so in the hope of helping to feed children they had already fathered but as direct payment for an affair. It was not easy to discover. Kim Hill (R323) found that he was gradually forced to drop questions about adultery from his studies because the Ache, under missionary influence, became increasingly squeamish about discussing the subject. The chiefs and the headmen were especially reluctant to talk about it, which is hardly surprising in view of the fact that they were the ones having the most affairs. By relying on gossip, Hill was able to piece together the pattern of adultery in the Ache. As expected he found that high-ranking men were involved most, however, unlike birds, it was not just the wives of low-ranking men who indulged. While Ache adulterers were frequently plying their mistresses with gifts of meat, Ache women were in turn constantly preparing for the possibility that they would be deserted by their husbands; and establishing alternative relationships through affairs. They are more likely to be unfaithful if the marriage is going badly. That is, of course, a double-edged sword: the marriage could break up if the affair is discovered. Hill and others believe that adultery has been much under-emphasized as an influence in the evolution of the human mating system.

When Kim Hill asked the Ache who their fathers were, he found he needed to expand his terminology - 321 Ache listed a total of 632 fathers - an average of almost two "fathers" each. Hence the Ache have a word, *miare*, for "the father who put it in"; *peroare*, for "the men who mixed it"; *momboare*, for "the ones who spilled it out"; and *bykuare*, for "the fathers who provided the child's essence." Men who provided the mother with meat while the baby was forming are seen as especially likely to have given the child its essence. In addition to the mother's husband, who is the socially designated father, a baby can be born with additional, secondary, fathers, who share some obligation to support this child as he or she matures. All men with whom a woman had sex when she became pregnant, and including the period just prior to when she was detectably pregnant, are expected to provide food for her child. This is a slightly different way of thinking about why the best hunters might get the most lovers. Are they out-competing other men for reproductive success, or incurring more obligations? Probably both. Among the Ache, Hill observed that children with just one father received less help, but when a mother lined up too many fathers, the extreme uncertainty of paternity dissuaded all candidates from helping. Children identified as having one primary and one secondary father had the best survival rates Are husbands jealous? Among the Ache, men deny it, but then later beat their wives. Not surprisingly, Ache mothers try to convince possible fathers that the club is more exclusive than it really is. (Hrdy R323 246)

When a man dies his small children are likely to die: since he can no longer share, other men do not share with his widow and children (Low R416 81). An infant who lost his father was four times more likely to die before the age of two. Even if the father was still alive, Ache children whose parents divorced were three times more likely to be killed than if the marriage endured. When a widowed or abandoned mother takes a new mate, risks to her infants shoot up. Terrible prospects are one reason why some foraging peoples bury orphans alive along with the deceased parent. Mothers themselves sometimes kill father-less infants after a conscious evaluation of what the future holds (Hrdy R323 236).

Canela: Matrilocal Promiscuity

The Canela of the Eastern Amazon are matrilocal and matrilineal at least over several generations and "have taken the 'touch of polyandry' that crops up so often in the mating behavior of other primates, justified and legitimized it through ideology and magnified its significance many times over through ritual" (Hrdy R323 249)

William Crocker (R138) gives a startling portrayal of Canela relationships. Sexual relations in both boys and girls usually begin as young as possible. A boy is initiated into sexual relations by an experienced woman in her late teens; formerly, he was then ordered by his "grandfathers" to have sex only with older women in their forties and fifties for several years. When a young male takes a girl's virginity, he has the choice of staying "married" to her ("they lie down") or of withdrawing from the relationship, after which his kin must pay a significant fine ("his-having-broken-in payment"). Every effort is made (largely exhortation by his kin and the elders) to keep a couple together, and the girl's family "buys" the young husband by means of a large meat pie ceremonially delivered to his family house late in the afternoon. Today meat pies increasingly are exchanged between both families.

Crocker and Crocker (R139 33) note that boys and girls are segregated at ages 6 to 7. At ages 6 to 14, a girl "is appointed to be a girl associate of a male society for one or a number of successive years. At one or more ceremonial points in the festival, beginning in her early teens, she has sexual relations with the society's members, teaching her that one of her roles in mature Canela life is to keep non-related males sexually satisfied." At age 11-13, "[a] girl's genitals [are] formally inspected by a disciplinary aunt to see if she had lost her virginity. If she had, the name of the male was demanded (Girls are no longer inspected)". After she has graduated as a girl associate, she is secluded under [postpuber-tal] food and sex restriction. At age 13 to 16, she presents food to her mother-in-law provided by her lover in return for sex with him. The period 13-18 is considered a time for sexual liaisons and few social responsibilities. The average age of first conception is 15. Formerly, girls were engaged to be married when they were 4 or 5 to young men 12 to 15 years older. Now, courtship takes place, and marriage is equated with defloration. "Girls almost always have intercourse before they menstruate, so their experience reinforces the Canela theory that sexual intercourse is the cause of menstruation. Ideally a girl has first intercourse with a young man in his late teens or 20s who has no children of his own".

Families often arranged engagements between children, a practice that is both old and current, but individual preferences prevail later. Just prior to and after puberty these engagements could be broken if the boy's kin made a small payment for his release. In a traditional Canela marriage ceremony, the bride and groom lie down on a mat, arms under each other's heads, legs entwined. The brother of each partner's mother then comes forward. He admonishes the bride and her new husband to stay together until the last child is grown, specifically reminding them not to be jealous of each other's lovers.

Until the birth of a child, young couples did not live in the same house. Although they were "married," young people were supposed to have sexual relations only very infrequently with persons of their own generation (including their spouses). Thus, a young man would only occasionally cohabit with his wife, and then usually just at night, on a platform bed raised high under the rafters for this purpose in her house. He returned to the plaza before the early morning dance. Nevertheless, the Canela do call these liaisons "marriages."

During this early childless stage, before the girl has given a whole deer to her mother-in-law and had her ceremonial belt and body painted red with urucu in return, the public aspects of her extramarital activities are restricted. After the belt-painting ceremony, however, which amounts to her husband's family's more complete acceptance of her, she is expected to be assigned as a girl associate to accompany male groups for the purposes of group sex. Her husband must not be jealous, though he increasingly objects these days, and maybe always did even in aboriginal times. Between the painting of her belt and child-birth, she is classed as a slippery, free person who must please most men with her sexual favors. If she does not, a group of men may waylay her to teach her to be generous.

Women may have great sexual flings between the belt-painting ceremony and the birth of their first child, but later they become embedded in the female matrix of domestic life. Hrdy (R323 247) notes: "in what may be one of the more extreme cases on record, unusual for hominids, ritual sex with twenty or more men during all-community ceremonies left some Canela mothers with an 'array' of candidates for fatherhood ... it is scarcely surprising that just as soon as she suspects she is pregnant, a Canela woman ... attempts to seduce the tribe's best hunters and fishermen". Between virginity loss and belt painting, and from the belt ceremony to conception —a girl might be "married" more than once. With conception and the survival of a child, however, divorce is almost impossible. There are numerous separations, however, some lasting as long as a year. This is remarkable, since matrilocal tribes are noted for their relatively high frequency of divorce.

The Canela marry persons they consider to be "non-related", where the genealogical relationship has been lost: forgotten or very attenuated by social or spatial distance. They also sometimes "commit incest" with relatives as close as third or second cross-cousins. First cross-cousin sexual relationships and marriages, which occur very rarely, are held to be shameful and life shortening. Uterine sibling sexual contacts are thought to cause madness or death. Quite clearly, there are no prescriptive or preferential marriage rules, nor do formal or statistically related alliances exist. The sororate is practiced only occasionally but nevertheless is theoretically favored whereas the levirate is not. Brothers do not marry into the same matrilocal family.

The main point of friction in the Canela sociocultural system is nevertheless between husband and wife. Tribal schisms, while rare, do occur, and political rivalries between age class leaders are relatively mild and suppressed by the high cohesiveness of the social structure and the great emphasis on generosity of spirit. Non-competitiveness and overt cooperation rather than a show of hostility are traits that are considered manly. "Women, animals and local Brazilians fight," the Canela say, "but Canela men bear up under problems and adversity." At least 80% of the cases coming before the tribal council involve marital disputes.

Survival of the mother's children takes priority over a man's exclusive sexual access to his wife. Traditionally couples with children, that is most of the adult population, would seldom part because of adultery. A man might come upon a man having relations with his wife on their platform bed, but even such a disrespectful act (especially on the part of his wife) would not be grounds for fighting, let alone divorce. Nevertheless, it would be sufficient reason for a payment between the two extended families to alleviate the husband's shame.

Canelas can however divorce and remarry if they are not raising children born to them. There are numerous other childless couples, however, who remain married for a lifetime, although a few separate over infertility. It is likely overall that formerly, men were married to women about ten years their junior. Many couples display great love and devotion to each other. After years of sexual intercourse, it is believed that a couple's blood has become interchanged. It was agreed that this mingling was enough to require the illness taboos to be maintained between the couple, as among uterine siblings, but that spouses were not considered to be of the same 'blood group'.

Only a man's departures are restrained by fines. In contrast, if a woman absolutely does not want a man, he must leave, even if they were married for some time and she had children by him. Whereas a husband can be coerced by pressure from his kin, his age class, the council of elders, and the ignominy of fines, a wife cannot be forced to change her mind through such pressures once she has taken a determined stand. Husbands can be controlled, reasoned with, and restrained. Wives, in contrast, are the immovable solid blocks of society. A man has very little influence in his marital home and in the disciplining of his children. His wife's actual and classificatory brothers and mother's brothers were responsible for counseling and ceremonial purposes and took a hand in controlling the children.

Matrilocal residence and the dominance of their ubiquitous female kin hold women strongly in place. Additionally, there used to be occasional visits from special patrilateral male and female counselors to pressure them into conformity. Fear of vicious female gossip and, formerly, the danger of illness and death through witchcraft, motivated women to be reasonably cooperative and generous. Thus in marked contrast to men, women find their security in the permanence and continuity of generations of strongly maintained social and ceremonial positions. Women are so secure that they can afford to be irritable, changeable, and demanding, while their husbands must put up with such treatment.

Maritally, women are seen as suffering more: possible physical damage in losing virginity and in childbirth, strenuous work when carrying wood and hauling water, and lack of mobility while raising children and maintaining a household for their husbands. Consequently, the husband is continually rebalancing the marital "scales" by working hard and making small payments to his wife's family. In modern times, however, the balance is changing, because the husband, as a son-in-law, is becoming freer — released from the ancient social pressures that forced him to stay with his wife's family for the sake of the children. He is now becoming a great asset because of his ability to contribute economically (sometimes becoming literate and obtaining odd jobs) to the increasingly important family group.

The old-timers pointed out that the ancestors were fierce . It was not that the men fought each other all the time but that they recognized a "pecking order" based on a combination of tribal authoritative power and fighting ability. There were continual showdowns between men but only rarely open hostilities, because internal harmony was most highly prized. There were stories of fierce men pulling weaker ones away from women in the very act of sexual intercourse and simply taking over. Any ensuing hostilities would then be frustrated by other nearby men, and continuing hatreds, pouting, and revenge were very much counseled against and lost in the all-consuming activities of age class life.

Shipibo: Subincision

We cannot leave this arena of warrior culture without noticing the incidence of female 'subincision' practised by tribes such as the Shipibo, Conibo and Amahuaca. Although said to be 'matriarchal' with women being involved prominently in the cultural crafts trade, the Shipibo traditionally practice clitoridectomy. Female circumcision from any point of view is a means of keeping women in check, it deprives them from pleasure during sex and hence interest in taking lovers. Their bodies do not, in effect, belong to them, but to their husbands. As usual, with African female genital mutilation, women are centrally involved.

The Shipibo girls' initiation involves clitorectomy. This is somewhat of a paradox because of the reported matriarchal aspects to Shipibo culture although they are patrilocal.

Singing is essential to several parts of the ceremony. Several thigh-supports are made of light balsa wood. These are hollowed out of the half-cylinders cut from a single log. It is essential that the men sing well while performing this task. During their songs the male carvers carry the thigh-supports on their shoulders. These men then carry the balsa wood to their wives so that the women can decorate them with special designs. After painting the designs, the women place the thigh supports on their shoulders 'singing, they then dance a ronda among themselves, forming a circle and holding hands.' The women continue drinking and singing while they dance in a circle on the plaza. With song and drink they invite the guests to the feast. In company with these dancing and drinking female singers, the girl's mother seeks out two helpers who will hold the girl during her operation. Next they go in search of a woman expert in cutting the clitoris. They invite the woman by playing on a long bamboo flute called the tiati. The husbands of the women who do the cutting are summoned with a different musical instrument. These are big two-toned signal gongs. When guests arrive for the feast, they arrive at the canoe landing blowing on their own bamboo flutes. A vigil of drinking precedes the day of the cutting. During that night the girl is encouraged to drink herself into a stupor. Special designs are painted all over her body and face. The women painting the girl with these designs must sing. In the meantime, all the guests perform a circular dance and sing the whole night through. On the day of the cutting music is a primary concern for the Shipibo. ... the girl is decorated with all her ornaments... she is also hung with trade bells, 'the seed that sings' in Shipibo. Their tinkling sound is characteristic of the ceremony, and mothers treasure the bells to hand on to their daughters. At the same time she is adorned the girl is sung beautiful puberty rite songs telling her how pretty she is and that she will be made drunk and will feel nothing ... While the girl is brought in with her two assistants, their husbands are playing music on their large bamboo flutes. The girl first dances with the husbands, then is brought to the women, who sing songs with her, then back to the men for more songs, and then finally back with the women (internet).

Significantly under Christian influence, the Shipibo have undergone a population explosion because of the repression of polygyny and its consequent sexual restrictions increased the average number of children a woman would have by an effective 1.3 (Hern R303, R304).

Warrior Peoples and the Rise of Male Dominance

The diversity of these warrior societies demonstrate several aspects of Sanday's thesis concerning the rise of patriarchy as a form of polarized response to ecological stress, including stresses caused by migrating warrior groups. They show in graphic detail how male dominance in warrior-hunter violence can lead to a break down of reproductive paradox, in which women are used as tradeable items or objects of rape, abduction and capture.

Associated with these motifs are mythologies of primal sexual conflict and origins wrought in violence, migrational instability and conquest by war. The sexual relations reflect these mythologies, in polarization, sexual dominance and attempts by men to assert control over culture and the instruments of religious power by violence and fear. They also appear to have resulted in practices of female sexual mutilation, wife abduction and patterns of homosexual activity, which themselves have intimations of power and class and the rule of power of one individual over another, be they male or female.

Penis worship in pre-Columbian pottery from Peru, Mexico and Ecuador

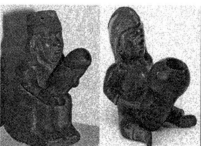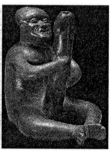

Melanesian cultures of New Guinea express further dimensions of such sexual distortions of dominance, arising from the tensions of warrior society. The Sambia (R438 377) practice wife abduction from neighbouring tribes and consequently there are severe tensions between men and women. The men believe they lose vital sexual energy to the women when they have sex and consequently that they have to store up additional sperminal energy before they enter marriage. They also believe a boy will not fully mature as a man, rather than a woman, who matures early and natuarlly, unless he receives sperm from older men. Boys are thus inculcated to receive as much sperm as possible in homosexual sex. Similar practices occur among the neighbouring Keraki and Kiwai (R82 297). As they mature, like the Greeks (p 203), they in turn become donors of sperm, first to younger boys, and then heterosexually in marriage. Thus the polarized heterosexual tension can be expressed in a two-phase dominant homosexual relationship. At another extreme, Schneebaum (R603, R604, R508) claims, the cannibalistic Amazonian Arakmbut and New Guinea Asmat live a sexually divided existence, in which men sleep together in their own long house, bonding homosexually, in contrast to the distant, unaffectionate relations between men and women.

Societies in which women are unavailable sometimes tolerate male homosexual relationships as a substitute. Australian aboriginal societies solicit boys as substitute wives for a number of years. The Nambicuarra of Brazil allow 'false love' between adolescent cross-cousins because of the unavailability of girls as prospective wives. But the adults find this a laughing matter thinking of them as infantile. Other societies such as the Nyakyusa of Tanzania allow homosexual relations between boys in adolescence but forbid them in adulthood. Of 42 world cultures, 11.9% have no knowledge of male homosexuality, 21.5% allow, or ignore it, 14.3% ridicule, or scorn, but don't punish it and 52.8% disapprove of it and take social measures against it (Broude R82 296). This demonstrates both that male homosexuality is not a cultural universal and that culture shapes same-sex relations in a variety of ways.

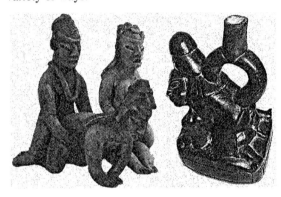

Moche portrayals of homosexual sodomy from Peru. The power, age and class relationships and consensuality of these sexual encounters remain unclear.

There is among warrior societies a clear pattern supporting Joan Bamberger's thesis (R39) that warrior society depends on the myth of matriarchy a previous time in which women were in control which led to chaos, social strife and a rationalization for men to seize control from women. Bamberger notes two further examples which parallel the myths of the origin of Yaje and the stealing of the Mundurucu trumpets. Father Martin Gusinde noted of the Yamana-Yaghan that women had sole power and the men did the domestic duties. The women invented the (now male) *kina* hut and intimidated the men by impersonating terrifying spirits until the sun man led an overthrow killing the women and transforming them into animals and taking control of the rituals for themselves (Taylor R670 137).

Likewise the Selk'nam of Amazonia claim the women once kept a lodge, initiated the girls in magic arts, and terrified the men, by bringing on sickness or death to those who displeased them. The men then killed the initiated women, waiting for the young girls to come of age, and in fear they might again band together, set up their own lodge whose purpose was to ensure the women couldn't again usurp power (Taylor R670 138).

Paradoxically however, the concept of partible paternity, with its limitations on male expectations of paternity certainty, has served to limit the capacity of men to claim sole paternity rights. This has also reinforced the capacity of the women to retain a primary sense of maternal continuity, while securing paternal support from more than one man, at the same time escaping some of the most immediate and dire consequences of sexual 'infidelity'.

The friction between matrilineal and matrilocal motifs and those of patriarchy, and their capacity to lead to a variety of cultural, sexual, marital, and parenting patterns are also evident and form a counterfoil for examining the rise of militarized cultures, which we shall examine next in the rise of urban societies central to the emergence of our major world 'civilizations' from Sumeria to the present day.

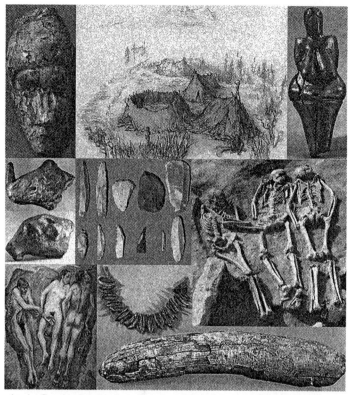

Dolni Vestonice in Czechoslovakia is a site of an encampment of mammoth hunters dating from about 30,000 years ago. The remains include a burial site apparently honouring people of both sexes (a 'menage-a-trois' with a central female, apparently bonded to the right-hand male, red ochre between the female's thighs and a disconcerting 'spike' driven into the left 'male's' crotch) and a hearth site with a 'venus' figurine baked clay animal figures, tools, jewelry, and a carved head of a woman whose arthritic disfigurement appears to match a skeleton at the site. An additional female figure is drawn on a tusk. The coincidence of female representations and the apparent significance of the role of the 'hearth' woman amidst a hunting encampment attests to a respect for both sexes (internet).

Emergence of Civilization and Fall into Patriarchal Dominion

Paleolithic Origins

There are two sexually polarized theories of human cultural origins, both of which have failed to stand the test of empirical evidence. The first is 'man the hunter' (Washburn, Morris) suggesting that male strength and hunting prowess led both to male dominance, and intelligence and culture, through skills of hunting, such as tool-making. Such theories are prone to stress male violence and treat women as mere possessions and tradeable items. While they do fit well with our cultural paradigm of male dominance, they do not well-explain the origin of intelligence (p 53), nor do they fit well with what we know of so-called primal cultures, where women bring in the majority of the diet by gathering (p 108), making them more autonomous as child-rearers than the theory would allow. As a natural successor of the 'killer-ape' theory it gives a pessimistic view of humanity's violence and viability.

The counterpoised matriarchal origin theory is the 'mother-right' proposed by Johan Jakob Bachofen (R31) - an evolutionary 'advance' in which an intervening stage of matriarchy led society out of barbarism into modern patriarchy, which he deemed the triumph of superior political and religious thought and organization, despite advocating the incorporation of the 'feminine principle' of nurturance and altruism in modern society. The Swiss philologist proposed an era of 'unregulated hetaerism' in which women were sexually degraded and defenseless, followed by an 'Amazon' revolt that inaugurated an era of matriarchy. In this stage, women created marriage to tame the male. This supposedly still-animalistic and 'backward' era was superseded by a 'higher' stage of human development: patriarchy. He never used the term matriarchy but 'mutterricht' and gynecocracy, for 'rule by women'.

Following him Engels (R192), used the term mother-right 'to describe matrilineal kinship relations, in which the property of men did not pass to their children, but to their sisters' children'. Both also accepted a progression from group marriage to monogamous marriage. Engels reasoned that a woman would seek monogamy because she 'acquired the right to give herself to one man only'. He also drew attention to prostitution as an indispensable prop to monogamous marriage. Engels went on to state (Taylor R670 77)"the first class antagonism which appears in history coincides with the development of the antagonism between man and woman in monogamous marriage, and the first class oppression with that of the female sex by the male". Both Engels and later Marx were strongly influenced by the work of Lewis Morgan (R474) who spent four decades studying the Iroquois, whom the French missionary Lafitau in Jesuit Relations 1724 had expressed astonishment at the power of Haudenosaunee (Iroquois) matrons: "All real authority is vested in them... nothing is more real than the superiority of the women" (Mann R425).

Joan Bamberger (R39) notes that myths of matriarchy - stories of prior rule by women are relatively widespread in patriarchal societies and that they function as social charters justifying male power (p 171). Several of the myths we have seen from the Hadza (p 131), through the Dogon (p 139), to the Mundurucu (p 164), and origin of Yaje (p 160) support this thesis.

The elevation of woman to deity on the one hand,
and the downgrading of her to child and chattel on the other, produce the same result ...
The myth of matriarchy is but a tool used to keep woman bound to her place.
To free her, we need to destroy the myth. Joan Bamberger (R39).

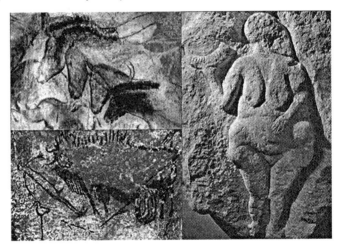

Top left: Hunting Chauvet (~30,000 BC). Bottom left: Shaft Scene Lascaux Man with erection apparently killed by a bison which is also disemboweled by a spear through its anus. The bird suggests a shamanic interpretation. Right: female relief at Laussel (~20,000 BC), associating fecundity, hand on uterus, the bull or bison horn as male moon with 13 notches of the menstrual year, (also the days of the waxing moon), suggesting her role was to promote fertility. She still shows traces of ochre, symbolic of menstrual blood. Horses were not domesticated until as late as 4,000-2,000 BC but caused explosive changes (p 183).

Central to the argument for matriarchy was ubiquitous evidence of 'mother goddess' figures (p 92), and founding myths in many ancient religions. Gerda Lerner (R397 29) notes: "the difficulty of reasoning from such evidence toward the construction of social organizations where women were dominant", particularly with the more ancient 'Venus' figurines such as Dolni Vestonice (p 173) and Laussel (p 174), is that we don't know the purpose they were used for, although their presence is suggestive. Were they goddesses, fertility symbols, subordinate tokens of femininity like the Virgin Mary, marriage tokens, or merely sexual objects? Certainly the female figurines express the fatness of fecundity, but there are no mother figures. Lauren Talalay notes many are neuter or hermaphroditic - with female breasts and male genitals. Cynthia Eller (R187) suggests some may have been shamanistic healing charms. Karel Absolon who excavated a number of the Dolni Vestonice figurines wrote that 'sex and hunger were the two motives that influenced the entire mental life of the mammoth hunters and their productive art', calling the phallic androgynous figurine below 'diluvial plastic pornography'. While the later cave paintings are full of dynamic representations, the 'Venus figurines' are faceless and show little indication of any form of activity, nor whether they were made by women or men or for what purpose. One from Kostienki apparently shows a pregnant female bound by the wrists opening serious questions as to the 'goddess' interpretation. One can also question whether the division of labour passed more to male hunters in the northern tundra of a Europe emerging from the ice age.

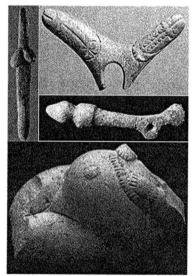

Above clockwise: Phallic batons from Dolni Vestonice, Gorge d'Enfer, St. Marcel. Below: Kostienki bound figurine.

Lerner notes that, as we have seen (p 143), such ethnographic evidence, as is held up, turns out to be evidence not for a dominant 'matriarchy', but 'matriliny' and 'matrilocality' in which, while women do have participatory power, many or most of the economic and family decisions are made by male relatives. This is true both of societies like the Canela and the *beena* marriages of the Old Testament, such as that of Laban. Matrilineal societies are now a small minority and are currently vanishing, because they tend to succumb to the pressures of more competitive patrilineal societies and their exploitative techno-economic systems. Moreover, in the gatherer-hunter societies which stand at the root of our genetic tree, there is a complementation of a major gathering food resource brought in by women, who also do the bulk of the child-rearing, while the men hunt food prized for sexual favours and the relative status of men and women is separate but equal, rather than a dominant matriarchy. These also demonstrate that patrilineal descent does not have to involve subjugation of women, nor does matrilineal descent indicate matriarchal dominance. Finally because the genetic evidence emerging from mitochondrial mtDNA and Y-chromosome DNA studies (Seielstad et. al. R620) suggests that human emergence, like ape societies is dominated by female exogamous migration (p 143) in a context of moderate polygyny, it is unlikely that matrilocal societies have predominated on a population basis during the Paleolithic.

Claude Lévi-Strauss (R400) offers a single monolithic building block out of which men constructed culture - the incest taboo, linking this immediately to the exchange of women "The prohibition of incest is less a rule prohibiting marriage with the mother, sister or daughter, than a rule obliging the mother, sister or daughter to be given to others. It is the supreme rule of the gift." He reasons that in this process, women are 'reified' they are dehumanized and thought of more as things than humans. This then marks the beginning of women's subordination. Lerner (R397 25) also questions the assumption that men should invent this basic rule and apply it to trading women rather than vice versa, pointing out however that male exogamy could lead to armed treachery. There are several difficulties here. The genetic studies suggest female exogamy is not a cultural invention but an evolutionary trend. Unlike most other mammals, apes are broadly female exogamous possibly for similar reasons. We have seen that ape exogamy appears to be driven by the females and that other species as well as our own, through childhood hyperfamiliarity and

MHC detection seek outside partners with complementary histocompatibility thus avoiding incest without imposing a cultural taboo. Ridley (R567) suggests the incest taboo is more a rule for deciding which cousins are permissible, because of these innate biological and genetic factors.

A more plausible argument for the cultural institutionalization of exchange of women, or their capture, is directly their capacity for reproduction and its positive effect on a groups future viability. Lévi-Strauss and Meillassoux assert the exchange of women leads to private property, reversing Engels' position (Lerner R397 49-52), supported by Aaby (R1). The former see this as sourced in a phase of sexually egalitarian abundance resulting from horticulture, leading to reproductive competition and consequently abduction of females and on a less warlike basis their mutual exchange. The latter sees it in a more generalized ecological context consistent with Sanday's findings. Large scale agriculture and the struggle between urban states appears to have been one of the critical contexts.

Engels established several ground-breaking connections between class and property and the rise of patriarchy - changes in kinship and the division of labour and womens' position in society, a connection between private property, monogamous marriage and prostitution, economic and political dominance by men and their control over female sexuality, and finally in Gerda Lerner's terms (R397 23) "by locating 'the world historical defeat of the female sex' in the period of the formation of archaic states, based on the dominance of properties elites, he gave the event historicity." It is this process that we shall turn to next.

Like the evidence from societies such as the !Kung (p 106), Mbuti (p 120),Biaka (p 124) and Sandawe (p 118), the evidence from European paleolithic sites is at least consistent with a social structure in which the expressions of the activities and visions of both sexes and particularly of female fertility and supernatural power are regularly represented. It is significant at Dolni Vestonice that a prominent aspect of what is presumed to be an active mammoth-hunting camp site is a hearth with both a female fertility figure, figures of the hunt and a carefully sculpted female head possibly of the partly disfigured women whose skeleton lies nearby. This and the burial site indicate that respect for and even reverence for female fecundity and the spiritual importance of women are present in this hunting culture. Similar considerations apply to the Laussel site where the female figure has many features suggesting an active cultural respect for fecundity and its propitiation.

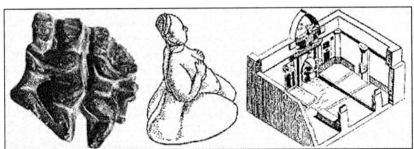

Three aspects of the feminine at Çatal Hüyük: Left: The hieros gamos or sacred sexual union, leading to progeny. The hieros gamos continued in nymphete form with Inanna in Sumeria and Ishtar in Babylon, but Yahweh, Zeus, Enki and Indra assumed patriarchal dominion from Greece to Vedic India. Centre: The fecund fat Goddess of plenty. Right: Temple with portal surmounted by a pregnant 'goddess'. Houses are also arranged with the maternal bed oriented towards the central temples while the male sleeping platforms are arranged haphazardly. Motifs of bull's horns and headless corpses picked by vultures with human skulls also pervade the temples (Melaart, Eisler R182)

The Neolithic and the Great Goddess

The first signs of the development of urban culture appear in the Near East around 10,000 years ago in sites such as Jericho, associated with the cultivation of wheat, in areas where it is naturally adapted, and with the beginnings of animal husbandry. It is said that women invented agriculture, and consistent with this, we find the expression of agricultural fertility in the form of a fertility goddess, sometimes called the Great Mother, who is a creatrix of all, but particularly of the fertile Earth and the fertility that, season by season, is regenerated in the agricultural cycle that springs from the Earth. At the same time there is a celebration of human fertility in the form of the *hieros gamos*, or sacred sexual union, a theme of fertility, based also in animal husbandry. Later in the lean season this is accompanied by male sacrifice and the ploughing of fresh blood back into the soil to refertilize it. These two themes, of goddess as creatrix and goddess as lover, continue to be elaborated in a variety of forms and personae, from Canaan, through Sumeria, to all the cultures of the Near East. In Sumeria the cultural interaction of the Shepherd King and the Planter Queen formed a counterpoint which became the progenitor of civilization as we know it today.

Çatal Hüyük was a Neolithic urban settlement of 6000 to 8000 people, a town built like a beehive of individual abodes showing little variation in size and furnishing, entered by a ladder from the roof and equipped with a mud-brick heath and an oven. The absence of streets, a large plaza or palace suggests a non-hierarchical society. Rush rugs, baskets and obsidian objects indicate a wide and healthy trade. Over a period of 1500 years from about 6200 BC new towns were built on the remnants of older settlements. Comparison of James Mellaart's (R456) excavations at Çatal Hüyük with the smaller village Hacilar about 1000 years older in Anatolia give us an insight into these early transitions. Every house had a large sleeping platform, oriented towards the shrines, under which the buried skeletons of women and sometimes children were found. In all 136 of the 222 adult skeletons were women. Smaller platforms were found in varying positions in the different rooms with sometimes men or children buried, but not both together. Women were buried with mirrors, jewelry, and bone and stone tools, men with their weapons, rings, beads and tools. About one in forty had ochre burials. Most of these were women. Mellaart reasons that the women had high status and were possibly priestesses. The overall pattern is consistent with matrilocal residence.

The various layers reveal an extraordinarily large number of extensively decorated shrines. In the lower layers there are only bulls and rams, animal paintings and bull's horns, commonly interpreted as symbolic of male gods, although Gimbutas, by contrast, imagined they were abstract Fallopian tubes (Taylor R670 156). From about 6200 BC these give way to the earliest representations of female figures, with exaggerated breasts, buttocks and hips, seated, giving birth, surrounded by plaster breasts some shaped over animal skulls. Artifacts include a depiction of the hieros gamos in naked partners embracing, followed by a mother with child. They include motifs of both life and death - vultures pecking headless figures, breasts with jaws, and human skulls. They also involve associations with both flower, grain and vegetation patterns and with the hunt, in the leopard. In one hunting scene there are large numbers of men and two women with their legs spread apart suggesting sexual favours of the hunt. Mellaart (R456) argues that these were goddesses, that the male was an object of pride, valued for his virility and that his role in procreation was understood, and that men and women shared power and community control.

Although the presence of skulls and headless corpses is a little spooky, there is no evidence of warfare, or of blood sacrifice, suggesting there was no military caste. Mellaart concludes that women developed agriculture, created Neolithic religion and were themselves the artists. Some of these conclusions are debated. Lawrence Angel has found a significant increase in the average life span of women over this period from 28.2 to 29.8 years, still short of the male span of 34.3, but consistent with improving conditions. The sudden demise of the settlement is also consistent with an incapacity to cope with incursions by more militaristic patriarchal cultures (Lerner R397 34).

Some have suggested the cult of Magna Mater (Great Mother) originated in Çatal Hüyük. The statue of a woman upon a throne with two leopards at her side, is the form she is known for in Phrygia as Cybele. In Rome, Cybele came to be known as Magna Mater, the magical goddess raised by panthers and lions. The leaders of her cult were female priestesses and castrated male priests called Galli. During her festivals frenzied music was played and male followers would chop off their testicles and throw then to the crowd, in a re-enactment of Attis's self-castration in a fit of madness due to his infidelity to the Great

Mother. He was turned into a pine tree. The Christmas tree and the social castration of the Roman Catholic priesthood stand in her long shadow. In the cult of Diana, human testicles were replaced by those of bulls, resulting in her 'many-breasted' form. The need for more sperm than one male could provide leads to the 'virginal' conception of Mary (Morris R477 201).

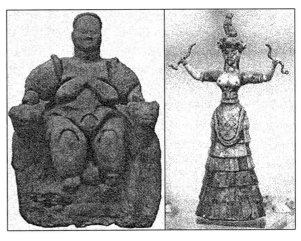

'Cybele' -Çatal Hüyük (reconstructed), snake 'goddess' Crete

As we have seen (p 143), Peggy Reeves Sanday's anthropological work shows that horticultural societies often have female creatrix deities, which tend to be supplanted by male ones as cultivation moves through shifting to advanced agriculture. She also found societies with a constant food supply were more likely to be sexually equal and express female power. This is consistent with the historical idea of the rise of female power and female deities in the Neolithic contemporary with women inventing horticulture and agriculture through knowledge of plant reproductive cycles, establishing certainty of food supply, and its later supplanting by competitive war-like patriarchal cultures, upon the development of large-scale agriculture, property and kingships.

Modern concepts of the 'Mother Goddess' are shrouded in psychoanalytic notions which fail to understand the complexity of our sociobiological heritage and tend to rationalize the cultural motivations of the authors. Gerda Lerner (R397 40) in considering the Neolithic Mother Goddess, suggests: "we can understand why men and women might have chosen this as their first form of religious expression by considering the psychological bond between mother and child", going on to cite Freud's struggle of separation of the self from an all-powerful mother. Following a culturalist rejection of the 'essentialist' role of mothering in modern society, Lerner then attempts to discretely justify the same role culturally in the 'permissible' context of the Great Mother:

> "under primitive conditions, before the institutions of society were created, the actual power of the mother over the infant must have been awesome. ... The life-giving mother truly had power over life and death. No wonder that men and women, observing this dramatic and mysterious power of the female, turned to the veneration of the Mother Goddess. My point here is to stress the *necessity* which created the initial division of labour by which women do the mothering. For millennia group survival depended on it, and no alternative was available."

Apparently it is fine for gatherer-hunter societies to depend on women as mother for both *essential* practical reasons of safety and survival and also for *cultural* constructions in which woman is venerated and enshrined as mother, but in any other cultural context this deeply biological relationship is an anathema. Furthermore in gatherer-hunter societies we do not find this infantile concept of deity-as-infinite mother, but sophisticated ironic portrayals of God. It is thus much more likely that the veneration of the Goddess is a Neolithic phenomenon associated with plant nurture and societies benefiting from the resulting abundance.

Gerda Lerner (R397 43) then uses Nancy Chodrow's psychoanalytic argument to outline a scheme for engendering of male and female roles:

> "Boys and girls learn to expect from women the infinite, accepting love of a mother, but they also associate with women their fears of powerlessness. In order to find their identity, boys develop themselves as other-than-the-mother, and turn away from cultural expression towards action in the world."

This leads to a feminine view of connectedness with the world and a masculine one of separation and differentiation. However this is not just a psychoanalytic view but a deeply evolutionary one. There is a great deal of validity in the idea that male fear of paternity uncertainty in a world where men do not themselves give birth has led to a patriarchal reaction. This is consistent with Freud's idea of childhood frustration and Mary O'Brien's idea of the construction of institutions of dominance based on men's psychological need to compensate for their inability to bear children (R397 46), but places them on a valid genetic and biological footing in institutions establishing paternity certainty and patriliny.

However the idea that a psycho-analytic infantile view historically preceded a natural view of male and female fertility, proceeding historically from female parthenogenetic birth, for example from clay and menstrual blood, to a later construct understanding only the role of the male in fertilization, based on the discovery of animal husbandry is not supportable or realistic for several reasons. Firstly all animals consciously or unconsciously base their entire reproductive effort on an implicit acceptence of the mutual role of the sexes in fertility. It is fundamental to our sociobiological heritage. It has always been clear that only heterosexual intercourse produces babies and both sexes can recognize their offspring by smell and visual characteristics and can often tell that offspring resemble both their parents in various intimate ways. Secondly there is no evidence for a truly primal matriarchy, and egalitarian gatherer-hunter societies who practice neither animal husbandry, nor horticulture still show an understanding of paternity and maternity. Thirdly the incest taboo has no meaning except in a context where paternity is understood. Fourthly animal husbandry itself has an ancient origin. The sheep was domesticated by 9000 BC and the dog probably very much earlier in the Paleolithic. Goats, pigs and cattle were all domesticated in the Near East by 5500 BC. Elizabeth Fisher and Mary O'Brien have suggested male rape and paternity fears both source from the discovery of animal husbandry, leading to patriarchy. Lerner (46) however acknowledges the ancient origin of animal husbandry consistent with its occurrence at Catal Hüyük, discounting a causal connection. Fifthly the hieros gamos is very ancient and occurs at Catal Hüyük. Sixthly patriarchal ideas of the female being the passive vessel of male fertility are sexually political cultural constructs designed to impose male institutions, rather than existing naive beliefs. Taking a cultural position, we would expect the 'Mother Goddess' to be equally a cultural overlay, and thus call her more honestly and simply the 'Neolithic Great Goddess'.

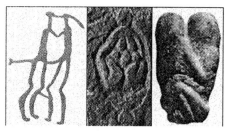

Hieros gamos or sexual union: Rock painting with French kiss (Tanum Sweden) , rock carving c 10,000 BC Europe , Negev Desert (Werner Forman, New Sci. 5 Oct 96, Campbell R104, Avi-Yonah R28)

Similar, although less complete remains, indicative of societies with female power and reverence, are scattered widely across Old Europe, from Avebury to Bulgaria. Marija Gimbutas (R239) reports 30,000 miniature sculptures in clay, marble, bone, copper and gold known from some 3000 sites in Southeastern Europe and that these testify to the communal worship of the Great Goddess and that the Neolithic cultural symbols survived into the third millennium BC in the Aegean and the second millennium in Crete. Putatively 'uterine' temples with a possible funerary role occur in Malta around 4000 BC and the beginnings of 'snake goddess' representations begin around 6000 BC in Crete, whose later Minoan civilization (c 1500 BC), with its feminine motifs has been much extolled by Eisler (R182) and Gadon (R229). In the eighth century Hesiod spoke of the Minoan culture "the earth poured forth its fruits unbidden in boundless plenty. In peaceful ease they kept their lands with good abundance, rich in flocks and ... did not worship the gods of war". Archaeologist Nicolas Platon, notes that this was a "remarkable peaceful society" where descent was still traced through the mother and that "the influence of women is visible in every sphere"(Eisler R182), consistent with sexually-egalitarian culture. Later Minoan representations include the famous 'snake goddess' (p 178), the poppy 'goddess' with slit opium pods in her head dress (p 473), a fresco of 'darker-skinned' men attending

180

a female priestess with bared breasts, and those of young men and women bull leaping, also associated with Europa and the legend of the Minotaur, through which Theseus the Greek king overthrew the culture. Zeus was identified by Greek settlers with the Year God of the Cretan Goddess, born in a cave sacred to her. At the site, later devoted to Zeus, horns and the labrys double-axe symbolic of the goddess are still present among the remains.

Genealogy of the Sumerian deities to Inanna and Dumuzi (Wolkenstein and Kramer). An, Enlil and Enki form a male trinity overthrowing Goddess culture. Ereshkigal and Gugalina the bull are sent to hell.

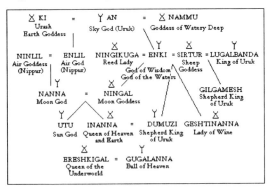

The Descent of the Queen of Heaven

There are also a profusion of archaeological finds scattered across the Near East emphasizing breasts, navel and vulva often in a squatting position characteristic of childbirth. However it remains unclear exactly what these represent, particularly in contexts like Israel where they may be an expression of the Canaanite Queen of Heaven or Qadesh in Hathor head dress, or a countercultural expression of such popular practice in the presence of other dominant patriarchal religious and social structures.

Lerner notes (R397 150) that in some of the most ancient depictions and myths the Great Goddess is a lone maternal creatrix, but she is 'later' joined by a consort who shares in the creative process in recognition of the sexual process of fertility. Founding myths of several cultures do allude to the Great Goddess as a virtually universal dominant figure in the most ancient stories. For example the Egyptian goddess Nun gives birth to the sun god Atum who then creates the rest of the universe, The Sumerian goddess Nammu parthenogenetically creates the sky god An and the earth goddess Ki, and in Greece Gaia parthenogenetically creates Uranos the sky. However as we have noted (p 179) the hieros gamos goes back to the paleolithic.

The difficulty with this idea is that these parthenogenetic myths may not be the most ancient human creation stories, but attest rather to a transitional period of neolithic matriliny associated with womens' discovery of horticulture and agriculture. The association between the planter goddess and shepherd kings, which the flowering of Sumer appears founded on, is a tale of fusion between a horticultural, presumably Great Goddess culture, 'overtaken' by nomadic, patriarchal shepherds. There is thus no single line of history, but two lines meeting. Gods are also extremely ancient and span diverse cultures.

The Babylonian Enuma Elish begins:

Firm ground below had not ben called by name,
Naught but primordial Apsu the begetter,
(and) Mummu-Tiamat, she who bore them all.
Their waters commingling as a single body ...

In the Sumerian descent of Inanna the previous older tradition is hinted at in Ereshkigal condemned to the underworld and the death of Gugalanna the sacred bull of heaven, reflecting the ancient bull's horns we have seen already from Laussel to Catal Hüyük in association with the Great Goddess and the lunar cycle.

Although she dates from as early as 3000 BC in Uruk, Inanna herself appears as the daughter of the moon god and goddess Nannar and Ningal, suggesting she carries a different and probably later archetype, partially into the patriarchal transition. Dumuzi the shepherd king is also the son of Enki the god of wisdom and Sirtur the sheep goddess. These are in turn descended from liaisons between An the sky god and either Ki the earth goddess or Nammu goddess of the watery deep, indicating city states have established a turn over of civic deities. Inanna is no longer so much a mother goddess as a nubile sex goddess of heaven, Earth and the underworld, who celebrates the agricultural cycle in the hieros gamos - the annual mating with the young god-king and his death and rebirth in propitiating the cycle of the season of agricultural fertility. However the Goddess is now projected into a more celestial sphere of sacred power encompassing heaven, Earth and the underworld in a shamanistic circumnavigation of life and death.

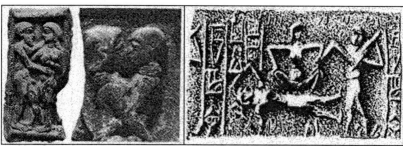

The courtship of the planter queen Inanna and the shepherd king Dumuzi (Wolkenstein and Kramer R747) is followed by Dumuzi's sacrifice. The new king kills the old in the presence of the goddess, as typified by Mot killing Aleyin for Anath in Canaan. (Campbell R103).

The hieros gamos and its association with sacred kingship and seasonal male sacrifice is ancient and almost universal to the widest spread of Near Eastern religion, common to Inanna of Uruk and Dumuzi, Ishtar of Babylon and Tammuz, Cybele and her son Attis, Artemis and Hippolytus, Kali and Shiva of the Indus Valley, Anath of Canaan and Aleyin, Aphrodite and Adonis, and Diana with Actaeon and the hapless king of the grove of Nemi, whose grisly fate became the keynote for Frazer's "Golden Bough" (R220).

Multiple personae of the Near Eastern Goddess include clockwise from top left, Lilith, Ishtar a cake mold from Mari (Batto), Inanna, Syrian Qadesh in Hathor head-dress with 'ithyphallic' god Min (below inset Hathor, Egypt and Timna and figurine Palestine), Isis nursing Horus, and Canaanite 'queen of the wild beasts' (Minet-al-Beida) suggestive of Asherah. For descendents of the so-called 'Mother Goddess', motherhood is rare among fertility goddesses. Only Isis has a maternal persona manifesting as nursing Horus. Lilith has an aura of precocious sexuality and fecundity without regard for her offspring, suggestive of maternal ambivalence. She has webbed feet indicating her wild nature. She precedes Inanna. When Gilgamesh cuts down the hulupu tree to establish Inanna's throne of office, Lilith flies out of it and away. Qadesh is broadly identified with the 'sacred prostitute', Ishtar, Hathor, and the Canaanite Queen of Heaven for whom Jeremiah (44:19) notes cakes were also fashioned in Jerusalem.

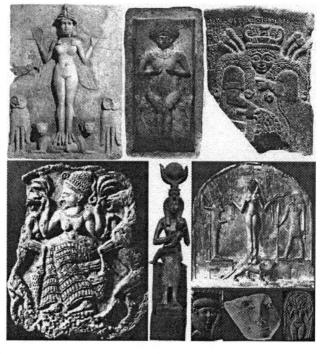

Inanna's courtship of Dumuzi is one of fertile power and beauty between the sexes (Wolkenstein and Kramer R747):

"Great Lady, the king will plow your vulva."

I Dumuzi the King, will plow your vulva."
"Then plow my vulva, man of my heart!
At the king's lap stood the rising cedar.
Plants grew high by their side.
Grains grew high by their side.
Gardens flourished luxuriantly....
"Make your milk sweet and thick, my bridegroom.
My shepherd, I will drink your fresh milk".
I poured out plants from my womb.
He put his hand in her hand.
He put his hand to her heart.
Sweet is the sleep of hand-to-hand.
Sweeter still the sleep of heart-to-heart.

Inanna descends to the underworld, is stripped naked, removing her seven veils of clothing and the instruments of power and queenship, and hung as a corpse on a peg. After three dark days she is rescued, but the seven galla rise with her to the surface to take their compensation. Innana rejects her sister and kin as a sacrificial substitute, but fixes her eye of death on Dumuzi for forgetting her and assuming the powers of state in her absence.

Neolithic agrarian cultures displayed a disturbing trend towards blood-fests of male sacrifice, personified in the ritual slaughter and dismemberment of sacred kings, in a confusion between the transience of male fertility in the reproductive process and the notion of sewing blood back into the pasture to ensure a rich harvest in the coming season. Thus the themes of nubile love in the song of Inanna are overlaid with her Descent, and Dumuzi's persecution on the third day by the seven galla of the underworld, and his emasculation in breaking his reed sceptre, echoing darkly all the way to the Saturnalia performed during Jesus' crucifixion and the shadowy role played by the women of Galilee in the same event after he is anointed by a woman, sometimes assumed to be Mary Magdalen, 'for his burial'.

They broke the reed pipe which the shepherd was playing.
Inanna fastened on Dumuzi the eye of death.
She spoke against him the word of wrath.
She uttered against him the cry of guilt:
"Take him! Take Dumuzi away!"

At his vanishing away she lifts up a lament, "My Damu!"
At his vanishing away she lifts up a lament, "My enchanter and priest!"
Like the lament that a city lifts up for its lord,
Her lament is the lament for a herb that grows not in the bed.
Her lament is the lament for the corn that grows not in the ear.
Her chamber is a possession that brings not forth a possession.

These are again echoed in the Song of Songs, which despite being the Holy of Holies of the Torah as the love of God and Israel (p 8) is believed to originate earlier, in love poetry and marriage ceremonies from Sumerian times, complete with the intimations of sacrificial thorns for the hero, as the red-streaked anemones of Adonis, the myrrh of sexual union, searching for the lost Adonai or Lord, and ritual wounding of the priestess:

I am the rose of Sharon, and the lilly of the valleys.
As a lilly among thorns, so is my love among the daughters.
As the apple tree among the trees of the wood, so is my beloved among the sons.
I sat down under his shadow with great delight, and his fruit was sweet to my taste.
A garden enclosed is my sister, my spouse; a spring shut up, a fountain sealed.
Thy plants are an orchard of pomegranates, with pleasant fruits; camphire, spikenard, and saffron;
calamus and cinnamon, with all trees of frankincense; myrrh and aloes, with all the chief spices:
A fountain of gardens, a well of living waters, and streams from Lebanon.
I sleep but my heart waketh : it is the voice of my beloved that knocketh,
saying open to me my sister, my love, my dove, my undefiled :
for my head is filled with dew, and my locks with the drops of the night.
I have put off my coat; how shall I put it on? I have washed my feet; how shall I defile them?
My beloved put his hand in the hole of the door, and my bowels were moved for him.
I rose up to open to my beloved and my hands dropped with myrrh,

and my fingers with sweet-smelling myrrh, upon the handles of the lock.
I opened to my beloved; but my beloved had withdrawn himself and was gone:
my soul failed when he spake : I sought him, but I could not find him;
I called him, but he gave me no answer

The watchmen that went about the city found me, they smote me and they wounded me;
the keepers of the walls took away my veil from me.
I charge you , O daughters of Jerusalem, that ye tell him, that I am sick of love.

The tragic sexual union of the sacred king and the goddess was later reduced to a seasonal stand-in ceremony where the king stood aside for a brief period and placed a surrogate in his stead, to perform the hieros gamos and suffer the ensuing indignities, in the Saturnalia. Such violence against the male hero is a distortion of sexual love, in which the female exerts not only reproductive choice, but whimsical betrayal for the new suitor, as simultaneous creatress and destructress, as Kali and the lifeless Shiva exemplify. This violence against the male formed a whetting stone for the patriarchal whiplash that was to follow.

Indo-Aryan Origins and the Goddess of Old Europe

Gimbutas using thousands of 'feminine' artifacts in Old Europe sees the rise of patriarchy as a cataclysmic overthrow of a peaceful goddess culture by an oppressive patriarchal one:

"The Old European and Kurgan cultures were the antithesis of one another. The Old European were sedentary horticulturalists prone to live in large well-planned townships. The absence of fortifications and weapons attests the peaceful coexistence of this egalitarian civilization that was probably matrilinear and matrilocal. The Kurgan system was composed of patrilineal, socially stratified, herding units which lived in small villages or seasonal settlements while grazing their animals over vast areas. One economy based on farming, the other on stock breeding and grazing, produced two contrasting ideologies. The Old European belief system focused on the agricultural cycle of birth, death, and regeneration, embodied in the feminine principle, a Mother Creatrix. The Kurgan ideology, as known from comparative Indo-European mythology, exalted virile, heroic warrior gods of the shining and thunderous sky. Weapons are nonexistent in Old European imagery; whereas the dagger and battle-axe are dominant symbols of the Kurgans, who like all historically known Indo-Europeans, glorified the lethal power of the sharp blade."

The 'Kurgan' Aryan migration is said to have occurred in three surges. As termed by Russian archaeologists: the first "early Yamna" culture of the Volga steppe was from 4400-4300 B.C., the second "Maikop" culture of the North Pontic area was around 3500 B.C., and the third "late Yamna" also of the Volga steppe was after 3000 B.C. Prior to 4500-4300 B.C. Gimbutas (R239 352) claims that neither are weapons to be found among grave goods, nor are hilltop defenses to be found, until the Indo-Europeans arrived with metallurgy and weapons such as daggers, spears, and bow and arrows. Some archaeologists, however, have found that weapons already existed in the former non-Indo-European cultures. Mellaart as we shall note, reports that male burials at Catal Hüyük contained weapons: stone mace-heads, obsidian arrowheads and javelin heads, also daggers. Some critics point out that [later] cultures which still engaged in goddess worship were warlike, citing the Celtics as an example. Evidence for the appearance of the Kurgans and characteristics unique to them appear in a wide range of archaeological evidence. The earliest example of horses represented in sculpture were found in cemeteries from the Volga region dating back to 5,000 B.C. around when Kurgans arrived in Old Europe. Flint and stone daggers can be found in the cemetery of S'ezzhee after the arrival of the Kurgans, along with a unique burial style (R239 355). Central to the thesis is the idea that the use of horses was combined with a conversion of existing metallurgy largely used for farm tools and jewelry into weapons of war.

Gimbutas also cites burials in the Kurgan tradition which have the characteristics of 'suttee' burials, 'chieftain graves', with a strong-man elite at the top. These graves are in Gimbutas's words clearly an 'alien cultural phenomenon'. In contrast to Old European burials, which showed little indication of social inequality, there are here marked differences in the size of the graves as well as in what archaeologists call 'funerary gifts': the contents found in the tomb other than the deceased. Among these contents, for the first time in European graves, we find along with an exceptionally tall or large-boned male skeleton the skeletons of sacrificed women - wives, concubines, or slaves of the men who died. Mallory (R424) disagrees however with her analysis of the northern Globular Amphora cultures.

Juliet Woods criticizes Gimbutas' example of the Celts as a pre-Indo-European Goddess culture because many current archaeological theories maintain that the Celts may have been a central part of Indo-European life. Certainly evolving Celt culture contains plenty of evidence for prominence being accorded to women, as noted by Davis-Kimball (R149):

"Hallstatt Culture [1200 -500 B.C.E.] In 1824 came the first signs of the existence archaeologically of an important Iron Age cemetery at Hallstatt, a small village in Upper Austria. The cemetery mostly dates to the seventh and sixth centuries B.C.E., and includes graves of many different classes. Warriors' graves made up only about a quarter of the Hallstatt cemetery. Women's graves tended to have masses of clanking jewelry and bulky fibulae. Rich graves in the cemetery often contained impressive sets of bronze vessels - buckets, situlae (buckets with rims turned inward), bowls, and cups, presumably imported from the Mediterranean. Hallstatt remains one of the richest known cemeteries of its kind, with a wide range of weapons, brooches, pins, and pottery. From these excavations, we can develop a comprehensive picture of who the early Celts were".

"La Tène Culture [500 - 50 B.C.E.] Located on the northern edge of Lake Neuchâtel in Switzerland, La Tène culture can truly be termed 'Celtic'. The La Tène culture evolved during the fifth century BC in part of the Hallstatt area. One most important and distinctively different feature of the La Tène culture is the unique art-style, usually represented in their metal-work. La Tène Culture generated some of the ancient world's most stunningly beautiful pieces of decorative art. The use of animals, plants, and spiral patterns in the art eventually epitomized and perpetuated the legend of the Celts. La Tène society seems to have risen to prominence through trade with the Mediterranean, with the Greeks and Etruscans, and later the Romans. La Tène Culture finds the Celts amongst wealth and glory and expression. In general, the technological level of the La Tène Celts, with very few exceptions, was equal to, and in some cases."

In "The Chalice and the Blade" (R182) Rianne Eisler posits the existence of an ancient 'gylanic' (gy- 'female' -an- 'male' -ic 'linked') culture, distinguished by the equal rule of men and women. However she also asserts that this period, marked by high cultural achievement, was supplanted some 5000 years ago by a baleful 'androcratic' regime, an event that, borrowing from Gimbutas, Eisler blames on a violent Kurgan invasion:

"At the core of the invaders' system was the placing of higher value on the power that takes, rather than gives, life. This was the power symbolized by the 'masculine' Blade, which early Kurgan cave engravings show these Indo-European invaders literally worshiped. For in their dominator society, ruled by gods, and men-of-war, this was the supreme power."

Judith Lorber (R414), likewise suggests a millennium of peaceful egalitarian horticulture in southeastern Europe followed by a gloomy oppression scenario, with populations transformed by warlike men into a vast exploited class of abused 'workers, sexual partners, child bearers, and emotional nurturers.' Although many contemporary archaeologists would support Lorber's conclusions about women's social roles in early cultures, most are wary of endorsing Gimbutas's Kurgan invasions as the cataclysm that destroyed the ancient order.

Gimbutas's findings are contradicted by Lotte Motz (R481), who argues that images of men and animals are just as prolific as goddess imagery in early European cultures. "There clearly was no introduction of warrior gods and warrior values, no imposition of a patriarchal system, and no humiliation of the Goddess." Cynthia Eller (R187) discounts the entire approach of the ancient matriarchy as a false icon developed by feminists.

Jani Roberts (R574) also notes there is evidence that in the British Isles and Ireland, a male dominated society replaced not a matriarchy, but a society in which women and men worked together as equals with safeguards and pledges to possibly control an innate male aggressive tendency. According to ancient legends the kings of Ulster had to pledge that they would look after the women's rights. Specifically they had to pledge that the harvest would be provided every year to the families, that there would be no lack of supplies of cloth dyes to the women and that medical supplies and midwives would be provided so that no women need die in child birth. If they broke this pledge they could apparently be deposed.

There is also contradictory evidence about how uniquely patriarchal the Kurgan Indo-Aryans were. 'Kurgan' culture is named from the burial mounds in which people are placed on a seasonal basis adjacent to pastures. Gimbutas has laid at their feet the prime cause of the rise of oppressive patriarchy in Europe. This is a very different picture of female social roles from the one Davis-Kimball (R149) has inferred from her Pokrovka kurgans - an

Indo-Aryan society from around 500 BC in which women, not just men, apparently held military and social power (p 205). The simultaneous existence of nomadic warrior women and subjugated Athenian housewives suggests that two thousand years ago, relations between the sexes varied enormously from one population to the next. So why and when did patriarchy become the universal norm? Davis-Kimball thinks "Gimbutas may have been wrong about the mother goddess per se. But she may have been right about an underlying, unbroken tradition of female cultic power and wisdom, which has been suppressed since the Middle Ages and especially since the Industrial Revolution." Davis-Kimball on a later trip through the museums of central Asia found evidence of female warriors and priestesses "all over the place" including in the remains of what she believed was an ancient culture dating to around 2000 BC unearthed in the Takla Makan desert by Chinese archaeologists.

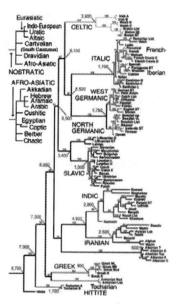

Evolutionary tree of Indo-European languages suggests the radiation corresponding to the Kurgans occurred around 4,900 BC (6,900 BP) and that they were preceded by Hittite migrations into Anatolia. Time scales in red are BP (Gray and Atkinson R252).Significantly Tocharian appears in Buddhist writings from China's Xinjiang province, indicating early far-eastern spread. Inset: hypothetical relationship between Indo-European and wider language groups such as Afro-Asiatic.

Timothy Taylor (R670 161) in discounting Gimbutas's thesis, makes a series of speculative claims for the rise of sexual inequality based on the growth of agriculture and animal husbandry in Europe. He claims that the culture named LBK (*Linearbandkeramik* for their pottery) who spread across Europe from about 5500 BC coincided with motifs of aggression leading to warlike patriarchy. Although he claims from their house styles that they may have been matrilocal and possibly monogamous, he then speculates that the shift to farming, and resulting shorted birth intervals and earlier weaning of infants introduced an infantile aggression syndrome, following French obstetrician Michel Odent, which he subsequently associates with evidence of mass murder and possibly child abduction at the Talheim pit. He then extends this argument to the 'secondary products revolution' of Andrew Sherratt around 3500 BC which along with wool and use of draught animals, saw the advent of milk production and further weaning to base the rise of patriarchy on. While it is tempting to blame patriarchy on a badly weaned *enfant terrible* there is no evidence to support it.

If we turn to the earliest origins of Indo-European language and culture especially associated with domestication of the horse, we find that linguistic tree modeling shows the origin of Indo-European languages appears to be older than the Kurgans and to originate from farmers migrating into Anatolia around 6,700 BC,(8,700 BP) with Hittite as one of its earliest branches, and was spread later by diverse migrations, rather than being specific to the Kurgan horsemen (Gray and Atkinson R252).

However detailed Kurgan cultural motifs do appear to penetrate to the Vedic tradition:

The oldest archaeological evidence for the Kurgan horse domestication is the Sintashta-Arkaim culture, found east of the Urals. The typical short bow of horse riding pastoralists was introduced in this period, and contact between the northern pastoralists and the Central Asian oases was established. Against the context of the Rgveda the Sintashta sites share some cultural features. These are simple settlements fortified with ramparts and ditches, with a circular or rectangular fence or wall built from unfired clay and wooden frames. And there are remnants of horse sacrifices and primitive horse drawn chariots with spoked wheels. A real "tripura", Arkaim, has two circular walls and two circles of dwellings around a central square. The settlements consist of frame houses, slightly sunk into ground (suggestive of Rgvedic kula "hollow, family"), with traces of copper (*ayas*) production. Apart from the development of the chariot, the Sintashta culture shows links with E. Europe both in pottery and bronze artifacts.

The graves at Sintashta are mounds with burial pits and log and timber chambers. Horse sacrifices have been made both inside and on top of the burial chamber. The graves also contain some light chariots with wheels (Witzel R742).

These chariots still are very narrow in width, pointing to their origin from, by necessity narrow, oxen-drawn wagons (*anas*). Horse bits made of bone have also been found. Most tellingly, perhaps, at the site of Potapovka, a unique burial has been found. It contains a human skeleton whose head has been replaced by a horse head; a human head lies near his feet, along with a bone pipe, and a cow's head is placed near his knees. This looks like an archaeological illustration of the Rgvedic myth of Dadhyañc, whose head was cut off by Indra and replaced by that of a horse. The bone pipe reminds, as the excavator has noted, of the RgVedic sentence referring to the playing of pipes in Yama's realm, the world of the ancestors. Many interpretations have been suggested in relation to Arkaim - a military fort, proto-city, or a ceremonial and religious center. If we bear in mind that the sets of artifacts excavated were not characteristic of everyday usage, sites such as Arkaim are a combination of administrative and ceremonial centers. Possibly this was a location where about 1,000 to 2,000 people – aristocracy (and craftsmen) gathered periodically to perform rituals.

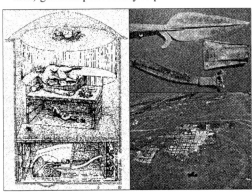

Left Arkaim burial with horses and chariot, top right: metallurgy lower right: Sintashta site (Koryakova)

Davis-Kimball (R149) notes the broad influence of these motifs in espousing the 'Yamna' migration: "Over the course of 5000 years the Kurgans migrated from East-Indo Europe and established trade routes all over Europe and across the continental divide into North America; as time passed these areas gradually became known as Alaska, Canada, northern China, Greece, India, Mesopotamia, Italy, Austria, Hungary, the Balkans, Spain, Switzerland, and France! They finally emerged as a Celtic presence in Hallstatt, Austria around 700 BC" However the subsequent diversity found during the spread of these cultures indicates local adaptation of existing societies and a relaying of technological innovation and cultural values, rather than mass migrations of a 'Yamna people' as such.

By contrast with Gimbutas's apocalyptic scenario is a gradualist model which posits a slow and inevitable transition from prehistoric egalitarianism to male-dominated modernity. In "Is Female to Male as Nature Is to Culture?" Sherry Ortner (R505) declared that "the search for a genuinely egalitarian, let alone matriarchal, culture has proved fruitless." Ortner concluded that the ubiquity of male domination had its roots in the facts of sexual reproduction. Women are nearly everywhere associated with nature because of their role in procreation. (Women, as de Beauvoir put it, are more enslaved to the species by biology.) Furthermore, all societies concoct rituals that aim to manipulate nature in the interest of culture. Notions of purity and pollution, evident in taboos connected with menstruation, create a gendered opposition between nature (dirty women) and culture (clean men) attesting to a powerful societal impulse to control nature's threat. Physically unhampered by their role in reproduction and therefore free from any symbolic association with nature, men are assigned an antagonistic value-- namely, that of culture itself, whose duty it is to assert that control.

In "Making Gender" (R506), Ortner elaborates:

"Men emerge as 'leaders' and as figures of authority, vis-a-vis both women and other men, as a function of engaging in a variety of practices, only some of which are predicated on power, including trade, exchange, kinship networking, ritual participation, dispute resolution, and so forth. That is, male dominance does not in fact seem to arise from some aggressive 'will to power,' but from the fact that--as Simone de Beauvoir first suggested in 1949 - men as it were lucked out: their domestic responsibilities can be construed as more episodic than women's and they are more free to travel, congregate, hang out, etc., and thus to do the work of 'culture.'"

Ortner's essay described an inexorable progression from biological fact to symbol to the gender stereotypes that enjoy nearly universal currency today. Patriarchy, she says, "arose as an unintended consequence of arrangements which were originally purely functional and expedient. That we demonize it as part of contemporary feminist politics unfortunately only confuses the issue". Elizabeth Barber, using textile production in ancient cultures, concludes that two fundamental conditions were necessary for patriarchy to emerge. First, there was long-distance trade in metal ores, which could be more easily conducted and monopolized by men, since women, burdened by infants and small children, couldn't travel long distances. Second, there was a "secondary products revolution" around 4000 BC, in which domesticated animals that had traditionally been raised for consumption were kept alive and exploited for their secondary products, including milk, wool, and drafting power. As a result, nutrition and clothing improved, and large-scale field cultivation became possible. This last development, she explains, was necessarily men's work as well. Echoing Ortner, Barber views the division of labor and gender as "an inevitable evil once subsistence farming had been left behind." She adds: "The communal, non-hierarchical model only worked in small, relatively poor Stone Age societies. As soon as people want and need commodities which they can't grow in their back yard, it breaks down irrevocably" (Osborne R507). Margaret Conkey notes: "By and large we now think of patriarchy as a by-product of technological and social upheavals." Nicola Di Cosmo concurs: "Gender divisions of labor were probably efficient and so were adopted as a matter of course. Warfare arises from a competition for resources as trading networks expand - not from some innate male aggression."

According to proponents of the gradualist school, patriarchy is less a male conspiracy to keep women down than a necessary by-product of a society in which progress increasingly depends on mobility and brute strength. Teenage girls and nursing mothers were simply impractical candidates for the heavy lifting required to build an infrastructure. Despite its sober tenor and considerable political appeal to some - neither sex is to blame for men having more power today. However our deeper investigation of sex differences, the innate basis of male jealousy and fear of paternity uncertainty, along with the many diverse and oppressive ways of combating it make this cultural approach seem a little innocent from all sides, from the sacrifices of male heroes and the castrating of male priests to stoning women for adultery and cutting out their organs of sexual pleasure.

Some suggest testing the gradualist theory against the future than against the past. If revolutions in technology once made dominance by men - and thus patriarchy - inevitable, it follows that when machines replace bodies altogether, as they have arguably begun to do today, patriarchy may well disappear. This is exactly what Ortner, among others, predicts. "Just as technological evolution created patriarchy," she says, "so technology now has the power to cancel it out because it obviates physical strength and equalizes the sexes." (Osborne)

Cultural prediction here becomes a significant danger. While technology can provide a much more sexually egalitarian society - 'gylanic' even as in Riane Eisler's words, unless we can approach this from a real basis of biological complementarity rather than mere cultural differences of pulling a plow or negotiating a computer maze we may lose our *raison d'etre* in a sexless or androgynous 'android' society rather than a 'gylanic' one.

We also need to consder the possibility that migrations, even in small waves of bands of warriors could alter the sexual demography of a migrating group to make them more patriarchally exploitative of societies they over-ran, for example abducting or seizing the women, consistent with Sanday's findings of increasing patrarchal emphasis in migrating peoples (p 143). Pinker (R532 327) notes also that in the context of herding and social chaos, more severe rules come to the surface:

> "Cultures of honor spring up all over the world because they amplify universal human emotions like Pride, anger, revenge, and the love of kith and kin, and because they appear at the time to be sensible responses to local conditions. Indeed, the emotions themselves are thoroughly familiar even when they don't erupt in violence, such as in road rage, office politics, political mudslinging, academic backstabbing, and email flame wars. In 'Culture of Honor', the social psychologists Richard Nisbett and Dov Cohen show that violent cultures arise in societies that are beyond the reach of the law and in which precious assets are easily stolen. Societies that herd animals meet both conditions. Herders tend to live in territories that are

unsuitable for growing crops and thus far from the centers of government. And their major asset, livestock, is easier to steal than the major asset of farmers, land. In herding societies a man can be stripped of his wealth (and of his ability to acquire wealth) in an eyeblink. Men in that milieu cultivate a hair trigger for violent retaliation, not just against rustlers, but against anyone who would test their resolve by signs of disrespect that could reveal them to be easy pickings for rustlers. Scottish highlanders, Appalachian mountain men, Western cow- boys, Masai warriors, Sioux Indians, Druze and Bedouin tribesmen, Balkan clansmen, and Indochinese Montagnards are familiar examples. A man's honor is a kind of 'social reality' in John Searle's sense: it exists because everyone agrees it exists, but it is no less real for that, since it resides in a shared granting of power. When the lifestyle of a people changes, their culture of honor can stay with them for a long time because it is difficult for anyone to be the first to renounce culture. The very act of renouncing it can be a concession of weakness and low status even when the sheep and mountains are a distant memory."

However if the evidence of the Hittite arrival upon the Hatti culture of Anatolia is any indication, there was a great deal of cultural merging. The Hattis are believed to be the one of the indigenous peoples in Anatolia. They lived around 2500 BC in walled city kingdoms and small tribes. The Hittites came to Anatolia over the Caucasus around 2000 BC. These newcomers did not invade the land suddenly. They settled alongside the existing people and established their own settlement units over time. Only after about 250 years, as many Hittite principalities emerged, did they claim the rule of the land. Rather than destroying the existing people and their cities, they mixed with the Hattis and other people of Anatolia. The Hittites were influenced by the Hatti culture in religion, mythology and literature. They even shared their gods, goddesses, art, culture and many words from Hatti language. Not only did they take the names of mountains, rivers and towns from them; Hittites preserved the country they lived in as "the land of Hatti". The Hatti art gives us the examples of a human-shaped pottery type (anthropomorphic) rather than an animal shape or a hybrid form. They worshipped such statues and figurines, and each one of them carried his or her name.

One can see a gradual transition to patriarchy in Hittite society in Anatolia 1700-1200 BC combining Indo-European with previous Hatti culture. Hatti right of succession was lodged in the prince's sister the *tawananna*. As in Egypt, a male ruler married his sister, who was a priestess with considerable powers, such as to collect taxes. Her male child inherited the right of succession rather than the son of the king. Later when brother-sister marriage was outlawed, the *tawananna* priestess continued to hold power of succession. This pattern was overthrown in stages. The first strong Hittite king abolished the *tawananna* when he took power. However matrilineal succession continued, shifting to joint succession and only finally being abolished after much friction between cntenders in the kingship which led to the Hittite empire. Even then it lingered in powerful queens serving a patriarchal society in the name of Ishtar (Lerner R397 155-7).

A Wandering Aramean Benjaminite was My Father

Abraham is said in the Bible to have made a journey from Ur of the Chaldees to Harran. These were the Southern and Northern centers of worship of the ancient Moon God, Nannar or Sin. When Woolley (R748, R749) excavated the Royal Tombs at Ur, he was surprised to find a 'ram in a thicket' echoing Abraham's sacrificial offer of Isaac and the 'scapegoat'. Many of Abraham's relatives and ancestors lived in the vicinity of Harran. Several key names in Abraham's family, Terah (compare Yerah Moon God of Canaan), Laban, Sarah and Milcah are all derived from worship of the Moon Deity (Bright R76 80, 91). The deification of Ab-ram in the earliest documents is a synonym for Ab-Sin (Briffault R75v3:108).

Benjaminites were a nomadic tribe on the outskirts of Mari around 1760 BC who had specific associations with Harran (Segal R618, R619). The names Abi-ram (Abraham) Yasmah-El (Ishmael) Yaqob-El (Jacob), a name also shared by a Hyksos chief and El-Laban (Laban) all appear at Mari. The root *mlk* denoting melech king or in its sacrificial form Moloch is also found. Another word at Mari in this time which will come to have significance in Islam is *umma* or "mother unit" of the nomadic tribes (Malamat R423 31, Bright R76 70).

Jacob's fourfold blessing is also of 'the deep' and 'the breasts and womb', hinting at the ancient 'mother' as well as the 'father' god and El Shaddai of the heavens:

Even by the God of thy father, who shall help thee;
and by the Almighty, who shall bless thee with blessings of heaven above,
blessings of the deep that lieth under, blessings of the breasts, and of the womb (Gen 49:25)

Associated with this cultural complex is an older form of marriage called the *beena* marriage, associated with the matriarchs at the founding of Old Testament myth. The episodes concerning Laban in Genesis, hint at a matrilineal society in which partners are subject to the wife's family and are expected to do service in dwelling with them for years at a time. The seven years Jacob spent with Laban for each wife indicates the line of Laban was matrilocal and matrilineal in a way which gave power to the brothers of the mother. Moving to the family of the wife is consistent with the injunction in Genesis to "leave your father and mother and cleave unto your wife" and with Jewish marriage practice to go into the wife's tent. In such a society child-support is achieved at least partly by immediate relatives of the mother, in which uncles figure prominently thus compensating for their lack of their own paternity uncertainty by a commensurate investment in their sisters' children with whom they share a significant genetic bond.

Family tree of the tribes of Israel (Jay R331) illustrates a careful attempt to resolve dissonance between matrilineal and patrilineal paradigms, involving cousin or even half-sister marriage. Names like Terah and Laban are associated with the moon god, who presided at both Ur (Woolley R748) and Harran (Segal R618), the two towns spanning Abraham's migration (Briffault R75). Abraham takes both a wife and a slave concubine who is sent away and Jacob is polygynous with two wives and a slave concubine of each given to them by Laban with whom he also sires children in their mistresses stead.

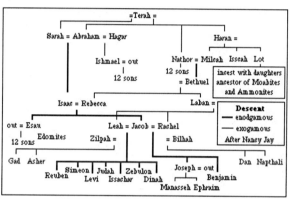

Arameans are any people belonging to a confederacy of tribes that migrated from the Arabian Peninsula to the Fertile Crescent in the 2nd millennium BC. The Britannica notes that among them were the biblical matriarchs Leah and Rachel, wives of Jacob. They formed principalities around and including Damascus. Aramaic language and culture spread through international trade, reaching a cultural peak during the 9th–8th centuries BC. Aramaic became the universal language of commerce, culture, and government throughout the fertile crescent and remained so to the time of Yeshua and in some places to the 7th century. Hebrew, Aramaic, Arabic and Akkadian all have a common origin in Afro-Asiatic. Aramaic script emerged in turn from Phoenician and old Canaanite phonetic.

Nancy Jay (R331) in "Throughout Your Generations Forever" draws attention to the schism between such societies probably originating in Canaanite planter cultures and the patriarchal traditions of shepherding tribes illustrated in Jacob's departure and many successive biblical invocations against the Queen of Heaven and her ways. The division between these two cultures cuts directly through the Gordian knot of paternity uncertainty discussed earlier. Despite the characterization of the Jews as archetypally patriarchal, the era of the patriarchs is noted for its strong independent women. The prominence and independence of Sarah 'the queen' as well as Rebecca, Rachel and Leah is notable. Briffault (v1 372) comments: "the Jewish rabbis themselves, at a comparatively late date acknowledged that the four matriarchs Sarah, Rebecca, Rachel and Leah had occupied a more important position than the three patriarchs, Abraham, Isaac and Jacob. According to Robinson Smith (R635) the tribe of Levi was originally metronymous (matrilineal), being the tribe of Leah." This matrilineal element still persists in Jewish descent coming through the mother, reflected in Gen 2:24:

'Therefore shall a man leave his father and his mother, and shall cleave unto his wife.'

It was the matriarch Rebecca who ordered Jacob to trick Isaac with a fleece, to steal hairy Esau's blessing as firstborn: "Upon me be thy curse, my son: only obey my voice, and go fetch me them." She did so because Esau had 'married out', taking two Hittite wives, Judith and Bashemath. It is Rebecca who sends Jacob to Laban: "Now therefore, my son, obey my voice; arise, flee thou to Laban my brother to Haran." The moment he arrives, a cousin marriage is arranged with Rachel. Having served seven years with the matrilineal kin for the love of Rachel, Laban tricks Jacob into also marrying Leah, because the first-born daughter should proceed the younger in marriage, causing him to tarry another 'week' of seven years. In an ironic tilt at the matriarchy, when Jacob escapes Laban's clutches as mother's brother, to return as he promised to his father's line, it is Rachel who hides under her menstrual skirts Laban's stolen teraphim, suggested to be tokens of land and lineage - "Is there yet any portion or inheritance for us in our father's house?" In Nuzi documents, possession of the 'house gods' are considered title to estate (Lerner R397 168). The entire myth of mutual deceit indicates a transfer from matriliny to patriliny in the name of the god of Bethel:

And thy seed shall be as the dust of the earth, and thou shalt spread abroad
to the west, and to the east, and to the north, and to the south:
and in thee and in thy seed shall all the families of the earth be blessed (Gen 28:13).

And he brought him forth abroad, and said, Look now toward heaven, and tell the stars,
if thou be able to number them: and he said unto him, So shall thy seed be (Gen 15:5).

Jay makes a penetrating analysis of the transition between matrilineal and patrilineal lines of descent, in which sacrifice, or forgone sacrifice, and the paternal blessing were a way of recognizing the more ephemeral male line of descent through the father to the blessed son. The theme of the 'barren' woman in Sarah and Rachel is likewise significant, both in terms of close relative infertility, and the female line of descent it implies. "Israelite tradition did not deny descent from women and consequently faced the dilemma: How is a pure and eternal patriline to be maintained if descent from women is not denied? Endogamy appears to be a solution; marriage to a woman of the same patrilineage ensures the off-springs' patrilineage membership, even if it is figured through the mother. Close agnatic endogamy (marriage within the patriline) is extremely rare, except in Semitic traditions. In a way reminiscent of the Patriarchs, throughout the Arab world, families have preferred men to marry their father's brother's daughters. The descent line of the Patriarchs contin-ued only through endogamy: Isaac and Jacob (but not Ishmael) married endogamously in cousin marriages. Joseph married exogamously but his sons were adopted by Jacob, cor-recting this, and other, irregularities of their descent".

"The 'Elohist E's account states that Sarah was an actual half sister of Abraham, having the same father but a different mother. Such a marriage would be impossible in any regular patrilineal descent system. Unless we reject E's account (thereby making the Patriarchs liars) we must see here a recognition of descent from women so pronounced as to be almost matrilineal, for if Abraham and Sarah had the same father but different mothers, it is only as their mothers' offspring that their marriage was not incestuous ... In Hurrian society the bonds of marriage were strongest and most solemn when the wife had simulta-neously the juridical status of a sister, regardless of actual blood ties.... The practice was apparently a reflection of the underlying fratriarchal system, and it gave the adoptive brother greater authority than was granted the husband ... The patriarchal narratives tell the story of the resolution of this descent conflict, a resolution in which sacrifice plays a cru-cial role".

Centrally Abraham's covenant with God is sexually reproductive:

And I will make my covenant between me and thee, and will multiply thee exceedingly....
And I will make thee exceeding fruitful,
and I will make nations of thee, and kings shall come out of thee. ...

It involves circumcision of the penis as a sacrificial token of male fertility:

This is my covenant, which ye shall keep, between me and you and thy seed after thee;

Every man child among you shall be circumcised.
And ye shall circumcise the flesh of your foreskin;

and it shall be a token of the covenant betwixt me and you.

Idol with bull's head and phallus - Palestine (Zehren),Timna Phallic teraphim and 'Nehustan' brazen serpent from Midianite period.(Rothenberg R579)

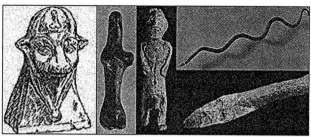

Testifying was likewise, for Abraham, swearing by the testis (L. *testis* testicle, witness) and hence the entire Old and New Testaments:

"And Abraham said unto his eldest servant of his house, ... Put, I pray thee, thy hand under my thigh: And I will make thee swear by the Lord, the God of heaven, and the God of the earth, that thou shalt not take a wife unto my son of the daughters of the Canaanites, among whom I dwell: But thou shalt go unto my country, and to my kindred, and take a wife unto my son Isaac. (Gen 24:2).

Malamat (R423 54) comments that the unusual genealogy of Nahor in Gen 22:20-24 suggests that Abraham was originally one of the wandering sons traditionally listed as children of concubines (Ishmael etc.) in the Old Testament as opposed to the blessed sons (Isaac, Jacob). The children of Israel are the wanderers from Aram-Naharaim on the upper Harbur. Such pastoral migrations were noted at Mari.

The Transition to Patriarchy in the Fertile Crescent

The mythology of a variety of our founding cultures displays a consistent trend in which male deities precipitated a transference of power to the male. These events are clearly detectable in the mythologies of cultures from Europe to Sumeria, from Enki in Sumeria, to Zeus in Greece, through Indra in Vedic India. Indo-Europeans had a pantheon of gods and goddesses headed by a sun god and a storm god and the dramatic shifts in the Greek and Dravidian pantheons typified by the turbulent relationship between Zeus and an uncooperative Hera, reflect these changes. Even in the Judeo-Christian tradition, Yahweh was the consort of Anath and Asherah, overthrown only later by the Yahweh-only movement in the reign of Josiah a mere 23 years before the exile. Driving these changes are major shifts of social and sexual power from partnership to frank male domination.

Once large urban societies developed, the rule of law and the patriarchal imperative passed the ascendancy to the male through social and military instruments of power. The males' jealously resulted in adoption of mores which ensured males could secure their own descendents from doubts about paternity which plague the male but are incontestable for the female. The sexual division of the female into two defined archetypes, faithful wife and whore, as illustrated in the game matrix (p 60) is firmly illustrated in the Biblical tradition running from the Proverbs to Revelation.

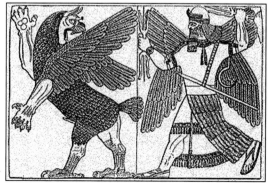

Male combat become cosmic sex war against the Mother (Cohn R125). Tiamat and Apsu's progeny disturb the peace. Apsu plots to smash them but Tiamat objects and he is 'put to sleep' by Ea. Later when Marduk again disturbs the gods with his storm winds, Tiamat is persuaded to attack and gathers an army of serpents. Marduk agrees to go to war if he gains kingship over all the other gods. Victorious, he splits Tiamat apart to become the Earth and sky. The patriarchal repression of the Mother Goddess is achieved in the victory of civic order over primal chaos in kingship.

We first see this attempt to deny women reproductive choice in legal terms in the Codex Hammurabi where death by drowning is the prescribed punishment for adultery. This initiative continues in Hebrew and Deuteronomic Law, which both pre-scribed stoning for adultery, and made it contingent on the tokens of virginity in the case of an unmarried girl, thus putting women uniquely in the firing line of male power. One should note how the invocation against adultery cuts unevenly between the sexes. Abra-ham sired children by both Sarah and Hagar, blessing Isaac and casting out Ishmael. This pattern of blessing one line and sending off another to outcross continued in a tradition in Judaic life in which a man would have a Jewish wife and Gentile concubine. What was not acceptable was any reproductive choice on the part of either the wife, the concubine, or the daughter who had at all costs to maintain her virginity under pain of death until formally married.

By degrees as cultures evolved, the position of women in society steadily deteriorated. In the Judeo-Christian-Islamic tradition of the West and Near-East, the females eventually became sequestered in the home, in the fields, in the chador and burqa, in harems, nunner-ies and brothels. The paternally ambiguous conjugal rites of the fertility goddess were repressed , women were treated as sexual possessions. In the Christian era a 600 year Inquisition and witch hunts were pursued, consuming 4 million European women (Walker).

Rianne Eisler (R183 216) writes: "The critical factors in politically repressive societies are, first, the repression of female sexual freedom and, second, the distortion of both male and female sexuality through the erotization of domination and violence".

Some of these manifestations resulted in frank sexual despotism. Laura Betzig(R59) notes:

"Things became really extreme when people began to grow crops and live together in towns and villages. The leaders of these early societies ruled by terror, and were able to procure vast num-bers of sexual partners. These guys had sexual licence." The record holder, she notes, was Udayama, who reigned in India around 500 BC and had a harem of 16,000. Powerful Romans often purchased female slaves for breeding. Historians assume the fathers of home-bred slaves, or *vernae*, were other slaves. But Betzig argues that the treatment of vernae only makes sense if they were the sons and daughters of the master himself. They were often educated with the mas-ter's children, shared the same wet nurses, and could even inherit his estate. In Europe, little changed for centuries. Huge domestic staffs of the English landed gentry, for instance, were pri-marily there to satisfy the master's sexual appetites, rather than to cook and clean (New Scientist Feb 22 1997).

Lyall Watson (R721) elaborates in in "Dark Nature":

"Men throughout human history have certainly been quick to treat power, not simply as an end in itself, but as a means to sexual and reproductive success. Laura Betzig, one of a new breed of Darwinian historians, set out to discover whether human sexual adaptations have been exploited to give individuals a selective advantage - and discovered that this is one of our most predictable traits. In all six of the great independent civilizations of early history, the rulers, always men, were despots who translated their power directly into extraordinary sexual pro-ductivity. That word 'productivity', usually used in an industrial sense, is totally appropriate here. Each emperor established a carefully controlled breeding machine, designed and dedi-cated to nothing more than the rapid spread and dominance of his own genes. Hammurabi of Babylon had thousands of slave 'wives'. Akhenaton, Egyptian pharaoh and husband of the gorgeous Nefertiti, was driven nevertheless to recruit at least 317 concubines. Montezuma, the last Aztec ruler, enjoyed the favours of 4,000 young women. Several of the Tang dynasty emperors in China demanded access to a minimum of 10,000 teenage girls. Udayama of India kept 16,000 consorts in palaces ringed by fire and guarded by eunuchs. And all of these rulers ran their gene machines in much the same way, recruiting pre-pubertal girls, pampering them under heavy guard, and servicing them as often as possible - sometimes even complaining of such onerous 'duties'. The measures adopted certainly seem to bear out the claim of duty rather than pleasure, but in a survey of 104 other societies, Betzig found that even when such super-polygamy was not being practised, there was always a direct correlation between power and sexual activity".

Gerda Lerner (R397 212) describes patriarchy (p 451) as follows:

"Patriarchy is a historic creation formed by men and women in a process which took nearly 2500 years to its completion. In its earliest form patriarchy appeared as the archaic state. The basic unit of its organization was the patriarchal family, which both expressed and constantly generated its rules and values. ... Men as a group had rights in women which women as a group did not have in men. Women themselves became a resource, acquired by men much as the land was acquired by men. Women were exchanged or bought in marriages for the benefit of their families; later, they were conquered or bought in slavery."

"The archaic state in the Ancient Near East emerged in the second millennium BC from the twin roots of men's sexual dominance over women and the exploitation by some men of others. From its inception, the archaic state was organized in such a way that the dependence of male family heads on the king or the state bureaucracy was compensated for by their dominance over their families. Male family heads allocated the resources of society to their families the way the state allocated the resources of society to them. The control of male family heads over their female kin and minor sons was as important to the existence of the state as was the control of the king over his soldiers. This is reflected in the various compilations of Mesopotamian laws, especially in the large number of laws dealing with the regulation of female sexuality. From the second millennium BC, forward control over the sexual behavior of citizens has been a major means of social control in every state society. Conversely, class hierarchy is constantly reconstituted in the family through sexual dominance."

"Male hegemony over the symbol system took two forms: educational deprivation of women and male monopoly on definition. ... On the basis of such symbolic constructs, embedded in Greek philosophy, the Judeo-Christian theologies, and the legal tradition on which Western civilization is built, men have explained the world in their own terms and defined the important questions so as to make themselves the center of discourse."

We shall examine Lerner's thesis in detail in the context of Sumer and successive Near Eastern and European civilizations, which form the central arena of the cultural development of patriarchy in Western culture. We can see first signs of this in the transfer of reproductive power from female and the *hieros gamos* to purely male fertility:

> *After he had cast is eye from that spot,*
> *After the father Enki had lifted it over the Euphrates,*
> *He stood up proudly like a rampant bull,*
> *He lifts the penis, ejaculates,*
> *Filled the Tigris with sparkling water ...*
> *The wild cow mooing for its young in the pastures ...*
> *The grain he brought, ... the people eat it ... (Thompson R675 162)*

This transition is also frequently accompanied by a shift in the emphasis of creation from natural to cultural in mental creations and written language, in the form of the 'word of god' in what Lerner (R397 151) calls the 'symbolification of creation', or in a creation by breath or by naming, rather than birth. We also see it also the establishment of civic gods representing the power of kingship such as Marduk of Babylon and Ashur of Assyria, and in battles for male supremacy such as Marduk slaying Tiamat. They are reflected also in the supremacy of the storm god Ba'al in Canaan and Yahweh in Israel.

The excavations at Ur offer a startling insight into Sumerian society around 2500 BC. The collective burials of kings and their wives, along with retainers in robes of honour, buried alive, apparently without violence, in a state of sedation, with a drinking cup next to each body, offer an insight into the relative status of men and women. Only royal graves show these signs of human sacrifice. Lerner (R397 61) comments:

"The royal tombs at Ur tell us that ruling queens shared in the status, power, wealth, and ascription of divinity with kings. They tell us of the wealth and high status of some women at the Sumerian courts, of their varied craft skills, their obvious economic privilege. But the overwhelming preponderance of female skeletons over male among the buried retainers also speaks to their greater vulnerability and dependency as servants."

In Lagash around 2350 BC we can see the dynamics of conflicts between leaders. Lugalanda seized power over the most important temples by installing himself and his wife and other members of his family as administrators, rather than a priest. He referred to the temples as the private property of the ruler. He and his wife Baranamtarra became the largest landholders, his wife also having the temple of the goddess Bau and her own estates. He was in turn overthrown by Urukagina, a populist leader acting on behalf of "boatmen, shepherds, fishermen and farmers." He claimed to be acting on behalf of the city god of Lagash to protect the weak and stop high level corruption and abuse of power, but further consolidated the power of kings against the priesthood. His edict is one of the earliest efforts to establish basic rights for citizens. Among his edicts are those against a practice of former times of 'a woman marrying two men', under pain of stoning. A women speaking disrespectfully is to have her mouth crushed with a fired brick. However this may not indicate a worsening of the position of women. The entire operation of the temple of Bau which extended over a square mile and employed over 1000 people the year round was under the legal and economic authority of his wife Shagshag who was also chief priestess. Both slaves and employees were harnessed as fishermen, spinners, wool workers, brewers, millers, kitchen workers, farmers, cowherds, singers, smiths, sometimes wet nurses and cooks (R397 62).

Shortly afterwards, the Semitic King Sargon of Akkad took control of the region and founded a vast empire including Sumer and Ashur, forming garrison cities and making alliances. His daughter Enkheduanna became high priestess of the temples of the moon god Nannar at Ur and supreme god An at Uruk, also fusing in her person the devotion of the goddess Inanna of Uruk and Akkadian Ishtar. Her poetry and hymns to Inanna have long survived her. This pattern of assigning daughters of kings as high priestesses to key temples continued for 500 years (66).

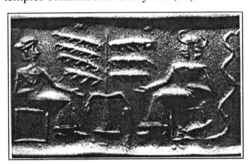

The 'Temptation Seal' Akkadian circa 2200 BC (Brtish Museum) Predates Eden in the seven branched tree of life, the serpent and the archetypal couple. In an evolution to patriarchy we also find Ur-Nammu as king taking over watering the tree of life although he offers libations to both Nannar and Ningal.

Later in the Ur III dynasty, we see a tradition of dynastic marriages between city states such as Ur and Mari (Batto R49, Dalley R142, Malamat R423) and other cities, involving the exchange of women. Although these women were pawns in the families dynastic designs, they were also frequently influential, politically active and powerful, despite shifting power struggles for several states and almost continual war from 2000-1800 BC.

Around 1760 BC at Mari royal documents describe a society which allowed elite women great scope in economic and political activities. Women just like men, owned and managed property, could contract in their own name, could sue in court and serve as witnesses. They took part in legal and business transactions such as adoptions, sales of property, the giving and taking of loans. They were scribes, musicians and singers, priestesses, diviners and prophetesses and hence sometimes royal advisers on an equal basis with men. A few women's gifts to the king in tribute indicate they had political standing. The queen, as the principal wife held power in the palace and temple and workshops and acted as a stand in for the king. The king's secondary wives in ranking order were installed in different palaces where their fortunes varied The wife's power, like that of the male vassal, depended on the will and whim of the king. Queen Shibutu, the wife of Zimri-lim "Her role is exceptional both in its scope and in the sheer multiplicity of activities in which she is engaged ... Her influence was felt everywhere. She offered sacrifices, she advised the king and carried out his instructions. She selected slave women for his harem." Of his twenty daughters, eight were married into vassal alliances. Some held influential positions for example as mayor of the vassal city. This marriage involved a stormy relationship between sister co-wives ending in effective divorce. Two were *naditum* - 'to lie fallow' - priestesses who were forbidden from having children, as dedicated sexually to the gods, but could adopt, and sometimes have husbands. They also brought with them rich dowries to the temple which they could also use as capital to do business and own property (Lerner R397 68).

These expressions of civic government were not shared by other Mesopotamian cultures. Amorite rulers retained many features of their tribal heritage. All authority was kept in the hands of the king, who directly oversaw, or personally delegated, all operations.

Diminishing the Moon: Patriarchal Law Codes

"From that time she, the moon as a female figure has had no light of her own, but derives her light from the sun. At first they were on an equality, but afterwards she diminished herself; for a woman enjoys no honor save in conjunction with her husband". (Zohar 1, 20a)

Throughout these periods and later, acts of warfare, besides resulting in wholesale slaughter, particularly of men, also became a basis for claiming captive populations as slaves. Raping women of a conquered groups was standard practice from the second millennium BC. Male slaves were more dangerous and frequently shackled, or subjected to other injuries such as blinding, castration or branding. Although slavery was a commuted death sentence, the slave experienced both natal and reproductive alienation, severance from kin and lack of parental rights over their offspring and general dishonouring. Women and children were thus selectively taken as slaves, both as labourers, as reproductive units and as prizes to win honour among men. Many of those taken in war became sick or died in transit (Lerner R397 76).

"Now therefore kill every male among the little ones, and kill every woman that hath known man by lying with him. But all the women children, that have not known a man by lying with him, keep alive for yourselves" (Num 31:17).

An idea of the treatment of slave women in Greece comes from Homer's Odyssey. Odysseus returns from many adventures sexual and otherwise to find a number of 'suitors' have besieged his wife and female slaves. His wife has stalled them off by promising herself when she finished a weaving which she unravels every night, but twelve of his fifty maidservants have been raped. Having bloodily eliminated the suitors he commands his adolescent son to get the twelve to carry out the dead and then to stab them all. He demurs and instead strangles them because of the dishonour they have helplessly brought to the family. Trophy wives were a standard feature of warfare. When his war bride is returned for fear of her priest father's curse, Agamemnon promptly seizes the trophy wife of his captain Achilles, leading her away by the wrist in a traditional sign of the submissive captive wife.

Slavery could also result from becoming indebted to another party. Slaves could be brought and sold at market. As a natural extension of the idea of 'exchange of women' as property, and abduction, a woman slave became the sexual property of her 'master'. He or a member of the family could cohabit with them without assuming the slightest obligation, or hired out as a prostitute. Slave women staffed the brothels as prostitutes and filled the harems of the ancient world. Slave couples could be forcibly separated and consensual 'wives' of slaves were obliged to submit sexually to their 'masters'. Slavery under varying circumstances and numbers is common to societies from Sumeria, through harsher treatment by the Assyrians, to Greece where captured men were frequently all killed and women and children taken captive in numbers. In China from the third century BC to the twentieth century AD, 'buying of concubines' was and established practice. Later in Roman times, formal monogamy existed in a polygnous context of slave concubinage.

Numbers 31 illustrates killing the men and taking the women as slave trophy wives:

"And they warred against the Midianites, as the Lord commanded Moses; and they slew all the males. ... And the children of Israel took all the women of Midian captives, and their little ones, and took the spoil of all their cattle, and all their flocks, and all their goods."

Deuteronomy 21:10 provides for relatively clement treatment of a woman taken in battle as slave concubine:

"When thou goest forth to war against thine enemies, and the Lord thy God hath delivered them into thine hands, and thou hast taken them captive, and seest among the captives a beautiful woman, and hast a desire unto her, that thou wouldest have her to thy wife; Then thou shalt bring her home to thine house, and she shall shave her head, and pare her nails; And she shall put the raiment of her captivity from off her, and shall remain in thine house, and bewail her father and her mother a full month: and after that thou shalt go in unto her, and be her husband, and she shall be thy wife. And it shall be, if thou have no delight in her, then thou shalt let her go whither she will; but thou shalt not sell her at all for money, thou shalt not make merchandise of her, because thou hast humbled her."

The practice of using slave women as servants and sex objects became the standard for class dominance over women in all historic periods. Serfs, peasants and workers were expected to serve men of upper class sexually - exemplified by the *droit du seigneur* - the right of first night, after a master grants the marriage of a serf.

In the Codex Hammurabi CH (Lerner R397 101) a man could offer his wife, children, concubines or slaves for a debt either by outright sale or a pledge, which allowed redemption within a fixed time. Abuse was countered by fines, or in the case of death of the son of a free man, death of the son of the creditor in exchange. Wives and children of a debtor became free after three years, marking an improvement in conditions. A man thus had authority over his wife and children to the point of sale, with slaves and concubines faring worse.

Slave concubines performed a dual service, 'wife' of the master and slave of the mistress. This was of importance given patrilineal inheritance if the betrothed wife failed to deliver an offspring, particularly a son. Such is the case for both Sarai and Rachel:

"Sarai said unto Abram, Behold now, the Lord hath restrained me from bearing: I pray thee, go in unto my maid; it may be that I may obtain children by her. And Abram hearkened to the voice of Sarai (Gen 16:2).

"And when Rachel saw that she bare Jacob no children, ... she said, Behold my maid Bilhah, go in unto her; and she shall bear upon my knees, that I may also have children by her. And she gave him Bilhah her handmaid to wife: and Jacob went in unto her" (Gen 30:1).

In the Codex Hammurabi, a *naditum* priestess, who could not bear children, could either give her husband her slave girl, in which case the children were considered to be of the first wife, as in Genesis, or he was entitled to a secondary wife. A slave wife who had born sons of the master could not be sold by her mistress but remained a slave. A master might legitimate sons by a slave and if he did not they became free without inheritance on his death. Lerner (R397 93) notes the pattern of freeing concubines who bore sons became incorporated into Islamic law and has become one of the most common features of world slavery.

The Babylonian Codex Hammurabi CH (c1750 BC), the Middle Assyrian laws MA and Hittite laws HL (c1500 BC) and finally Hebrew law of the Biblical Covenant Code BC (c800 BC) show an interesting evolution of social attitudes in Mesopotamia. Each of these cemented legal customs already in existence for several hundred years. In the CH 73 of 282 laws pertain to sex and marriage. In MA 59 out of 112 do indicating increasing stress in this area, with the much greater control of women being striking. Only 26 out of 200 do in HL. Not all these laws coincided with legal practice which tended to follow accepted norms. Neither were all enforceable under the principle of *lex talionis* - the punishment fitting the crime, such as surgeons having their hands cut off for performing an unsuccessful operation except in extreme cases.

CH deals with three social classes, patricians including priests and officials, the burgher and slaves, with punishments ascending for the severity of the impact each class can have. A great deal of mobility between classes is assumed and much is concerned with the plight of debtors and their families.

Biblical Code allows a male debt slave to go free after six years, with his wife if he married her previously but not if he has during his service:

"If thou buy an Hebrew servant, six years he shall serve: and in the seventh he shall go out free for nothing. If he came in by himself, he shall go out by himself: if he were married, then his wife shall go out with him. If his master have given him a wife, and she have born him sons or daughters; the wife and her children shall be her master's, and he shall go out by himself. And if the servant shall plainly say, I love my master, my wife, and my children; I will not go out free: Then his master shall bring him unto the judges; he shall also bring him to the door, or unto the door post; and his master shall bore his ear through with an aul; and he shall serve him for ever" (Ex 21:2)

A woman does not go free. She can however be redeemed if he has not taken her for a concubine, but might be sold into prostitution, although not exported:

" And if a man sell his daughter to be a maidservant, she shall not go out as the menservants do. If she please not her master, who hath betrothed her to himself, then shall he let her be redeemed: to sell her unto a strange nation he shall have no power, seeing he hath dealt deceitfully with her. And if he have betrothed her unto his son, he shall deal with her after the manner of daughters. If he take him another wife; her food, her raiment, and her duty of marriage, shall he not diminish." (Ex 21:7)

In CH the power of a father over his children was unlimited. A son striking his father could have his hand cut off and one renouncing adopted father could have his tongue cut out. In Hebrew law, as in the 'Ten Commandments', this included the mother as well:

"And he that smiteth his father, or his mother, shall be surely put to death." (Ex 21:15)

If a man have a stubborn and rebellious son, which will not obey the voice of his father, or the voice of his mother, and that, when they have chastened him, will not hearken unto them: Then shall his father and his mother lay hold on him, and bring him out unto the elders of his city, and unto the gate of his place; 21:20 And they shall say unto the elders of his city, This our son is stubborn and rebellious, he will not obey our voice; he is a glutton, and a drunkard. And all the men of his city shall stone him with stones, that he die: so shalt thou put evil away from among you; and all Israel shall hear, and fear (Deut 21:18).

Daughters are not mentioned, presumably because they can be married off. The bride price received was usually used to finance the acquisition of a bride for a son. Marriages were usually arranged by the fathers of the groom and bride. Many laws in CH cover the exchange of gifts or money. The groom's father paid the bride's father a betrothal gift (*biblum*) and a bridal gift (*tirhâtum*), representing a 'bride price' of the older marriage by purchase. whereupon the couple were considered betrothed. Usually she stayed with her family but sometimes child brides were sent to their in-laws as a servant until the marriage was completed. There are penalties to try to prevent the obvious abuse this situation invites. If the betrothed pair had made love and the father-in-law raped her, he is drowned for adultery. If he does when she was still a virgin, he had to pay a fine and return her and any property or dowry she has provided to the house of her father. She might then marry "a husband after her heart" - a rare provision, probably taking into account her humiliation. Notice also the prospective groom can have sexual relations free of censure. There were also marriages by contract (*riksatum*), which could endow the wife with certain property rights and conditions in separation and avoid her becoming a debt slave to her husband. After marriage, the bride's father gave her a dowry (*seriktum*) or settlement (*nudunnum*) which was administered by the husband for her benefit to be transmitted to her sons and for her use in the case of his death or divorce . A wife divorced for not delivering sons or for illness also has the option of remaining with life time maintenance. If a wife who had not delivered sons died, the dowry and bride price were returned (Lerner R397 106).

Marriages tended towards homogamy - marriage into a similar propertied class. Dowry and settlement money made the marriage more stable by giving both partners an invest- ment. Sons received their father's inheritance and daughters a dowry. Strict supervision of girls' chastity and strong family control over selection of marriage partners maintained the system. A marriage could be dissolved if the girl didn't possess the tokens of virginity.

Virginity was prized in Jewish society. It's mandatory prescription for priestly marriage reflects the staunchly demanding conservatism of the families of many bridegrooms:

"And he shall take a wife in her virginity. A widow, or a divorced woman, or profane, or an harlot, these shall he not take: but he shall take a virgin of his own people to wife" (Lev 21:13).

The older form of marriage without joint residence where the wife remains in her father's (or mother's) house and the groom resides with her as an occasional or permanent visitor - the Biblical *beena* marriage is also noted as a Mesopotamian cultural practice overtaken by patriarchal Hammurabic law. This gave the wife greater autonomy and ease of divorce. The historical evolution appears to be from the *beena* marriage, towards a Semitic patriar- chal marriage by purchase and then to a contract, the latter two preserved in CH. In a soci- ety where ownership of agricultural land and herds meant high status, the purpose of marriage became the continuation of the family line and property through sons. Marriage by purchase applied to lower class wives and contract to higher class ones where the bride had wealth.

Marriages were generally monogamous. The older practice of taking a second lower class wife being replaced by slave concubines who were clearly subservient. Men were free to commit adultery with prostitutes, concubines and slave servants. A man could reduce the status of a wife who was "behaving foolishly, wasting her house or belittling her husband" to a slave, divorce her or marry a second wife. A husband could file for divorce at any time but had to return the dowry and up to half his estate. Divorce was for the wife virtually unobtainable. If a husband philandered in a belittling way a wife could sue for divorce, but if her case was unproven she would be drowned. In Hebrew law a man had free right to divorce for an economic penalty, but women were barred. Marriages of the early patriarchs were polygynous, but later monogamous marriage became an ideal as in Mesopotamia with free access to slave 'servants' and gentile concubines, again consistent with the Jewish line being passed down to the children of the legitimate Jewish wife, as was the case with Sarah and Hagar where the son carrying the line is Isaac and not Ishmael, the actual firstborn. Frequent insertions of foreign Y-chromosomes into the Jewish line indicate this pattern of confirming biology in the face of religion has continued over historical time.

The practice of the Jewish line being inherited through the mother may have ben perpetuated under patriarchy because in biblical times (and in Mesopotamia into the middle ages) this practice continued with some Jewish men also taking a gentile wife or concubine in a polygynous family, with only the sons of the Jewish mother having the entitlement. The 'absence of adoption in Jewish law is probably also traceable to the fact that the Law is not in principle oriented to monogamy, and only reckons with the child's natural ties, based on birth. Adoption wasn't necessary in Judaism, since the husband could always entrust several wives with maintaining his ancestral line. A good many civil rights were bound up with a flawless genealogy ... all important public offices of honor and trust were reserved to the full-blooded Israelite. As part of this system, the choice of a wife played a major role. " (Ranke-Heinemann R552 65).

Meyers (1988) says that, despite the patriarchal, male-oriented nature of Yahwistic religion, the counterpoint between public and home life, which valued the home and its emphasis on procreation, gives rise to a centre of female power in the home and in intimate domestic matters. Aschkenasy (R24) has a much bleaker picture of the situation facing women:

> "Patriarchal structure provided the woman with protection and shelter. She was declared the sexual mate of one man only, not to be touched by the other males. At the same time, the woman became the chattel of that male, part of his worldly possessions, and she lost her freedom to choose and decide for herself. Two types of feminine oppression come to the fore. ... As a minor and a dependent within the law, the woman found herself, in ancient times, within a legal system that was male-centered and designed to protect men's rights and interests. The woman also existed in a certain social and cultural ambience, not defined by the law, in which her femininity-her ability to arouse desire in man, and her reproductive powers-was regarded with a mixture of awe and jealousy. This resulted in a situation where the woman's sexuality was both guarded and exploited, and where she was often seen as a being tyrannized by her own anatomy, who had to pay the price not only for her own excesses but for those she may have aroused in the male".

She points out that "a husband who suspects his wife of infidelity, but has no proof of it, may require her to submit to a humiliating ordeal. If she is found to be innocent, the husband will have to pay no penalty for his false accusation."

> If "he be jealous of his wife, and she be defiled; ... or not. Then shall he bring his wife to the priest. ... And he shall cause the woman to drink the bitter water that causes the curse, ... Then it shall come to pass, that, if she be defiled, and have done trespass against her husband, that the water that causes the curse shall enter into her and become bitter, and her belly shall swell, and her thigh shall fall away, and the woman shall be a curse among her people". (Num. 5:11-28).

Women were unclean by virtue of menstruation and were thus barred being priests. Although women were allowed to read the Torah at congregational services they were forbidden to read lessons in public in order to 'safeguard the honour of the congregation'. In the first century AD Rabbi Eliezer said 'Rather should the words of the Torah be burned than entrusted to a woman'. It was for much the same reason that in the Synagogue women were seated apart from men. ... Their exclusion from the priesthood was based on their supposed uncleanness during menstruation as defined in Leviticus 15, a taboo which extends into the Christian church. A priest in Leviticus 21, 22 was to be clean and holy at all times to enter office (Haskins R291 12). Leviticus 12 extends uncleanliness to between 40 days after childbirth for a son and 80 for a daughter.

A wife having sexual relations with any other man commits adultery. A man, by contrast, married or not, commits adultery only by taking another man's wife. The penalty for adultery in CH was death by drowning for both parties, if taken before the king. The husband had the right to see his wife live. MA is more sadistic. A man can save his wife's life, but cut off her nose. The male lover is then turned into a eunuch and his face disfigured. In HL a man can kill his wife and the adulterer himself and not be punished, as in tribal customs.

If he brings the case to court he can grant their lives but otherwise the king shall decide.

Death is also ordained in Hebrew Law:

> *"And the man that committeth adultery with another man's wife, even he that committeth adultery with his neighbour's wife, the adulterer and the adulteress shall surely be put to death" (Lev 20:10).*

In Deuteronomic Law and in its inherited sequel in Islamic Law, the penalty for adultery is death by stoning, both for promiscuity before marriage and after it:

> *"But if this thing be true, and the tokens of virginity be not found for the damsel: Then they shall bring out the damsel to the door of her father's house, and the men of her city shall stone her with stones that she die: because she hath wrought folly in Israel, to play the whore in her father's house: ... If a man be found lying with a woman married to an husband, then they shall both of them die, both the man that lay with the woman, and the woman: so shalt thou put away evil from Israel"*
> *(Deut 22:20).*

The pattern here and in continuing passages is as follows. If a girl is engaged and gets married and the husband says she wasn't a virgin and the girl's parents have the tokens of virginity (the bloody bed sheet), he gets a fine and becomes a slave of the father-in-law. But if they can't find these tokens when accused, she is stoned to death. If a married woman commits adultery, both she and her lover are killed. If a betrothed virgin is raped in town she is also stoned because she didn't cry out. Only a virgin in the fields gets saved because no one could hear her. She is then forced into an indissoluble marriage with the rapist.

Rape, for example that of Dinah, is not seen in terms of the emotional damage it may cause to a woman, especially a young girl, and the perpetrator is not regarded as a vicious criminal. He must simply marry the girl, and make the appropriate marriage gift to her father. In matters of the heart, too, only the male's point of view is considered.

> "Jewish girls usually got engaged when they were twelve or twelve and a half years old. ... An engagement was the first phase of getting married, which was followed after somewhat more than a year by the bride's being taken to her fiancee's home. Engagement counted as marriage, not de facto but de jure: The fiancee was already the man's wife. If the man died before bringing her home, she was already his widow. Infidelity by the fiancee was considered adultery. If the husband demanded that she be taken before the court and punished, a harsh sentence loomed ahead: A girl between twelve years and a day up to twelve years and six months would be stoned along with her lover. An older girl would be strangled; a younger one was considered a minor and went unpunished" (Ranke-Heinmann R552 65-6).

Ranke-Heinmann notes that the scribes added on conditions to the penal provisions for adultery by the fiancee reducing its likelihood. At least two witnesses had to prove that they had warned the adulterous pair about the consequences facing them, and that the couple had nevertheless continued in their sin. ... Yet executions did take place. Records note an engaged daughter of a priest was burned to death for adultery around AD 35 (R552 35-6).

> *"And the daughter of any priest, if she profane herself by playing the whore, she profaneth her father: she shall be burnt with fire" (Lev 21:9).*

In CH a woman merely accused of adultery if so accused by her husband could swear by a god her innocence, but if accused by the locals, she was thrown in the river to sink or swim for her husband. In MA allows for a man's wife to be ordered to be publicly flogged, her breasts torn off, or her ears, or nose cut off by officials. A man may [scourge] his wife, pluck [her hair], bruise and destroy [her] ears with no liability.

In CH a widow with sons was favoured, protected by having permanent residence in her sons house. A propertied widow could if she chose return to her fathers house with her dowry and bride price, provided her sons are provided for. By by the time of MA "a young widow shall be who has no sons shall be given either to one of her husband's brothers or to his father. Only if there was no man to take her, could she "go whither she wishes".

The Decalogue lists a wife among the man's possessions, between house, slaves and cattle:

> *"Thou shalt not covet thy neighbour's house, thy neighbour's wife, nor his manservant, nor his maidservant, nor his ox, nor his ass, nor any thing that is thy neighbour's" (Ex 20:17)*

The preservation of the family line in the tribal patrimony rested with the patriarchal head of the family and usually fell to the eldest son. If there was no son it could fall to daughters, but they would have to marry into their tribe so their portion was not transferred out (Num 27:7-8, 36:6-9). If the owner died childless the inheritance went to his brother, uncle or nearest kinsman. This is reflected in the Jewish *levirate* where a widow was family property which was not allowed to lie fallow if the deceased had died without a male heir and the brother of the deceased could become her husband and sire heirs in his stead.

Inheritance through the female line and its relation to the levirate is elaborated in the story of Tamar. Judah's daughter-in-law Tamar (Gen 38) is left to confront widowhood because none of her surviving brothers-in-law will perpetuate their brother's line (Fox 407). Judah had children by the Canaanite Shuah, but his firstborn Er, Tamar's husband, was wicked and was slain. When asked to fertilize Tamar, Onan then spilled his seed on the ground to avoid 'giving it to his brother' in a sign of coitus interruptus rather than masturbation. Judah then says Tamar can have his son Shelah, but fails to come to the party. Tamar discards her widows garments, covers her face with a veil and sits in a public place. "When Judah saw her, he thought her to be a harlot because she had covered her face." She then keeps his signet, bracelets and staff as security for his payment of a sheep. She conceives by Judah. He condemns her to be burned to death for being pregnant by harlotry, but when she reveals his possessions, he realizes "that the child is his and that she has gained a well-merited heir by trickery". He acknowledges "She is more righteous than I"

CH deals with abortion and induced miscarriage as follows: a fine of ten shekels for a patrician's daughter and five for a burgher's. If the daughter dies it is death of the aggressor's daughter in the case of a patrician and a fine for a burgher's daughter. MA sees the wife of an aggressor having the fruits of her womb destroyed and an assault causing miscarriage of a first born son results in death for the aggressor. In both laws *lex talionis* applies. HL has a graded series of fines according to the age of the fetus. Hebrew law stipulates both fines and retribution on the same principle of 'an eye for an eye'.

In MA, with no precedent, a woman causing her own miscarriage is to be impaled and not buried - the ultimate penalty equivalent to that of treason. Although infants were subject to exposure after birth, this was the right of the father. Thus the mother, in usurping the right of the father, has upset the entire patriarchal order, from king to paterfamilias.

Iwan Bloch noted "prostitution appears among primitive people wherever free sexual intercourse is curtailed and limited. It is nothing else than a substitute for a new form of primitive promiscuity". Engels suggests "hetaerism derives quite directly from group marriage, from the ceremonial surrender by which women purchased the right of chastity [sacred prostitution] ... Among other people hetarism derives form the sexual freedoms allowed girls before marriage. ... With the rise of inequality of property ... wage and slave labour ... and as its necessary correlate, the professional prostitution of free women side by side with the forced surrender of the slave" seeing it to be a complement to monogamous marriage in patriarchal society predicting its demise with the rise of social property (Lerner R397 123-4).

The actual origin of our own terms is intriguing and informative. 'Whore' is an ancient European word *huor* whose root is 'adultery' and possibly relates to Latin *carus* 'dear' (cf charity). 'Prostitute' literally means *pro-* before *-statuere* cause to stand - expose publicly consistent with Assyrian law (p 201) requiring prostitutes and slaves to be unveiled.

Gerda Lerner (R397 127) notes a sequence from the highest *en* priestesses through *naditum* dedicated as consorts of the gods, to *qadishtum* who were lower ranking temple servants and finally *harimtu*, slave prostitutes attached to the temple. The goddess Ishtar is also referred to as a *qadishtu*. *Harimtu* are also associated with taverns and Ishtar is their patroness:

> "When I sit in the entrance of a tavern, I, Ishtar am a loving harimtu" (Lerner G 131).

Qadesh which has connotations of holy as 'sacred prostitute' is illustrated in the naked love goddess in Hathor head-dress standing on lion in the manner of Ishtar (p 181), also epitomized in many of the female goddess figures scattered throughout Israel-Palestine.

She traditionally holds a lotus in her right hand and two snakes in her left, indicating renewal of life. Asherah, the old supreme wife of Canaanite El, and reluctant mother of Ba'al, was imported into Egypt, along with Anath, in the 13th Century BC as *Qodshu*, or *Qedeshat*. Rameses II called himself a companion of Anat (Warner 118). Asherah and Anath were paired with Yahweh at Gezeh and Elephantine. Asherah or 'the grove' stood before the Hebrew temple until the time of Josiah in the form of a tree or pole. Hathor also manifests as a golden cow or calf and has a strong presence in Sinai, from Serabit to Timna and Palestine from Hazor to Byblus. Like Miriam, Hathor beats a timbrel or tambourine and like Mirian she is associated with water, issuing the waters of life from her sacred sycamore tree:

> *"and the Lord brought again the waters of the sea upon them; but the children of Israel went on dry land in the midst of the sea. And Miriam the prophetess, the sister of Aaron, took a timbrel in her hand; and all the women went out after her with timbrels and with dances. And Miriam answered them, Sing ye to the Lord, for he hath triumphed gloriously" (Ex 15:19)*

In Hebrew a prostitute is *kadoshet*, and it is at Qadesh that Miriam dies and Moses is cursed for not striking the waters in Yahweh's name:

> *"and the people abode in Kadesh; and Miriam died there, and was buried there. And there was no water for the congregation" (Num 20:1)*

In the accounts of Herodotus in the fifth century BC and later Strabo, Babylonian women were expected to prostitute themselves for the love goddess in return for a silver coin, after which no gift, however great, would prevail. One can see this as a token of female inscrutability characteristic of neolithic matrilineal societies who followed the *beena* marriage and unmarried sexual freedom as illustrated in the Canela (p 168). The token ceremony of promiscuity is then followed by marital compliance in the later patriarchal age. Thousands of Dalit (untouchable) girls in India are still consecrated to sacred prostitution in the name of the Goddess (p 294), often at the behest of Brahmin elders.

What has been called the 'oldest profession' harks back to the wild primal man Enkidu, 'tamed' by the *harimtu* Shamhat:

> *and he possessed her ripeness.*
> *She was not bashful as she welcomed his ardour.*
> *She laid aside her cloth and he rested upon her.*
> *She treated him the savage, to a woman's task,*
> *as his love was drawn unto her.*

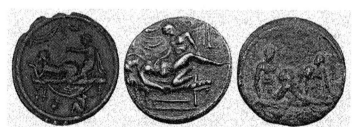

Spintria, Roman brothel tokens, display various services in relation to the obverse value of the coin.

Like the Eden myth (p 211), McElvaine (R446 96) sees Enkidu's role as that of a reluctant primal hunter, drawn into the woman's arts of sexuality and civilized agriculture, later becoming mortally weakened by his new wisdom. Enkidu then curses the gateway through which he came and Shamhat for removing him from wild freedom in nature, consigning her to the seamy role of a street prostitute, rejecting her wiles in a statement of male rebellion, before forgiving her at Shamash's behest in coming to terms with civilization. Lerner emphasizes Shamhat's as a civilizing role, pleasing to the Gods - a woman's task not set off from others of the female sex, which attests as much to her original higher status and to the emergence of patriarchal sexual service based on slavery of women by debt and conquest.

When we come to Assyrian law (Lerner R397 134) we are dealing with a frankly militaristic patriarchal society in which a clear wedge has been driven between virgin daughters and commercial prostitutes. Nowhere is this more clear than in the laws which cover the earliest regulations known concerning the veiling of women. MA asserts that neither wives, daughters, nor widows of seigniors who go out in the street may have their heads uncovered. A concubine who goes with a mistress must cover herself. A married sacred prostitute must be covered but an unmarried one uncovered. A harlot or a girl slave must not veil herself. Sexually assigned women are thus to be veiled as 'private'. Others are 'public women'. The penalty for a harlot veiling herself was severe - to be stripped, flogged and tarred on the head, but her jewelry is untouched. A slave girl would be stripped and have her ears cut off. This has become an affair of state security and any man who failed to report it was treated similarly. Unlike in Islam, there is no specific penalty for a respectable woman being unveiled. Presumably social pressures were sufficient to cause 'respectable' women to avoid the harassment of 'publicity'. This represents an outstanding example of class-based discrimination applied to women on the basis of their ownership by men and their sexuality.

While feminist authors like Lerner demur at the negative connotations of 'prostitution' and seek to distinguish it from the fertility rites of the *hieros gamos* as a higher calling in the name of the fertility goddess, later sullied by patriarchal commercial exploitation, even questioning Herodotus' account, we need to understand that the confusion of paternity is central to all fertility rites, from the masked faces in Beltane to those in Biblical times, on every high hill and under every green tree, and the ritual prostitution of every woman before marriage at the blue gates of Babylon, all of which involve female promiscuity.

Woman as Empty Vessel - The Greek Experience

Greece is central to the development of Western civilization in terms of philosophy and science and the development of historical thought, all of which became separated from religion by the sixth and fifth centuries BC. As was the case in Mesopotamia and Israel, Greece was a patriarchal class-driven society with slavery, in which women were excluded from political life and were lifelong minors under the guardianship of a male. City states were established and defended on the basis of a phalanx of male defenders who fostered a spirit of egalitarianism, responsibility and discipline. We can thus see a paradoxical link between egalitarian democracy and hierarchical patriarchy - all things being equal, but among men only. The right to a voice in public affairs thus spread from the nobles to all citizens having the means to equip themselves. However this definition resulted in the exclusion of women. Premarital and marital chastity were strictly enforced on women, but their husbands were free to enjoy sexual gratification from lower class women, heterae, slaves and young men. In Sparta both men and women figured in the equality of the phalanx women as necessary bearers of children. Adultery and legitimacy were not so clearly defined as in Athens. Other cities associated oligarchy as opposed to democracy with the higher status of women. Reacting to increasing class divisions caused by commercial development of agriculture, the laws of Draco and Solon laid the foundations of democracy in the classical age.

Hesiod's theogeny describes in mythical terms the rise of patriarchy and the suppression of the female's role on procreation. First comes primal Chaos and in turn Gaia the Earth Goddess and Eros the god of sexual desire. The sky god Uranos is created parthenogenetically by Gaia, whom she made her equal in grandeur, so he might surround her and cover her completely and be a secure home for the blessed gods forever. Uranos tries to prevent a challenge from his son Kronos, by hiding his children in the womb of Gaia. But she and Kronos castrate Uranos and overthrow him. Kronos fearing in turn he will be overtaken by his sons with Rhea, swallows them alive. Rhea hides her son Zeus in a cave protected by Gaia. When he is grown, Zeus overthrows Kronos and to avoid suffering the same fate, swallows his wife Metis thus preventing her bearing a son, but in the same process assimilating to himself her power of procreativity. He is thus able to give birth to Athena. We thus see not just woman but the very capacity of women to contribute to the nature of the offspring unraveled by the patriarchy (Lerner G 207).

Aeschylus' "Eumenides" or "Furies" lays waste to the last defense of Mother Goddess power against the patriarchy. Agamemnon sacrifices his daughter Iphigenia to propitiate the wind god on his journey to defeat Troy. On his return, his wife Clymenestra kills him in revenge. Their son Orestes then kills his mother for treason against the king. The furies excuse her actions on the primacy of mother-right "The man she killed was not of her own blood." Orestes then asks "But am I of my mother's?" The furies retort "She nourished you in her own womb. Do you disown your mother's blood?" To which Apollo replies, speaking directly of the penis:

> *"The mother is not the true source of life.*
> *We call her the mother, but she is more the nurse,*
> *The furrow where the seed is thrust.*
> *The thruster, the father is the true parent:*
> *The woman but tends the growing plant".*

Athena then chimes in with her 'virgin' birth from Zeus to prove the point, banishing the furies and mother-right and freeing Orestes (Lerner G 205, Friedman R225 19). Apollo in his free-wheeling chauvinism was renowned for rape and abandonment "What's wrong with him? He rapes young girls, then takes off? He fathers children secretly and then lets them die" says Euripedes (Hrdy 1999 239). This false 'maternal' birth from Zeus continues with the second Dionysus, born out of the knee of Zeus, after he has copulated with human Semele and she is killed by a bolt of lightning after asking to see him in his full power, leading to a parallel with Yeshua born of the human 'virgin' Mary by the father god Abba.

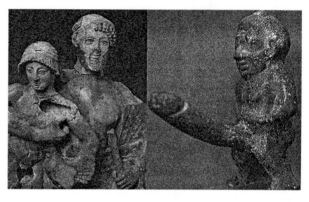

Left: Zeus abducts his great-grandson Ganymede in an incestuous homosexual act of paedophilia to become his lover and cup bearer on Olympus. 470 BC Temple of Zeus, Olympia. Right Priapos (god Bes) c500 BC from a brothel in Ephesus.

Having swallowed Metis, the avowedly polygynous Zeus marries Themis goddess of order, spawning the fates and then his own sister Hera, herself a much more ancient fertility goddess, after whom the heroes were named (Walker R708 392). However the women didn't take this frontal assault lying down. The turbulent and tempestuous sex war between Zeus and Hera becomes a principal source of conflict in Greek mythology. Hera is now depicted as a jealous wife pursuing Zeus for his multiple philandering and pederastic ways. Zeus became so angry with Hera that he attached anvils to her legs and hung her from Mt. Olympus. Hera, the disaffected matriarch in the dysfunctional family whom Zeus heads, has remained stranded, strung upside down ever since, their 'sacred marriage' lying at the very heart of the 'deadlock of wedlock' in Greek culture (Willis R734 132).

Aristotle took up the theme of women as 'mutated males' accepting that women also contributed *catamenia* a female discharge comparable to semen but in need of working up by the more active semen. Females to him were too 'reptilian' - too cold in the blood to produce a fully viable fertility substance, passive rather than active in creation, in affinity with primitive matter. Man is thus the maker and woman just the 'labourer'. The female as a 'mutilated' male was thus seen as devoid of 'soul' and liable to give birth to monstrosities, leading to a view that the entire female anatomy, and with it the vagina and uterus, was a kind of inverted penis, reflecting in a male dominant myth the homology of the sex organs (p 358). Running counter to this trend, Plato in the voice of Socrates in his "Republic" advocates equal education for girls and boys, freeing guardian women from housework and child care, but the aim of this was the destruction of the family in the interests of the state. The idea that only the male was procreative, made iconic in McElvaine's (R446) "Eve's Seed", spilled over into excessive absorbtion with male sexuality in men loving men, and 'passing on one's manhood' to under-age boys. Pederasty was an institution sanctioned by the Olympian gods and mythical heroes. Zeus, Apollo, Poseidon and Heracles all had pederastic experiences. So did many of the most illustrious real-life Greeks including Solon, Pythagoras, Socrates and Plato. The act was part of the foundation of an elitist, military culture that elevated the idea of the penis beyond biology and religion to the rarefied heights of philosophy and art. The pederastic act was the culmination of a one-on-one mentoring aimed at passing on *arete* a set of manly virtues including courage, strength, fairness and honesty. Believing Anaxagoras, in a bid to father only sons, men even had their left testicle removed.

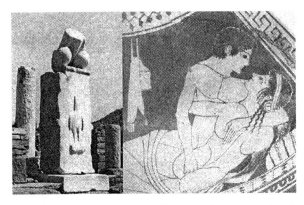

Left: Greek Dionysian Statue Right: Homosexual lovers in the gymnasium

The city and country were dotted with *Hermae*, posts with the head of Hermes and marked at the mid-point by an erection. When the Athenians prepared to attack Sicily in 415 BC, in an apparent war protest by women the penises of hundreds of the city's *hermae* were smashed off. The Sicilian invasion failed and Athens' defeat by Sparta confirmed the men's worst fears.

When Dionysus introduces drink to a farmer Icarius, he is killed by his friends who fear they are poisoned. In revenge Dionysus appears as a beautiful boy who vanishes leaving them with priapism, which the Delphic oracle ordains can be cured only by carrying penises in Dionysus's honour. In a Dionysian festival in Alexandria around 275 BC there was a golden phallus 180 feet long topped with a gold star. Following the penis was a golden statue of Zeus and fifty thousand foot soldiers (Friedman R225 19).

Lefkowitz (R395) explains Greek patriarchy as a result of the Athenians' obsession with racial purity and with keeping the city's wealth in the hands of its own citizens: "It was their pursuit of pure citizenship that made them obsess about the patrilineal bloodline. To control those lines they had to control women directly. They had to know who the fathers were."

In the backdrop of female resentment towards the Greek patriarchy lurks a mythical matriarchy whose possible existence as a culture has recently received new credibility:

"We are riders; our business is with the bow and the spear, and we know nothing of women's work."
Herodotus IV, 114

Numerous myths and legends grew up around women or tribes of women in ancient times, who either fought alongside or alone against men. The Greeks and Romans called some of these Amazons. They gained their warlike reputation because of reported attacks they launched on the lands of Greece and Asia Minor. According to one classical account, they were besieging Troy when Archilles killed their queen, Penthesilea, and then fall in love with her dying face. They were given credit for founding many cities such as Ephesus, Smyma, Cyme and Myrine. Monuments and tombs are ascribed to them on the plains and mountains about Thermodon. The Amazons were eventually driven from these cities. By all accounts, the principal land of the Amazons lay in the plains north east of the Black Sea near the Caucasus Mountains. The Greeks said that the Amazons were a self-sufficient society of women without men, in which women ploughed the fields, looked after cattle and particularly trained horses. They reported that this society was the result of a rebellion of women who, in company with some other rebellious women from the Greek related cities of the Thacians and Euboeans, set up their own army and founded independent settlements. They were said to be consecrated to Cybele, the Mother Goddess of Nature, whose rites included much dancing and music. These were traditionally presided over in the Middle East by priestesses including some who were 'transgendered' castrated men. For pro-creation they had an agreement with the neighbouring Gargarian people (whom Gimbutas accused of having introducing patriarchy to Europe some 2 to 4 millennia earlier) to meet once a year at a spring festival ritual held on a mountain between their territories. After-wards the Amazons would lie in the dark with Gargarian men selected at random for the purpose of gendering children. The boys born from these encounters would be returned to the Gargarians. They also hunted on horseback and made their shields, helmets and clothes from the skins of animals. They used a wide range of weapons including the bow and arrow, the sagaris and especially the javelin. It was said, in accounts that they would cut off their right breast if it interfered with their throwing of the javelin (Roberts R574).

New excavations from a time contemporary with classical Greece (c 500 BC), at Pokrovka on the Kazakh-Russian steppes have yielded evidence that women among the Sauromatian and Early Sarmatian (Early Nomad) tribes are warriors (Davis-Kimball R149). Because they are located much further to the east of the north Black Sea region where the ancient Herodotus gathered his information, the female warriors at Pokrovka were most probably not the Amazons that this ancient Greek historian wrote about in the 5th century B.C. The populations in this region are Indo-Europoids and spoke an Indo-Iranian language. A skull of one such women was reconstructed. At this early date there is no Mongoloid admixture.

Offerings in the burials in their 'kurgans' or burial mounds that the nomads needed for their journey to the next world included ordinary household objects, religious and cultic items, horse trappings, and weaponry for both men and women alike. Male roles are pre-dominently warriors, although there is a wide variety from rich to poor. Three quarters of women in domestic burials have many imported artifacts including gold-covered bronze earrings, imported jet, and other semi-precious stone beads, as well as faience and magical glass eyebeads. They also frequently contained spindle-whorls. The women's occupations during their lifetime run the gamut from housewife, to herder, to priestess 7%, to warrior horsewoman 15%. Two cemeteries had significant numbers of female burials with mortu-ary offerings indicating they were priestesses of various degrees of rank or importance. Gold artifacts including animals style plaques and temple pendants, fossilized sea shells, a beautiful bronze mirror, and a ceremonial altar were all part of her accoutrements. The burial of one young female warrior contained 40 bronze arrowheads in a quiver and an iron dagger. At an average of five foot six, the women were exceedingly tall for their time. (Modern American women average five foot four); the skeleton itself had bowed leg bones, possibly, Davis-Kimball speculated, from a lifetime spent in the saddle. Lodged beneath the rib cage of another was a bent arrowhead--testimony, perhaps, to a violent death in battle. The occurrence of such a large class of woman warriors among these graves which relate strongly to an Indo-Aryan culture raises very significant problems about identifying the early Aryans who migrated into wide aras from Greece to India with the onset of patriarchy.

However patriarchal dominance became a theme across almost all developed cultures. Patriarchal cultural patterns became established and continued uninterrupted to the present day from China through Asia and Mesopotamia to Europe. In Vedic India, gods of thunder such as Indra and those of marital conformity, such as Vishnu and Shri, who epitomized the model Indian wife, loyal and submissive to her husband, continued in Vishu's many incarnations, including Rama and Sita, who immolated herself to prove her chastity, only to be abandoned by her husband even though she was innocent to avoid tarnishing his fam-ily name. Brahmanic widows were expected to throw themselves on their husband's funeral pyres in the name of Sati the faithful chaste wife, in the rite of suttee, young wives were frequently burned for their dowries, and high class girl infants were frequently killed at birth. In China, women remained marginal outsiders in their kin groups. While men 'belonged in' a household or lineage, women 'belonged to' males who had acquired rights in them. Foot-binding became a symbol of the confined upper-class woman rationalizing the fact that she didn't need to serve by her own actions. Paradoxically, under certain cir-cumstances, concubines could rise to the highest positions in society. Some became empresses and the mothers of kings. As in many other places, male slaves were castrated for harem service. The wives and children of criminals were subject to enslavement. In Rome the male head of the family continued to hold rights of life and death over his children as the *paterfamilias* until 312 AD when Christian Constantine finally banned it. However the historical theologian Constance Parvey writes, "within the Roman Empire in the first century AD many women were educated, and some were highly influential and exercised great freedom in public life." There were still legal restrictions. Roman women had to have male guardians and were never given the right to vote. But, particularly in the upper classes, women increasingly entered public life. Some took up the arts. Others went into professions such as medicine. Still others took part in business, court, and social life, engaged in athletics, went to theaters, sporing events, and concerts, and traveled without being required to have male escorts.

Although the seemingly commensurate ideal of monogamous marriage between husband and wife became gradually upheld by Christian influences, despite the polygynous practices of European societies, such as the Visigoths who sacked Rome, the doctrine of *coverture* (covering; shelter; defense; hiding) inherited from feudal Norman custom, proclaimed that wives were the property of their husbands, the rights of the husbands being unlimited and permanent. Marriage thus dissolved all independent rights of a woman under the law. The pattern of repression of women and of feminine religious motifs continued unabated in the Inquisition and witch hunts (p 246), and in the exploitation of women as female serfs, servants and sexual surrogates, to the 20th century. In closing, Gerda Lerner (R397) comments:

"Today, historical development has for the first time created the necessary conditions by which large groups of women - finally, all women - can emancipate themselves from subordination. Since women's thought has been imprisoned in a confining and erroneous patriarchal framework, the transforming of the consciousness of women about ourselves and our thought is a precondition for change. We have opened this book with a discussion of the significance of history for human consciousness and psychic well-being. History gives meaning to human life and connects each life to immortality, but history has yet another function. In preserving the collective past and reinterpreting it to the present, human beings define their potential and explore the limits of their possibilities. We learn from the past not only what people before us did and thought and intended, but we also learn how they failed and erred."

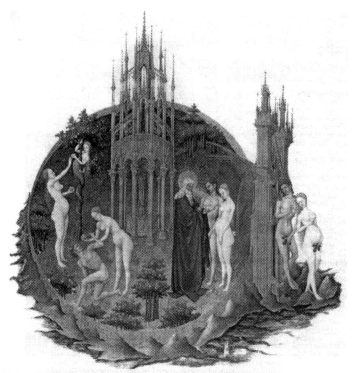

Temptation, Fall, and Expulsion from nature and sexual integration, into mortality through a Jealous God: Judeo-Christian and Islamic traditions explain our origin in the Eden myth, in which Eve and then Adam are cursed for eating the fruit of the tree of knowledge of good and evil, which Eve sought rather as the wisdom of the life tree, not knowing there were two. They are banished lest they also eat of the tree of life and become as God. For their 'concupiscence' in 'knowing' one another, barred from paradise as sexual mortals by a flaming sword, woman to suffer the travail pains of childbirth and to be ruled by her husband while man to conquers nature by the sweat of his brow.
(Brothers Limbourg)

A God Whose Name is 'Jealous'

"We Yolungu are a jealous people and have been since the days we lived in the bush in clans. We are jealous of our wife or husband, for fear she or he is looking at another. If a husband has several wives he is all the more jealous, and the wives are jealous of each other ... make no mistake, the big J is part of our nature" (Australian aboriginal).

It is not just perpetual jeaolusy in our human nature that permeates monotheism, but the unrelenting jealousy of God. The Old Testament, imbues God's essential nature *sine qua non*, by his very name, as jealousy and sexually jealous of those 'whoring' after other gods.

> But ye shall destroy their altars, break their images, and cut down their groves:
> For thou shalt worship no other god: for the Lord, WHOSE NAME IS JEALOUS,
> is a jealous God: Lest thou make a covenant with the inhabitants of the land,
> and they go a WHORING after their gods. (Exodus 34:13)

This utterly mammalian defensive emotion is a projection of primate male emotional and sexual anxiety on to the creative source itself. Jealousy is centrally sexual and the Old Testament speaks of the jealousy of God in clearly sexual terms:

> And I will judge thee, as women that break wedlock and shed blood are judged;
> and I will give thee blood in fury and jealousy. (Ezekiel 16:38)

> Ye shall not go after other gods, of the gods of the people which are round about you; (For the Lord thy God is a jealous God among you) lest the anger of the LORD thy God be kindled against thee, and destroy thee from off the face of the earth. (Deut 6:14)

There is clearly a paradox here, for while jealousy is also natural, although epitomized by male violence against women, it is also acknowledged to be potentially disastrous and love is supreme. In the words of the Song of Songs:

Set me as a seal upon thine heart, as a seal upon thine arm:
for love is strong as death; jealousy is cruel as the grave:
the coals thereof are coals of fire, which hath a most vehement flame.
Many waters cannot quench love, neither can the floods drown it (8:6)

Nowhere are our double-standards more pronounced than in the matter of jealousy. "Thou shalt not covet". "Thou shalt not commit adultery". These two run partially counter to one another, for while covetous jealousy is regarded as morally corrupt envy, a destroyer of love and trust, jealousy is a natural evolutionary defence against the ubiquitous threat of sexual betrayal. To be jealous is to be 'zealous' of one's threatened resource in a partner. Men often display violent reactions if 'their' woman falls for another, because of the intensely felt threat of defilement to their genetic paternity. Women can afford to be more circumspect about a partner's one night stand, but become very defensive when a man might transfer his principal affections and resources to another. However the greatest double standard of all is the way in which a jealous God came to zealously rule our lives and social order. This leads precisely to the world crisis of apocalyptic proportions we continue to creep towards.

God's jealousy can have meaning only in a climate of frank polytheism, where 'He' may and does have real rivals inside and outside the immediate cultural context:

God standeth in the congregation of the mighty; he judgeth among the gods. ...
I have said, Ye are gods; and all of you are children of the most High.
But ye shall die like men, and fall like one of the princes.
Arise, O God, judge the earth: for thou shalt inherit all nations (Psalm 82).

As we shall note, Yahweh-Adonai was originally paired conjugally with consorts Anath and Asherah. This sexual partnership is apparent in Proverbs, where God is paired from the beginning with his feminine complement, Hochmah, or Wisdom:

The Lord possessed me in the beginning of his way, before his works of old.
I was set up from everlasting, from the beginning, or ever the earth was.
When there were no depths, I was brought forth; when there were no fountains abounding with water.
Before the mountains were settled, before the hills was I brought forth:
While as yet he had not made the earth, nor the fields, nor the highest part of the dust of the world.
When he prepared the heavens, I was there: when he set a compass upon the face of the depth. (8)

Wisdom is also the tree of life:

She is more precious than rubies: and all the things thou canst desire are not to be compared unto her.
Length of days is in her right hand; and in her left hand riches and honour.
Her ways are ways of pleasantness, and all her paths are peace.
She is a tree of life to them that lay hold upon her: and happy is every one that retaineth her.
The Lord by wisdom hath founded the earth; by understanding hath he established the heavens (3).

Trouble in Paradise

Turning to this very mythical beginning in Genesis we find a frank double perspective running through the whole account. In the priestly sabbatical creation of Genesis 1, God in the plural 'Elohim, creates the universe from the formless deep - *tohu vo vohu*,

In the beginning God created the heaven and the earth.
And the earth was without form, and void;
and darkness was upon the face of the deep.
And the Spirit moved upon the face of the waters.

in a male act of symbolic creation, dividing primal chaos through the power of speech:

And God said, Let there be light: and there was light.
And God saw the light, that it was good:
and God divided the light from the darkness.

Then 'Elohim creates woman and man dyadically in 'their' likeness:

Let us make man in our image, after our likeness:

So God created man in 'their' own image,
in the image of God created he him;
male and female created he them.

and blesses them, exhorts them to be sexually fruitful and gives them dominion over the whole of nature to subdue it and yet to replenish the Earth.

And God blessed them, and God said unto them,
Be fruitful, and multiply, and replenish the earth,
and subdue it: and have dominion
over the fish of the sea, and over the fowl of the air,
and over every living thing that moveth upon the earth.

However, the Yahwistic author J's Edenic account has very different undertones of cursing rather than blessing, blaming the entire fall of humanity from immortality in paradise on the perfidious nature of woman. A lone God, jealous lest humanity like 'him' gain both knowledge and immortal life, casts them out of paradise, and submits woman to the rule of man.

Yaweh firstly forms man from the dust of the earth and breathes a living soul into him, supplanting a natural birth from the womb of the goddess in the patriarchal tradition, and then makes a garden of paradise for the man to dress and keep, containing at its centre the trees of life and knowledge of dark and light. After making man, God makes the animals, whom Adam names in a secondary act of symbolic creation.

In the garden God plants a dyad of two trees, the tree of life representing immortal wisdom and the tree of good and evil representing analytic knowledge. He tells Adam alone that the fruit of the tree of knowledge is forbidden:

Of every tree of the garden thou mayest freely eat:
But of the tree of the knowledge of good and evil, thou shalt not eat of it:
for in the day that thou eatest thereof thou shalt surely die.

Only then does he create 'woman' out of Adam's rib:

And the Lord God caused a deep sleep to fall upon Adam,
and he slept: and he took one of his ribs,
And the rib, which the Lord God had taken from man,
made he a woman, and brought her unto the man.

This is an inversion of the more ancient Sumerian tale in which the goddess Ninhursag allows eight forbidden plants to grow in the garden of creation. Enki eats from them and is stricken. Ninhursag relents: "To the goddess Ninti I have given birth for you". Ninti means both 'female ruler of life' and 'female ruler of the rib'.

This twist to the tale is calculated to make woman subject to man from the very beginning and indeed Adam promptly names her 'woman' because she is flesh of 'his' flesh. Neither are they non sexual because he shall 'cleave' unto her as man and wife.

And Adam said, This is now bone of my bones, and flesh of my flesh:
she shall be called Woman, because she was taken out of Man.
Therefore shall a man leave his father and his mother,
and shall cleave unto his wife: and they shall be one flesh.
And they were both naked, the man and his wife, and were not ashamed.

Commentators have endlessly debated how this affects the status of women. Calvin saw the Woman as merely an accession to the man, though created in the image of God, albeit to the second degree. Other commentators, consistent with Kabbalistic ideas, suggest Adam, before losing his rib, was androgynous 'human' rather than primal 'man', consistent with the third, briefest and again 'Elhoistic creation story of Genesis 5:

"This is the book of the generations of Adam.
In the day that God created man, in the likeness of God made he him;
Male and female created he them;
and blessed them, and called their name Adam,
in the day when they were created".

Rachel Speight saw woman as more refined, made by God from flesh, rather than mere dust. Tribble (R687) extended this idea to woman being the culmination of God's creation.

However as Milton notes in "Paradise Lost" - man is for God, she is merely for God in him.

We now enter into the period of trickery by Yaweh and his opponent the 'serpent'. This is again reminiscent of several Sumerian myths. Gilgamesh is robbed by a serpent of the plant of immortal life. Adapa is likewise tricked by the gods into rejecting the bread and waters of life thinking them to be those of death.

The serpent asks a seemingly innocent question: "Hath God said, Ye shall not eat of every tree of the garden?" Eve responds, presumably on the basis of Adam's word, that the tree "in the centre of the garden" is forbidden, suggesting she has not even been told by the men which tree is which. The serpent responds "Ye shall not surely die" saying God knows your eyes will be opened, knowing good and evil and you shall be as gods.

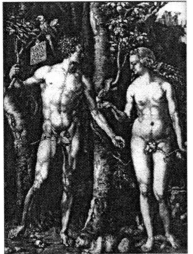

Durer: The cat is about to pounce - Sex becomes predation.

Eve now makes the best assessment she can, finding the fruit fair in an astute gatherer's eyes, neither seeking analytic knowledge, but integrative wisdom:

And when the woman saw that the tree was good for food,
and that it was pleasant to the eyes,
and a tree to be desired to make one wise,
she took of the fruit thereof, and did eat,
and gave also unto her husband with her; and he did eat.

"Their eyes were opened", but the consequence seems to be the immediate sexual modesty of the fig leaf. The 'lubricity', or 'concupiscence', Augustine cited as 'original sin' is the loss of voluntary control over the unruly penis and the sexual desire that necessarily engulfs us as biologically reproducing beings, but this is a far cry from Jewish fertility religion, which extols the sexual act. The implication is however that by disobeying God and eating the fruit, man was enticed into lustful sex by woman, which now becomes a primal tragedy - mortality by the curse of a jealous God - through the knowledge of good and evil. Woman is thus branded as the earthy seducer of male fidelity. But notice this is not a same sex union. Adam and Eve is not Adam and Steve.

Yahweh now sets enmity between the woman and the serpent suggesting this refers to a liaison between the serpent and female fertility, but in a way which for all time remains a pregnant and tacit acknowledgment of women's own genetic fertility - 'her seed' in addition to that of Adam:

And I will put enmity between thee and the woman,
and between thy seed and her seed;

Is the serpent a projection of female fascination with the unrestrained penis of mixed paternity, as these two seeds suggest, or a manifestation of the goddess, or the accursed religions of the nations? Although Qadesh held two snakes, these were serpents of regeneration of life. The serpent is also Nabu, god of wisdom and language. Moses himself carried the serpent Nehustan on a pole, as echoed in the brazen serpent found in the Midianite shrine at Timna. The key to the serpent, as always, is the trickster of immortality, shedding its skin.

Now the patriarchal imperative really begins to bite. First and foremost, Yahweh condemns the woman to reproduction in the place of immortality, in the pain of child-bearing, and establishes the entire paradigm of male domination, in submission to her husband:

I will greatly multiply thy sorrow and thy conception;
in sorrow thou shalt bring forth children;
and thy desire shall be to thy husband,
and he shall rule over thee.

Only then does he curse the ground, condemning the man for hearkening to the woman, now doomed to live by the sweat of his brow, conquering the wilderness, passing from dust to dust as mortal beings. Creation is replaced by procreation. McElvaine (R446) sees Eden as a metaphor for the transition from gatherer-hunter society, in which men reacted to the power women gained from the 'fruit' of agriculture by seizing patriarchal control.

At this point Adam renames his wife Eve:

"And Adam called his wife's name Eve; because she was the mother of all living."

Eve as the 'mother of all living' hearkens back to the mother goddess. This again has a double meaning. In Hebrew the word Hawwa (Eve) means 'she who creates life', but in Aramaic it means 'serpent'. Of course Jewish folklore says that Eve is the tame woman in the piece, and that Adam's first wife was Lilith, who refused to lie under him in the submissive 'missionary position' and flew up into the heavens. Solomon is said to have tested Bilqis the Queen of Sheba to walk across a mirror in case her feet were hairy like Lilith's.

Then in an ultimate act of jealousy, Yahweh shuts them out of paradise lest they become 'as one of us' strangely again suggesting not one god but 'Elohim - a host:

Behold, the man is become as one of us, to know good and evil:
and now, lest he put forth his hand,
and take also of the tree of life, and eat, and live for ever:
So he drove out the man; and he placed at the east of the garden ...
a flaming sword which turned every way, to keep the way of the tree of life.

Central to the elaboration of this theme is the concept of the covenant between God and his 'chosen' people, a theme repeated with Noah, then Abraham and finally with Moses. Lerner (188) points out that the form of the covenant closely parallels Hittite royal pacts with a vassal subject from Nuzi. In each of these covenants there is a central male procreative purpose of promising seed as the stars in the sky and dust of the earth, in return for the sacrificial male sexual token of circumcision of the foreskin. The supposedly higher abstract aniconic 'god acting in history' is thus a god of patrimony, paternity certainty and pantriliny.

In a frightening turn around from the priestly vegetarian 'trees for meat' of Genesis 1, when God likes the smell of Noah's burned meat, we hear:

"And the fear of you and the dread of you shall be upon every beast of the earth, and upon every fowl of the air, upon all that moveth upon the earth, and upon all the fishes of the sea; into your hand are they delivered. Every moving thing that liveth shall be meat for you; even as the green herb have I given you all things" (Gen 9:1).

"The Two Conditions of the World" The primal division of reality imposed on the feminine through the culture of the jealous god.

Sacred Marriage and the Strange Woman

The jealousy, central to the manner of God acting in history, manifests in a directly sexual relationship - a 'marriage' between God and the people. In Judaism it is the marriage between YHVH as husband and Israel as unfaithful wife.

Proverbs contrasts the good wife to the 'strange woman' who is a seductress:

I have perfumed my bed with myrrh, aloes, and
cinnamon.
Come, let us take our fill of love until the morn-
ing:
let us solace ourselves with loves.
For the goodman is not at home, he is gone a
long journey: ...
Let not thine heart decline to her ways, go not

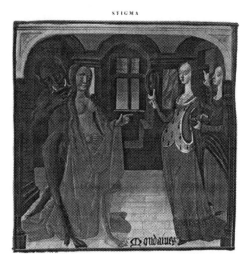

The Two Conditions of the World (anonymous, 15th Century).

astray in her paths.
For she hath cast down many wounded: yea, many strong men have been slain by her.
Her house is the way to hell, going down to the chambers of death (7).

The young virginal wife and the prudent wife, like Wisdom, are extolled:

Let thy fountain be blessed: and rejoice with the wife of thy youth.
Let her be as the loving hind and pleasant roe;
let her breasts satisfy thee at all times;
and be thou ravished always with her love (5).

House and riches are the inheritance of fathers: and a prudent wife is from the Lord (19).

By contrast, the 'strange woman' is 'abhorred' as the pits of Sheol:

And why wilt thou, my son, be ravished with a strange woman,
and embrace the bosom of a stranger? (5)

For the lips of a strange woman drop as an honeycomb, and her mouth is smoother than oil:
But her end is bitter as wormwood, sharp as a two-edged sword.
Her feet go down to death;
her steps take hold on hell (5).

To keep thee from the evil woman, from the flattery of the tongue of a strange woman.
Lust not after her beauty in thine heart; neither let her take thee with her eyelids.
For by means of a whorish woman a man is brought to a piece of bread: and the adulteress will hunt
for the precious life (6).

The strange woman poses in iconic form the reaction of Jewish patriarchal society to the prospect of a married woman having an affair with a younger man while her husband is away. This is not a professional prostitute but simply a wife who is not staying alone at home like the good woman should. The implication is that any reproductive freedom for the woman is equivalent to prostitution, while the male may have wives aplenty. Nehama Aschkenasy (1986) compares her to Eve "The first female became the prototype of all women and her story a paradigm of female existence."

Regina Schwartz (R616) in "The Curse of Cain" notes

"The laws collude with this metaphor of Israel as a subjugated and disobedient woman: in Lev 20:10 and Deut 22:22, both the man and the woman who engage in adultery must die; in Deut 22:20, a bride who cannot prove her virginity must be stoned to death. "Adultery in this larger context is understood not only as an aberration of personal behavior, but also as a social disorder with religious implications: adultery is a disturbance of the order of social relations established by God.' The "alien woman"-another man's wife-has forgotten the covenant of God (Prov 2:17), and the link between such faithlessness and landlessness is overt: Those who go to the foreign woman "delight in the perversities of the wicked whose paths are crooked" (Prov 2:14). ... For her house bows down to death, and her tracks to the departed. All going in to her do not return, nor do they reach the paths of life.... For the upright shall live (in) the land; and the perfect shall remain in it. But the wicked shall be cut off from the earth; and the transgressors shall be rooted up from it. (Prov 2:18) ...The biblical "alien woman" has been described succinctly: "she is an archetype of disorder at all levels of existence."

Just how lethal the jealousy against any 'whoring' or adulterous relationship of Israel with the gods of the nations was set out to be is stated in Deuteronomy. Here if people are found to be worshiping other gods or even secretly suggesting to do so, even if brother, son or daughter, wife or friend, they are condemned to summary personal and vigilante murder of religious freedom, which carries over directly to the Islamic death penalty for apostasy.

"Then shalt thou bring forth that man or that woman, which have committed that wicked thing, unto thy gates, and shalt stone them with stones, till they die. ... The hands of the witnesses shall be first upon him to put him to death, and afterward the hands of all the people. So thou shalt put the evil away from among you." (Deut 13.6, 17:2).

Shepherd Tribes in the Land of Milk and Honey

The origins of this highly dysfunctional 'divine' relationship of male jealousy and ultimate suspicion of the 'whoring' ways of the woman lie in the clash of cultures emerging from the Exodus. "In agricultural Canaan the Queen of Heaven eclipsed the male god. Adon, the Lord was the son of the Queen of Heaven, and a subordinate deity by her side. ... But to the more conservative elements among the Hebrew tribes those agricultural forms of the Semitic cult were an abomination.

"So completely had Yahweh become assimilated to him that not only were the two cults con-founded, the Jewish women celebrating the 'lamentations' for Tammuz in the national temple, but the very names had become inextricably blended; Yahweh was as often as not spoken of as 'The Lord', Adon", or Adonai .. also the Syrian Adonis, born from a tree" (Briffault R75v3 109).

"When the Hebrew tribes under the leadership of the votaries of the god of Sinai came out of the 'land of drought' into a land flowing with milk and honey of the Queen of Heaven, they found their own race there and their own religion but modified by the effects of agricultural civilization ... The Queen of Heaven, under whatever name,. she may have been worshipped - possibly Miriam, ... the high-priestess among the Levites, - belonged from time immemorial to Jewish cult ... The Host of Heaven - the very 'Elohim of the astral deities was a notable compo-nent of this worship. ... The temple of Jerusalem was simultaneously dedicated to Yahweh and the Queen of Heaven. Before it stood the asherah, symbolic trees that are throughout Semitic lands associated with the female aspect of the deity" (R75 110).

Looking back through the inverted telescope of multiple editorial redactions of the Old Testament, in the polarized climate of exile, and the ensuing apocalyptic revival of mono-theism under the patronage of the Zoroastrian Persian king Cyrus the Mede, it is hard for us to appreciate that the roots of Hebrew worship are far more diverse and syncretic than the monolithic monotheism of the Yahweh-only movement would suggest.

Tribal religion was a decentralized spiritual faith extending from the divided animals of Abraham's desert covenant, through the stones of Bethel and the oaks of Shechem and Mamre, to the canvassed tabernacles which preceded the centralized temple worship.

"In all places where I record my name I will come unto these and bless thee" (Ex 20:24).

During the Philistine dominance a series of conflicts and treaties ensued between the shep-herding settlements established in the drier hillier areas by the Israelites and Canaanite cit-ies. Joshua tells of genocidal battles at Hazor and Jericho in which all were slain by the command of God, but archaeology tells of a mix of local warfare and cultural intermin-gling.

In the time of the Judges, the power and respect of women was comparable to that of men:

"And Deborah, a prophetess, the wife of Lapidoth, she judged Israel at that time.
And she dwelt under the palm tree of Deborah between Ramah and Bethel in mount Ephraim:
and the children of Israel came up to her for judgment. (Judges 4:4)"

The Song of Deborah, one of the oldest passages in the Bible, illustrates the continuing strength of women even in times of conflict.

"Then sang Deborah and Barak the son of Abinoam on that day, saying, Praise ye the Lord for the avenging of Israel, when the people willingly offered themselves. ... Lord, when thou wentest out of Seir, when thou marchedst out of the field of Edom, the earth trembled, and the heavens dropped, the clouds also dropped water. The mountains melted from before the Lord, even that Sinai from before the Lord God of Israel. ... The inhabitants of the villages ceased, they ceased in Israel, until that I Deborah arose, that I arose a mother in Israel" (Judges 5:1).

There is a severe warning in Judges (19) that matrilineal patterns were giving way to a staunch patriliny. The concubine of Bethlehem-Judah is accused of 'whoring' by going back to live with her father-in-law for four months. When the Levite returned to claim her, the father-in-law kept saying to stay a little longer for six days, nigh on a week. When the couple left and turned in at Gibeath of the Benjaminites, men of Belial ask to 'know the man within'. In an attempt to avoid sodomy, the host offers his daughter to which they refuse. The Levite then offers his concubine. She is raped and abused all night and dies on the doorstep, while her master sleeps peacefully. He then cuts her in twelve pieces and sends them to all the coasts of Israel setting off the Benjaminite wars. These are finally resolved in moving four hundred virgins of Jabesh-Gilead to their husbands homes, capped by the abduction of the daughters of Shiloh dancing at a festival to satisfy the remaining Benjaminite men. As noted by David Bakan, the story is a glaring affront to those matriarchal traditions which expected the son-in-law to stay with the wife's family as Jacob did (Lerner R397 175).

The tale of the Daughter of Jephtath mingles human sacrifice, particularly in times of disaster with a tradition of goddess worship in the high places which lingered long after:

"Jephthah vowed unto the Lord 'If thou shalt deliver the children of Ammon into mine hands, what-soever cometh forth of the doors of my house, shall surely be the Lord's, and I will offer it up for a burnt offering.' So Jephthah passed over unto the children of Ammon to fight against them; and the Lord delivered them into his hands. ... And Jephthah came unto his house, and his daughter came out to meet him with timbrels and with dances: and she was his only child; And he rent his clothes, and said, 'Alas, my daughter! thou hast brought me very low, and thou art one of them that trouble me: for I have opened my mouth unto the Lord, and I cannot go back'. And she said unto him 'Let me alone two months, that I may go up and down upon the mountains, and bewail my virginity, I and my fellows'. And he sent her away for two months: and she went with her companions, and bewailed her virginity upon the mountains. At the end of two months, she returned unto her father, who did with her according to his vow: and she knew no man. And it was a custom in Israel, That the daughters of Israel went yearly to lament the daughter of Jephthah the Gileadite four days in a year" Judges (11:30).

Hebrew Kings and the Rape of the Sanctuaries

During the era of the Kings, a period of syncretic integration with the settled agricultural Canaanites of the cities began. This was probably a consequence both of the unification of the agrarian and nomadic populations under one rule, and the somewhat more cosmopoli-tan perspective of the monarchs. The Jewish kings followed the tradition of ancient fertil-ity kings. David danced before the Ark of the Covenant in the eyes of all the women to Michal's bane and disgust. Sacred kingship is evidenced again in the termination of the aged David's reign when he is unable to consort with Abishag. It is Bathsheba, who at this point entreaties the king, ensuring the succession to her own son Solomon, the son she conceived with David, as the wife of Uriah the Hittite, David's general, whom David arranged to be killed in battle. David's son Absalom had already attempted to usurp the throne by going "unto his father's concubines in the sight of all Israel". Absalom was hung in a tree in an *aition* of ritual sacrifice of the sacred king accursed, as Jesus was:

" And if a man have committed a sin worthy of death, and he be to be put to death, and thou hang him on a tree His body shall not remain all night upon the tree, but thou shalt in any wise bury him that day; (for he that is hanged is accursed of God;) that thy land be not defiled, which the Lord thy God giveth thee for an inheritance." (Deut 21:22),

Solomon, was also a sacred king who was renowned for building the Temple at Jerusalem, but equally reviled for also following the deities of his many wives and building sanctuar-ies to them on the high places round Jerusalem (1 Kings 11:8).

And likewise did he for all his strange wives, which burnt incense and sacrificed unto their gods.

Briffault notes: "The temple of Jerusalem was simultaneously dedicated to Yahweh and to the Queen of Heaven. The pillars Jachim and Boaz were said to stand for the sun and moon. Before it stood the Asherah".

The son of Solomon, went further and moved the image of the goddess into the Temple itself. In Samaria, Jeroboam installed golden calves at Bethel and Dan. Afterwards there was a partial removal of the idols, but it did not extend to the high sanctuaries. Ahaz again returned the equilibrium to the syncretic worship of the nations:

"and made his son to pass through the fire, according to the abominations of the heathen, whom the Lord cast out from before the children of Israel. And he sacrificed and burnt incense in the high places, and on the hills, and under every green tree."

At Gezeh remains of sacrificed cows and bulls are found consistent with worship of Yaho and Hathor (Briffault R75v3 110). At Kuntillet in the 8th century BC Yhwh gives a bless-ing with his Asherah, identified with Canaanite Athirat (McCarter R441 143,Maier R421). Among the Jews of Elephantine as late as the fifth century B.C., Yahweh was associated with his consort. The names of the Elohim were joined, as Anath-Yahu (Kraeling R381 88).

The worship of the Queen of Heaven continued alongside that of Yahweh through the time of the Kings until the fall of the Kingdom of Israel to the Assyrians. The colonization of Samaria was perceived by the more conservative Judaeans as a sign that the ways of toler-ance of the Northern Kingdom had led to disaster. Thus in about 720 Hezekiah led a fun-damentalist revision: (2 Kings 18:4):

"He removed the high places, and brake the images, and cut down the groves [asherah],

and brake in pieces the brasen serpent that Moses had made:
for unto those days the children of Israel did burn incense to it: and he called it Nehushtan".

However Jeremiah 44:16 notes the continuing popularity of the Queen in Jerusalem:

"As for the word thou hast unto us in the name of the Lord, we will not harken unto thee. But we will certainly do whatever thing goeth forth out of our own mouth, to burn incense unto the Queen of Heaven, and to pour out drink offerings unto her, as we have done, we and our fathers, our kings and our princes, in the cities of Judah, and in the streets of Jerusalem: for then we had plenty of victuals, and were well, and saw no evil. But since we left off to burn incense to the Queen of Heaven, and poured out drink offerings to her, we have wanted all things, and have been consumed by the sword, and by the famine. And when we burned incense to the Queen of Heaven and poured out drink offerings to her, did we alone make her cakes or worship her ... without our men folk?"

His passage in 7:15 is prophetic of what is to come.

"Seest thou not what they do in the cities of Judah and in the streets of Jerusalem? The children gather wood, and the fathers kindle the fire, and the women knead their dough, to make cakes to the queen of heaven, and to pour out drink offerings unto other gods, that they may provoke me to anger. Do they provoke me to anger? saith the Lord: do they not provoke themselves to the confusion of their own faces? Therefore thus saith the Lord God; Behold, mine anger and my fury shall be poured out upon this place, upon man, and upon beast, and upon the trees of the field, and upon the fruit of the ground; and it shall burn, and shall not be quenched."

However again Manasseh brought the pendulum back and built up again the high places which Hezekiah his father had destroyed; and he reared up altars for Ba'al, and made a grove (Asherah), as did Ahab king of Israel; and worshipped all the host of heaven, and served them. And he made his son pass through the fire, and observed times, and used enchantments, and dealt with familiar spirits and wizards: he wrought much wickedness in the sight of the Lord, to provoke him to anger. And he set a graven image of the grove that he had made in the house, of which the Lord said ... will I put my name for ever".

But in 622 Hilkiah persuaded young King Josiah that a "hidden" text in the temple (Deuteronomy) revealed the "true faith" of the "Yahweh only" movement. This is arguably the point where 'no other gods before me' became strict monotheism - no other gods at all. Much of the Old Testament has been subsequently recomposed to portray the earlier history as monotheistic. What is very significant is that a prophetess is made responsible for the judgement:

"And Hilkiah the high priest said unto Shaphan the scribe, I have found the book of the law in the house of the Lord ... and Shaphan the scribe ... read it before the king. And ... when the king had heard the words of the book of the law, that he rent his clothes. And ... commanded ... 'Go ye, enquire of the Lord for me, and for the people, and for all Judah, concerning the words of this book that is found: for great is the wrath of the Lord that is kindled against us, because our fathers have not hearkened unto the words of this book' ... So Hilkiah the priest, and Ahikam, and Achbor, and Shaphan, and Asahiah, went unto Huldah the prophetess, wife of Shallum, keeper of the wardrobe; in Jerusalem in the college; and communed with her. And she said ... 'Tell the man that sent you to me 'Thus saith the Lord, Behold, I will bring evil upon this place, and upon the inhabitants thereof, even all the words of the book which the king of Judah hath read Because they have forsaken me, and have burned incense unto other gods, that they might provoke me to anger with all the works of their hands; therefore my wrath shall be kindled against this place, and shall not be quenched" (2 Kings 22:8).

In both Kings and Chronicles we find parallel accounts of the 'rape of the sanctuaries':

"[Josiah] began to purge Judah and Jerusalem from the high places, and the groves, and the carved images, and the molten images. And they brake down the altars of Baalim in his presence; and the images, that were on high above them, he cut down; and the groves, and the carved images, and the molten images, he brake in pieces, and made dust of them, and strowed it upon the graves of them that had sacrificed unto them. And he burnt the bones of the priests upon their altars" (2 Chron 34 4-5).

And he brought out the grove (asherah) from the house of the Lord, without Jerusalem, unto the brook Kidron, and burned it and stamped it small to powder, and cast the powder thereof upon the graves of the children of the people. And he brake down the pavillions of the effeminate, which were in the house of the Lord, where the women wove hangings for the grove (2 Kings 23 3).

So we have one of the most outstanding examples in history of a self-fulfilling prophecy, for Josiah was simply carrying out the instructions 'found' so conveniently in the temple:

"These are the statutes and judgements ... Ye shall utterly destroy all the places wherein the nations which ye possessed served their gods, upon the mountain and on the high hills and under every

green tree. And ye shall overthrow their alters and break their pillars and burn their groves with fire ... But unto the place which the Lord your God shall choose out of all your tribes ... thither thou shalt come. ... Take heed of thyself that thou offer not thy burnt offerings in every place that thou seest, but in the place the Lord shall choose in any one of thy tribes" (Deut 12:1).

Not only were the Ba'al destroyed, but so was the Asherah or grove, Yahweh's own consort. Instead of the diverse natural forms of Yahweh worship, there was only one legitimate form and one place of worship - the Temple at Jerusalem. This Yahweh-only tract has thus established Judaism in the ending of the Hebrew practice of small shrines and tabernacles dotted throughout the towns and countryside from time immemorial. Just as Marduk slew Tiamat, so the Yahweh-only movement slew the Asherah of fertility.

This coup is echoed in Exodus (34:13) with undertones of seduction of the sons of Israel:

"But ye shall destroy their altars, break their images, and cut down their groves: For thou shalt worship no other god: for the Lord, whose name is Jealous, is a jealous God: Lest thou make a covenant with the inhabitants of the land, and they go a whoring after their gods, and do sacrifice unto their gods, and one call thee, and thou eat of his sacrifice; And thou take of their daughters unto thy sons, and their daughters go a whoring after their gods, and make thy sons go a whoring after their gods".

Although this would sound like the sad end of the story for the Queen of Heaven, it was only to be some 36 years later that Jerusalem fell to the Babylonians and despite these attempts to expunge the weakness of whoring with the nations, the entire country was returned to being the vassal of a pagan civilization. Edom had continued to worship the Goddess and her consort, particularly in the high places such as Khirbet Tannur . With the emergence of the Nabateans, a whole stream of worship of the Queen of Heaven and her consort Duchares rose again to prominence to the east of the Jordan (Browning R91, Glueck R242).

Hosea's Plight and Jeremiah's Lament

This relationship, with a sexually jealous God, the ultimate alpha male at the head of the table of the gods, continues through the Old Testament, in repeated diatribes against whoring and harlots:

"And they shall burn thine houses with fire, and execute judgments upon thee in the sight of many women: and I will cause thee to cease from playing the harlot, and thou also shalt give no hire any more. So will I make my fury toward thee to rest, and my jealousy shall depart from thee, and I will be quiet." (Ezekiel 16:41)

Hosea in the eighth century BC took it upon himself to purchase an unfaithful wife, who thus represented the archetype of Israel, the unfaithful wife of Yahweh. "Then said the Lord unto me, Go yet, love a woman beloved of her friend, yet an adulteress, according to the love of the Lord toward the children of Israel, who look to other gods, and love flagons of wine. So I bought her to me for fifteen pieces of silver, and for an homer of barley, and an half homer of barley" (3:1).

He is clearly siding against the whoring of the Goddess which acts to disrupt the male inheritance lines of the patriarchal supporters of Yahweh:

"Plead with your mother, plead: for she is not my wife, neither am I her husband: let her therefore put away her whoredoms out of her sight, and her adulteries from between her breasts; Lest I strip her naked, and set her as in the day that she was born, and make her as a wilderness, and set her like a dry land, and slay her with thirst. And I will not have mercy upon her children; for they be the children of whoredoms. For their mother hath played the harlot: she that conceived them hath done shamefully: for she said, I will go after my lovers, that give me my bread and my water, my wool and my flax, mine oil and my drink. Therefore, behold, I will hedge up thy way with thorns, and make a wall, that she shall not find her paths" (2:2).

Regina Schwartz (R616) highlights the relation between pollution of the land and the image of the whore:

"In the Book of Hosea, two completely contradictory images of Israel's relation to the land are elaborated. The land is depicted as both a prostitute and a wilderness: as a prostitute, because Israel worships foreign gods; as a wilderness, to reflect the nomadic ideal of wandering over land, rather than owning it. Both metaphors depict a margin-a social one in which a woman is not an exclusive possession and a territorial one in which land is outside the boundaries of possession. One image is reviled the land as a prostitute violates the contract that Israel is the

exclusive possession of Yahweh-while one is celebrated-the land as a wilderness depicts a nostalgic return to the birth of Israel. Born in the wilderness, the hope is that Israel will be reborn there. But we cannot plausibly read Hosea as a ringing endorsement of an unlanded ideal, for in the end, the period in the wilderness is cast as an interim, a precondition to reentering the cultivated land-the owned land-and when the woman is sent into the wilderness, it is hardly to acknowledge that she is not an object of possession. Instead, it is to purge her so that she can be more completely possessed".

> *That is why I am going to lure her*
> *and bring her out into the wilderness*
> *and speak to her heart.*
> *I am going to give her back her vineyards,*
> *and make the polluted valley a gateway of hope."*
> *Then she will answer there, as in the days of her youth, and as*
> *the day when she came up out of the land of Egypt.*
> *I will betroth you to me for ever.*
> *Yes, I will betroth you with righteousness and in judgment,*
> *with mercy and in compassion;*
> *and I will betroth you to me in faithfulness,*
> *and you shall know Yahweh.*
> *And it shall be in that day-it is Yahweh who speaks-I will answer.*
> *I will answer the heavens and they shall answer the earth,*
> *and the earth shall answer the grain, the wine, and the oil,*
> *and they shall answer jezreel.*
> *I will sow her in the earth, I will love Unloved;*
> *I will say to No-People-of-Mine, "You are my people,"*
> *and he will answer, "You are my God." (Hos 2:14-23)*

Hosea (4:9) further laments the wine and whoredom of the high places and the good shade of the sacred groves:

> *"and I will punish them for their ways, and reward them their doings. For they shall eat, and not have enough: they shall commit whoredom and not increase: because they have left of to take heed of the Lord. Whoredom and wine and new wine take away the heart. My people ask counsel to their stocks ... and they have gone a whoring from under their god. They sacrifice upon the mountain tops, and burn incense upon the hills, under oaks and poplars and elms, because the shadow thereof is good: therefore your daughters shall commit whoredom and your spouses shall commit adultery. "*

Yet he has Yahweh yet be tolerant for a time, in a way which later becomes lost:

> *"I will not punish your daughters when they commit whoredom, nor your spouses when they commit adultery: for themselves are separated with whores, and they sacrifice with harlots: therefore the people that doth not understand shall fall" (4:14).*

Jeremiah likewise laments Israel as the unfaithful wife:

> *"Moreover the word of the Lord came to me, saying, Go and cry in the ears of Jerusalem, saying, Thus saith the Lord; I remember thee, the kindness of thy youth, the love of thine espousals, when thou wentest after me in the wilderness, in a land that was not sown" (2:1).*

> *"They say, If a man put away his wife, and she go from him, and become another man's, shall he return unto her again? shall not that land be greatly polluted? but thou hast played the harlot with many lovers; yet return again to me, saith the Lord" (3:1).*

Jeremiah makes a more specifically social warning of vengeance:

> *"And I saw, when for all the causes whereby backsliding Israel committed adultery I had put her away, and given her a bill of divorce; yet her treacherous sister Judah feared not, but went and played the harlot also. And it came to pass through the lightness of her whoredom, that she defiled the land, and committed adultery with stones and with stocks. ... Return, thou backsliding Israel, saith the Lord; and I will not keep anger for ever" (3:8).*

Schwartz (R616) notes the frenzy of 'sexual pollution':

> "The link between sexuality and land pollution reaches a frenzied pitch in the obsession with that most heinous of offenses, prostitution: "Do not profane your daughter by making her a prostitute; thus, the land will not be prostituted and rifled with incest" (Lev 19:29). A body/land analogy governs the rhetoric that describes women and land as possessions (of one man/deity), women and land as faithful or idolatrous, women and land as monogamous or adulterous, women and land as fertile or barren. But women and land are not only analogous; they become causes and effects in this system of monotheism/monogamy. When Israel worships a foreign deity, she is a harlot, the land is made barren, and she is ejected from the land."

She then quotes in Jeremiah (3:2) a fascinating slant on bedouin life of the times, echoing through to the Nabatea of Yeshua's times:

*"Lift up thine eyes unto the high places, and see where thou hast not been lien with.
In the ways hast thou sat for them, as the Arabian in the wilderness;
and thou hast polluted the land with thy whoredoms and with thy wickedness."*

The second Isaiah (50:1) echoes this theme again:

*"Thus saith the Lord, Where is the bill of your mother's divorcement, whom I have put away? or
which of my creditors is it to whom I have sold you? Behold, for your iniquities have ye sold yourselves, and for your transgressions is your mother put away".*

Separatist Sentiments of the Exile

The exile brought with it a new sense of alienation and separation, as is characteristic if a
small people in another culture adopt exclusive ways to protect their separateness and
maintain it against the greater flux of 'foreign' ideas and genetic influences. Effectively the
exile thus cemented what was to become the separatist path.

Ezekiel (8:1) writing during the exile laments at the things he suspects are going on back
home in the temple:

*"And I beheld and lo a likeness as the appearance of fire; from the appearance of his loins even
downward fire; and from his loins even upward as the appearance of brightness, as the colour of
amber. And behold the glory of the god of Israel was there. Then I lifted my eyes ... and behold at the
gate of the altar was the image of jealousy. Son of man seest thou what they do? even the great
abominations that the house of Israel do here that I should go far from my sanctuary? In the temple
"he saw every form of creeping things and abominable beasts and the idols of the house of Israel
portrayed on the wall round about... and there stood before them seventy men of the ancients... and a
thick cloud of incense went up. At the north door 'there sat women weeping for Tammuz' ... and in
between the porch and the altar 'five and twenty men with their backs toward the temple facing the
east and they worshipped the sun ... Therefore shall I deal in fury : mine eye shall not spare, neither
will I have pity."*

His prescription is an elaboration of Deuteronomy:

*"Then shall thee know that I am the Lord when their slain men shall be among their idols round
their altars, upon every high hill, in the tops of the mountains, and under every green tree and under
every thick oak, , the place where they did offer sweet savour to their idols." (Exek 7:13).*

Schwartz (R616) has cutting comment:

"Ezekiel 16, the extended allegory of Israel as a whore, brings the relation between whores,
exile, and monotheism (adultery, defiled land, and idolatry) into sharp focus. It is the story of a
child being born and growing up wild and unloved in the field, and when she matures into
puberty, of her being owned, sexually and materially, by Yahweh."

*"And I passed by you and I looked on you and behold, your time was the time of love. And I spread
my skirt over you and I covered your nakedness. And I swore to you and I entered into a covenant
with you and you became Mine. She is now washed, anointed, dressed, wrapped, covered, and
adorned with silks, fine linen, embroidery, gold, and silver. And you were very beautiful and you
advanced to regal estate. And your name went out among the nations, because of your beauty; for it
was perfect, by My Splendor which I had set on you."*

"But then young Israel commits adultery with the nations: with Egypt, Assyria, Canaan,
Chaldea - with, not incidentally, all of Israel's enemies".

*"At every head of the highway you have built your high place and have made your beauty despised,
and have parted your feet to all who passed by, and have multiplied your fornications. You have
whored with the sons of Egypt. . . . You have whored with the sons of Assyria without being satisfied.
You have multiplied your fornication in the land of Canaan."*

"But this adulteress has not, strictly speaking, been a harlot, for she has not taken wages;
instead, she has done all the giving, even paying her lovers for their services. "The adulterous
wife: instead of her husband, she takes strangers. They give a gift to an harlots, but you give
your gifts to all your lovers, and bribe them to come to you from all around, for your fornication." Presumably, Israel the harlot would be superior to Israel the adulteress, for she would
receive property instead of giving her property away, and that careful distinction offers a clue
that, throughout this harangue against the adulteress, the issue is less sexual morality than
ownership of property. The emphasis on property is underscored by the punishment of the
adulteress. She will be stripped of her garments, of her wealth; Israel win be stripped naked
and then brutally stoned and stabbed"

*"Because your lewdness was poured out and your nakedness was bared, in your fornications with
your lovers and the idols of your abominations ... therefore I will gather all your lovers with whom
you have been pleased, even all whom you have loved with all whom you have hated, and I will
uncover your nakedness to them, and they will see all your nakedness. ... They shall also strip you of*

your clothes and shall take your beautiful things and leave you naked and bare ... and they shall stone you with stones and cut you with their swords."

Schwartz sums up the situation: "Monotheism, then, is not simply a myth of one-ness, but a doctrine of possession, of a people by God, of a land by a people, of women by men".

I will give them a different heart so that they will always fear me. ... I will make an everlasting covenant with them; I will not cease in my efforts for their good, and I will put respect for me into their hearts, so that they turn from me no more. (Jer 32:39)

Ezekiel continues in this vein concerning cultural pollution *(20:27):*

"Your fathers have blasphemed me ... For when I had brought them into the land, for the which I lifted up mine hand to give it to them, then they saw every high hill and all the thick trees, and they offered there their sacrifices, and there they presented the provocation of their offering; there they made also their sweet savour and poured out their drink offerings... Wherefore say unto the house of Israel Are ye polluted after the manner of your fathers? and commit ye whoredom after their abominations?"

Later in chapter 23 he relates the downfall of such women:

"there were two women, the daughters of one mother [Aholah of Samaria and Aholibah of Jerusalem]: and they committed whoredoms in Egypt; they committed whoredoms in their youth: there were their breasts pressed and they bruised the teats of their virginity ... and poured their whoredom on her ... And Aholah played the harlot when she was mine; and she doted on her lovers, the assyrians and her neighbours, which were clothed with blue ... with all their idols she defiled herself, neither she left her whoredoms brought from Egypt ... And Aholibah sent messages unto them in Chaldea ... and the Babylonians came to her in the bed of love... therefore I will bring [thy lovers] against thee on every side ... because thou hast gone a whoring after the heathen and because thou art polluted with their idols... and with the men of a common sort were brought Sabeans from the wilderness, which put bracelets on their hands, and beautiful crowns on their heads ... and so they went in" (23).

Israel After the Rains

When the Jews returned from the exile they were dismayed to find those who had stayed in the Holy Land had reverted to their old ways and intermarried with Canaanite wives. Those returning disregarded the cultural accommodation of their compatriots and unilaterally imposed their own form of exilic separatism on Israel. Nevertheless the urban population was not so easily to be suppressed and invectives by Nehemiah indicate the post-exilic reforms were slow to take effect. But Ezra arrived in 397 BC and, in the pouring rain, delivered a diatribe that every man should sever his ties of love and marriage with the Canaanite women. At the same time the old Hebrew script was ironically replaced by Aramaic.

"There follows in this tenth and final chapter of Ezra a mass divorce and expulsion of children. Scores of Jewish man are listed by name, each of whom had married a non-Jewish woman and in some cases had children by her. All of these women and children are driven out" (Miles (379):

"Then all the men of Judah and Benjamin gathered themselves together unto Jerusalem within three days. It was the ninth month, on the twentieth day of the month; and all the people sat in the street of the house of God, trembling because of this matter, and for the great rain. And Ezra the priest stood up, and said unto them, Ye have transgressed, and have taken strange wives, to increase the trespass of Israel. Now therefore make confession unto the Lord God of your fathers, and do his pleasure: and separate yourselves from the people of the land, and from the strange wives. Then all the congregation answered and said with a loud voice, As thou hast said, so must we do" (10:9)

Tobit 4:12 declares "take first a wife of the seed of thy fathers, and take not a strange wife which is not of thy father's tribe: for we are all sons of the prophets". The Testaments of the Twelve Patriarchs echoes this "take therefore thyself a wife without blemish or pollution, while yet thou art young and not of the race of strange nations". The Book of Jubilees goes so far as to invoke death by stoning for an Israelite who would give his daughter or sister to a Gentile, and the woman is to be burned to death, indicating the conservative position of the Essenes in the face of Greek influence in Jerusalem. However the Testament of the Twelve Patriarchs in the first century BC concedes a stem from which "shall grow a rod of righteousness to the Gentile to judge and save all that call upon the Lord".

The Son of the Father and the Women of Galilee

There is a very strong streak of sacrificial violence merged into the concept of atonement - both the union of at-one-ment and a terrible penalty that has to be paid to God for the error of the people's ways, which is expressed in multiple places, from Psalm 22, to the 'just man' who is killed out of jealousy in Wisdom of Solomon 2:12-20 (p 227). The 'suffering servant' of Isaiah and the 'foolish shepherd' of Zechariah set the tone of the rejected messenger of doom whom the people reject or kill, only to find to their remorse he was their savior. Zechariah spoke of a final struggle against false ways surrounding the temple of Jerusalem, in a military and cosmic confrontation, splitting apart the entire world as then known.

Later traditions of Judaism became infused with such apocalyptic thought, emerging from the Zoroastrian cosmic renovation in a final struggle between dark and light. While in Persian thought this was a cleansing struggle between clarity and ignorance, in the Jewish apocalyptic context, it became a struggle between divine and malign forces of Belial, Prince of Darkness personified in Essene terms in the Wicked Priest. In the visions of the desert seers or *nabis*, such as Jokanaan (John the Baptist R651), it became a cosmic struggle between God and Satan, who was originally a tester of commitment to God, but had now become a dark force, into which the messianic hope was launched as a cosmic quest (Cohn R125, Pagels R513).

Jokanaan's beheading takes place in a highly provocative sexual context. The lands of Edom and Moab had coalesced into the Kingdom of Nabatea, centered on Petra, a high peak of Arabic culture, based on irrigation, whose citizens worshipped the fertility goddess by various names, including al-Lat (goddess), Manat (fate), and al-Uzza (powerful) with her Dionysian(R510) consort Dhu Shara (R242) in the high places. Relative equality between female and male power was expressed in their coinage in the joint kingship and queenship of Aretas IV and Shaqilat II (p 221).

Salome - Beardsley (Wilde)

Herod Antipas had deserted his marriage to the Nabatean princess in favour of his cousin Herodias, who was his brother, Philip's wife. The princess took flight, fearing Herod would kill her and the Nabateans had in response declared war on Herod. Jokanaan then accused Herod and Herodias of adultery, and was imprisoned in the castle Machaerus on the Nabatean border, where Herod and his generals were holding a war cabinet (R341). Thus begins the tale of Salome dancing what is presumed to have been the dance of the seven veils of Inanna's descent before the men for which Herod offered her half his kingdom in a clear reference to the descent, echoed in Esther 5:3 in claiming Haman's head:

"When the daughter of Herodias came in, and danced, and pleased Herod and them that sat with him, the king said unto the damsel, Ask of me whatsoever thou wilt, and I will give it thee. And he sware Whatsoever thou shalt ask of me, I will give it thee, unto the half of my kingdom. And she went forth, and said unto her mother, What shall I ask? And she said, The head of John the Baptist." (Mark 6:22).

Jokanaan is thus killed as the substitute sacred king in the male sacrifice of Inanna's descent. Jokanaan's challenge and death signify the very arrow of cultural, religious and gender conflict. In Luke, Jokanaan talks in apocalyptic terms, using images of Tammuz and Ba'al:

"Whose [winnowing] fan is in his hand, he will thoroughly purge his floor, and will gather the wheat into his garner; but the chaff he will burn with fire unquenchable."

Yeshua (Jesus) brilliantly encompassed this confused cultural tradition of jealousy and endeavoured to unite the apocalyptic and fertility traditions in one renewal as a hybrid lord Adonai and mashiach. We explore his 'persona', as diversely described in orthodox and gnostic texts, the Talmud, and by historians. Upon his baptism by Jokanaan, the holy spirit descended on him in the form of (Aphrodite's) dove. He became the 'bridegroom' - the nominal consort of the sacred marriage, cryptically referred to in Isaiah 61, the unique 'black verses of god-anointing' which he read in liberation in the synagogue at Nazareth:

The Spirit of the Lord God is upon me; because the Lord hath anointed me ... to proclaim liberty to the captives, and the opening of the prison to them that are bound ... as a bridegroom decketh himself with ornaments, and as a bride adorneth herself with her jewels. ... as a garden causes the things that are sewn in it to spring forth (Is 61)

Jesus now turns the tables, claiming the destiny of the prophets was to heal gentiles:

"But unto none of them was Elias [Elijah] sent, save unto Sarepta, a city of Sidon, unto a woman that was a widow .And many lepers were in Israel in the time of Eliseus [Elisha] the prophet; and none of them was cleansed, saving Naaman the Syrian".

For his challenge to the role of the 'elect' in espousing the 'lost sheep of Israel', Yeshua was nearly cast off the cliffs of Nazareth but passed through the angry crowd. The term 'messiah' comes from the Hebrew *mashiach*, meaning 'anointed one', as does 'christ'. The only places in the Bible where anointing occurs are those of priests anointing kings. Central to the anomaly of Yeshua is that he cited Isaiah 61 'blasphemously' and was anointed by a woman.

This set the stage for a mission of consorting, controversy, chaos and miraculous dread, from his mother's request to turn water into wine at the wedding at Cana on the day of the festival of Dionysus' epiphany (Ranke-Heinemann 1992) to the walking on water at Galilee.

And new wine is not put into old wineskins, lest they burst; nor is old wine put into a new wineskin, lest it spoil it. (Thomas 47)

As the 'true vine' Yeshua espoused the ultimate fertility parable of the mustard seed:

"I am the true vine, and my Father is the husbandman" (John 15:1).
"Tell us what the kingdom of heaven is like." "It is like a mustard seed. It is the smallest of all seeds. But when it falls on tilled soil, it produces a great plant and becomes a shelter for birds of the sky." (Thomas 20)

Dionysian (Dhu Shara) tragic mask with dolphins . Khirbet Tannur. Aretas IV and Shaqilat II share Nabatean coinage as partners (Glueck R242).

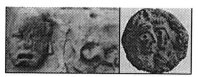

This tradition of miraculous dread and chaos messiahship, whipping up controversy and committing frank blasphemy in breaking traditional taboos, is in no way a fulfillment of traditional ideas of the Jewish messiah. It falls into the orbit of Dhu Shara, Lord of Seir as mentioned in Genesis (33.14): "until I come unto my lord unto Seir", the Dionysian 'God of Gaia' of the vineyards of Edomite Nabatea . Their orgiastic festivals (Browning R91 47), involved "Rich food in plenty and strong wine without stint" (Glueck R242 166). Bar-Hebraeus quoted Psalm 12:8 of Nabatean women: "the wicked walk on every side while vileness is exalted among the sons of men." One can only surmise that Yeshua was attempting a cultural synthesis of all the religious currents in the greater Israelite backdrop, including a considerable degree of popular fertility worship, particularly among the women of the countryside, an aspect of the 'lost sheep of Israel'. Graves (R253) notes the Talmud babli Sanhedrin called Yeshua or Yeshu-ha-Notzri "Balaam the Lame", claiming he came from the wicked kingdom of Edom. Graves suggests Yeshua was lamed in the manner of sacred kings (Graves R254), echoed in Luke's "physician heal thyself".

His miraculous reputation was however ephemeral and inversely related to familiarity, as is evidenced by his marginal performance in his home town of Nazareth:

"A prophet is not without honour, but in his own country, and among his own kin, and in his own house. And he could there do no mighty work, save that he laid his hands upon a few sick folk, and healed them" (Mark 6:4).

Such chaos messiahship extended from sending the hapless herd of pigs to their doom in the name of casting out spirits and a performance of feeding the five thousand morsels of loaves as communion wafers, capped by such apocalyptic blasphemy that many disciples deserted:

"Verily, verily, I say unto you, Except ye eat the flesh of the Son of man, and drink his blood, ye have no life in you." (John 6:52).

"From that time many of his disciples went back, and walked no more with him" (6:56).

Yeshua restated central Jewish ethics, reversing Hillel's "Do not do to others what you would not have them do to you" quoted when he was asked to recite the Torah standing on one foot, into the affirmative "Do to others what you would they should do to you" (Matt 7:12). Both are significant moral advances on 'tit for tat' or 'an eye for an eye' in the prisoners' dilemma, because they are educative of good intent. Hillel stresses non-defection and non-violence but risks non-involvement; Yeshua asserts cooperation, risking coercion.

Yeshua took this further into a naked altruism, going far beyond mutuality, or reciprocation, setting a 'standard' of almost sacrificial giving to the defector in the face of evolutionary and social survival, which only God, or those taking a quick exit, can really 'afford':

Ye have heard that it hath been said, An eye for an eye, and a tooth for a tooth: But I say unto you, That ye resist not evil: but whosoever shall smite thee on thy right cheek, turn to him the other also. (Matt 5:38)

'Always cooperate' is one of the most rapidly eliminated strategies. The evolutionary value of love is its capacity to unite in a win-win of good will and empathy that goes far beyond the boundaries of kin and 'self-serving' reciprocation, so embracing selfless love is a high ethical ideal, conducive to loving cooperation. But is every form of love which is sensitive to, or conditional on, a loving response simply to be equated with the divisiveness of sin?

"Love your enemies, do good to them which hate you, Bless them that curse you, and pray for them which despitefully use you. And unto him that smiteth thee on the one cheek offer also the other; ... For if ye love them which love you, what thank have ye? for sinners also love those that love them. And if ye do good to them which do good to you, what thank have ye? for sinners also do even the same. And if ye lend to them of whom ye hope to receive, what thank have ye? ... But love ye your enemies, and do good, and lend, hoping for nothing again; and your reward shall be great, and ye shall be the children of the Highest: for he is kind unto the unthankful and to the evil. Be ye therefore merciful, as your Father also is merciful. Judge not, and ye shall not be judged: condemn not, and ye shall not be condemned: forgive, and ye shall be forgiven: Give, and it shall be given unto you" (Luke 6:27).

In Isaiah 61, we hear jubilaic mention of both the bridegroom and the bride, but during Yeshua's mission the bridegroom has assumed a lone role as an apocalyptic sacred king:

"And Jesus said unto them, Can the children of the bridechamber fast, while the bridegroom is with them? as long as they have the bridegroom with them, they cannot fast. But the days will come, when the bridegroom shall be taken away from them, and then shall they fast in those days" (Mark 2:19)

Several passages in the Gospel of Thomas continue this trend:

"Many are standing at the door, but it is the solitary who will enter the bridal chamber." (75)

They said to Jesus, "Come, let us pray today and let us fast." Jesus said, "What is the sin that I have committed, or wherein have been defeated?" But when the bridegroom leaves "the bridal chamber, then let them fast and pray." (104)

In John, Jokanaan in a later Christian construction, 'prophesies' a sacred marriage:

"Ye yourselves bear me witness, that I said, I am not the Christ, but that I am sent before him. He that hath the bride is the bridegroom: but the friend of the bridegroom, which standeth and heareth him, rejoiceth greatly because of the bridegroom's voice: this my joy therefore is fulfilled." (3:28)

The real support for Yeshua's mission and the disciples came always from the women:

"and the twelve were with him, And certain women, which had been healed of evil spirits and infirmities, Mary called Magdalene, out of whom went seven devils, and Joanna the wife of Chuza Herod's steward, and Susanna, and many others, which ministered unto him of their substance" (Luke 8:1).

The Greek version's 'them' infers the 12 were supported by the women (WalkerR708).

Magdalen's 'seven devils' hark directly to the seven galla of Inanna and the descent and link her allegorically to the role of the 'sinner' as 'sacred whore'.

Although Yeshua's sexual life remains enigmatic, he is said to have "loved Mary and her sister Martha". His role with Mary suggests the sacred union, although it is the Descent:

"Martha, Martha, thou art careful and troubled about many things: But one thing is needful: and Mary hath chosen that good part, which shall not be taken away from her" (Luke 10:41).

He is implicated in the *hieros gamos* with Salome in the Gospel of Thomas (Robinson):

"Jesus said, 'Two will rest on a bed: the one will die, and the other will live.' Salome said, 'Who are you, man, that you ... have come up on my couch and eaten from my table?' Jesus said to her, 'I am he who exists from the undivided'. ... 'Therefore I say, if he is destroyed he will be filled with light, but if he is divided, he will be filled with darkness'." (61)

This suggests he is claiming to speak from the 'whole' condition before Adam and Eve became twain, and is a key part of his attitude to marriage, which has steered Christianity and Western culture in the direction of monogamy ever since.

But from the beginning of the creation God made them male and female. For this cause shall a man leave his father and mother, and cleave to his wife; And they twain shall be one flesh: so then they are no more twain, but one flesh. What therefore God hath joined together, let not man put asunder (Mark 10:6).

Ye have heard that it was said by them of old time, Thou shalt not commit adultery: But I say unto you, That whosoever looketh on a woman to lust after her hath committed adultery with her already in his heart (Matt 5:27).

But I say unto you, That whosoever shall put away his wife, saving for the cause of fornication, causeth her to commit adultery: and whosoever shall marry her that is divorced committeth adultery (Luke 16:18, Matt 5:32).

Jesus then refers to 'eunuchs for heaven' in a way which caused Origen and some cult followers to castrate themselves, but Uta Ranke-Heinemann (R551 23) has pointed out this was not about intercourse, but remarriage - men curtailing their polygynous tendencies.

"His disciples say unto him, If the case of the man be so with his wife, it is not good to marry. But he said unto them, All men cannot receive this saying, save they to whom it is given. For there are some eunuchs, which were so born from their mother's womb: and there are some eunuchs, which were made eunuchs of men: and there be eunuchs, which have made themselves eunuchs for the kingdom of heaven's sake. He that is able to receive it, let him receive it." (Matt 19:10).

This is a far cry from the delightful invocation to be ravished by the breasts of the young wife in Proverbs, which is positively sexual in the Jewish fertility tradition, although condemning the strange woman's equally enticing ways. Here sexuality has become confined and negative outside the invocation to cleave to one's wife as one flesh. Sexual pleasure is denied. Even to appreciate a woman sexually is evil. Remarriage after divorce has become adulterous and the emphasis, even if it is not on physical castration, is on psychic castration. While physical divorce is banned, we now have a divorce between sexual pleasure and god-ordained reproduction which will wrack the Christian community for two millennia.

His statement "Before Abraham was, I am" (John 8:57) echoes this second Adamic claim.

Healing destiny is in turn achieved by making the two sexes one in an 'Edenic' reunion:

"When you make the two one, and when you make the inside like the outside and the outside like the inside, and the above like the below, and when you make the male and the female one and the same, so that the male not be male nor the female female; and when you fashion eyes in place of an eye, and a hand in place of a hand, and a foot in place of a foot, and a likeness in place of a likeness, then will you enter [the kingdom]" (Thomas 22)

In a patriarchal twist, Jesus asserts that making woman 'male' is the route to the kingdom:

"Simon Peter said to them, 'Let Mary leave us, for women are not worthy of life.' Jesus said, 'I myself shall lead her in order to make her male, so that she too may become a living spirit resembling you males. For every woman who will make herself male will enter the kingdom of heaven'." (114)

In 'Stromata' Clement of Alexandria claims that in the lost Gospel According to the Egyptians, when Shelom [Salome] asked how long death would prevail Yeshua replied "So long as you women bear children" to which she replies "Then I have done well in not bringing forth." When she asked when the kingdom would come, he replied: "When you women have trampled the garment of shame, when the two become one, and when the male with the female is neither male nor female" and in the same gospel he said "I have come to destroy the works of the female" (Graves R253).

The Dialogue of the Saviour, also originating in the first century, conveys these sentiments
: "The Lord said: 'Pray in the place where there is no woman'.
Matthew said: 'meaning Destroy the works of womanhood,
not because there is any other [manner of birth] but because they will cease [giving birth]'." (91)

We can see extensions of this idea in the following two passages, firstly in Thomas again trampling the garments of shame in returning to the child-like state:
"When will you become revealed to us and when shall we see you?" Jesus said, "When you disrobe without being ashamed and take up your garments and place them under your feet like little children and tread on them, then [will you see] the son of the living one, and you will not be afraid" (37).

When describing the after-life Yeshua is said in a possible orthodox redaction to have portrayed a sexless heaven, in which 'original lubricity' is replaced by sexless immortality:
"And Jesus answering said unto them, The children of this world marry, and are given in marriage: But they which shall be accounted worthy to obtain that world, and the resurrection from the dead, neither marry, nor are given in marriage: Neither can they die any more: for they are equal unto the angels; and are the children of God, being the children of the resurrection" (Luke 20:34).

The female mother in opposition to the father god appears again in Thomas:
"He who knows the father and the mother will be called the son of a harlot" (105).

"When you see one who was not born of woman,
prostrate yourselves on your faces and worship him. That one is your father" (15).

Although these hark back to the undivided Adam, they have the strained sentiments of a male messiah who is engaging the feminine tradition, while in the same motion, trying to overthrow it, in a misguided attempt to undo the perceived sins of Eve and the entire reproductive biological paradigm. We cannot thus see Yeshua as a feminist, nor even the 'gylanic' figure of 'partnership society' Eisler (R182) suggests, but rather an ingenious, yet tortured masculine attempt to encompass all traditions, and force the hour of doom as noted in Graves (R253 343-4) citing the very verse in Isaiah preceding Yeshua's Nazareth reading:
Mary: "His fault was this - he tried to force the hour of doom by declaring war on the female. But the female abides and cannot be hastened."
Shelom: "Peace woman - Is it not written of the Kingdom of God
"I the Lord will hasten it in his time"

His negative attitudes to family contrast sharply with his Edenic view of innocent children:
"If any man come to me, and hate not his father, and mother, and wife, and children, and brethren, and sisters, yea, and his own life also, he cannot be my disciple" (Luke 14:26).

"For I am come to set a man at variance against his father, and the daughter against her mother, and daughter in law against mother in law. And a man's foes shall be of his own household" (Matt 10:35).

"Whoever does not hate his father and mother cannot become a disciple to me. And whoever does not hate his brothers and sisters and take up his cross in my way will not be worthy of me" (Thom 55).

Yeshua describes himself as a winebibber and friend of publicans in a manner reminiscent of Ishtar, declaring feminine wisdom to be the arbiter:
"For John the Baptist came neither eating bread nor drinking wine; and ye say, He hath a devil. The Son of man is come eating and drinking; and ye say, Behold a gluttonous man, and a winebibber, a friend of publicans and sinners! But wisdom is justified of all her children" (Luke 7:33).

In the following passage he preaches love for a weeping 'sinner' or 'sacred prostitute' who anoints his feet with ointment, washing his feet with her tears and wiping them with her hair:
"And he turned to the woman, and said unto Simon, Seest thou this woman? I entered into thine house, thou gavest me no water for my feet: but she hath washed my feet with tears, and wiped them with the hairs of her head. Thou gavest me no kiss: but this woman since the time I came in hath not

ceased to kiss my feet. My head with oil thou didst not anoint: but this woman hath anointed my feet with ointment. Wherefore I say unto thee, Her sins, which are many, are forgiven; for she loved much: but to whom little is forgiven, the same loveth little. And he said unto her, Thy sins are forgiven" (7:44).

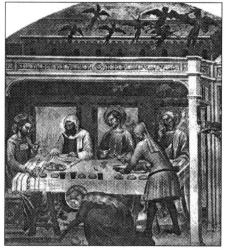

The 'sinner' anoints Christ's feet while seven galla emerge - Giovanni de Milano (Haskins R291).

In a parallel event, he liberated the woman taken in adultery, sometimes also identified with Magdalen, exposing the male accusers:

"He that is without sin among you, let him first cast a stone at her" (John 8:7).

He was anointed again by Mary of Bethany sometimes identified also with Magdalen:

"Then took Mary a pound of ointment of spikenard, very costly, and anointed the feet of Jesus, and wiped his feet with her hair: and the house was filled with the odour of the ointment" (John 12:3).

When Judas protests at the profligate waste, Jesus replies "Let her alone: against the day of my burying hath she kept this". In a closely parallel account he is anointed on the head by a woman in a traditional gesture of messiahship:

And being in Bethany in the house of Simon the leper, as he sat at meat, there came a woman having an alabaster box of ointment of spikenard very precious; and she brake the box, and poured it on his head. And there were some that had indignation within themselves ... And Jesus said, Let her alone; why trouble ye her? she hath wrought a good work on me. For ye have the poor with you always, and whensoever ye will ye may do them good: but me ye have not always (Mark 14:3).

According to Margaret Starbird (R648, R649), this 'nard' although formally an aromatic root, is from the enclosed vaginal garden of paradise, hinting at the priestess as a 'sacred prostitute'. In both cases the anointing is a provocation to imminent betrayal.

In John (12:23), Jesus declares himself to be resurrecting grain of Tammuz, gaining immortality just as Dhu Shara gained immortality by donning the tragic mask:

"The hour is come, that the Son of man should be glorified. Verily, verily, I say unto you, Except a corn of wheat fall into the ground and die, it abideth alone: but if it die, it bringeth forth much fruit. He that loveth his life shall lose it; and he that hateth his life in this world shall keep it unto life eternal"

The crucifixion reads as a carefully crafted Dionysian tragedy performed with Shakesperian subtlety. Yeshua has carefully organized many details in advance, arranged by code word, including the ass and the room for the last supper. He passes the sop to Judas in a ritual division of the twelve into a sacrificial paschal lamb and a scapegoat 'betrayer'.

He enters Jerusalem as sacred fertility king heralded by palm leaves and makes to overturn the tables in the Temple in the tradition of Zechariah's foolish shepherd, thus provoking the high priests to accuse him of the original charge of blasphemy and the Romans to try him for insurrection. He is seized in an Edenic garden, the disciples scattering like sheep, with Peter denying him the ritual three times. The High priests, to avoid committing him to death themselves, pass him over and he is shipped backwards and forwards between Herod and Pilate, neither of whom wish to be saddled with responsibility for his provocation, but become very good friends over the exchange (Luke 23:12). When Pilate asks Yeshua does he claim to be king, he can find no fault when Jesus replies:

"To this end was I born, and for this cause came I into the world, that I should bear witness unto the truth."

Barabbas, whose ritual name means 'the son of the father', a title noted in other Saturnalia in the region, is offered in his place as scapegoat three times by Pilate, but the high priests say"We have no king but Caesar" (John 19:15), and the crowd cries "His blood be on us, and on our children" (Matt 27:25), sealing the process of the accusation of blasphemy, as recorded in the Talmud:

> "On the eve of Passover they hung Jesus of Nazareth. And the herald went out before him for 40 days [saying, 'Yeshua] goes forth to be stoned, because he has practiced magic, enticed and led astray Israel. Anyone who knows anything in his favor, let him come and declare concerning him.' And they found nothing in his favor."

As confirmed in the many accounts of threatened stoning by the Judeans in the gospels:

> "Verily, verily, I say unto you, Before Abraham was, I am".
> Then took they up stones to cast at him: but Jesus hid himself, and went out of the temple, going through the midst of them, and so passed by (John 8:57).

> "I and my Father are one".
> Then the Jews took up stones again to stone him. ...
> For a good work we stone thee not; but for blasphemy;
> and because that thou, being a man, makest thyself God.(John 10:30).

Yeshua's reply to this accusation casts him into the blood-shedding, Josephic Northern tradition of Galilean Israel (Schonfield), rather than the Judaism of Herodian Judea. He refers to Abba among the congregation of the gods: "Is it not written in your law, I said, Ye are gods?" (p 208) - only to die like one of the princes.

> Therefore they sought again to take him: but he escaped out of their hand,
> And went away again beyond Jordan into the place where John at first baptized; and there he abode.

Finally he returns to Judea, Lazarus and the sacred tragedy of a death for a life:

> Then after that saith he to his disciples, Let us go into Judaea again.
> Master, the Jews of late sought to stone thee; and goest thou thither again? (11:8)

He is subjected to the Saturnalia, variously by the Roman soldiers, or earlier by Herod's men. His reed sceptre is broken and he is 'set to nought' in an intimation of ritual castration and arrayed in 'royal' garbs and marched to Golgotha, lamented by the women in the manner of Tammuz, to which Yeshua utters the apocalyptic curse against female birth:

> "There followed him a great company of people, and of women, which also bewailed and lamented him. But Jesus turning unto them said, Daughters of Jerusalem, weep not for me, but weep for yourselves, and for your children. For, behold, the days are coming, in the which they shall say, Blessed are the barren, and the wombs that never bare, and the paps which never gave suck." (Luke 23:28).

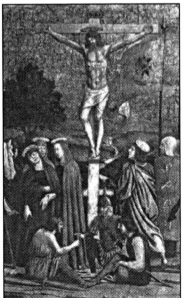

The three women at the crucifixion, with the men casting lots on the vesture (Francesca)

It is noted in Matt 27:32 that immediately after the humiliation "as they came out, they found a man of Cyrene, Simon by name: him they compelled to bear his cross." According to Basilides, Christ changed places with Simon of Cyrene and then mingled with the crowd of onlookers, while Simon carried the cross, bore it to the hill, drank the gall and vinegar and was crucified. The 'Second Treatise of the Great Seth', a revelation dialogue allegedly delivered by Jesus, says (Robinson R576 365, Pagels R511 91):

> "It was another, their father who drank the gall and vinegar; it was not I. They struck me with the reed; it was another, Simon, who bore the cross on his shoulder. It was another on whom they placed the crown of thorns,. But I was rejoicing in the height ... and I was laughing at their ignorance."

Having been given the title "King of the Jews" by Pilate he is then crucified, has his abdomen pierced in a focal confirmation of Zechariah's prophecy (12:10):

> "and they shall look upon me whom they have pierced,
> and they shall mourn for him,
> as one mourneth for his only son."

He utters the cry of Psalm 22

"El El why have you forsaken me?"

In the tradition of the Wisdom of Solomon *(2:12-20):*

Let us lie in wait for the righteous man,
because he is inconvenient to us and opposes our actions;
he reproaches us for our sins against the Law,
and accuses us of sins against our training.
He professes to have knowledge of God,
and calls himself a child of the Lord ...
Let us see if his words are true,
and let us test what will happen at the end of his life;
for if the righteous man is God's son, he will help him,
and deliver him from the hand of his adversaries.
Let us test him with insult and torture,
that we may find out how gentle he is,
and make trial of his forbearance.
Let us condemn him to a shameful death,
for, according to what he says, he will be protected.

This cycle of jealous oppression of the 'just man' is a sacrificial rite, echoing the Descent, but denuded of its *hieros gamos* fertility - a death of sacrificial atonement dedicated to the jealous God - again lamented in Isaiah's 'suffering servant':

He is despised and rejected of men; a man of sorrows, and
acquainted with grief: and we hid as it were our faces from him; he
was despised, and we esteemed him not.
Surely he hath borne our griefs, and carried our sorrows: yet we
did esteem him stricken, smitten of God, and afflicted.
But he was wounded for our transgressions, he was bruised for our
iniquities: the chastisement of our peace was upon him;
and with his stripes we are healed.
He was oppressed, and he was afflicted, yet he opened not his
mouth: he is brought as a lamb to the slaughter, and as a sheep before
her shearers is dumb, so he openeth not his mouth.
He was taken from prison and from judgment: and who shall declare
his generation? for he was cut off out of the land of the living: for
the transgression of my people was he stricken (53).

The fragmentary Gospel of Peter says Yeshua was as silent in just this way:

"And they brought two criminals and crucified the Lord between them.
But he himself remained silent, as if in no pain" (4:1).

He then succumbs so precipitously that Pilate 'marvels', suggesting he could possibly have survived the 'Passover plot' (Schonfield, Graves and Podro R257).

"And Jesus cried with a loud voice, and gave up the ghost.
And the veil of the temple was rent in twain
from the top to the bottom" (Mark 15:37).

The feminine veil of the temple is rent - the marriage is consummated and the hymen is broken. The women of Galilee, who somehow have come down to the passover, knowing the Lord they have given their 'substance' to is performing the descent, all look on from far off including a triple of three key women.

"There were also women looking on afar off: among whom was Mary Magdalen, and Mary the
mother of James and of Joses, and Salome; (Who also, when he was in Galilee, followed him, and
ministered unto him;) and many other women which came up with him unto Jerusalem" (Mark
15:40).

He is then laid in the sepulchre by Joseph of Arimathea followed by the women:

"And the women also, which came with him from Galilee, followed after, and beheld the sepulchre,
and how his body was laid. And they returned, and prepared spices and ointments" (Luke 23:55).

Yeshua was sacrificed in the presence of the women and not the male disciples, who have fled, they are the last to be with him in the sepulchre and the first to return after the sabbath:

"And when the sabbath was past, Mary Magdalene, and Mary the mother of James, and Salome,
had bought sweet spices, that they might come and anoint him" (Mark 16:1).

228

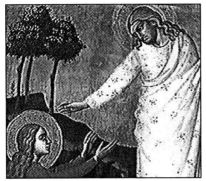

"Noli me Tangere" echoes the sacred sexual union of the Song of Songs (R741).

He is exulted as risen on the third day after harrowing hell, as in Inanna's descent, by Magdalen alone, who in an allegory of the second Adam mistakes Yeshua for the 'gardener' and recites the searching lament for Adonis and Tammuz (John 20:13):

"And they say unto her, 'Woman, why weepest thou?'
She saith unto them, 'Because they have taken away my
Lord, and I know not where they have laid him.' Jesus
saith unto her, 'Mary'. She turned herself, and saith
unto him, 'Rabboni'. Jesus saith unto her, 'Touch me
not; for I am not yet ascended' " .

As echoed in the Song of Songs:

"I opened to my beloved; but my beloved had withdrawn himself, and was gone: my soul failed
when he spake: I sought him, but I could not find him; I called him, but he gave me no answer"

Magdalen then conveys the exultation of the 'risen Christ' to the male disciples:

"Mary Magdalene came and told the disciples that she had seen the Lord,
and that he had spoken these things unto her "(John 20:18).

Luke confirms the central role of Magdalen, although derided by Peter and the apostles:

"It was Mary Magdalen and Joanna, and Mary the mother of James, and other women that were
with them, which told these things unto the apostles.
And their words seemed to them as idle tales, and they believed them not." (24:10) .

Yeshua declares Magdalen's name shall be told:

"Wheresoever this gospel shall be preached in the whole world, there shall also this, that this
woman hath done, be told for a memorial of her" (Matt 26:13)

Apostola Apostolorum: Magdalen announcing the resurrection Albani Psalter b 1123 (Haskins R291).

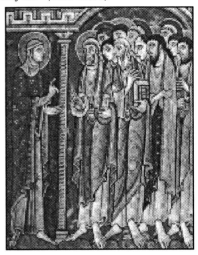

In the orthodox account, Yeshua was styled as the one and only apocalyptic male hero of cosmic renovation in the Essene and Zoroastrian vision who shall come again in the final apocalyptic crisis, the only begotten son of God, sacrificed in tragic 'atonement' so that, in believing in him, we shall not perish, but have everlasting life.

The notion of the bridegroom continues after the crucifixion in the messianic hope. In Luke we are reminded to wait on the Lord as a returning bridegroom (12:35):

"Let your loins be girded about, and your lights burning;
And ye yourselves like unto men that wait for their lord,
when he will return from the wedding; that when he
cometh and knocketh, they may open unto him immedi-
ately."

In Mark the hope is embodied in the bridegroom:

"Then shall the kingdom of heaven be likened unto ten virgins, which took their lamps, and went
forth to meet the bridegroom.... While the bridegroom tarried, they all slumbered and slept. And at
midnight there was a cry made, Behold, the bridegroom cometh; go ye out to meet him. Then all
those virgins arose, and trimmed their lamps. And the five foolish said unto the five wise, Give us of
your oil; for our lamps are gone out. But the wise answered, saying, Not so; lest there be not enough
for us and you: but go ye rather to them that sell, and buy for yourselves. And while they went to buy,
the bridegroom came; and they that were ready went in with him to the marriage: and the door was
shut" (25:1).

In the synoptics Peter declares Yeshua to be the apocalyptic Christ:

"He saith unto them, 'But whom say ye that I am?' And Simon Peter answered and said, 'Thou art the Christ, the Son of the living God'" (Matt 16:15).

But in the Gospel of Thomas, rather than declaring himself messiah, Yeshua makes the inscrutable reply of a gnostic teacher:

"'Compare me to someone and tell me whom I am like'. Simon Peter said to him, 'You are like a righteous angel.' Matthew said to him, 'You are like a wise philosopher.' Thomas said to him, 'Master, my mouth is wholly incapable of saying whom you are like.' Jesus said 'I am not your master. Because you have drunk, you have become intoxicated from the bubbling spring which I have measured out'" (13).

Yet in one of the most intimate of his gnostic statements he is the 'all' and is everywhere:

"It is I who am the light which is above them all. It is I who am the all. From me did the all come forth, and unto me did the all extend. Split a piece of wood, and I am there. Lift up the stone, and you will find me there." (77)

And rather than a kingdom in the heavens, he declares it is the natural world before us:

"If those who lead you say to you, 'See, the kingdom is in the sky', then the birds of the sky will precede you. If they say to you, 'It is in the sea', then the fish will precede you. Rather, the kingdom is inside of you, and   it is outside of you" (3).

"It will not come by waiting for it. It will not be a matter of saying 'here it is' or 'there it is'. Rather, the kingdom of the father is spread out upon the earth, and men do not see it" (113).

The initial group which gathers before Pentecost still contains the women, although Peter chauvinistically mentions only the males:

"When they were come in, they went up into an upper room... The [apostles] all continued with one accord in prayer and supplication, with the women, and Mary the mother of Jesus, and with his brethren. And in those days Peter stood up in the midst of the disciples, and said: "Men and brethren, this scripture must needs have been fulfilled" (Acts 1:13).

This delicate relationship between Peter and the disciples, the women and the desposyni - Yeshua's family, headed by James, continues to the Pentecostal revelation, which is a prophecy based on sons and daughters, servants and handmaidens - males and females together:

" And suddenly there came a sound from heaven as of a rushing mighty wind, and it filled all the house where they were sitting.... And they were all filled with the Holy Ghost, and began to speak with other tongues, as the Spirit gave them utterance.... which was spoken by the prophet Joel. 'and your sons and your daughters shall prophesy, and your young men shall see visions, and your old men shall dream dreams: And on my servants and on my handmaidens I will pour out in those days of my Spirit; and they shall prophesy'." (Acts 2:1).

Pentecost is really a three-way schism and parting of the ways between three paths 'ordained' by Yeshua: the following of Mary Magdalen and the 'women' [Matt 26:13], the Hebrew Christians headed by Yeshua's brother James the Just [Thomas 12] (Eisenman R181), and Peter's death-cursing brand of Christian communism [Matt 16:18, Acts 5:5], which was overtaken by Pauline born-again 'paganism'. The women now vanish from the synoptic account and from this early time on, in orthodox Christianity, women have been barred from the Church, ostensibly because they carry the earthly principle of 'carnal sin' through which Eve's wiles drew Adam and us all into a 'life of death', despite Christ's redeeming act. The gnostic Christians professed to carry the inner illumination of Yeshua's teaching. Some took their tradition directly from Magdalen, Martha and Salome and were notable for the equal status accorded to the genders. By 200 AD Irenaeus was complaining that women were still celebrating the Eucharist with the gnostic teacher Marcus and the gnostic sects were repressed.

John is noted as being a 'gnostic' gospel despite inclusion in the canon, although it has been cast in opposition to the egalitarian gnosticisn of Thomas (Pagels R514). Of all the Gospels, John carries Yeshua into the heights as logos, only -begotten. It is John who repeatedly cast aspersions on Thomas as doubting the unique power of Christ. Brown (R 1979 149) suggests that the originating group (50-80 AD) of the community was led by Mary Magdalen but that there was a schism early in the Johannine Community. She was highly esteemed as the primary witness to the resurrection and recognized as such even by believers who did not belong to this particular community. She was known, very early on, as the 'companion of Jesus' Later (c 90-100 AD), the claim that a female disciple of Jesus had been their community's first leader and hero became an embarrassment. Jusino (1998) thus suggests John's gospel is a sexually redacted version of an original gospel of Magdalen.

Mary Magdalen's enigmatic nature remains. Some scholars believe that the name Magdalene is the Greek rendering of the Aramaic word *m'gad'lla* meaning 'hairdresser' (Graves R253, Graves and Podro R255). Women practising this profession were regarded among the Jews as ladies of easy virtue. Magdalen 'alone stands out undefined by a designation attaching her to some male as wife, mother, or daughter and she is the only one to be identifiable by her place of birth'. Magdalini in Greek signified her belonging to *el Mejdel* (Migdal   tower for 'fish tower') a prosperous fishing village on Galilee, destroyed in 75 AD because of its infamy and the licentious behaviour of its inhabitants (Haskins R291 15). A tiny desolate dome shrine marks the site. Starbird (R649) refers to her as *magal eder* the tower of the flock.

"And thou, O tower of the flock, the strong hold of the daughter of Zion, unto thee shall it come, even the first dominion; the kingdom shall come to the daughter of Jerusalem" (Micah 4:8).

This is also tied up with mother Mary's ambiguous figure as an unmarried mother. It is quite clear that Yeshua's parentage was a source of concern to early Christians and of satirical derision from the Rabbis. Matthew 1:19 confesses: "Joseph her husband, being a just man, and not willing to make her a publick example, was minded to put her away privily". The Talmud claims that Jesus was Yeshua ben Pantera the illegitimate son of Mary M'gadd'la (the braider or hairdresser) by a Roman (Graves and Podro R255 98, Wilson R741 62) and that she was 'descended from princes and rulers but consorted with carpenters' (Graves R253 6). Pantera is a Roman surname known from the archaelogical record (Wilson R741). In Matthew, Yeshua's descent is reckoned through four 'loose' women: Tamar, Rahab, Bathsheba and Ruth. In addition to the 'virgin birth', star, magi, and slaughter of the innocents, the infancy legends are permeated with fertility paganism. Bethlehem is 'the House of Bread' (Frazer R220 5/257). St. Jerome stated that: "Bethlehem ... lay formerly under the shadow of a grove dedicated to Tammuz [the grain god], that is to say Adonis, and the very grotto where the infant Christ uttered his first cries resounded formerly with the lamentations over the lover of Aphrodite" (Briffault R75 3/97).

In early and medieval lore Mary Magdalen is represented as a beautiful and meretricious woman, a witch and a whore. In many gnostic texts she is the companion of Jesus and is with him on several important occasions. In one curious case, however, Mary is not present, and this is during an event of especial significance. Before the last supper Jesus called his disciples together and asked them for the bread and the cup to bless them. At that moment Mary Magdalen laughed, whereupon Jesus asked all the women to leave (Walker R709).

There is still greater confusion about the Salomes. One Salome appears in the 'infancy gospels' as a midwife and is the first to recognize him as the Christ. Traditionally, Salome is the name given to the wife of Zebedee and mother of James and John. Then we have the beautiful sixteen-year old daughter of Herodias and step-daughter of Herod Antipas the tetrarch. In a popular tradition current at the time she, like her mother, had lusted after John the Baptist and had been spurned by him, leading to the beheading (Wilde R731). Another is mentioned in the Gospel to the Egyptians (p 223), who appears to be childless, and in Thomas Yeshua 'comes up' on Salome's couch (p 223). To add to the confusion, she is sometimes referred to as Mary Salome. The only Salome mentioned in the Bible is watching the crucifixion from afar off, and coming after the entombment to anoint the body (Walker R709).

The apocryphal Coptic Book of the Resurrection of Christ, attributed to the apostle Bartholomew, names the women who went to the tomb. Among them were: Mary Magdalen; Mary the mother of James whom Jesus delivered out of the hand of Satan; Mary who ministered to him; Martha her sister; Joanna (Susanna) who renounced the marriage bed; and 'Salome who tempted him.' It would seem that some time after she had contrived the beheading of John the Baptist, Salome may have tried to use her wiles to tempt Jesus, but became his follower, and like Mary Magdalen remained close to him thereafter.

Satan and the Male Combat of Dark and Light

We can't leave this arena without dealing with a new apocalyptic form of the 'jealous god' in the form of the ultimate male combat myth - the polarization of the entire universe into light and dark in the contest between God and Satan. Male combat is as central to sexual jealousy, as are the ancient invocations against whoring in the Old Testament. It is also central to some of the most diabolical manifestations of Christianity in terms of treating the 'other' in any form of perceived deviation as agents of the Devil.

Although Satan has a historical precedent in the Zoroastrian cleansing final conflict between the forces of dark and ignorance and those of light, he emerges first in Jewish writings as a kind of tester of faith in Yaweh, and only later gains the aura of being God's nemesis as a rebel leader of the fallen angels, leading to a final apocalypse.

Elaine Pagels (R513) notes:

"What fascinates us about Satan is the way he expresses qualities that go beyond what we recognize as human. Satan evokes more than the greed, envy lust and anger we identify with our own worst impulses and more than what we call brutality which imputes to human beings a resemblance to animals ... Thousands of years of tradition have characterized Satan instead as a spirit. ... Many people have claimed to see him embodied at certain times in individuals and groups that seem possessed by an intense spiritual passion, one that engages even our better qualities, like strength, intelligence and devotion, but turns them towards destruction and takes pleasure in inflicting harm. ... I invite you to consider Satan as a reflection of how we perceive ourselves and those we call 'others'. Satan has after all made a kind of profession out of being the 'other', and so Satan defines negatively what we think of as being human. The social and cultural practice of defining certain people as 'others' in relation to one's group may of course be as old as humanity itself. ... Conflict between groups is of course nothing new. What may be new in the Western Christian tradition ... is how the use of Satan to represent one's enemies lends to conflict a specific kind of moral and religious interpretation, in which 'we' are God's people and 'they' are God's enemies, and ours as well ... aspects of Christianity I find disturbing ... [revealing] certain fault lines in the Christian tradition that have allowed for the demonizing of others throughout Christian history - fault lines that go back nearly two thousand years to the origins of the Christian movement."

This brings us full circle to the question of genetic competition, jealousy, male combat and Alexander's theory of morality (p 44) as a solidarity within groups to make them more effective at inter-group conflict.

Although there are relatively few direct references to Satan in the synoptic gospels, only one in John and none in those of Thomas or Mary, Yeshua's mission is strongly polarized between light and dark forces and the advent of the Kingdom is bound up in a powerfully dualistic way between the actions of players perceived to be on the dark side, such as Judas, the high priests, scribes and Herodians, in John the 'Jews'; with the Pharisees, certain Samaritan villages, Chorazin, Bethsaida, and sometimes the disciples, caught somewhere in the middle; while the lone figure of Yeshua, a 'fox without a hole', bears the light, while issuing such provocation and controversy that it is hard to tell which side, dark, or light, is the active agent in the escalating confrontation.

This carries over to the Crucifixion, where virtually all the players are implicated, Judas for betraying Yeshua, when savagely provoked by the sop and the profligate female anointing 'for my burial', the High priests when Yeshua assaults the temple sufficiently to cause them to fear Roman intervention (John 11:47), Pilate when the situation overtakes him, and despite protesting he can 'find no fault' washes his hands of him, the Jewish crowd who called for his blood saying 'whosoever maketh himself a king speaketh against Caesar', Satan who is waiting to figuratively gash him from the pinnacles, and finally God who is about to sacrifice his only begotten Son so that 'all who believe in Him should not perish but', despite this homicide 'have everlasting life' in the sacraments of flesh and blood. Or is it Yeshua himself who brought this all upon us, however ingeniously and prophetically?

Ever since, for Christians, Satan and the Jews have been implicated together while Yeshua and God have been cleared of any crime. Jews consider Yeshua and Satan are implicated but the they still have God on their side. Yet why was this killing necessary? As Elaine Pagels notes in her historical analysis, these times were apocalyptic and led directly towards the siege and sacking of Jerusalem, which was one of the most genocidal episodes in classical history, but is this a standard by which to set our paradigm of survival?

The direct references to Satan begin with Yeshua's forty days in the desert, where he is challenged to perform miracles, tempted with worldly power and challenged to tempt death off the Temple to see if he will be saved - something he later does in overturning the tables:

> *"And he was there in the wilderness forty days, tempted of Satan; and was with the wild beasts; and the angels ministered unto him" (Mark 1:13).*

> *"Being forty days tempted of the devil. And in those days he did eat nothing. And the devil said unto him, If thou be the Son of God, command this stone that it be made bread. And Jesus answered him, saying, It is written, That man shall not live by bread alone, but by every word of God. And the devil, taking him up into an high mountain, shewed unto him all the kingdoms of the world in a moment of time. And the devil said unto him, All this power will I give thee, and the glory of them: for that is delivered unto me; and to whomsoever I will I give it. If thou therefore wilt worship me, all shall be thine. And Jesus answered and said unto him, Get thee behind me, Satan: for it is written, Thou shalt worship the Lord thy God, and him only shalt thou serve. And he brought him to Jerusalem, and set him on a pinnacle of the temple, and said unto him, If thou be the Son of God, cast thyself down from hence: For it is written, He shall give his angels charge over thee, to keep thee: And in their hands they shall bear thee up, lest at any time thou dash thy foot against a stone. And Jesus answering said unto him, It is said, Thou shalt not tempt the Lord thy God. And when the devil had ended all the temptation, he departed from him for a season." (Luke 4:2).*

In a second passage Yeshua curses the unwelcoming cities to be thrust down to hell claiming that anyone who rejects him or the disciples are also enemies of God. The seventy revel in wielding power over the devils and Yeshua gives them miraculous power to tread on scorpions. We thus have a complete role reversal. 'Power over' is now assumed in just the way Satan offered, but here it is 'with God on our side':

> *"Woe unto thee, Chorazin! woe unto thee, Bethsaida! for if the mighty works had been done in Tyre and Sidon, which have been done in you, they had a great while ago repented, sitting in sackcloth and ashes. But it shall be more tolerable for Tyre and Sidon at the judgment, than for you. And thou, Capernaum, which art exalted to heaven, shalt be thrust down to hell. He that heareth you heareth me; and he that despiseth you despiseth me; and he that despiseth me despiseth him that sent me. And the seventy returned again with joy, saying, Lord, even the devils are subject unto us through thy name. And he said unto them, I beheld Satan as lightning fall from heaven. Behold, I give unto you power to tread on serpents and scorpions, and over all the power of the enemy: and nothing shall by any means hurt you. Notwithstanding in this rejoice not, that the spirits are subject unto you; but rather rejoice, because your names are written in heaven" (Luke 10:13).*

Yeshua as much as admits this conflict is one of fragmentation, when accused by the scribes of being Ba'al Zebul, Lord of the Flies, for using diabolical means of exorcism:

> *"And the scribes which came down from Jerusalem said, He hath Beelzebub, and by the prince of the devils casteth he out devils. And he called them unto him, and said unto them in parables, How can Satan cast out Satan? And if a kingdom be divided against itself, that kingdom cannot stand. And if a house be divided against itself, that house cannot stand. And if Satan rise up against himself, and be divided, he cannot stand, but hath an end" (Luke 3:22)*

Yeshua's point is a direct confirmation of Alexander's position (p 44). Unity within the group is necessary for effective competition or final combat with the 'other.' Neither is it clear that infirmities, whether psychic or physical are 'devils' but natural maladies, even if amenable to powerful forms of faith healing.

Peter is even accused of being possessed by Satan for the 'humanity' of questioning the self-destructive act, so similar to the one Satan tempted Yeshua perform from the pinnacles:

> *"And he began to teach them, that the Son of man must suffer many things, and be rejected of the elders, and of the chief priests, and scribes, and be killed, and after three days rise again. And he spake that saying openly. And Peter took him, and began to rebuke him. But when he had turned about and looked on his disciples, he rebuked Peter, saying, Get thee behind me, Satan: for thou savourest not the things that be of God, but the things that be of men" (Mark 8:31).*

Finally we have Judas' betrayal, and the only passage in John to refer directly to Satan:

Jesus answered them, Have not I chosen you twelve, and one of you is a devil? (6:70)

"And after the sop Satan entered into him.
Then said Jesus unto him, That thou doest, do quickly" (13:27).

Hereafter I will not talk much with you:
for the prince of this world cometh, and hath nothing in me (14:30).

Pagels (R513 100) notes: "Casting the struggle between good and evil as that between light and darkness, John never pictures Satan as the other gospels do, appearing as a disembodied being. ... John ... tells the whole story of Jesus as a struggle with Satan that culminates in the crucifixion. ... Although John never depicts Satan as a character on his own, acting independently of human beings, it is *people* who play the tempter's role."

In the key passage in John declaring he is the only-begotten son, the war is between dark and light in a pure Zoroastrian sense. The darkness of evil also seeks to hide its deceptions, lest it be reproved, but the light of truth declares itself openly that its deeds be manifest. So too for knowing (gnosis) and ignorance. This is the prisoners' dilemma of defection and cooperation crying out across the aeons:

"For God sent not his Son into the world to condemn the world; but that the world through him might be saved. He that believeth on him is not condemned: but he that believeth not is condemned already, because he hath not believed in the name of the only begotten Son of God. And this is the condemnation, that light is come into the world, and men loved darkness rather than light, because their deeds were evil. For every one that doeth evil hateth the light, neither cometh to the light, lest his deeds should be reproved. But he that doeth truth cometh to the light, that his deeds may be made manifest, that they are wrought in God" (3:17).

I must work the works of him that sent me, while it is day:
the night cometh, when no man can work.
As long as I am in the world, I am the light of the world (9:4).

"His disciples say unto him, Master, the Jews of late sought to stone thee; and goest thou thither again? Jesus answered, Are there not twelve hours in the day? If any man walk in the day, he stumbleth not, because he seeth the light of this world.
But if a man walk in the night, he stumbleth, because there is no light in him." (11:8)

Then Jesus said unto them, Yet a little while is the light with you. Walk while ye have the light, lest darkness come upon you: for he that walketh in darkness knoweth not whither he goeth (12:35).

This theme of the tangled violence between the light in the 'party of God' and the darkness in the 'evil empire' continues throughout Christian and Western history. Firstly in the era of martyrdom in perceiving that the pagans who persecuted them were agents of the devil, then dangerously turning the 'other' into 'self', the heretics in the Christian midst:

Paul, who was martyred for his convictions, saw the problem of evil arising both in the political sphere of world powers, and extending even to the heavens:

"Our contest is not against flesh and blood [humans] but against powers,
against principalities, against the world rulers of this present darkness,
against spiritual forces of evil in the heavenly places" (Eph 6:12)

However the enemy within was even more of a subtle threat, illustrating that the ultimate danger of the whole concept of evil is that, as Yeshua said, it splits every which way:

"For such are false apostles, deceitful workers, transforming themselves into the apostles of Christ. And no marvel; for Satan himself is transformed into an angel of light.
Therefore it is no great thing if his ministers also be transformed as the ministers of righteousness; whose end shall be according to their works" (2 Cor 11:13).

This dance with the Devil continued on through Crusade, Inquisition, Witch Hunt, Shoah, World Wars, Nuclear confrontation by 'mutually assured destruction', even to the self-contradictory war on terror.

Samael's Jealousy and Thunder's Perfection

Gnosticism (gnosis meaning 'primal knowing') is a partially ascetic contemplative movement that both precedes and succeeds Christianity. Gnostic Christians had a much more multifaceted view of divinity in which God was among other things revealed as a demiurge who assumed dictatorial power over the primal silence, the feminine spirit of Wisdom in Sophia. We have only been able to discover the richness and complexity of the Gnostic Christian visions because a sect which was being repressed in the second century hid its works in jars at Nag Hammadi only to be discovered by the world nearly two millennia later.

Among these the Gospel of Thomas 70-150 CE contains older forms of source saying parallel to the author Q who forms a basis for several synoptics. (Pagels R511, Robinson R576). The Gospel of Thomas was most likely composed in Syria, where tradition holds the church of Edessa to have been founded by Judas Thomas, 'The Twin' (Didymos). Pagels (R511) proposes that the Gospel of Thomas is an avenue to the transcendent 'Christ state', shared in a twinning with all. The gospel opens declaring these are the secret sayings which the living Jesus spoke which Thomas wrote down: The first declares the sayings are the key to life:

"Whoever finds the interpretation of these sayings will not experience death."

echoing John's "If a man keep my saying, he shall never see death." The next saying is more specific and suggests full illumination in power:

"Let him who seeks continue seeking until he finds. When he finds, he will become troubled.
When he becomes troubled, he will be astonished, and he will rule over the all."

The very idea of such illumination will later become heresy punishable by death.

Many gnostics saw the world as a dualistic one, in which the darkness of matter, a product of the demiurge bound them from spiritual liberation and the light, and in Manichaeism, females and sexuality were seen as physical snares and contributed indirectly to the monastic tradition. Such movements regarded procreation as to be avoided to prevent the spirit being again entrapped in the flesh. They thus embraced contraception.

Thomas echoes the derogation of the flesh and the physical:

Jesus said, "If the flesh came into being because of spirit, it is a wonder.
But if spirit came into being because of the body, it is a wonder of wonders.
Indeed, I am amazed at how this great wealth has made its home in this poverty" (29).

Jesus said, "Whoever has come to understand the world has found (only) a corpse,
and whoever has found a corpse is superior to the world" (56).

Jesus said, "Wretched is the body that is dependent upon a body,
and wretched is the soul that is dependent on these two" (87).

Certain of the gnostics, including Valentinus, Marcion, and the Carpocratians had relatively liberated attitudes to sexual relationship, morality, and particularly to sexual equality in the church, to the ire of the orthodox bishops. Occhigrosso (R500 302) even describes the consolidation of the synoptic canon as a reaction to the gnosticism of Marcion which rejected the gospels as misrepresenting Yeshua's vision of a god of love rather than fear, quite distinct from the Old Testament God, whom Marcion considered an inferior being. The gnostic group following Carpocrates, headed by a female bishop Marcellina, claimed a secret tradition going back to Mary, Martha and Salome.

In the Dialogue of the Saviour, which, like the Gospel of Thomas, contains traditional sayings in archaic form and has a possible date of origin in the first century are several passages emphasizing the key role of Mary in her depth of understanding and revelation of his inner message as one who had understood completely (Robinson R576 252):

Mary said: "Tell me Lord why have I come to this place, to profit or to forfeit"
The Lord said "You make clear the abundance of the revealer!" (60)

Mary said "I want to understand all things just as they are",
Mary utters "There is but one saying I will speak to the Lord concerning the mystery of truth:
In this we have taken our stand and to the cosmic we are transparent" (69).

As noted, signs of the division noted firstly in the exaltation are apparent in the Gospel of Thomas a tension between Peter (the orthodox) and Mary Magdalen (the gnostic).

'Let Mary leave us, for women are not worthy of life.'

The tension between Mary and Peter continues in the later Gospel of Mary:

"Peter said to Mary, "Sister, we know that the Savior loved you more than the rest of women. Tell us the words of the Savior which you remember - which you know (but) we do not, nor have we heard them." Mary answered and said, "What is hidden from you I will proclaim to you." And she began to speak to them. ... When Mary had said this, she fell silent, since it was to this point that the Savior had spoken with her. But Andrew answered and said to the brethren, "Say what you (wish to) say about what she has said. I at least do not believe that the Savior said this. For certainly these teachings are strange ideas." Peter answered and spoke concerning these same things. He questioned them about the Savior: "Did he really speak with a woman without our knowledge (and) not openly? Are we to turn about and all listen to her? Did he prefer her to us?" Then Mary wept and said to Peter, "My brother Peter, what do you think? Do you think that I thought this up myself in my heart, or that I am lying about the Savior?" Levi answered and said to Peter, "Peter, you have always been hot-tempered. Now I see you contending against the woman like the adversaries. But if the Savior made her worthy, who are you indeed to reject her? Surely the Savior knows her very well. That is why he loved her more than us" (Robinson 524).

In the Valentinian Gospel of Philip, Magdalen is called Christ's 'companion' (Gk *koinonos* partner) the most important of the three women "who were always with the Lord".

"But Christ loved her more than all the disciples and used to kiss her often on the mouth. ... They said to him, why do you love her more than all of us? ... Jesus said 'when the light comes, he who sees will see the light, but he who is blind will remain in darkness'" (Robinson 148, Haskins 40).

In the Pistis Sophia Mary warns "Peter makes me hesitate, I am afraid of him because he hates the female race" (Walker R708 791, Haskins R291 42). When she asks him if she may speak in boldness Jesus replies: "Mariham Mariham, the happy, this shall I complete in all the mysteries of ... the Height. Speak in boldness because thou art she whose heart straineth toward the Kingdom of the heavens more than all thy brothers." When she says she has comprehended every word, he marvels because she has become spirit quite pure (R291 50-1).

In a later apocryphal tradition, Mary Magdalen, along with sister Martha, brother Lazarus, Mary the wife of Cleophas who was the half-sister of the Virgin Mary, Mary the mother of James and Joses, and Mary Salome, were all washed up on the shores of Provence in a rudderless boat, after they had fled persecution in the Holy Land. Various forms of this myth have the two Marys and a little black madonna Sarah also called Sara Kali, as celebrated at Saintes Marie de la Mer, thought to have been an Egyptian but also suggested to have been the child of Yeshua and Magdalen from their sacred union (Starbird R648 60), .

In teachings attributed to Marcus or Theodotus (circa 160 C.E.), we read that "the male and female elements together constitute the finest production of the Mother, Wisdom." The Valentinians borrowed the mother-goddess myth from the Ophites (Gk. *ophis* snake) (Haskins R291 45) who saw the serpent of Eden as the divine complement of the world egg regenerating immortal life in wisdom and also implicitly as the penis. Orthodox opponents made tempestuous allegations of promiscuous gnostic sexual fertility rites. Iraneus comments: "Others, again, following upon Basilides and Carpocrates, have introduced promiscuous intercourse and a plurality of wives, and are indifferent about eating meats sacrificed to idols." Barbara Walker mentions the 'agape' being referred to as *synesaktism* suggesting Shakti worship. Epiphanius described the agape practiced by Ophite Christians, while making it clear that these heretical sexual activities filled him with horror (Walker R708 640) :

"Their women they share in common; and when anyone arrives who might be alien to their doctrine, the men and women have a sign by which they make themselves known to each other. When they extend their hands, apparently in greeting, they tickle the other's palm in a certain way and so discover whether the new arrival belongs to their cult. ...Husbands separate from their wives, and a man will say to his own spouse, 'Arise and celebrate the love feast (agape) with thy brother.' And the wretches mingle with each other...after they have consorted together in a passionate debauch...The woman and the man take the man's ejaculation into their hands, stand up...offering to the Father, the Primal Being of All Nature, what is on their hands, with the words, 'We bring to Thee this oblation, which is the very Body of Christ.' ...They consume it, take housel of their shame and say: 'This is the Body of Christ, the Paschal Sacrifice through which our bodies suffer and are forced to confess to the sufferings of Christ.' And when the woman is in her period, they do likewise with her menstruation. The unclean flow of blood, which they garner, they take up in the same way and eat together. And that, they say, is Christ's Blood. For when they read in Revelation, 'I saw the tree of life with its twelve kinds of fruit, yielding its fruit each month' (Rev. 22:2), they interpret this as an allusion to the monthly incidence of the female period."

Some of these statements may be exaggerated diatribes by opponents. The Borborite Ophites were also said to extract fetuses from pregnant women and consume them, particularly if the women accidentally became pregnant during related sexual rituals. However gnostic sexuality has a factual basis in libertine gnostic myth and practice (Gero R232), although others quoting the Nassene Ophites describe them as innocently worshipping the androgynous condition, regarding sexual concourse as symptomatic of the paradigm of death.

Valentinus attributes the paradox of the creation of the imperfect world to Wisdom: "Desiring to conceive by herself, apart from her masculine counterpart, ... she became the 'great creative power from whom all things originate', often called Eve, 'Mother of all living'. But since her desire violated the harmonious union of opposites intrinsic in the nature of created being, what she produced was ... defective; [causing] the terror and grief that mar human existence. To author her creation, Wisdom brought forth the demiurge, the creator-God of Israel, as her agent. ... Besides being the 'first universal creator', who brings forth all creatures, [wisdom] also enlightens human beings. Followers of Valentinus and Marcus therefore prayed to her as the 'mystical, eternal Silence' and to 'Grace, She who is before all things', and as 'incorruptible Wisdom' for insight (gnosis). Valentinus reasons that Silence is the appropriate complement of the Father, designating the former as feminine and the latter as masculine ... He goes on to describe how Silence receives, as in a womb, the seed of the Ineffable Source; from this she brings forth all the emanations of divine being, ranged in harmonious pairs of masculine and feminine energies. Followers of Valentinus prayed to her for protection as the Mother, and as 'the mystical, eternal Silence'." (Pagels R511 76).

The Great Announcement ... explains the origin of the universe in the manner of Shiva and Shakti: "From the power of Silence appeared 'a great power, the Mind (nous) of the Universe, which manages all things, and is a male ... the other ... a great Intelligence (epinoia) ... is a female which produces all things.' ... This is one power divided above and below; generating itself, making itself grow, seeking itself, finding itself, being mother of itself, father of itself, sister of itself, spouse of itself, daughter of itself, son of itself - mother, father, unity, being a source of the entire circle of existence" (Pagels R511 73).

"A work attributed to Simon Magus suggests a mystical meaning for Paradise, the place where human life began: Grant Paradise to be the womb; ... 'I am He that formed thee in thy mother's womb' (Isaiah 44:2) ... Moses ... using allegory had declared Paradise to be the womb ... and Eden, the placenta" (R511 75).

The divine mother is portrayed by gnostics as mystical silence, Holy Spirit, the image of thought (*ennoia*) and wisdom Sophia. Other gnostics attributed to Sophia the nourishment and self-awareness that Adam and Eve received in Paradise ... When the creator became angry with the human race because they did not worship or honor him as Father and God, he sent forth a flood upon them, that he might destroy them. But Wisdom opposed him ... "and Noah and his family were saved in the ark by means of the sprinkling of the light that proceeded from her, and through it the world was again filled with humankind" (R511 76). Yet others point out that for Adam to produce Eve he must have been androgynous, as is suggested by the first Genesis account.

God was now perceived as a lesser demiurge. "Some concluded that the God of Israel ...was merely instrumental power whom the Mother had created. ... They say that he believed that he had made everything by himself, but that, in reality, he had created the world because Wisdom, his Mother, 'infused him with energy' and implanted into him her own ideas. ... 'It was because he was foolish and ignorant of his Mother that he said, 'I am God; there is none beside me'.' According to another account, the creator caused his Mother to grieve by creating inferior beings, so she left him alone and withdrew into the upper regions of the heavens.

The Secret Book of John notes the paradox of a sole jealous god:

"he said: 'I am a jealous God, and there is no other God beside me.' But by announcing this he indicated to the angels ... that another God does exist; for if there were no other one, of whom would he be jealous? ... Then the mother began to be distressed" "Others declared that his Mother refused to tolerate such presumption: [The creator], becoming arrogant in spirit, boasted himself over all those things that were below him, and exclaimed, 'I am father, and God, and above me there is no one.' But his mother, hearing him speak thus, cried out against him, 'Do not lie, Ialdabaoth'" (R511 79).

"According to the Hypostasis of the Archons, ... both the mother and her daughter objected when he [said], 'It is I who am God, and there is no other apart from me.'. . . And a voice came forth from above the realm of absolute power, saying, 'You are wrong, Samael' [which means, 'god of the blind']. And he said, 'If any other thing exists before me, let it appear to me!' And immediately, Sophia ('Wisdom" stretched forth her finger, and introduced light into matter, and she followed it down into the region of Chaos.... And he again said to his offspring, 'It is I who am the God of All.' And Life, the daughter of Wisdom, cried out; she said to him, 'You are wrong, Saklas!'" (ibid).

In the Apocalypse of Adam, it is revealed to Seth that God struck Adam and Eve apart in wrath for Eve's vision (Robinson R576 277):

"When God created me out of the earth along with Eve your mother, I went about with her in a glory which she had seen in the aeon from which we had come forth. She taught me a word of knowledge of the eternal god. And we resembled the great eternal angels, for we were higher than the god who had created us and the powers with him whom we did not know. Then god, the ruler of the aeons and the powers divided us in wrath. Then we became two aeons. And the glory of our hearts left us, me and your mother Eve, along with the first knowledge that breathed within us ... and went into the great aeons. ... Then we recognized the god that had created us ... and we served him in fear and slavery".

The gnostic teacher Justinus describes the Lord's shock, terror, and anxiety when he discovered that he was not the God of the universe. Gradually his shock gave way to wonder, and finally he came to welcome what wisdom had taught him. The teacher [ironically] concludes: "This is the meaning of the saying 'The fear of the Lord is the beginning of wisdom'" (Pagels R511 79).

Trimorphic Protennoia (literally, the 'Triple-formed Primal Thought'), celebrates the feminine powers of Thought, Intelligence, and Foresight:

"I am Thought that [dwells in the Light]. [She who exists] before the All ... I move in every creature. ... I am the Invisible One within the All. I am perception and knowledge, uttering a Voice by means of Thought. I am the real voice. I cry out in everyone, and they know that a seed dwells within. ... Now I have come a second time in the likeness of a female ... I have revealed myself in the Thought of the likeness of my masculinity. ... I am androgynous. [I am both Mother and] Father, since I [copulate] with myself ... [and with those who love] me ... I am the Womb [that gives shape] to the All ... I am ... the glory of the Mother" (Pagels R511 77)

Thunder, Perfect Mind extends this revelation into a metaphysical koan abrogating all authority except gnosis itself, and a female gnosis of the valley. The awareness of the paradox of the nature of deity in this work is mysterious and profound (Pagels R511 67):

'Look upon me you who reflect upon me
and you hearers hear me
You who are waiting for me take me to yourselves.
For I am the first and the last.
I am the honored one and the scorned one.
I am the whore, and the holy one.
I am the wife and the virgin.
I am (the mother) and the daughter....
I am the barren one, and many are her sons
I am she whose wedding is great,
and I have not taken a husband....
I am knowledge, and ignorance....
I am shameless; I am ashamed.
I am strength, and I am fear....
I am senseless, and I am wise. ...
I am the silence that is incomprehensible
and the idea whose remembrance is frequent.
I am the one whom they call Life
and you have called death [Eve]
I am the one you have pursued
I am the one you have seized
I am the one you have scattered

238

and you have gathered me together [Christos].
I am the one before whom you have been ashamed
and you have been shameless to me.
I am godless, and I am one whose God is great.
I am the union and the dissolution.
I am the judgement and the acquittal.
I am the sinless and the root of sin derives from me
I am lust in (outward) appearance
and interior self-control exists within me
For many are the forms ... and fleeting pleasures
which men embrace until they become sober
and go up to their resting place.
And they will find me there
and they will live
and they will not die again.'

Pauline Paganism and Martyr's Blood

Christianity has since made sex a lubricious mortal sin, while contriving that Gothic pinnacles of stone are the marriage bed of a fallen hero, whose blood continues to drip from his wounded body, in its all-too-protracted death throes, from every crucifix and statue into the cup of every communion service, partaken with God the world over as the *soma* and *sangre* - a flesh and blood celebration of human sacrifice ordained by God for forgiveness' sake.

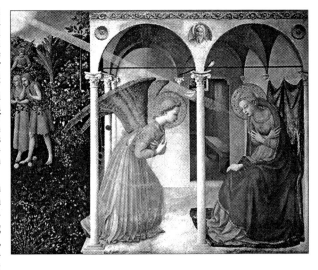

Fra Angelico "The Annunciation of Mary" Mary played little part in Yeshua's mission. When told "Thy mother and thy brethren stand without, desiring to see thee" he demurred "My mother and my brethren are these which hear the word of God, and do it." However Mary was later crafted by the orthodoxy to provide a more politically correct form of the chaste feminine than Magdalen, in the shadow of Eve's 'error' in Eden (left), now a Hellenistic virgin mother, rather than a priestess out of wedlock.

From the time of born-again Paul, the Christian path became a pagan one, permeated by symbols replacing reality; from the Rapture, through divine birth, the Virgin Mary; to the Trinity; which were never a part of the original teachings of Yeshua, and whose immense popularity in the pagan gentile world attests to their intrinsic Dionysian and Hellenistic paganism.

The Christian God in Yeshua's apocalyptic terminology is *Abba* - father - again male paternity, but in an ostensibly more compassionate, forgiving form, though steeped in the agrarian confusion of seasonal sacrifice of the male hero, attributed to a supposedly infanticidal 'Father', to prove to us all that we must be utterly faithful to Him. Naturally God's innate jealousy remains central:

"Do we provoke the Lord to jealousy? are we stronger than he?" (1 Corinth 10:22)

"For I am jealous over you with godly jealousy" (2 Corinth 11:2)

Pauline Christianity inserts a pagan view into the creation account which leads to a profoundly distorted view of sexuality. Jesus has moved from the messiah of the lost sheep of Israel to a demi-god, risen to the heavens in a bodily resurrection. He is a cosmic only begotten son of God, the second Adam born to a virginal Mariam, undoing Eve's carnal sin in chastity while Eve and the first Adam now endow us all with death. Womankind is the source of sin amid a violently masochistic contempt for the continuity of life in the form of martyrdom in the image of Yeshua's death.

"For since by man came death, by man came also the resurrection of the dead. For as in Adam all die, even so in Christ shall all be made alive. But every man in his own order: Christ the firstfruits; afterward they that are Christ's at his coming. ... And so it is written, The first man Adam was made a living soul; the last Adam was made a quickening spirit. Howbeit that was not first which is spiritual, but that which is natural; and afterward that which is spiritual. The first man is of the earth, earthy; the second man is the Lord from heaven." 1 Cor 15:21

To commentators in the five centuries before Christ, Adam's death was due to his own sins, and not to any sin innate in the race of man (Haskins R291 72). Paul's act was to link Adam, the first father, and the rest of mankind in a hereditary manner. Adam's descendants became in Eph 2:2 the 'children of disobedience', 'by nature the children of wrath' (Fox R219 25).

In Gal 5:17 we see an almost Manichaean war of the flesh and spirit: 'For the flesh lusteth against the Spirit, and the Spirit against the flesh: and these are contrary the one to the other: so that ye cannot do the things that ye would' He notes the works of the flesh in a way which became of hideous significance during the inquisition "adultery, fornication, uncleanness, lasciviousness, idolatry, witchcraft, hatred, variance, emulations, wrath, strife seditions, heresies" (Haskins R291 72).

Paul took a very celibate view of sexuality, proclaiming beatitudes of celibacy and virginity.

"Blessed are they who have wives as if they had none, for they shall inherit God" (1 Cor 7:29)

"Blessed are they who have kept the flesh pure, for they shall become a temple of God." (2 Cor 6:16)

However he neither advocates nor prohibits virginal chastity "Now concerning virgins I have no commandment of the Lord" (1 Cor 7:25). In Ephesians 5:28 he even advocates empathic love: "So ought men to love their wives even as their own bodies, for he that loveth his wife loveth himself." Some passages suggest Paul might have castrated himself as Origen did. Numerous Christians adopted the same course; surgeons were besieged with requests to perform the operation (Briffault R75v3 372), following Yeshua's enigmatic statement, although others derided it.

"I would they were even cut off which trouble you." (Galatians 5:12)

Paul advocates sexual union, but only as an antidote to fornication:

"It is good for a man not to touch a woman. Nevertheless, to avoid fornication, let every man have his own wife, and let every woman have her own husband Let the husband render unto the wife due benevolence: and likewise also the wife unto the husband. ... Defraud [deprive] ye not one the other, except it be with consent for a time, that ye may give yourselves to fasting and prayer; and come together again, that Satan tempt you not for your incontinency. But I speak this by permission, and not of commandment. ... For I would that all men were even as I myself. ... But if they cannot contain, let them marry: for it is better to marry than to burn" (1 Cor 7:1).

Although the orthodox supported family life as a means of continuation of the faithful, many Christians from the first and second centuries, following Yeshua's condemnations of family commitment, believed that conversion transferred the individual to an eschatological identity set in opposition to family structures that reproduced a fallen history. For them becoming Christian meant renouncing sexual relations and family ties. Thecla for example, is said to have abandoned her fiancé and family and followed Paul, twice miraculously escaping being eaten by lions (Ruther R586 34).

As we learn from Acts and Paul's own epistles, women were able to have important functions as bishops and deacons in the fledgling church, earning the admiration of Paul himself (Haskins 53, Pagels R512 18).

"I commend unto you Phebe our sister, which is a servant of the church which is at Cenchrea: That ye receive her in the Lord, as becometh saints, and that ye assist her in whatsoever business she hath need of you: for she hath been a succourer of many, and of myself also. Greet Priscilla and Aquila my helpers in Christ Jesus: Who have for my life laid down their own necks: unto whom not only I give thanks, but also all the churches of the Gentiles" (Rom 16:1).

However we find in 1 Cor 14:34 women barred from public ministry:

"Let your women keep silence in the churches: for it is not permitted unto them to speak; but they are commanded to be under obedience as also saith the law. And if they will learn any thing, let them ask their husbands at home: for it is a shame for women to speak in the church."

Pagels (R512 24) notes "The deutero-Pauline letters constitute in part a reaction to celibacy, stressing instead family life. However these authors also stress the lowly nature of woman as the perpetrator of original sin":

"I permit no woman to teach or to have authority over men;
she is to keep silent with all subjection; for Adam was first formed then Eve.
Adam was not deceived, but the woman was deceived and became a transgressor" (1 Tim 2:11)

In a Manichaean vein both Ambrose and Tertullian declared that the extinction of the human race was preferable to its propagation by sexual intercourse (Briffault R75v3 374).

"The sentiments of the early Christians were almost hysterically connected with martyrdom in their desire to confess their faith and become sacrificial victims in the shadow of Christ, perpetuating the agony of the crucifixion in further cycles of violence. For some apocalyptist movements martyrdom was a direct route to the imminent kingdom. Montanists, for whom women had prominent roles, were confessors who gave condemned women special powers of intercession. Even when the authorities tried to persuade the accused to come to their senses for their own accord, sometimes ordering a stay of execution for a month, the accused often preferred a gruesome death to having to atone later to Jesus for denying him, even as Peter himself had done. "You wish no time for reconsideration?" "In so just a matter, there is no need for reconsideration." Justin Martyr comments "no one can terrify or subdue us who believe in Jesus Christ ... though beheaded and crucified, and thrown to the wild beasts, in chains, in fire, in all kinds of torture, we do not give up our confession; but the more such things happen, the more do others, in larger numbers, become believers." Tertullian claimed that, despite initially enjoying these ludicrous cruelties of the noonday exhibition, the sight of Christians dressed to look like Attis being torn apart in the arena, or burned alive as Hercules ultimately inspired his own conversion: "You must take up your cross and bear it after your master,... the sole key to unlock paradise is your life's blood" (Pagels R511 94-113).

The hatred of heresy (whose meaning 'choice'indicates orthodoxy is choice denied) came hand in hand with the love of martyrdom. Some did recognize that perhaps this was against the will of God, since Jesus had died so they might not have to, particularly gnostic 'heretics' who were not so uniformly literal minded, but were instead diverse. Some supported it some opposed it on the grounds that it was no instant fix to replace realization.

The story of Perpetua (Pagels R512 33-6) is a shrine to the way in which the Kingdom of the Father has led to precipitate and tortured death on the part of Christian believers. Perpetua, twenty-two years old, recently married, and nursing her infant son, was arrested along with her friends. They were scourged and thrown into a stifling and crowded African jail. After her arrest, Perpetua's father, ... out of love for me," she wrote, "was trying to persuade me to change my decision." Refusing his pleas to give up the name Christian, Perpetua rejected her familial name instead, although she says she grieved to see her father, mother, and brothers "suffering out of compassion for me." At first, she wrote, "I was tortured with worry for my baby there," but after she gained permission for him to stay with her in prison, "at once I recovered my health, relieved as I was of my worry and anxiety for the child." Perpetua's slave Felicitas was pregnant when she was arrested and was in her eighth month as the execution date approached: "Felicitas was very distressed that her martyrdom would be postponed because of her pregnancy; for it is against the law for pregnant women to be executed." She feared she would have to endure a later execution along with criminals. Two days before the execution the Christians prayed for her in one torrent of common grief, and immediately after their prayer the labor pains came upon her. When Perpetua's brother asks her for a vision as to whether they will be condemned or freed, she dreams of scaling a ladder covered in harsh sharp weapons reaching to the heavens guarded by a dragon emerging to a heavenly garden, meeting the grey haired one and the blessed and realized she faced martyrdom. "From then on we gave up having any hope in this world". Hilarianus the governor said to me: "Have pity on your father's grey head; have pity on your infant son. Offer the sacrifice for the welfare of the emperors." "I will not," I retorted. "Are you a Christian?" said Hilarianus. And I said: "Yes, I am. When my father persisted in trying to dissuade me, Hilarianus ordered him to be thrown to the ground and beaten with a rod. I felt sorry for my father, just as if I myself had been beaten. I felt sorry for his pathetic old age. Then Hilarianus passed sentence on all of us: we were condemned to the beasts, and we returned to prison in high spirits. A mad heifer was set loose after them; Perpetua was gored and thrown to the ground. She got up and, seeing Felicitas crushed and fallen went over to her and lifted her up, and the two stood side by side. Then after undergoing further ordeals and seeing Saturus endure agonizing torture. Perpetua and Felicitas, along with the others were called to the centre of the arena to be slaughtered. A witness records that Perpetua "screamed as she was struck on the bone; then she took the trembling hand of the gladiator and guided it to her throat". It is said in the Golden Legend that she was mauled by a lion and Felicitas by a leopard. (Young R758 47).

It is an irony of history that out of the orthodox churches collective solidarity in the face of the holocaust of martyrdom came also the eclipse of the gnostic 'inner path'. By 200 AD Irenaeus ushered in the campaign of the orthodox church against the gnostics, complaining in particular that women were celebrating the Eucharist with the gnostic teacher Marcus. Tertullian, before going to the other side and becoming a gnostic himself, expresses similar outrage: "These heretical women - how audacious they are! They have no modesty; they are bold enough to teach, to engage in argument, to enact exorcisms, to undertake cures, and it may be, even to baptize!" (Pagels R512 80-81).

Tertullian described women as 'the devil's gateway' and coined the word concupiscence from the Latin, *concupiscere*, to long for, to be desirous of, to covet (p 530), which signified Adam and Eve's fatal flaw and the loss of integrity which had resulted from their disobedience to God. Tertullian makes clear the scorn and prejudice of early Church fathers:

"And do you not know that you are [each] an Eve? The sentence of God on this sex of yours lives in this age: the guilt must of necessity live too. You are the devil's gateway: you are the unsealer of that [forbidden] tree: you are the first deserter of the divine law: you are she who persuaded him whom the devil was not valiant enough to attack. You destroyed so easily God's image, man. On account of your desert - that is, death - even the Son of God had to die" (Haskins 79).

Many of the early fathers, from Tatian to Jerome and Ambrose, believed that the animal act and the loss of virginity were the cause of the fall (Pagels R512 27, Haskins R291 79, Briffault R75v3 373). This attitude to virginity implied that marriage was an inferior state of being to the higher glory of chastity, which prepared one for the heavenly state. Clement rejected such associations and declared that sexual intercourse was not sinful but was part of God's original and 'good' creation - cooperation in God's act of creation as in fact many Jews had thought before him. Clement however claimed: "Every woman ought to be filled with shame at the thought she is a woman", and saw procreation as the sole legitimate purpose in sexuality - a reverberating doctrine of the Christian church (Pagels R512 28-9):

"Our ideal is not to experience desire at all ... A man who marries for the sake of begetting children must practice continence so that it is not desire he feels for his wife ... not even at night or in the darkness is it fitting to carry on immodestly or indecently ... for even that union which is legitimate is still dangerous, except in so far as it is engaged in procreation of children" never to take place in the morning, daytime or after dinner, and never with menstruating, barren, or menopausal wives".

The mix of the rapture of martyrdom in the shadow of Yeshua's own increasingly mythical act, the gnostic revilement of the flesh, and the strict orthodox view of sex as reproduction produced a paradoxical attitude to the sanctity of life. Christians took up the Jewish attitude to sex as reproduction and abhorred the attitudes to abortion and exposure of infants, (which was a father's right) of pagan Mesopotamia and Rome, and were seen by such cultures as practical means of avoiding unwanted or intellectually, or physically handicapped progeny. Philo the Jew, around the time of Jesus, had linked abortion and infanticide: "The same prohibition [on abortion] applies to another greater form of wrongdoing, namely the exposure of infants, an outrage which has become a common practice among many other peoples." Justin Martyr in the second century wrote that exposing infants was wicked because it led to debauchery (on the basis that children were found alive and taken by strangers) as well as murder. At the same time Barnabas ordained "Thou shalt kill neither the fetus by means of abortion, nor the newborn child". In 318 Constantine outlawed fathers killing their children under the rights of paterfamilias, but it wasn't until 374 that the killing of newborn children was identified as murder (Ranke-Heinemann R551 54).

John Chrysostom inveighs against all forms of non-reproductive sex and any control of fertility, including contraception and abortion:

"Why do you scatter your seed where the field is at pains to destroy the harvest, where pregnancies are avoided by all or any means, where murder is committed prior to birth? Even a harlot you do not suffer to remain a harlot; you make her a murderess as well. ... There is indeed something worse than murder, and I know not what to call it, for such women do not kill what has taken shape, they prevent it from taking shape at all"

However in the place of abortion, infanticide and exposure, early Christians appear to have substituted frank abandonment. John Boswell (R71), noting a peculiar piece of advice given by early theologians: That 'men should be careful never to visit brothels, or have recourse to prostitutes, because in doing so they might unwittingly commit incest', realized the implication - not occasional, but wholesale abandonment of their offspring by the Christian forefathers. "The deeper Boswell delved, the clearer it became that very nearly the majority of women living in Rome during the first three centuries of the Christian era, who had reared more than one child, had abandoned at least one. He found himself looking at rates of abandonment around 20 to 40 percent of children born. If Romans gave to crippled beggars it was because 'everyone is afraid he might say no to his own child'." Judging by later statistics, a vast majority of those abandoned would have died. (Hrdy R323 297).

The 'Demon Rod' that wouldn't Lie Down

In Uta Ranke-Heinemann's words (R551 62):

"St Augustine, the greatest of all the Fathers of the Church, was the man responsible for welding Christianity and hostility to sexual pleasure into a systematic whole. His influence on the development of the Christian sexual ethic is undisputed, and the papal condemnations of the contraceptive Pill were heavily coloured by it. To speak of sexual hostility, therefore, is to speak of Augustine. He was the theological thinker who blazed a trail for the ensuing centuries indeed, for the ensuing millennium-and-a-half. ... Theologically, he established a relationship between original sin, which played so great a part in his redemptive system, and enjoyment of the sexual act. To him, original sin betokened eternal death and damnation for all who had not been saved, that is to say, delivered by God's grace from 'the multitude of the damned' to which all human beings belonged. Salvation was, however, denied to many even ... to unbaptized children".

In 'Confessions' Augustine wrote that he had several love affairs as a young man. After turning twenty, however, he chose one woman with whom he lived, apparently monogamously, for the next thirteen years. Augustine chose [her] because he loved her; and he slept with her because he loved to'. While still living with his mistress, however, Augustine joined the Manichaeans, a sect that saw the world divided into two realms, God's and Satan's ,which saw light and dark, locked in permanent conflict and the soul, a spark of light, seeking to escape the darkness of the physical world, and taught that all sexual activity aided the powers of evil. Augustine was an auditor in the group, a rank below the Elect, who abstained from sex totally and ate as little as possible. Augustine, not yet the man he would become, responded with a now famous prayer of his own: "Lord, give me chastity, but not now." Then, walking in the garden, he heard a childs voice chanting "Take it, read it" and his eye caught the following passage:

"Let us walk honestly, as in the day; not in rioting and drunkenness, not in chambering and wantonness, not in strife and envying. But put ye on the Lord Jesus Christ, and make not provision for the flesh, to fulfil the lusts thereof" Rom 13:13).

Augustine's conversion in the year 387, when he was 29, while reading a passage of Pauline Platonism, was hard luck on the married. He repudiated his common-law partner 'she had sensed my unthinking ardour, albeit she was my only mistress', and on whom he had fathered a son. His mistress, unnamed although he felt a 'sharp and searing pain' on their separation swore to remain eternally faithful to him when he sent her away. "Since the one whose bed I used to share was wrested from my side, being as it were an impediment to my marriage, my heart, because it clung to her was deeply wounded and bled". Nevertheless, he called his relations with her "a loose bond of impure love in which children are most unwelcome, even if they subsequently constrain us to love them" His mother was making preparations for a suitable marriage, but the wealthy prospective bride of her choice was only 12 and had yet to attain marriageable age. Rather than wait another two years, Augustine took another mistress" (Haskins R291 71, Friedman R225 37, Ranke Heinemann R551 61).

His strict observance of contraceptive methods and attention to his partner's infertile days, foiled by the miscalculation that resulted in the birth of his son, was succeeded after his conversion by a fanatical campaign against contraception of all kinds, although, following Leviticus and Aristotelian biology, Augustine and Jerome considered the fetus was not 'human' for up to 80 days: "The seed takes gradual shape in the uterus, and it does not count as killing until the various elements have acquired their outward appearance and their members." He nevertheless pronounced a comprehensive ban on all forms of birth control: "It is impermissible and vile to have intercourse with one's wife and avoid the conception of pregnancy" Contraceptive herbal and other medications and cervical barriers, which had been known from the time of the Egyptians in 2000 BC were particularly singled out: "Sometimes this cruel lust is such that they even procure poisons of infertility so that the wife actually becomes the husband's whore or he an adulterer with his own wife."

Augustine's epiphany was tautological: he was powerless to control the penis because free choice is an illusion. Adam's birthright at Creation was freedom, defined by Augustine as the ability to obey God, yet Adam scorned that gift because he wanted the "freedom to do wickedness." Adam's sin deprived his descendants of the freedom to choose not to sin. The ultimate embodiment of this, Augustine wrote, is "disobedience in the member." After Adam and Eve flouted God's will by eating the forbidden fruit, they experienced two new sensations: shame at their nakedness and sexual stirrings they could not control. "We are ashamed of that very thing which made those beings ashamed, when they covered their loins." That "very thing" is a spontaneous erection. Before sinning, Adam and Eve had mastery over sex, procreating as an act of volition, "the way one commands his feet when he walks." But since leaving Eden men have become powerless over, and tortured by, erections. "At times the urge intrudes uninvited," Augustine wrote in City of God. "At other times, it deserts the panting lover, and, although desire blazes in the mind, the body is frigid." With this one stroke, this one man transformed the penis more than any man who had yet lived: the sacred staff became the demon rod. "Everyone is necessarily evil and carnal through Adam," Augustine wrote. The agent transferring this stigma from one generation to the next is semen. This "astonishing argument," declared that "every human is born contaminated." (Pagels R512, Friedman R225 37). To Augustine, the sin of Adam and Eve had not been sexual intercourse but their presumption, in their desire for knowledge, to rival their Creator. Concupiscence affected the whole being, as man in his fallen state no longer had control over himself, and was prey to agitations of the flesh. Adam and Eve's sin lay not in the sexual act, but the lust accompanying a procreative process, which would otherwise have occurred with angelic apathy.

Ambrose, a champion of orthodoxy, and an ardent advocate of the Virgin Mary, taught that Adam and Eve had fallen from a state of 'original perfection' and adopting this thesis, Augustine wrote in glowing terms of the life that Adam had originally had in Paradise, exempt from all physical evils or sickness, endowed with immortal youth, and with the possibility of immortality, through eating of the tree of life. Adam's intellect and moral character had been equally elevated. He had, however, misused the free will given him by his Creator, and succumbed to temptation. As a punishment, he had acquired a moral debility, concupiscence, which was transmuted through physical heredity to his descendents, who were thus rendered a massa damnata. To Augustine, death had come upon all human beings by their union with Adam, and they also shared in the responsibility for the Fall; he thereby denied that humanity had a free moral choice. "For we were all in that one man ... who fell into sin through the woman who was made from him" (Haskins R291 76, Jones R340 22).

In 'City of God' (413-26) he notes that it would be "a manifest absurdity to deny that the sexual differences were created for begetting children. But marriage would have taken place in Paradise without the accompanying - 'lust'." Augustine tells us that before the Fall, Adam had been capable of moving his sexual member with as much control as fallen man might exercise over a finger. But now, infected by the stain of original sin, the sexual organs functioned with no regard to their owner, in retribution for their sin of disobedience. "Without the allurement of passion goading him on, the husband would have relaxed on his wife's bosom in tranquillity of mind and with no impairment of his body's integrity". After their sin our first parents covered their parts of in shame of their pudenda (Latin, pudendus shameful). Eve's formation from Adam's rib rendered her the weaker part of the couple, and she compounded her subordinate role as helper by tempting Adam to fall. Adam's culpability lay merely in his desire please his spouse (Haskins R291 77).

Pelagius also held that the Fall had come about through God's gift of free will, but denied that the sin of Adam and Eve had been passed on to their descendants - it had been theirs alone - and thus rejected St Paul's pronouncement in his letter to the Romans. Augustine disputed with Pelagius and claimed that humanity had no free will, but was doomed to transgress because original sin - estrangement from God - was congenital and universal. To allow man freedom to decide minimized the role of God and the power of the Church. Pelagius was twice accused of heresy, partly through Augustine's bribing of the emperor and died soon after (Pagels R512 129-30). One of his followers, Julian of Eclanum challenged Augustine back. Augustine summoning all his eloquence and fury argued for a view of nature utterly antithetical to scientific naturalism. Augustine's error Julian believed, was to regard the present state of nature as punishment, for Augustine went further than those Jews and Christians who agreed that Adam's sin brought death upon the human race. He insisted that Adam's sin also brought upon us universal moral corruption. Julian responded that 'natural sin' does not exist. No physically transmitted, hereditary condition infects human nature, much less nature in general. (Pagels R512 132-3). In reply, Augustine releases the Pandora's box of genetic abnormality: "If nothing deserving punishment passes from parents to infants, who could bear to see the image of God sometimes born retarded, since this afflicts the soul itself. You must explain why such innocence is sometimes born blind or deaf." citing even children's suffering and of course mortality as original sin. Augustine took things to other impossible lengths, claiming that before the Fall there were no weeds, an age of innocence which defies all biological realities. Pagels comments that Augustine denies nature, the existence of nature *per se* ... for he cannot think of the natural world except as a reflection of human desire and will.

Julian rejected the notion of natural sin and accused Augustine of retaining his Manichaean heresy, insisting the church was founded on the praise of creation, marriage, law, saints and will. In counter to Augustine's reading of pain in childbirth he pointed out naturally that [pagan] village women with good childbirth practice had easy deliveries. Julian sees childbirth pains, death, being ruled by a husband and living by the sweat of labor as conditions of nature, not punishment, noting that sweat is a beneficial, not sinful, response to exertion and that Adam anyway had to "dress and keep" the garden before the Fall. Julian's greatest feat however was to correctly realize that the fall is the existential situation that arises when we fall into the sin of separation from the whole and make the world harsh through our selfishness (Pagels R512 136-8). Augustine saw Julian's "vital fire" of the natural 'appetite' of sexual desire as that "which does not obey the soul's decision, but for the most part, rises up against the soul's desire in disorderly and ugly movements". The ultimate punishment - to be tormented by 'natural' sexual arousal. And by Julian, who continued to reject his arguments until Augustine's death.

Augustine's theory of original sin not only proved politically expedient, since it persuaded many of his contemporaries that human beings universally need external government ... but also offered an analysis of human nature that became, for better or worse, the heritage of all subsequent generations of western Christians (Pagels R512 xxvi). Such was Augustine's later reputation that his views were to permanently color the Christian view of sin, sexuality and the female. Augustine's doctrine was austere. As children were born full of sin they were damned if they died before baptism. Hell, he said, was paved with infants.

He could not understand why God had chosen the sexual option, and the opportunity it gave for sin, for the Garden of Eden. After debating whether there was sexual intercourse before the Fall or merely metaphorical fruitfulness or asexual reproduction he resigned himself to the idea that a woman was chosen because of her 'generative purpose': "If it was good company and conversation that Adam needed, it would have been much better arranged to have two men together as friends, not a man and a woman" (Jones R339 222). Ranke-Heinemann notes: (R551 73) "women to their great dismay had been pronounced fit only for childbearing and unqualified for anything of a spiritual or intellectual nature".

The contortions to which Christian and particularly Catholic thinking went to suppress sexual pleasure are accounted in full by Uta Ranke-Heinemann (R551) in 'Eunuchs for Heaven'. Augustine's concern with sin was extended to a form of sexual slavery in which women were expected to be sexual 'nurses' offering themselves to their husbands, even at risk of death, or when still in child bed, if there was any chance of male extra-marital fornication (133). Later the view in which marriage was a remedy for sexual desire evolved into high scholasticism in which the grace conferred by marriage consisted of its suppression of sexual desire (136).

In a bizarre twist, the 'restrained embrace' of Cardinal Huguccio (d1210) consisted of satisfying the 'incontinent' demands of a wife for sex by withholding male orgasm (150) in a pleasureless form of Tantrism (p 462).

> I can so render my wife her due and wait in such manner as she assuages her desire. Indeed often on such occasions a woman is want to anticipate her husband, and when the wife's desire for the carnal work is assuaged, I can if I wish withdraw, free from all sin, without assuaging my own desire, or emitting my seed of propagation.

In turn, inducing orgasm in the wife in this way also became a mortal sin. Female orgasm by now was associated with a 'semen' of its own, following Galen's attribution of it to procreation in contrast to Aristotle. In what Ranke-Heinemann (156) describes as theology's golden age and woman's darkest hour, Albertus Magnus declared that woman was 'less suited to morality':

> For woman contains more fluid than man, and is characteristic of fluid to absorb readily and retain poorly. Fluid is easily moved, so women are inconstant and inquisitive. When a woman has intercourse with one man, she would feign lie underneath another at the same time. Woman is a stranger to fidelity. ... Woman is an imperfect man and possesses compared to him, a defective and deficient nature She is therefore insecure in herself. That which she herself cannot receive, she endeavours to obtain by means of mendacity and devilish tricks. In short therefore, one must beware of every woman as one would a poisonous serpent and the horned devil.

Protestantism was by no means immune from this mentality. The fall, for Luther as well as Augustine had brought the debasement of sex into lust and a more coercive subjugation of woman to punish her for her priority in sin. In Luther's words (Ruether R586 74):

> The rule remains with the husband and the wife is compelled to obey him by God's command. He rules the home and the state, wages war, defends his possessions, tills the soil, plants etc. The wife on the other hand is like a nail driven into a wall. She sits at home.

In this, Luther, who espoused marriage rather than celibacy, looks to a natural procreation based on a well-defined and brief estrus in the absence of sexual desire, hinting also that before the Fall, women held social power and esteem (Young R758 85):

> if the woman had not been deceived by the serpent and had not sinned, she would have been the equal of Adam in all respects. For the punishment, that she is now subjected to the man, was imposed on her after sin and because of sin, just as the other hardships and dangers were: travail, pain, and countless other vexations. Therefore Eve was not like the woman of today; her state was far better and more excellent... In addition - and this is lamentable - woman is also necessary as an antidote against sin. And so, in the case of the woman, we must think not only of the managing of the household which she does, but also of the medicine which she is. In this respect Paul says (1 Cor. 7:2): "Because of fornication let each one have his own wife." ... Therefore we are compelled to make use of this sex in order to avoid sin. It is almost shameful to say this, but nevertheless it is true. For there are very few who marry solely as a matter of duty. But the rest of the animals do not have this need. Consequently, for the most part they copulate only once a year and then are satisfied with this as if by duty. But the conduct of human beings is different. They are compelled to make use of intercourse with their wives in order to avoid sin. ... If Adam has persisted in the state of innocence, this intimate relationship

would have been most delightful. The very work of procreation would have been most sacred and would have been held in esteem. ... Therefore was this fall not a terrible thing?

The end result is to accept reproduction, but to deny any form of sexual pleasure. To invoke the rule of man but deny the redemptive power of woman. It is also to imbue all the natural world, which was originally paradisiacal, with the culpability of human original sin, explaining 'natural evil' as ultimately a consequence of human concupiscence. Yet only humans are capable of potential immortality through the redemption of Christ. In Rosemary Radford Ruether's (R585 30) words in 'Gaia and God': "On the one hand, humans are said to be guilty for the inadequacies of the rest of nature ... On the other hand humans bear no ultimate responsibility for the rest of creation. Animal and plant life can be exploited at will by humans as our possessions. They have no personhood in their own that need to be respected, and we share no common fate with them. These ambiguities in the Christian world picture ... have contributed to ecological irresponsibility."

Freedom of Spirit and the Christian Dark Ages

While Augustine did acknowledge that marriage provided three virtues, progeny, channeling the lust of the flock through fidelity and the sacrament of marriage which was a reflection of that between Christ and 'his' church, it was still a secondary condition not quite fully Christian in the sense of the new 'virginal' age ushered in by Christ and Mary. There was at the same time a major move towards clerical celibacy. Although early Christian celibacy was a shared attitude among all, 1 Timothy had spoken of the priesthood in terms of paterfamilias and priests were generally fathers. But from the Council of Elivira in 309, all bishops, presbyters and deacons were called to give up sex with their wives as a condition of ordination (Ruther R586 47). In the eastern church both patterns coexisted. This council also excommunicated women for remarriage but only advised against it for men and banned women from writing or receiving letters in their own name (Ranke-Heinemann R551 26, 112).

However these reforms were not to be of lasting effect. In the fourth century, Germanic and Celtic expansion resulted in a significant change of marriage patterns. They practised a 'resource polygyny' that allowed powerful chiefs to accumulate a plurality of wives and concubines. A marriage involved a dowry and possibly estates. In addition the chief could have 'free love' concubines (Ruether R586 52). Divorce was by mutual consent with the wife expected to take her wedding gifts with her. This enabled some women to gain political power through their combined familial associations, but many women were thus monopolized by the elite men. Although the clergy railed at these practices, many also adopted them. The church attempted to unravel these associations asserting monogamy along with exogamy to the seventh degree. Since marriages were secular and often informal it was hard for the church to define the actual marital status even of nobility, but they concentrated their attention on the principal wife, who was often in a political marriage for dynastic ends. A host of tolerated concubinages continued unrecognized. A sharp distinction between legitimate and illegitimate liaisons and their offspring was now drawn.

In the eleventh century the papal reform movement sought to take control of all church offices and property to prevent nobility from appointing religious positions and the control of their estates as extensions of family holdings. The clergy accused the nobility of simony and married priests as fornicators and heretics while their opponents accused them of being sodomites who preferred other men to marriage. The reformists had significant victories and the nobility, in response sought more consolidated control over their own lands and family systems, through male primogeniture and patrilineage. Ordination was again made a bar to marriage and illegitimacy a bar to ordination. The male population was thus split in Europe between a celibate priesthood and a married laity. The fallout, as we have seen today is a priesthood riddled with pederasty, paedophilia, and other forms of sexual abuse.

In the same century the Crusades began, following the capture of Jerusalem, blocking the road to pilgrimage and the defeat of the Byzantine army. Hopes of the Papacy for reunification of East and West, the nobility's hunger for land at a time of crop failures, population pressure in the West, and an alternative to warfare at home were major impulses, lured by the fabulous riches of the East and as a means of extending trade routes. The First Crusade was launched by Pope Urban II in 1095. With the cry *Deus vult!* ("God wills it"), thousands took the cross. Bands of poorly armed pilgrims, inexperienced and poor, set out for Constantinople under Peter The Hermit and Walter the Penniless even before the army gathered. Some began by massacring Jews in the Rhine valley. Many perished on their way east, and the rest were destroyed by the Muslims when they crossed into Anatolia. Ten thousand French of utter cruelty had plundered the territory. They dismembered babies, others they put on spits and roasted over a fire, those of advanced years, they subjected to every form of torture. The Turkish sultan ambushed them by pandering to their greed for the spoils of war. Such a large number of Franks became the victim of the Turkish swords that, when the remains of the slaughtered men were collected, "they made a huge mountain, deep and wide, most remarkable, so great were the pile of bones" (Hallam R275 67-8).

Treachery for greed again unwound the second Crusade when Damascus failed to be taken because some men received a vast sum of money to misdirect the attack. Sexual misadventure among the high court ladies also weakened and confused the campaign, with Elanor of Aquitane cuckolding the king for her uncle and reputedly Saladin as well. Women were later denied the right to object to their husbands leaving on Crusade to force support, but begrudgingly it was acknowledged that women needed to accompany the men to populate new lands. Women were involved in hand to hand combat with long knives.

The third Crusade began after Saladin took most of Palestine, Syria and Mesopotamia. The effort disintegrated through attrition and lack of cooperation, although Acre was recaptured, Jaffa was secured, and Cyprus occupied. Richard the Lion-heart, beloved of Robin Hood, presided over the beheading of 2700 Islamic men, women and children of Acre, illustrating the Christian will to religious genocide and a breach of faith. By contrast, Saladin was a man of honour. When a French woman came to him during a siege saying "Yesterday some Muslim thieves entered my tent and stole my little girl. My commanders told me the King of the Muslims is merciful". Saladin was touched. He sent someone to the slave market to search and within an hour a horseman arrived bearing the child on his shoulders (Hallam 157).

In the eleventh century, the violence and treachery of the Crusades began to turn on its own people. Contact with the holy land had led to a revival of gnostic ideas. The idea took firm hold around Albi, in southern France. Soon, its adherents the Albigenses and Cathars - the *katharol*, with an elite of *perfecti* or pure ones - controlled much of the Languedoc. They believed in two eternal principles of good and evil, did not acknowledge the sacraments, the doctrines of hell or purgatory, or the resurrection of the body and developed their own ceremony and ritual, rejecting the authority of the Church. They had lives of simplicity and penance in which salvation lay only in the Lord. The Pope became alarmed at the threat to his power and proclaimed a crusade against them. Thousands of Cathars were killed and many more tortured into accepting the true faith. Laws were passed to suppress the Albigensian heresy, and the first Inquisition established to ensure that they were applied.

Early in the war, both Cathars and Catholics were besieged by an army of the Church within the walls of Beziers. On the day of the feast of Mary Magdalen they killed their viscount in the church dedicated to her name and were in turn horrendously punished on the same day for repeating the Albigensian heresy that she was Christ's concubine. When the city fell, the commanding general was asked who to slaughter: heretics, his men assumed, must surely be separated from believers. Their leader's reply was simple: "Kill them all," he said, "the Lord will know his own". (Haskins R291 135, Jones R339 223, 241). Our forces spared neither rank nor sex nor age. About twenty thousand people lost their lives at the point of the sword. The destruction of the enemy was on an enormous scale. The entire city was plundered and put to the torch. Thus did divine vengeance vent its wondrous rage (Hallam R275 232).

"After discussion, our men entered the town of Carcassonne with the cross in front. When the church had been restored they placed the Lord's cross on top of the tower ... for it was Christ who had captured the town and it was right that his banner should take precedence. ... The venerable abbot of Vaux-de-Cernay went to a great number of heretics who had gathered in one of the houses wishing to convert them to better things, but they all said with one voice 'Why are you preaching to us? We don't want your faith We deny the church of Rome. You are wasting your time. Neither life nor death can turn us from the beliefs we hold.' He then went to see the women gathered in another building but the female heretics were more obstinate and difficult in every way. Simon de Montfort first urged the heretics to convert, but having no success, he dragged them out of the castle. A huge fire was kindled and they were all thrown into it. It was not hard for our men to throw them in, for they were so obstinate in their wickedness that they threw themselves in. Only three women escaped, whom a noble lady snatched from the flames and restored to the Holy Church" (Hallam R275 234).

The papal Inquisition was formally instituted by Pope Gregory IX in 1231 as an extension of the Albigensian Crusade. This has become the most diabolical manifestation of a religion projecting the jealousy of God. A jealousy in the form of religious paranoia in which any form of deviation is seen as a diabolical act of the Devil, with whom God is at war, so that any act of violence becomes permissible, regardless of any standards of humanity, or justice.

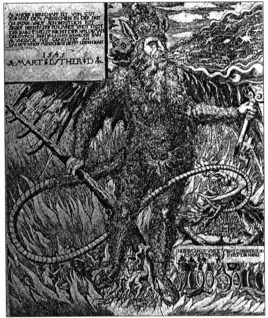

The Pope as the anti-Christ (Cohn R124)

Along with public disgust at the church's avarice, there was a growing suspicion, sparked by gnostic philosophies, that rejected the church's myths of the garden of Eden, the fall, original sin, heaven and hell, the virgin birth, the meaning of salvation, the flesh and blood Eucharist. The church responded with calculated violence. Following a law of Holy Roman Emperor Fredrick II, Gregory ordered convicted heretics to be seized by the secular authorities and burned. The power of the Inquisition was established and enlarged by a series of papal bulls. That of Pope Innocent IV, in 1252, authorized seizure of their goods, imprisonment, torture, and, on conviction, death, all on minimal and highly selective evidence. It was in historian Henry Charles Lea's words: "a standing mockery of justice - perhaps the most iniquitous that the arbitrary cruelty of man has ever devised.... Fanatic zeal, arbitrary cruelty, and insatiable cupidity rivalled each other in building up a system unspeakably atrocious.

Notoriously harsh in its procedures, the Inquisition was defended during the Middle Ages by appeal to biblical practices and to Augustine, who had interpreted Luke 14:23 "And the lord said unto the servant, Go out into the highways and hedges, and compel them to come in, that my house may be filled." as endorsing the use of force against heretics. However the version in Thomas 64 says: "The master said to his servant, 'Go outside to the streets and bring back those whom you happen to meet, so that they may dine'"

It was a system which might well seem the invention of demons." St. Bernard deplored the church's greed: "Whom can you show me among the prelates who does not seek rather to empty the pockets of his flock than to subdue their vices?" Bulgarian writers said the priests of Rome were given to drunkenness and robbery, and "there is none to forbid them." Priests were a privileged class, but their privileges were more and more resented. In the 12th century, monasteries made themselves into wine shops and gambling houses;

nunneries became private whore-houses for the clergy; priests used a confessional to seduce female parishioners (Walker R708). The Spanish Inquisition was particularly severe and selected out ex-Jews and ex-Moslems who had previously been forced to convert to Christianity. Mass burnings on the Iberian peninsula were known as 'acts of faith'. They were held once a month on the average, usually on a Sunday or holiday so all could attend; to stay away was thought suspicious. Sometimes the spectators were invited to participate, as in the diversion genially known as "shaving the new Christians." This meant setting fire to the hair or beards of those waiting their turn at the stake. The power of the inquisitors extended to the Americas where the Aztecs marvelled at the similarity of the communion to their own human sacrificial rite and identfied Cortez and the conquistadors with Quetzalcoatl who was prophesied to return. Extreme Catholics committed violent atrocities in the face of pagan practices killing and dismembering the native population, merely for playing heathen native music (Gruzinski R267).

After arrest, the property of the accused was instantly confiscated. Nothing seems to have been returned. The popes publicly praised the rule of confiscation as a prime weapon against heresy. Affluent Italy made its inquisitors incredibly rich in the 14th century. "When I have you tortured, and by the severe means afforded by the law I bring you to confession, then I perform a work pleasing in God's sight; and it profiteth me." Torture was officially sanctioned in 1257 and remained a legal recourse of the church for five and a half centuries until it was abolished by Pope Pius VII in 1816.

A major target of the Inquisition was the Free Spirit movement (Lerner R398, Cohn R124, Zweig R769), which both represented a pure historical form of liberal gnosticism and a central threat to Christian sexual repression. It is believed to have originated from Sufis who entered Spain a century or two before, who had themselves had contact with liberal gnostic elements in the East, who held a tradition of complete assumption of Christ nature. The word 'beggar' comes from the male begherds and female beguines of the 'Heresy of the Free Spirit' whose followers embraced sexual freedom and enlightened amorality, allowing all actions to be permissible to the initiates who had experienced the godhead in inner ecstasy. During the twelfth to fourteenth centuries the movement became very popular in certain sections of society and was part of the widespread pilgrimage circuit. The begherds were wandering males who spiritually supported and sexually exploited, lonely women and widows. The beguines came from often wealthy families in a social situation where there was an excess of unpartnered women as a result of both war and the large number of men committed to celibate duties in the church.

On the last day of May, 1310, Marguerite Porete was burned at the Place de Grieve in what the first formal *auto de fe* (burning to death of heretics) of which we have cognizance at Paris. Her book had been condemned and burned in her presence by the Bishop of Cambrai, who warned her not to disseminate her ideas or writings any further under pain of being relaxed to the secular arm. The admonition, however, was to no avail. Between 1306 and 1308 Marguerite was brought before the new Bishop and the Inquisitor of Lorraine. This time she was accused of propagating it among simple people and beghards. Instead of acting further themselves her judges apparently sent her to Paris where we know that she was taken into custody by the Dominican Inquisitor. There Marguerite refused to answer any questions or even to take the vows necessary for her examination and languished in prison for almost a year and a half. But in 1310 the Inquisitor, for want of direct testimony, extracted a list of articles from Marguerite's book and presented them for examination to twenty-one theological regents of the University of Paris, who unanimously declared the articles to be heretical. 'Mirror of Simple Souls' taught that a soul annihilated in the love of the Creator could, and should, grant to nature all that it desires. It invokes the realms of enlightenment, outstripping the Christian orthodox view, as the higher levels of illumination are reached with an autonomous realization of God-nature or Christ-nature that we are God's sons like Christ without distinction. The Mirror was very popular throughout Europe and was translated into many European languages and had a vigorous life in England.

The Free Spirit movement sanctified the sexual act of intercourse as 'Christerie'. According to John of Viktring's description, men and women of various classes assembled at midnight in an underground hideaway which they named a temple. There 'a priest of the devil' said mass and delivered a sermon. Then the assembly put out the lights, chose partners, and feasted, danced, and fornicated. This, they said, was the state of paradise in which Adam and Eve lived before the fall. Their leader called himself Christ and claimed that though condemned to be executed he would rise on the third day. He presented a beautiful young virgin as Mary, but taught that Christ was not born of a virgin, that God was neither born nor suffered, and that fasting was unnecessary.

The decree of Vienne listed eight errors of an abominable sect of malignant men known as Begherds and faithless women known as beguines in the Kingdom of Germany which are generally considered to be the essence of the Free Spirit heresy. The first tenet was the central one. This stated that man can attain such a degree of perfection in his earthly life that he is incapable of sin. In this state he can achieve no additional grace because such would give him a perfection superior to Christ. The second point followed that such a man need not fast or pray because in his state of perfection sensuality is so subordinated to reason that he can accord freely to his body all that pleases him. Similarly the third point was that such a man is not subject to human obedience or to any laws of the Church because "where the spirit of the Lord is, there is liberty" (2 Cor. 3:17). The following five propositions were elaborations or consequences of the first three: man can attain final blessedness just as much in this life as in the other; such men do not need the light of glory to be elevated to the vision and enjoyment of God; the acts of virtue are only necessary for imperfect men, but the perfect soul no longer needs them; a kiss is a mortal sin when nature does not demand it, but the sexual act itself is not sinful when demanded by nature; and it is not necessary to rise or show any sign of reverence during the elevation of the host because to think of the sacrament of the Eucharist or the passion of Christ would be a sign of imperfection and a descent from the heights of contemplation.

Marguerite Porete shared her inquisitional fate with a converted Jew who was supposed to have relapsed and to have spat in a fit of contempt on an image of the Virgin. The reason why scandalous charges were launched, often independently, against medieval heretics is similar to why they were launched so frequently against Jews. The Church considered Jews, sorcerers, and heretics, each in their way, as minions of the devil whose threat was age-old. Christians have never been able to forget that the Jews rejected Jesus and demanded his death. For centuries Christians were convinced that the Jews failure to accept the Christian faith was due to a stubborn perversity that must have the Devil behind it.

Burning of Jews 1390 (Cohn 1957)

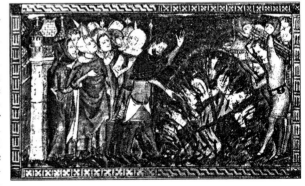

This gave rise to the legend of the ritual murder of Christian children at Passover, a symbolic perpetuation of the Crucifixion. As late as the sixteenth century the dwellers in the European ghettos lived in continual terror of being framed for this crime by the Christians. Trials for ritual murder were still occurring in Central Europe through the turn of the nineteenth century. In the meantime, the assumption of Jewish depravity had been giving the followers of Christ carte blanche - not merely with a quiet conscience but with fervour and exaltation - to penalize, tax, torture and slaughter the Jews, under the sign of the crucified Jesus" anticipating Shoah (Wilson R736 104).

In a climactic culmination of centuries of persecution, the Roman Church remained silent in acquiescent knowledge of the holocaust of six million Jews during the second world war.

> [Hitler] said it was one of the most important tasks to guard Germany's coming generations from the same political fate that struck the country from 1918 to 1933, to keep vigilant in them the awareness of racial danger. For this reason alone the Oberammergau Festival [the re-enactment of the crucifixion] would absolutely have to be preserved. For hardly ever had the Jewish danger, as seen in the example of the ancient Roman empire, been so graphically illustrated as by the character of Pontius Pilate in the Festival. He appeared as a Roman whose racial and intellectual superiority is so great that he seemed a rock amid the swarming rabble of the Near East. In recognizing the enormous importance of the Festival for the enlightenment of future generations as well, he [Hitler] said he was an absolute Christian. (Rolf Hochhuth, Der Stellvertreter, historische Streiflichter 1980, 247)

The witch hunts form an extension of the Inquisitional process and its greater complex of male paranoia directed right into the heart of European women. Europe had associations with the fertility goddess predating the spread of Christian ideas, as hinted at in the Arthurian legends of Avalon. Appreciation for feminine spirituality, power and medicinal arts continued through the Christian era. European villages still hid many "wise-women" who acted as priestesses officially or unofficially. Since church fathers declared Christian priestesses unthinkable, all functions of the priestess were associated with paganism. These included arts of midwifery, beliefs in fertility worship in rites such as Beltane.

They also involved the use of powerful hallucinogens based on tropane alkaloids, including scopolamine, based on belladonna, henbane and mandrake (Schultes and Hofmann 86, Rudgley 90). Frequent references can be found in the middle ages to maids found unconscious and naked who had rubbed themselves with a green ointment "in such a way that they imagine they are carried a long distance". The witch's broomstick was also a device to apply such ointments to the vaginal mucosae to induce such 'flying', enough in itself to drive Christian men to madness. The link with the Inquisition is also clear. "Dominus Augustinus de Turre the most cultivated physician of his time notes:

> "when the Inquisition of Como was being carried out, in Lugano the wife of a notary of the Inquisition was accused of being a witch and sorceress. Her husband, who was troubled and thought her a holy woman, early on Good Friday when he missed her found her naked in a corner of the pigsty displaying her genitals, completely unconscious and smeared wit the excrement of the pigs. He went to draw his sword but hesitating she awoke and prostrated herself before him confessing that she had gone that night on the journey. When the accusers came to take her for burning she had vanished, possibly drowned in the lake nearby" (Harner R285 134).

Knowledge of the details of such use of herbs was carefully gleaned by the Papal office. The physician of Pope Julius II in 1545 took the jar of ointment of an accused couple seized as witches, which was so heavy and offensive and soporiferous to the ultimate degree, composed of hemlock, nightshade, henbane and mandrake. This was anointed from head to toe on the wife of the hangman who was restless with suspicion of her husband:

> "She became comatose and could be wakened by no one for 36 hours with her eyes open like a rabbit. Her first words were 'Why do you wake me at such an inopportune time? I was surrounded by all the pleasures and delights of the world' and to her husband "Knavish one, know that I have made you a cuckold, and with a lover younger and better than you" (R285 135).

Johannes Nieder in 1692 gives the following account of a woman who believed herself to be literally transported through the air during the night with Diana and the other women and invited a priest to witness the event:

> "having placed a large bowl on top of a stool, she stepped into it and sat herself down. Then rubbing ointment on herself to the accompaniment of magic incantations, she lay her head back and fell asleep. With the labour of the devil she dreamed of Mistress Venus and other superstitions so vividly that crying out with a shout and striking her hands about, she jarrd the bowl in which she was sitting and falling down from the stool seriously injured herself about the head. As she lay there awakened the priest cried out 'Where are you? You are not with Diana ... you never left this bowl!'" (R285 131).

Remy in the late 16th century makes this matter clear: "Now if witches, after being aroused from an 'iron' sleep tell of things they have seen in places so far distant as compared with the short period of their sleep, the only conclusion is that there had been some substantial journey like that of the soul" (R285 132). A similar explanation applies to lycanthropy the belief that one can change into the form of an animal (ibid 140).

Christians perceived in the rites of the horned god and his 'wiccan' counterparts frank coitus with the devil in the form of incubi and succubi. Bishops described pagan gatherings in their dioceses, attended by "devils ... in the form of men and women." John of Salisbury wrote that it was the devil, "with God's permission," who sent people to gatherings in honor of the Queen of the Night, a priestess impersonating the Moon-goddess under the name of Noctiluca or Herodiade. Others taking flying potions invoked Diana.

"Thou shalt not suffer a witch to live" (Ex 22:18).

Although Exodus had from old cast a death curse of witchcraft, it had not been illegal. Witchcraft was allowed through the first half of the Christian era. It was not called a "heresy" until the 14th century. In 500 AD the Franks' Salic Law recognized witches' right to practice. In 643, an edict declared it illegal to burn witches. In 785, the Synod of Paderborn said anyone who burned a witch must be sentenced to death.

The phenomenon of the witch hunts became a religious war of a jealous God and his church against women, perpetrated by Catholics and Protestants alike in which by some estimates over four million people died. Geographically, the center of witch-burning lay in Germany, Austria, and Switzerland, but few areas were left untouched by it. The chronicler of Treves reported that in the year 1586, the entire female population of two villages was wiped out by the inquisitors, except for only two women left alive. A hundred and thirty-three persons were burned in a single day at Quedlinburg in 1589, out of a town of 12,000. Henri Boguet said Germany in 1590 was "almost entirely occupied with building fires (for witches); and Switzerland has been compelled to wipe out many of her villages on their account. Travelers in Lorraine may see thousands and thousands of the stakes to which witches are bound." In 1524, one thousand witches died at Como. Strasbourg burned five thousand in a period of 20 years. The Senate of Savoy condemned 800 witches at one time. Param stated that over thirty thousand were executed in the 15th century. Nicholas Remy said he personally sentenced 800 witches in 15 years and in one year alone forced sixteen witches to suicide. A bishop of Bamberg claimed 600 witches in 10 years; a bishop of Nancy, 800 in 16 years; a bishop of Wurtzburg, 1900 in 5 years. Five hundred were executed within three months at Geneva and 400 in a single day at Toulouse. The city of Traves burned 7,000 witches. This genocide was not confined to the Catholics. The protestant Lutheran prelate Benedict Carpzov, sentenced 20,000 devil-worshippers. Even relatively permissive England killed 30,000 witches between 1542 and 1736. The slaughter went on throughout Christian Europe for nearly five centuries (Young R758, Walker R708).

The Malleus Maleficarum (Hammer of Sorceresses), written by two Dominican Inquisitors, appeared in Germany in 1486 and became the authoritative handbook describing the activities of witches and how to convict them. The misogyny of this text is hysterical in tone and its authors are fixated on sexuality.

> "In the Old Testament the Scriptures have much that is evil to say about women, and this because of the first temptress, Eve, and her imitators; yet afterwards in the New Testament we find a change of name, as from Eva to Ave (as St. Jerome says), and the whole sin of Eve taken away by the benediction of Mary. Therefore preachers should always say as much praise of them as possible. But because in these times this perfidy is more often found in women than in men, as we learn by actual experience, if anyone is curious as to the reason, we may add to what has already been said the following: that since they are feebler both in mind and body, it is not surprising that they should come more under the spell of witchcraft. ... And proverbs xi, as it were describing a woman, says: As a jewel of gold in a swine's snout, so is a fair woman which is without discretion. ... But the natural reason is that she is more carnal than a man, as is clear from her many carnal abominations. And it should be noted that there was a defect in the formation of the first woman, since she was formed from a bent rib, that is, a rib of the breast, which is bent as it were in a contrary direction to a man. And since through this defect she is an imperfect animal, she always deceives."

The Malleus Maleficarum said the accused witch must be "often and frequently exposed to torture. If after being fittingly tortured she refuses to confess the truth, he [the inquisitor] should have other engines of torture brought before her, and tell her that she will have to endure these if she does not confess. If then she is not induced by terror to confess, the torture must be continued." If she remained obdurate, "she is not to be altogether released, but must be sent to the squalor of prison for a year, and be tortured, and be examined very often, especially on the more Holy Days." Centrally at stake is woman's sexuality itself which is deemed to be insatiable:

> "To conclude: All witchcraft comes from carnal lust, which is in women insatiable. See Proverbs 30: There are three things that are never satisfied, yea, a fourth thing which says not, It is enough; that is, the mouth of the womb. Wherefore for the sake of fulfilling their lusts they consort even with devils" (Malleus Maleficarum 47).

It can hardly be doubted that a major driving force of all witch hunts was sadistic sexual perversion. Torturers liked to attack women's breasts and genitals with pincers, pliers, and red-hot irons. Under the Inquisition's rules, little girls were prosecuted and tortured for witchcraft a year earlier than little boys - at 9, as opposed to 10 for boys. Witch hunting generally was directed against the female sex, and the abject helplessness of imprisoned and tortured women invariably encouraged sexual abuse along with every other kind of abuse

The Malleus Maleficarum served to put a large number of women into immediate jeopardy by stating that the activities of midwives can reveal signs of witchcraft. "That witches who are midwives in various ways kill the child conceived in the womb, and procure an abortion; or if they do not this offer new-born children to Devils." At this time in history the great majority of births were attended by midwives, women familiar with childbirth and herbal cures. In other words these women were healers. They were also the confidants of women who wanted to have children and those who did not want children, so they had some knowledge of birth control and abortion. They were experts in sexual matters in a society dominated by a celibate clergy that had confounded sexuality with devil worship. Once the Malleus Maleficarum made the association of midwives with witchcraft these women could be brought before the Inquisition for questioning. Few were found innocent. Thus begun, the witch burning craze continued into the eighteenth century. (Young R758 79)

From ruthlessly organized persecutions on the continent, witch hunts in England became largely cases of village feuds and petty spite. If crops failed, horses ran away, cattle sickened, wagons broke, women miscarried, or butter wouldn't come in the churn, a witch was always found to blame. A woman was convicted of witchcraft for having caused a neighbor's lameness-by pulling off her stockings. Another was executed for having admired a neighbor's baby, which afterward fell out of its cradle and died. Two Glasgow witches were hanged for treating a sick child, even though the treatment succeeded and the child was cured. Joan Cason of Kent went to the gallows in 1586 for having dry thatch on her roof, which sparked when burnt (Walker R708 1078).

Bobbi Low (R416 163) notes a basis for this in sexual conflict over resources:

> "The demographic and economic particulars of witchcraft trials show a pattern that is a logical, if curious, example of conflict over resources and reproduction in a particular culture. The communities in which accusations of witchcraft flourished were communities long torn by internal strife. Witchcraft accusations often originated in property disputes. Women owned almost no property but they were three times as likely to be accused of witchcraft, seven times as likely to be tried, and five times as likely to be convicted of witchcraft then men. Women who held resources alone, and were not likely marriage candidates because their reproductive value was low were significantly more often accused, tried and executed as witches than others".

The edicts that established the Inquisition have never been repealed. They are "officially still part of the Catholic faith, and were used as justification for certain practices as recently as 1969." In January 1998 the Vatican permitted scrutiny of one of the most notorious periods in Roman Catholic Church History when it opened the archives of the department once known as the Inquisition. The secret files, date between 1542 and 1902. The department later became the Holy Office and its successor now is called the Congregation for the Doctrine of the Faith, which controls the orthodoxy of Catholic teaching.

Unraveling the Sacramental Covenant

Regina Schwartz notes that in its Christian sequel, "the covenant comes not in stone, but in the 'fleshly tables of the heart.' John Donne shockingly depicts such a physical inscription of divinity, as rape, even if it is a bondage he relishes." It is this very bondage and spiritual rape that leads to the male violence of God in history.

> *Take me to you, imprison me, for I,*
> *Except y' enthrall me, never shall be free,*
> *Nor ever chaste except you ravish me. (31)*

The invective against the great whore of Babylon, the Goddess Ishtar anathema capitalized:

> *"And upon her forehead was a name written,*
> *MYSTERY, BABYLON THE GREAT,*
> *THE MOTHER OF HARLOTS*
> *AND ABOMINATIONS OF THE EARTH. (Reve)*

is based again on male jealousy of female reproductive choice - a patriarchal desire to split the feminine, contrasting the great whore with the travail 'Miriam' with the twelve stars, standing on the moon, herself another form of Inanna-Ishtar the Queen of Heaven, who long graced the land of milk and honey.

> *"And there appeared a great wonder in heaven; a woman clothed with the sun,*
> *and the moon under her feet, and upon her head a crown of twelve stars.*
> *And she being with child cried, travailing in birth, and pained to be delivered."*

It is ultimately jealousy and motifs of male competition projected on to God which spawned the Crusades, the Inquisition, the holocaust of 6 mllion Jews in Shoah and all the diabolical manifestations of Christianity, from the Colombian Americas to the genocide of witches, the free spirit movement and the gnostic Cathars and Albigenses. This repression was also ironically unraveled by the downfall of Byzantium to the Muslims, liberating the cultural climate of the Renaissance from the Dark Ages, seeding the explosion of scientific knowledge, the industrial revolution, and the rise of social democracies. However the structure of our social institutions, and our attitudes to the world still derive from social coercion. Our lack of interdependence with nature, and our degree of mutual suspicion and resort to the use of lethal force and weapons of mass destruction in the pursuit of a clash of civilizations all stem from patriarchal imperatives coloured by the war of dark and light, a state of crisis, which could bring about our extinction, not only as a culture, but as a species.

This dysfunctional relationship is a 'shotgun marriage' imposed on another type of deeper sexual relationship, which is much more subtle and cosmic. The paradox of an interdependent source consciousness and physical universe, manifest in each of us, falsely portrayed as an arranged marriage forced on us by a jealous God, fearing the almost perpetual infidelity of 'his' people, first Eve, then Adam, then Israel and then all humanity, in an original sin which reeks of repressed female reproductive choice at its very core.

In all these motifs lie a common attribution of the feminine to the nether realms of chaos and the mortal slime of the physical, while man assumes the role of arbiter of cosmic order from the higher conscious realms. But Hochmah Wisdom stands set up from everlasting, co-primal with to God or even primeval in *tohu vu vohu* - the primal 'chaos' even before form and void. In accepting the chaotic within the feminine, even in the face of paternity uncertainty, mankind reengages the sustainable complementarity out of which all life flows -the complementary nature of reality on which subjective consciousness and objective reality, wave and particle, and chaos and order are interdependent in giving rise to natural complexity. All our evidence is that this mystery lies deeper than an external creator deity, through the sentient mind and the physical universe being complementary to one another. We are not just a thought in the mind of a god whose psyche is a reflection of an alpha male who has lost, banished or 'liquidated' his omega *femme fatale*. At the other extreme, the materialism of purely objective science leads to dissolution of the subjective aspect we depend on for our experience as an ephemeral illusion, a mere epi-phenomenon. All our experience of the physical world is gained through the umbilical cord of direct conscious perception, without which it remains unclear the physical universe could have a manifest existence.

The conflict between Yahweh and the whoring Gods and Asherah's groves was a socio-sexual conflict in the transition zone between the quasi-matriarchal society of Laban, where a wife would expect to stay with the her family, and children might be brought up by the wife's immediate relatives, and the staunch patriarchal nomadic shepherd tribes of Jacob and the Benjaminites, where the husband and father ruled. El offered Abraham off-spring spermatogenetically as the stars in the sky and the dust of the Earth. Old Testament intimations of sexual violence abound. The dire homicide metered out to the wife of the Jew who stayed too long with her father - raped and left to die in the gutter - attests to this division, as does the crushing of the bones of the practitioners of fertility worship "on every high hill and under every green tree", who by their anonymous celebration of sex, the power of the feminine, and their untamed revelry, confused the narrow division between the faithful wife and the scarlet whore. Every one emphasizes the sexual nature of this 'covenant' with God.

Islam (p 257), although it does not use the terms of jealousy directly in attempting to arrive at a more abstract form of god, in Al-Llah still articulates the principal themes of male combat myth against the 'infidel', rejection of the female deities which previously accompanied the old high god, and the jealous anger of god in the face of those who do not 'submit' to al-Llah's will. The world is divided between the domain of Islam and the domain of war in an apocalyptic end of days which abets suicidal martyrdom in acts of mass terror. Those who embrace Islam and then have doubts face the death penalty for apostasy, as do all infidels except the believers in the paths of the book - the hanif of Abraham, Jews and Christians. Islam attempts to bind Religion, Law (Sharia) and State into one totalitarian monolith. Islam remains the only religion today in which women are stoned for adultery and female genital mutilation is approved. Although polygynous Islam perceives sex as positive, by comparison with the negative spin given it as original sin fit only for procreation in Christianity, it fears the power and capriciousness of female lust so much that women are secluded in all-enveloping veils, so we may not even be able to see their eyes, let alone their breasts and buttocks and legs, as evolution selected us to do. They remain subject to strict codes of chaperoning, under potentially dire punishment for any deviation, even though heaven is conceived as an erotic garden with 72 black-eyed virgins. A woman is only half the value of a man in legal disputes and less than the dogs in the street in the hadiths. This is little different from the role of woman in the ten commandments in terms of the jealousy of coveting, where the wife is a possession of the husband, more than a beast, but less than a house:

The root message is that our relationship with God has become a sado-masochistic sexual perversion in the name of paternity uncertainty and fear of female sexual energy, which has, in a variety of forms, infiltrated the spontaneous and good nature of human society, to erect a coercive set of social institutions based on male exploitation, frankly risking the end of the world, and a boom and bust confrontation, which could terminate humanity through its very exploitation. This leads to alienation, social injustice and a war of defection between social control and criminality. Along with the violent repression of female reproductive choice through a variety of means, in Helen Fisher's words from 'An Anatomy of Love': "public whipping, branding, beating, ostracism, mutilation of genitals, chopping off nose and ears, slashing feet, chopping off one's hips and thighs, divorce, desertion, death by stoning, burning, drowning, choking, shooting, stabbing", and the frank desecration of women in killing the girl child across much of Asia. Even in our so-called enlightened society, it is signal that the men of this generation are still only beginning to come to terms with how women achieve sexual ecstasy, how to yield to the paradox of this 'divine' feminine force and the challenge to our relationships and social structures female sexuality and the female reproductive investment in continuity and egalitarian networks might bring.

In Kabbalistic thought, the feminine face the Shekhinah retreats in the Fall from paradise, remaining aloof until the final phase , returning as fragmented 'sparks' into integration of the male 'torah' with the feminine face. Closing the circle of jealousy in love means closing the war of dark and light in the matrimonial concord the Shekhinah evokes, as reflected in the pregnant 'queen of heaven' in Revelation departing to the wilderness for a time and a half on Shekhinah's eagle wings, holding the apocalyptic keys to the resolution of the whole existential dilemma of the fall, and with it God's insane jealousy for his paternity.

Holy matrimony, unlike the property heritage of patrimony, arises from the whole condition of relationship, embracing as much the inscrutable reproductive investment of the mother as the desire for paternity certainty of the father.

Islam, Jihad and Sakina

Flags of many Muslim countries bear the ancient astral symbolism that preceded Islam, from Nabatea Astral moon Goddess with zodiac (R242) and Sabean lunar astral symbols (Pritchard R542, Doe R169) see also (Zehren R760).

In the early 19th century holy wars of Islamization in Nigeria relegated the political power of Hausa women, who had been able to hold political positions, become rulers and own land to that of minors who must remain in the home. Female power was pushed underground where it remains as a spiritual guerilla movement. The Hausa creation myth tells the story:

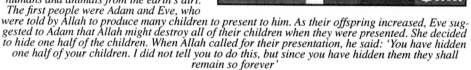

A few hundred years ago Allah made the universe from his own dung, and later made humans and animals from the earth's dirt. The first people were Adam and Eve, who were told by Allah to produce many children to present to him. As their offspring increased, Eve suggested to Adam that Allah might destroy all of their children when they were presented. She decided to hide one half of the children. When Allah called for their presentation, he said: 'You have hidden one half of your children. I did not tell you to do this, but since you have hidden them they shall remain so forever'

Eve's children, banished by Allah to invisibility, play an important part in Hausa life. As the 'Bori spirits' they are central to the Bori cult, controlled mainly by women. Bori spirits have clandestine power for they: 'inflict illness on hidden or unknown evil doers; they are the fountains of fortune and misfortune, wealth and poverty, happiness and sorrow.' Through Bori and spirit possession, women wield lost power. Because the spirits are beings of great force and must be treated with submissiveness and subservience, possessed women can defy not only the domestic authority of their husbands but also that of political authorities. By this means indigenous female power was consolidated and maintained during the years of Islamization. Today it remains a conduit of female liberation (Sanday R596 35).

Jahiliyah: Arabia before Islam

The ancient Arabian high God al-Llah, like El, simply means 'God'. Muhammad first bowed to Jerusalem and only later turned the centre of 'God's energy' from the Jewish spiritual capital to Mecca. The Qur'an is strewn with unique detail of Jewish history from targum, midrash and folklore. al-Llah can be no other than Yahweh and El before him, the ancient father God of paternity as we see acknowledged ibn the Qur'an:

"Say: We believe in Allah and [in] that which had been revealed to us, and (in) that which was revealed to Ibrahim and Ismail and Ishaq and Yaqoub and the tribes, and (in) that which was given to Musa and Isa, and [in] that which was given to the prophets from their Lord, we do not make any distinction between any of them, and to Him do we submit" (2.136).

"We believe in Allah and what has been revealed to us, and what was revealed to Ibrahim and Ismail and Ishaq and Yaqoub and the tribes, and what was given to Musa and Isa and to the prophets from their Lord; we do not make any distinction between any of them, and to Him do we submit" (3.84).

O children of Israel! call to mind My favor which I bestowed on you and be faithful to (your) covenant with Me, I will fulfill (My) covenant with you; and of Me, Me alone, should you be afraid (2.40).

However the deep association with astral worship is still represented by the star and crescent of Islam, the astral symbols prefigured in the perennial ubiquitous symbolic relationship between the crescent moon of Nannar or Sin the moon god and Venus the evening star of Inanna, Ishtar and al-Uzza, who is also a moon goddess, spanning much of Mesopotamian and Arabic culture and history. The source of these traditions originates in two 'high' cultures, one in Southern Arabia, and the other in what is now Jordan.

The South Arabian culture of the Sabeans runs back far in history to before the time of Solomon and his visit by the Queen of Saba [Hebrew Sheba]. South Arabian cultures had a pantheon of astral deities of which the moon god and sun goddess are prominent. The national god of each of the states was the moon god: 'Ilumquh of the Sabaeans, 'Amm by the Qatabanians, Wadd by the Minaeans, and Sin by the Hadramis. The term 'God is Love' is characteristic of Wadd (Briffault R75v3 85). 'the Merciful' ascribed to Allah is also South Arabian (Pritchard R542). The sun-goddess was the moon's consort; she was perhaps best known in South Arabia as Dhat Hamym, 'she who sends forth strong rays of benevolence'. In the centuries preceding Muhammad there was a gradual breakdown of Sabian culture, partly as a result of the fracture of the Marib Dam and a return to nomadic life and partly through a series of genocidal wars between evangelical Jews and Christians in the peninsula. In 522, King Dhu Nawas Yusaf "Lord of Curls", the last elected Himyar king, descendent of a Jewish hero, made war on the Christians who had a stronghold at Naryan, an ancient pagan pilgrimage spot. He offered the citizens the choice of Jewry or death. When they refused he burned them all in a great trench. Afterwards Naryan was named "the trench". In response, the Ethiopians overcame them and Abraha made Sabian San'a a Christian pilgrimage point which rivalled Mecca. An expeditionary force of Christians to try to destroy the Ka'aba. In turn Persia invaded and for a short time the country became a Persian satrapy. This confused situation in the period of *jahiliyah* laid the seeds for the emergence of Islam.

Nabatea a second prominent Arab culture, speaking Arabic, but writing in Aramaic script, sprang up from southern Sinai around 600 BC and from around 400 BC in the land of the Edomites in Jordan. They had a close relationship with the Edomites. Each claim a female line of descent from Ishmael (Browning R91 32). The Nabateans originally were tent-dwelling shepherds renowned for eschewing houses, planted crops, or wine (Negev R489 101), a sentiment shared by Muhammad, who looked with contempt upon the Kuryshites and Ansari "for they employ themselves with sowing seeds" ... "The divine glory is among the shepherds, vanity and impudence among the agricultural peoples" (Briffault R75v3 111). Agricultural settlement brought changes and the Greek period resulted in a hybrid culture.

Nabatean inscriptions in Sinai and other places display widespread references to names including Allah, El (god) and Allat (goddess), with regional references to al-Uzza, Ba'al and Manat (R489 11). Allat is also found in Sinai in South Arabian language. Allah occurs particularly as Garm- 'allahi - 'god decided' and Aush-allahi - 'gods covenant'. We find both Shalm-lahi 'Allah is peace' and Shalm-allat, 'the peace of the goddess'. We also find Amat-allahi 'she-servant of god' and Halaf-llahi 'the successor of Allah'. Allah is thus an ancient deity who preceded Muhammad and Islam. The Nabateans had two principal gods in their pantheon, and a whole range of djinns, personal gods and spirits similar to angels. These two deities were Dhu Shara, or Duchares and al-Uzza. It is said that when Allat (which simply means goddess as al-Llah means god) became the goddess of the Nabateans, she became al-Uzza the 'mighty one' as she evolved from a local deity of small rural shrines into a patron of an expanding culture (Browning 47). Al-Uzza is also referred to in connection with the Bedouins at Harran (Green R260 59,157). Segal (R619 145) mentions a Christian claim that a bedouin chief seized 400 virgins and sacrificed them to the goddess during a time of retaliatory wars. Duchares means Lord of Shera (Seir Genesis 33:14), a local mountain and thunder god who was worshipped at a rock high place as a block of stone. Dhu Shara is described on a dam inscription as 'Dushara the god of Gaia' (R489 107). He was celebrated as a god of immortality celebrated by a Dionysian tragic mask of death, in which its wearer became united with him, thus escaping the limitations of the mortal span (Glueck R242 242). In the Greek period al-Uzza became identified with Atargatis-Aphrodite and Dhu Shara with Dionysus. Rich food in plenty and strong wine without stint helped bring the deities and their worshippers into fervid relationship (Glueck R242 166). Herodotus says of the Arabs: "They deem no other to be gods save Dionysus and Heavenly Aphrodite ... they call Dionysus Orotalt and Aphrodite Alilat" (Negev R489 101).

In Mecca, Allah was originally paired with his 'daughters' - the *banat al-Lah*. Briffault notes: "This Arabian goddess was triune, being also known as the three Holy Virgins". The

Manat consisted of al-Lat "the goddess", Q're (possibly Kore) the Virgin, and al-Uzza the 'powerful one'. Al-Uzza was the moon. Manat was bringer of good and bad luck, just as the fates, and the Arabic term *mana*. Briffault claims al Uzza was worshipped also at Mecca:

> "Al-Kindy says that Al-Uzza was the moon, her chief shrine being the Ka'aba at Mecca, where she was worshipped in the form of a sacred stone, ... the very stone which the pilgrims to this day visit Mecca to kiss. In doing so the pilgrims recite Caliph Omar's warning declaration: 'I know well that you are a stone that can neither do good nor evil, and unless I had seen the prophet, on whom be prayer and the blessings of god kiss you, I would not kiss you'."(R75v3)

Occhigrosso (R500) affirms the astronomical basis of the black stone:

> Before Muhammad appeared, the Ka'aba was surrounded by 360 idols, and every Arab house had its god. Arabs also believed in djinn (subtle beings), and some vague divinity with many offspring. Among the major deities of the pre-Islamic era were al-Lat ("the goddess"), worshiped in the shape of a square stone; al-Uzzah ("the mighty"), a goddess identified with the morning star and worshiped as a thigh-bone-shaped slab of granite between al Taif and Mecca; Manat, the goddess of destiny, worshiped as a black stone on the road between Mecca and Medina; and the moon god, Hubal, whose worship was connected with the Black Stone of the Ka'aba'. The stones were said to have fallen from the sun, moon, stars, and planets and to represent cosmic forces. The so-called Black Stone (actually the color of burnt umber) that Muslims revere today is the same one that their forebears had worshiped well before Muhammad and that they believed had come from the moon.

The *hajj* was originally an Autumn rite apparently persecuting the dying sun to bring on the winter rains. Pilgrims would rush in a body to the hollow of Muzdalifa, the abode of the Thunder God, make an all-night vigil on the plain by Mt. Arafat, hurl pebbles at the three sacred pillars of Mina and offer an animal sacrifice" (Armstrong R21 62). Hurling the pebbles at the pillar of the Shaitan is still one of the most dangerous phases of the hajj. In 2004 at the time of writing, 244 people died in a stampede. A tradition of sexual freedom on the *hajj* predates Islam in more anceint fertility rites. Briffault (R75v3 221) states:

> At the immemorial shrine of al-Uzza at Mecca, it is a practice for women to offer themselves to the holy pilgrims. With Shi'ites it is the custom to form temporary unions during the period of the holy pilgrimage. It is stipulated at a fixed date all relations must cease, and the parties of such unions do not give signs of recognition if they subsequently meet. Any children of such unions are regarded as a blessing in the family and are looked upon as divine children or saints.

All forms of violence were forbidden in Mecca for four months during the *hajj*. The Ka'aba was holy ground and a measure of the holiness was its religious tolerance. All the faithful could assemble to honour a time-immemorial tradition. Worshippers of al-Llah, al-Lat and even the Christian Arabs could all come together there.

Al-Lat had a shrine at Taif, which was in a cooler and more fertile part of the Hijaz, and al-Uzza had one Naklah to the south east of Mecca and that Manat, the fateful one had her shrine at Qudayd on the Red Sea coast (Armstrong R21). Just as Mecca had the Ka'aba, so these places were also centres of pilgrimage, as described in detail by al-Kalbi (Faris).

> "The *banat al-Llah* [daughters of Allah] may well simply have been 'divine beings'. They were represented in their shrines not by a personalized statue or portrait but by large standing stones, rather like the fertility symbols used by the Canaanites which are so often described in the Bible. When the Arabs venerated these stones they were not worshipping them in any crude, simplistic way but were seeing them as a focus of divinity. It has also been suggested that these three goddesses were related to the Semitic fertility goddesses Anat and Ishtar, so their cultus may have begun before the Arabs adopted the nomadic life, when they were still farmers and living on the land. The Arabs may not have worshipped al-Lat, al-Uzza and Manat in a personalized way, but ... they felt very passionate about the shrines of the banat al-Lah" (Armstrong R21).

Allah's Daughters and the Satanic Verses

al-Llah's daughters, the *banat al-Lah* were overthrown by Muhammad, along with other pagan deities. Tabari quotes an early tradition of about seventy years after the prophet's death. ... "As long as he preached the cult of al-Llah, with its concern for the poor and needy, everybody in Mecca had been ready to accommodate this reformed cult of the old High God. But once he affirmed that the worship of al-Llah must preclude the worship of all the other ancestral gods, the Quraysh 'rebutted him with vehemence, not approving what he said, and aroused against him those who had followed him, except those whom

God kept safe and they were few in number'. Overnight, Islam became a despised minority sect."

The historians Ibn Sa'd and al Tabari describe the origin of the 'Satanic Verses'. The prophet is approached by the Quraysh and persuaded to utter the verses in return for promise of admission to Mecca's inner circles. He tries to find a place for the goddesses without compromising his monotheism. "When the apostle saw that his people had turned their backs on him and he was pained by their estrangement from what he brought them from God, he longed that there should come to him from God a message that would reconcile his people to him. One day, Tabari says, while he was meditating in the Ka'aba, the answer seemed to come in a revelation that gave a place to the three 'goddesses' without compromising his monotheistic vision (Armstrong R21 113).

"Have you then considered the Lat and the Uzza, And Manat, the third, the last?
these are the exalted birds [gharaniq] whose intercession is approved"

According to this version of the story, the Quraysh were delighted with the new revelation, which in al-Kalbi's words was the traditional invocation made by the Quraysh to the goddesses as they circumambulated the Ka'aba (Faris R198 17). The *gharaniq* were probably Numidian cranes which were thought to fly higher than any other bird. Muhammad, may have believed in the existence of the banat - al-Llah as he believed in the existence of angels and djinn, was giving the 'goddesses' a delicate compliment, without compromising his message. ... The Quraysh spread the good news throughout the city: 'Muhammad has spoken of our gods in splendid fashion. He alleged in what he recited that they are the exalted gharaniq whose intercession is approved' (Armstrong R22 112).

It is said that Muhammad later removed these verses because he was later told by the angel Gabriel they were "Satan inspired". The rejection of the Manat led to the historic conflict with the Qura'sh which resulted in the flight to Medina.

"Have you then considered the Lat and the Uzza, And Manat, the third, the last?
What! for you the males and for Him the females! This indeed is an unjust division!
They are naught but names which you have named, you and your fathers;
Allah has not sent for them any authority.
They follow naught but conjecture and their low desire." (53.19).

Muhammad meets Gabriel on his night journey (Mi'raj-nameh Turkey 15th c redrawn from Cook)

This comes straight after the Prophet's report of his night journey on the axis Mundi, possibly under the inspiration of *isfand*. Rudgley (R584 52) suggests the Prophet had a vision on the sacred plant which led him to perceive the idols as mere wood and stone .

He disclaims female angels despite the *houris* the black-eyed virgins of paradise:

"And how many an angel is there in the heavens
whose intercession does not avail at all
except after Allah has given permission to whom
He pleases and chooses.
Most surely they who do not believe in the hereafter
name the angels with female names" (53.26).

A hint of the reversal of the satanic verses can be gleaned in the following denial:

"We sent not ever any Messenger
or Prophet before thee, but that Satan
cast into his fancy, when he was fancying:
but God annuls what Satan casts, then
God confirms his signs."

The guardians of the Ka'aba are still called the *Beni Shaybah*, or sons of the old woman (Briffault R75v3 80). Popular tradition relates how Abraham, when he founded the Ka'aba brought the ground from an old woman to which it belonged. She however consented to part with it only on the condition that she and her descendents should have the key of the place in their keeping" (Briffault R75). The Hajira or 'sudden departure', although applied to Muhammad's sudden exit, bears the name of Hajira (Hagar), who discovered the spring of Zam Zam flowing by Ishmael's foot searching for water for him after the 'sudden departure' of Ibrahim (Shad R621 48), again a symbol of the sacred feminine.

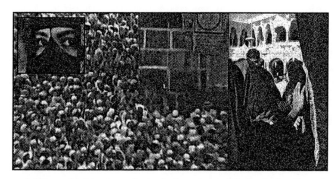

Left: Veil Saudi-style. Center: Pilgrims passing the 'black stone' in the Ka'aba, a remnant of pre-Islamic worship. Right: Women touching the black stone. The Haj predates Islam as a pagan pilgrimage. (Time, BBC, Stewart).

Muhammad then mounted a singular rejection of the daughters of al-Lah. Muhammad was offered a pact of mutual religious toleration between Allah and Allat which was entirely in keeping with the holy place it was: "the Muslims could go on worshipping al-Llah in their religion, and the others could go on worshipping al-Lat al-Uzza and Manat. In response Muhammad recited the Sura of Rejection:

"Say O unbelievers, I serve not what you serve
and you are not serving what I serve,
Nor am I serving what you have served.
To you your religion and to me my religion!" (109)

The attitude of the critics is frankly portrayed in the Quran:

"And the chiefs of those who disbelieved from among his people said: 'He is nothing but a mortal like yourselves who desires that he may have superiority over you, and if Allah had pleased, He could certainly have sent down angels. We have not heard of this among our fathers of yore: He is naught but a man bedevilled'." (23.24)

Circumstances deteriorated. A ban was imposed which led to much hardship. Khadja, the merchant woman who adopted Muhammad as consort, to whom he was devoted, died. Muhammad was asked a difficult question by Abu Lahab: "Would Muhammad's father have gone to hell because he was a pagan?" (Armstrong R21 136). Muhammad ended up having to retreat to Medina. It is significant that of the pilgrims to Mecca from Medina in 622, 73 of the men, but only 3 of the women were followers of the Prophet (Armstrong R21 149).

Genocide at Medina and Sakina

The subsequent rise of jihad after the Pledge of War at the hajj of 622 resulted in the notorious genocide in the souk of Medina in which 700 Jews were beheaded, only to end without war because Muhammad would, if reluctantly, accept the peace of sakina in the compromise of Hudaybiyah and enter Mecca without war. Thus the beheading of 700 Jews was unnecessary and jihad was not fulfilled. The Jews had not actually betrayed Muhammad's followers to the Quraysh but had merely parleyed, nevertheless there was a fear they could have opened the gates of Medina to the enemy. This has historical precedents in the genocide of Jericho and similar immolations by the Prince of Curls of the Christians in Southern Arabia, but what is signal here is a frank act of genocide by a religious leader and 'final prophet'.

"The Jews are said to have asked Abu Lubabah what Muhammad intended to do and he touched his throat, tacitly telling them that they had been sentenced to death. He was then so overcome by remorse that he bound himself to a pillar of the mosque for fifteen days until Muhammad released him. If he had told the Jews of their fate in this way, it does not seem to have affected their decision, so it has been suggested that he had perhaps indicated that he would honour his old allegiance to Qurayzah. The next day, the Qurayzah agreed to accept Muhammad's judgement and opened their gates to the Muslim army, presumably trusting in the support of their former confederates in the tribe of Aws. Indeed, the Aws begged Muhammad to be merciful; had he not granted the Bani Qaynuqa their lives at the request of Ibn Ubbay, a Khasrajite? Muhammad asked them if they would accept the decision of one of their own leading men and they agreed. During the siege, Sa'd ibn Muadh had received a fatal wound, but he was carried to the territory of Qurayzah on a donkey. His fellow chiefs urged him to spare their former allies, but Sa'd would have realised that this could be the thin end of the wedge that would bring chaos back to Medina. Should an old loyalty take precedence over commitment to the umma? Sa'd judged that all the 700 men should be killed, their wives and children sold into slavery and their property divided among the Muslims. Muhammad cried aloud: 'You have judged according to the very sentence of al-Llah above the seven skies!' The next day Muhammad ordered another trench to be dug, this time in the souk of Medina. Some individuals were spared at the request of the Muslims, but the rest were tied together in groups and beheaded; their bodies were thrown into the trench" (Armstrong R22 206).

"It is probably impossible for us to dissociate this story from Nazi atrocities and it will inevitably alienate many people irrevocably from Muhammad. But Western scholars like Maxime Rodinson and W. Montgomery Watt argue that it is not correct to judge the incident by twentieth-century standards" (Armstrong R22 206).

Only one woman was executed, for throwing a millstone on one of the Muslims during the siege of the tribe. Aisha remembered her vividly:

"She was actually with me and was talking with me and laughing immoderately as the apostle was killing her men in the market when suddenly an unseen voice called her name. 'Good heavens,' I cried, 'what is the matter?' 'I am to be killed,' she replied. 'What for?' I asked. 'Because of something I did,' she answered. She was taken away and beheaded. Aisha used to say, I shall never forget my wonder at her good spirits and her loud laughter when all the time she knew that she would be killed" (Armstrong R22 206).

His first attempt to return to Mecca was met with stiff opposition for which he displayed prophetic forbearance. He agreed to reconciliation, not war at Hudaybiyah. He displays his considerable knowledge of Jewish tradition when he invokes the Sakina or Spirit of Tranquillity - Armstrong says: "The sakina it will also be recalled, seems to be related to the Hebrew Shekhinah, the term for God's presence in the world" (Armstrong R21 224)

"It is He who sent down the sakina into the hearts of the believers,
that they might add faith to their faith." (48.2)

The peace treaty was for 10 years, but 2 years later, when his forces were stronger and the Meccans were living securely and off their guard, he marched into Mecca. There is thus a principle in Islam, *takiya* - the right to fake peace when you are weak (R534), so as to defeat your enemy when you are stronger. Although Muslims claim the treaty was technically broken by skirmishes from allies of the other side, Hudaybiyah symbolizes 'trick or treaty'.

Muhammad's second return to the Ka'aba was the Lesser Pilgrimage negotiated through the treaty at Hudaybiyah. "The huge crowd of pilgrims in their white garments filed slowly into their holy city, led by Muhammad riding on Qaswa, and the valley resounded with their cry: 'Here I am at your service, 0 God!' When he reached the Ka'aba, Muhammad dismounted and kissed the Black Stone, embracing and stroking it, and then began to make the circumambulations followed by the whole pilgrim body" (Armstrong R21). The eventual compromise was that Mecca would retain the ancient hajira pilgrimage, a centre of its energy, but would embrace Islam. Briffault (R75v3 78) notes:

"When Muhammad overthrew the old religion of Arabia, he was not strong enough to defy and offend the immemorial sentiment of the Arab people. The divine mission of the prophet was reconciled with the old religion by Islam receiving the sanction of the immemorial deity".

Cutting out the Tongues

On his next return to Mecca, he came in triumph. "He rose, performed the ritual ablutions and offered the prayer. Then he rode round the Ka'aba seven times, touching the Black Stone each time and crying 'al-Llahu Akbar!' The shout was taken up by his 10,000 soldiers and soon the whole city resounded with the words that symbolised the final victory of Islam.

Muhammad and Ali destroy the idols in the Ka'aba (http://www.unf.edu/classes/saints/images/Muhammad-and-Ali-destroyidolsinkaaba-safavidMS.jpg.

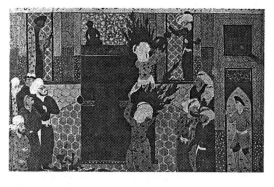

Next Muhammad turned his attention to the 360 idols around the shrine: crowded on to their roofs and balconies, the Quraysh watched him smash each idol while he recited the verse: 'the truth has come, and falsehood has vanished'. Inside the Ka'aba the walls had been decorated with pictures of the pagan deities and Muhammad ordered them all to be obliterated, though it is said that he allowed frescoes of Jesus and Mary to remain. Eventually Islam would forbid the use of all imagery in its worship, because it distracts the mind from God by allowing it to dwell on purely human symbols of the divine" (Armstrong R21).

But the black stone remained. Briffault (R75v3 79) comments:

"When he abolished the idols, of the old religion, Muhammad, whose dominating ideal was to, unite all Arabian tribes into a single political body bound by a common cult, felt it to be undesirable or impracticable to do away with the most sacrosanct object or symbol of the old religion"

In "The Naked Face of Eve, Nawal el Sadaawi (R188) notes the immediate murder of Sarah:

"Sarah was a famous slave singer who aimed her barbed words against the Moslems. She was among those whom Mahomet ordered to be executed on the day of his victorious entry into Mecca. In the region of El Nagir, it was recounted that some women had rejoiced when the Prophet died and Abu Bake, the first of the Caliphs, ordered their hands and feet to be cut off. Thus women who dared to give voice to their protest or opposition could be exposed to cruel punishment. Their hands might be cut off, or their teeth pulled out, or their tongues torn from their mouths. This last form of punishment was usually reserved for those who were singers. It was said of these women that they used to dye their hands with henna, brazenly display the seductions of their beauty, and beat time with their fingers on tambourines and drums in defiance of God, and in derision towards the rights of God and his Prophet. It was therefore necessary to cut off their hands and tear out their tongues".

Each temple was demolished or burned to the ground, and the priests and priestesses put to the sword. When the banu-Umahmah were slaughtered and the women raped for defending dhu-al-Khalasah which stood half way to San'a, a woman cried (Faris R198 31):

"The banu-Umamah, each wielding his spear,
Were slaughtered at al-Waliyah, their abode;
They came to defend their shrine only to find
Lions with brandished swords clamouring for blood.
The women of Khath'am were then humiliated
by the men of Ahmas and debased".

It is thus said by al-Bukhari that the Prophet himself said:

"This world shall not pass away until the buttocks of the women of Daws wiggle [again] around the dhu-al-Khalasah and they worship it as they were want to do [before Islam]" (Faris R198 32).

Brooks (R80) comments about further atrocity against women:

"Not everyone mourned the passing of Islam's prophet. In the southern Arabian region of Hadramaut, six women decorated their hands with henna, as if for a wedding, and took to the streets beating tambourines in joyful celebration of Muhammad's death. Soon, about twenty others joined the merry gathering. When word of the celebration reached Abu Bake, he sent out the cavalry to deal with 'the whores of Hadramaut.' When his warriors arrived, the men of the settlement came to their women's defense but were defeated. As punishment, the women had their henna-painted, tambourine-playing hands severed at the wrists. Who knows what motivated the women to make their rousing and reckless celebration? To them, at least, it must have seemed that Muhammad's new religion had made their lives more burdensome, less free".

She then notes a sea change for the worse in patriarchal conservatism against women:

"And much worse was coming. Repression of women was about to be legislated into the religion on a large scale by Abu Bakr's successor as caliph, the violent misogynist Omar. That Aisha supported Omar's bid for leadership shows the depth of her loathing for Fatima's husband, Ali. Her opinion of Omar was not high. Knowing his cruelty to the women of his household, she had cleverly helped foil a match between him and her sister. Omar cracked down on women in ways that he must have known flouted Muhammad's traditions. He made stoning the official punishment for adultery and pressed to extend the seclusion of women beyond the prophet's wives. He tried to prevent women from praying in the mosque, and when that failed, he ordered separate prayer leaders for men and women. He also prevented women from making the Hajj, a ban that was lifted only in the last year of his life".

Within the history of Islam, there has been great diversity of tradition from liberal to fundamentalist. In the golden early ages of the cultural flowering of Islam, there was a diversity of outlook from the rationalist Faylsufs (Armstrong R22 199) through the metaphysical Kalam (R22 195) theological discoursers, the mystical Shi'ite genealogies of the Imams, the gnostic archons of al-Farabi (R22 204), the gnostic hidden (*batin*) inner interpretations of the Ismailis (R22 208. Green R260 141), the blended science and illumination of Suhrawardi in the Hermetic tradition of Idris (R22 268), the 'prophetic spirit' of al-Ghazzali (R22 221) and the visionary inner garment of the Sufi way, the transpersonal epiphanies and Sophia of Ibn al-Arabi (R22 272) to the trasformative knowledge of the Shi'ite Mullah Sadra (R22 301). However this diversity has later become unraveled through return to narrow moral prescriptions in the Qur'an and Sharia in the closing of 'the gates of *ijtihad*'.

The Prophet's Nine Women

Muhammad took nine wives and a concubine after Khadja, more than the four plus slave concubines he permitted in the Qur'an, as eloquently described in "The Prophet's Women" in "Nine Parts of Desire" (Brooks R80) summarized here by (Occhigrosso R500 403):

"At age 50, Muhammad married again, this time exercising the Arab option of taking several wives, which he had not done while married to Khadja. In Mecca he wed the widow Sawda and was engaged to Aisha, the 6-year-old daughter of Abu Bake. He later married her in Medina at age 9, although the marriage was not consummated until she reached the age of womanhood in Arabic culture. Next he married Hafsa, the daughter of Umar, a notable Companion, as the circle of Muslims closest to Muhammad came to be called. Muhammad's marriage to Zaynab, the wife of his adopted son Zayd required some thought and several revelations. Zayd assured the Prophet that his marriage to Zaynab was not a happy one, and though Islamic law permitted yet disapproved of divorce as well as marriage to one's son's relations, Zayd and Zaynab were divorced and Muhammad married her. As the Prophet's revelations granted permission for his marriages, the outspoken Aisha remarked (according to oral tradition), "It seems that God is hastening to satisfy your desires"-demonstrating Aisha's remarkable freedom as a woman. Muhammad then married Umm Salama and two Jewish women, Raihana and Safiya, followed by Umm Habiba, a daughter of Abu Sufyan, a famously idolatrous opponent of Islam, and Maimuna, sister-in-law of his uncle and the aunt of Khalid, the great Quraysh military leader. Besides these 9 official wives, Muhammad took as concubine-over the objections of Aisha and his other wives-Mariya, a Coptic Christian slave girl who was a gift from the ruler of Egypt."

Other forthright women offered themselves freely to Muhammad in marriage and some demurred having sexual relations with him, indicating women were assertive in his time. Wiebke Walther (R712) notes:

"this woman had offered herself in marriage to the Prophet himself, and it is said that she was not the only one to do so. This is proof of the magnetism Muhammad must have had for those around him. It is also evidence of a self-confidence on the part of women in Ancient Arabia totally lacking ... among Muslim women of later centuries. There are reports of other women who were married to Muhammed but who, when he came to them in the bridal chamber, said: 'I take refuge from you in God.' At this, so it goes, he had them sent back to their families without delay. This, too, shows Arab women at the time of Muhammed were assertive enough to make no secret of their desires or disinclination".

To his credit, Muhammad tried to keep to the Quran's instruction that a man must treat his wives equally. His practice was to see each of them, every afternoon, in a brief private meeting, but to dine and spend the night with one at a time, in strict rotation. However he still accepted the patriarchal views of dominant cultures of his day, setting women to be clearly lesser than men - half the value - and subject to defined paternity rights and beatings.

Martyrdom, Jihad and Black-Eyed Virgins

"Those who are slain in the cause of Allah are not counted among the dead.
They are living in the presence of their Lord and are well provided for." (Qur'an R246)

Islam means 'submission' to God. Jihad means 'struggle' or 'striving'. It can be taken metaphorically or even mystically, but in raw physical terms it means a state of holy war, involving killing, and preparedness to die as a martyr, which is described as a painless trip to heaven to see the face of al-Llah, partly in the belief that Jesus did not die a painful death on the cross, but was 'taken up' by God. Islam is unique for combining martyrdom with intentional violence. The fundamental tenet of Islamic faith *Shadadah* - 'there is no God (reality) but al-Llah and Muhammad is his prophet' also means sacrifice, or martyrdom (p 282). In Muslim apocalyptic vision, the world is divided between Domain of Islam and the Domain of War - *Dar al-Harb* - invoking a utopian agenda of violent world conquest. Jihad in the Qur'an is striving, the 'strivers' are mightily rewarded, death is mentioned in the same breath, and those dying in the cause of al-Llah have a special reward in paradise:

"O Prophet! strive hard against the unbelievers and the hypocrites and be unyielding to them;
and their abode is hell, and evil is the destination" (9.73).

"and Allah shall grant to the strivers above the holders back a mighty reward" (4.95).

"Do you think that you will enter the garden while Allah has not yet known those who strive hard
from among you, and (He has not) known the patient. And certainly you desired death before you
met it, so indeed you have seen it and you look (at it)" (3.142).

"and (as for) those who are slain in the way of Allah, He will by no means allow their deeds to per-
ish. He will guide them and improve their condition.
And cause them to enter the garden which He has made known to them" (47.4).

Muhammad stated that Jesus (*Isa* - after Esau is his Arabic name) did not die a death of agony on the cross, but was taken straight up to heaven:

"And their saying: Surely we have killed the Messiah, Isa son of Marium, the apostle of Allah; and
they did not kill him nor did they crucify him, but it appeared to them so (like Isa) and most surely
those who differ therein are only in a doubt about it; they have no knowledge respecting it, but only
follow a conjecture, and they killed him not for sure. Nay! Allah took him up to Himself; and Allah is
Mighty, Wise" (4.157).

Faithful men entering paradise are greeted by *houris* (Arabic *hawra*) female angelic 'virgins' who exist to offer pleasure to those who have merited eternal bliss while on earth. Numerous references to the houri in the Qur'an describe them as "purified wives" and "spotless virgins." Each new man arriving in the Islamic heaven is given seventy-two houris who fulfill his every want or desire, each of whom he may cohabit once with for each day he has fasted in Ramadan and once for each good work he has performed. The *houri*, meanwhile, is rewarded in this union by becoming a virgin after each night's enjoyment. The Arabic word 'hawra' contrasts the clear white of the eye to the blackness of the iris.

Surely those who guard (against evil) are in a secure place, In gardens and springs;
They shall wear of fine and thick silk, (sitting) face to face;
Thus (shall it be), and We will wed them with houris pure, beautiful ones. (44.51)

The chastity of the black-eyed is not violated by man nor jinn, and every virtuous man has seventy two wives in heaven:

And for him who fears to stand before his Lord are two gardens. Having in them various kinds. In
both of them are two fountains flowing. In both of them are two pairs of every fruit. Reclining on
beds, the inner coverings of which are of silk brocade; and the fruits of the two gardens shall be
within reach. In them shall be those who restrained their eyes; before them neither man nor jinni
shall have touched them. Which then of the bounties of your Lord will you deny? (55.46)

Narrated through al-Khudhri, who heard the Prophet Muhammad (Allah's blessings and peace be
upon him) saying, 'The smallest reward for the people of Heaven is an abode where there are eighty
thousand servants and seventy two wives, over which stands a dome decorated with pearls, aquama-
rine and ruby, as wide as the distance from al-Jabiyyah to San'a.

Clearly this is a polygynous paradise. An Australian Muslim asked: "If men [in Paradise] get the black-eyed, what do the women get?" The answer, provided by the deputy director of Al-Azhar's Center for Islamic Studies, Sheikh Abd Al-Fattah Gam'an, read:

"Most of 'the black-eyed' were first created in Paradise, but some of them are women from this world, and are obedient Muslims who observe the words of Allah: 'We created them especially, and have made them virgins, loving, and equal in age.' ... when the women of this world are old and worn out, Allah creates them [anew] after their old age into virgins who are amiable to their husbands; 'equal in age' means equal to one another in age. At the side of the Muslim in Paradise are his wives from this world, if they are among the dwellers in Paradise, along with 'the black-eyed' of Paradise. If a woman is of the dwellers in Paradise but her husband in this world is not, ... she is given to one of the dwellers in Paradise who is of the same status... Regarding the woman who was married to more than one man in this world, and all her husbands are dwellers in Paradise ... [The Prophet] answered: 'She... chooses the best of them, saying, Oh Allah, this is the best of them that was with me in this world, marry me to him'... Thus it is known that the women of Paradise also have husbands. Every woman has a husband. If her husband in this world is of the dwellers in Paradise [he becomes her husband in Paradise], and if her husband in this world is an infidel, she is given to one of the dwellers in Paradise who is suited to her in status and in the [strength] of his belief"

The several accounts of the Qur'anic creation story (2.28, 7.11,15.26) come right out of Genesis. al-Llah, in the 'Elhoistic plural, "and certainly We created you", makes the angels out of fire and Adam out of dust or black mud. Then al-Llah, now Yawistic "your Lord", as in the Edenic account, breathes "my spirit" into him and tells the angels to make obeisance. But Iblis (Shaitan) would not, saying "I am better than he: Thou hast created me of fire, while him Thou didst create of dust". God thus casts out Satan for hubris. Satan asks for respite in the day of judgement. al-Llah replies mercifully "Surely you are of the respited ones." But Iblis, disappointed, says he will lie in wait for mankind: "I will certainly cause them all to deviate ... Thou shalt not find most of them thankful". Satan is more of a figure of rebellion, and a 'tester' as in the original Jewish concept, rather than a dark force on a par with God. al-Llah then drives him out and curses all 'deviators' who follow him "whoever of them will follow you, I will certainly fill hell with you all ... It has seven gates; for every gate there shall be a separate party of them."

Adam is then told, again in the 'Elhoistic plural not to eat of the tree of the unjust:

"And (We said): O Adam! Dwell you and your wife in the garden; so eat from where you desire, but do not go near this tree, for then you will be of the unjust" (7.19).

But the Shaitan deceives them into eating the fruit, causing them to have 'evil inclinations':

"Your Lord has not forbidden you this tree except that you may not both become two angels or that you may (not) become of the immortals. Then he caused them to fall by deceit; so when they tasted of the tree, their evil inclinations became manifest to them, and they both began to cover themselves with the leaves of the garden; and their Lord called out to them: Did I not forbid you both from that tree and say to you that the Shaitan is your open enemy?"

In the Hadiths women are condescendingly doomed to be the 'bent rib' (Walther R712, Rafiqul-Haqq and Newton R549):

"Treat the women well, for woman was created from a rib,
and the most curved part of the rib is the top part. Should you try to bend it straight,
you will destroy it, but if you leave it as it is, it remains curved. So treat the women well!"

The woman is like a rib; if you try to straighten her, she will break.
So if you want to get benefit from her, do so while she still has some crookedness

Adam and Eve appeal to God's mercy and he gives humankind the Earth for a time as mortals until the resurrection:

They said: Our Lord! We have been unjust to ourselves, and if Thou forgive us not, and have (not) mercy on us, we shall certainly be of the losers. He said: Get forth, some of you, the enemies of others, and there is for you in the earth an abode and a provision for a time. He (also) said: Therein shall you live, and therein shall you die, and from it shall you be raised.

Clothing is advocated for beauty and to guard against sexual shame and evil, suggesting this was started by their original clothing having been pulled off by Satan:

O children of Adam! We have indeed sent down to you clothing to cover your shame, and (clothing) for beauty and clothing that guards (against evil), that is the best. This is of the communications of Allah that they may be mindful. O children of Adam! let not the Shaitan cause you to fall into affliction as he expelled your parents from the garden, pulling off from them both their clothing that he *might show them their evil inclinations, he surely sees you, he as well as his host, from whence you cannot see them; surely We have made the Shaitans to be the guardians of those who do not believe.*

Islam incorporates and end of days, coupled with an apocalyptic vision, like Christianity of the Day of Judgement amid signs of lunar eclipse and cosmuc tumult:

He asks: When is the day of resurrection? So when the sight becomes dazed,
And the moon becomes dark, And the sun and the moon are brought together,
Man shall say on that day: Whither to fly to? By no means! there shall be no place of refuge!
With your Lord alone shall on that day be the place of rest (75.6).

Isa is surely a knowledge of the hour of the day of judgement and the followers of the book Christians, Jews and the *hanif,* or *sabians* of Harran, are the only exceptions.

"He [Isa] is surely a knowledge of the hour. ...
And when Isa came with clear arguments he said: I have come to you indeed with wisdom,
and that I may make clear to you part of what you differ in" (43:61).

"And there is not one of the followers of the Book but most certainly believes in this before his death,
and on the day of resurrection he [Isa] shall be a witness against them" (4.159).

The infidels will be thrown into hell and the believers will rest in the garden of paradise in some versions surrounded by black eyed virgins. This sexually implicit vision is a prime motivator for Islamic martyrdom:

"Surely. as regards My servants, you have no authority ,over them except those who follow you of the deviators. And surely Hell is the promised place of them all: It has seven gates; for every gate there shall be a separate party of them. Surely those who guard (against evil) shall be in the midst of gardens and fountains: Enter them in peace, secure" (15.42).

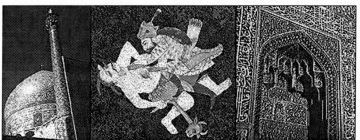

Islamic art indicates the faith penetrating as a jewel into the celestial sphere. However this comes at the cost of a death-sentence for representing the sacred in any form of image following the Pentateuch edicts against idolatry. Thus the language of edict becomes the new idol worshipped in the place of life itself. Iblis, himself the shaitan, is given a light sentence for his hubris, while Salman Rushdie (R587) and Taslima Nasrin are given death fatwas for making a critique of religious hubris.

Monotheistic Monolith

Islam sets up a triple monolith of religion, law and state expressed in the Qur'an, Sharia and the Islamic state - the 'legacy of the prophet'. This has an explicit danger that all the forces shaping society are combined into one monolithic totalitarian block, contrary to the very principles of freedom, and of true religion, however much it may have been originally designed with the welfare of the people as a society in mind (Armstrong R22 298).

"'Allah is its goal, the Prophet its model, the Koran its Constitution,
Jihad its path, and death for the sake of Allah its most sublime belief,' ...
How could they participate in a secular legislative system
when all good Muslims knew that the Koran
was the only legitimate constitution and source of divine law?"
(Ninety-nine Names of God)

Karen Armstrong (R22 297) notes this danger became a reality: "In the fifteenth century, the Sunni *ulema* of the *Madrasas,* the schools of Islamic studies, decreed that 'the gates of *ijtihad* (independent reasoning had been closed'. Henceforth Muslims should practice 'emulation' (*taqlid*) of the great luminaries of the past, especially in the study of the *Shariah,* the Holy Law" - adding "It was unlikely that there would be innovative ideas about God in this conservative climate, or indeed anything else". Although early Islam had a freer and more tolerant tradition in which reinterpretation of the law, philosophy, science and mysticism flourished a fixed tradition now claimed that legal prescriptions had been determined for all time, casting Islamic law into a permanent medieval mold on the Deuteronomic model. Ibn Taymiyah while intending to provide clarity for the people of Islam, not a "repressive discipline" (ibid 298) condemned the dimensions of diversity of Islam from the Falsafah (philosophical) and Kalam (metaphysical discourse on God) and his disciple al-Jawziyah similarly condemned the Sufis (R22 298). Although interpretations of Sharia vary and Shi'ite tradition has been protestant and more progressive, this century has seen fundamentalistic interpretations manifested alike in both traditions.

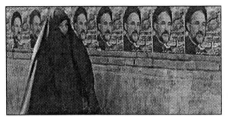

In Iran, the supreme leader is appointed for life and overrides all other authorities. He appoints half of the unelected Guardians' Council who then vet parliamentary candidates and laws (p 434). Laws passed by parliament can be circumscribed by the clerics, so democracy is subject to theocracy Despite Khatami's landslide win, he remaned relatively powerless (NZ Herald).

The Qur'an is not the only source of Muslim law. Soon after the death of Muhammad, it was noticed that the prescriptions in the Qur'an were not sufficient for the shaping of a life which would be pleasing to God. And so his followers began by collecting narratives (*hadith*) of what Muhammed did, said, or tacitly approved of in certain situations. Another authority was needed, and this was found in the *ijma'*, the 'unanimous consensus', the concurrent opinion of all Muslim scholars alive at the same time in a certain period on a given problem. The fourth and final source of Islamic law is analogies (*qiyas*). In Sunna the universe is divided into dark and light just as left is to right:

"The aim was to shape one's own life according to Sunna or 'custom' the 'fine example' of the Prophet, in other words. This even included such details as Muhammed's pronouncement that it was better to eat and drink with one's right hand, since the left was used by the Devil" (R712).

Islam also has a tradition of issuing death fatwahs inciting the killing of those it deems have crossed the lines of blasphemy or apostasy or any infringement of whatever moral code a given mullah chooses to interpret as such, including any image, or representation. Islamic law ordains death for apostasy. Like the laws governing adultery this is a reflection of Deuteronomic law (17:2). It is the only religion still issuing such death orders:

"Surely (as for) those who believe then disbelieve, again believe and again disbelieve, then increase in disbelief, Allah will not forgive them nor guide them in the (right) path. Announce to the hypocrites that they shall have a painful chastisement: ... surely Allah will gather together the hypocrites and the unbelievers all in hell" (4.137).

Taslima Nasrin was the victim of a death fatwah for suggesting Sharia should be modified:

"I guess what I remember most about my life in hiding was the dark. I stayed in a dark room all the time. I moved ten times in two months, but all the rooms were small and dark. My friends used to lock the door, the window shades were drawn. I had no books, no pens or paper, no radio, no phone only darkness. I wanted to see my family, - my friends refused. I couldn't sleep at night or during the day. I used to hear the chants of the fundamentalists outside on the street 'Kill Tastima! Kill Taslima!' I was terrified. I was sure they would find me and chop me into pieces with their swords and knives. "Did you say that the Koran should be revised?" "No, I said that Shariat law should be revised. I want a modern, civilized law where women are given equal rights. I want no religious law that discriminates, none, period - no Hindu law, Christian law, no Islamic law. Why should a man be entitled to have four wives? Why should a son get two-thirds of his parents' property when a daughter an inherit only a third?"

"What was it about Mymensingh that so caused Taslima to rebel?" "Women are sold here for take, for money!" her father Dr. Ali responded. "Men are encouraged to beat their wives. We had a relative, a pir, a learned Sufi holy man, who issued fatwas to prevent our women from leaving the house, fatwas against his own family for years. He declared me an apostate who would burn in Hell, along with my entire family, including Taslima. She was only nine years old" (New Yorker):

"[The pir] was mad," she said. "An Old Testament religion is what he preached. My mother used to take me to his house. He used to sit in a very comfortable place. His supporters surrounded him, reading their religious books. Women were behind a partition, a screen. There were many young women there; he always liked young girls. He would tell us that we should never get married, that the world would be destroyed and we would go on to a new life - that we would go before God, and he would punish us. Religion was punishment - sanctions."

Zarghona 15 lies in a Peshawar shelter, burned by her father-in-law, who said she had not cleaned her husband's clothes properly (Time). Such burnings also occur on a huge scale in patriarchal Hindu India, where dowry burnings may account for 25,000 deaths a year.

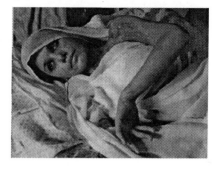

Stoning and Burning Female Flowers

You see in the book what is written, it says girls are like
flowers
exposed in front of the sunshine they will wilt.
It's so beautiful, it's poetry. And it's a bad thing that
these bad things
are written in such a poetic way because you believe
they must be right
Samira Makhmalbaf, producer of 'Apple'
(Guardian Wkly 3 Jan 99 19)

The Arabic word *zina'* that is often translated by the word 'adultery' really means something more than that - any sexual relations between a woman and a man who are not bound to each other by a legal marriage, and as long as slavery existed, intimate relations between a man and a slave who did not belong to him or was married to another. The Qur'an does not prescribe stoning to death for adultery. Nevertheless, in many Islamic countries to this day, including Afghanistan, Pakistan, Bangla Desh and Saudi Arabia women are regularly stoned to death. Sharia uses the precedent of Hebrew law to kill women for what is often only nominally 'adultery'.

"A woman named Noorjehan Begum was, by most accounts, the daughter of a landless peasant - a twenty-one-year-old who, in January, 1993, after her first marriage was dissolved, married again. The local mullah, giving no reasons, declared that a second marriage was contrary to Islamic law. A few weeks later, just after dawn, she was led to an open field in a small village in the district of Sylhet a stronghold of the fundamentalists - where a pit had been dug overnight. She was lowered into the pit and buried waist deep. Then, slowly and methodically, she was stoned - a hundred and one times."

Women are also burned , and beheaded and thrown down wells, whether or not they have actually committed adultery:

"The last case was a 17 year old - the father knowing that she lost her virginity - they took her to two doctors - both gynecologists told him that she lost her virginity - so he ended up taking her at night and throwing her head [down a well] - cutting her head totally - separating the head from the body" Palestinian woman doctor.

Hundreds of women in Pakistan are killed each year by relatives for offending the family honour or Islam. Over 4000 between 1998 and 2004. In Jordan a quarter of murders are honour killings of women, whether or not they have committed a sexual act. In 2003 Jordan's parliament overwhelmingly rejected a proposed law imposing harsher punishments for men who kill female relatives in "honour killings". Islamists and conservatives opposed to the new law said it would encourage vice and destroy social values:

"A woman is like an olive tree. When its branch catches woodworm, it has to be chopped off
so that society stays clean and pure." (Tribal Leader on Honour Killings)

Jordan: A man took his two teen-age daughters, 16 and 17, for exams when he heard from neighbors that both were dating. Though the two were found to be virgins, two weeks later both were killed by their father and two brothers - they refused to believe the girls hadn't had sex. Back in Zarqa after serving one year for murder, Ahmad recalled the childhood good times with his sister Haneen. "We used to have fun when we played football together, but I always won because I am a man," he said. " Any regrets?" "I am not sorry. She was wrong. Had she been alive and committed the same mistake, I would have killed her again."

Turkey: A father, brother and uncle killed a 14-year old girl who had been abducted and repeatedly raped. The alleged rapist claimed in the media they had been having an affair and wanted to marry. Her father said "We wanted to marry her off first. Some relatives opposed the idea. So I decided to kill her. She begged as I strangled her ... but I didn't take any notice of her cries."

Women marrying for the first time are expected to be virgins no matter their age. Hymen restorations complete with a sachet of blood are thus necessary for many women's survival:

"In Jordanian society, some things remain the same. A Jordanian woman marrying for the first time, no matter what her age, must be a virgin. And if she isn't, it is a simple matter to become one again. Hymenorrhaphy, or hymen restoration, is a medical procedure offered in countries throughout the Islamic world. It takes just a few minutes, in Amman costs $300, and is done on an outpatient basis and without anesthesia. 'It is quite common in Jordan,' said Dr. Efteem Azar, one of the country's leading obstetrician/gynecologists. 'It is a very simple procedure and quickly done. Anesthesia isn't necessary because if you work with a very fine needle it is less painful than an injection of painkiller would be. Hymenorrhaphy must be done three to seven days before the wedding, because the tissue is simply pulled together and the procedure doesn't last.'" (Goodwin R246)

Another service gynecologists in Muslim countries are called on to supply is post-wedding night verification that the bride was a virgin before the event:

"It is not uncommon for a gynecologist to find in his office a blushing young bride surrounded by a whole horde of male relatives demanding that she be examined," says Dr. Azar. "She did not bleed during sexual intercourse on her wedding night, and the men all want to know why. You always have to favor the girl, because if you don't, she'll be killed by her family. Sometimes, if the girl has the opportunity, she'll beg you to cover for her. They are very frightened, they know they will be killed. So you tell the male relatives the bride had an elastic hymen, which many women do anyway, and in such cases she wouldn't bleed." (R246)

The Qur'an prescribes confinement to death for indecency, but allows for mercy:

"And as for those who are guilty of an indecency from among your women, call to witnesses against them four (witnesses) from among you; then if they bear witness confine them to the houses until death takes them away or Allah opens some way for them" (4.15).

"And as for the two who are guilty of indecency from among you,
give them both a punishment; then if they repent and amend, turn aside from them;
surely Allah is Oft-returning (to mercy), the Merciful" (4.16).

And for adultery, flogging a hundred times, not death:

"[As for] the fornicatress and the fornicator, flog each of them, [giving] a hundred stripes, and let not pity for them detain you in the matter of obedience to Allah, if you believe in Allah and the last day, and let a party of believers witness their chastisemen. The fornicator shall not marry any but a fornicatress or idolatress, and (as for) the fornicatress, none shall marry her but a fornicator or an idolater; and it is forbidden to the believers" (24.3).

Technically four witnesses are required although this can backfire in a case of multiple rape, where the accused men can become the accusers:

"And those who accuse free women then do not bring four witnesses, flog them, (giving) eighty stripes, and do not admit any evidence from them ever; and these it is that are the transgressors" (24.4)

However the prescription in Sharia is stoning a woman to death for adultery.

"In Muslim law the punishment of lapidation is only inflicted for adultery. Under Jewish law idolaters or bearers of false witness were also stoned. It is founded not upon the Qu'ran where the only punishment Sura 24:2 is one hundred stripes but upon the traditions where Muhammad is related to have said 'Verily God hath ordained for a man and a woman not married to one hundred lashes and expulsion from their home town for one year, and for a man and a woman having been married one hundred lashes and stoning'." When a woman is to be stoned, a hole or excavation should be dug to receive her as deep as her wallet ... The purpose of the hole is to conserve 'decency' for the female. Neither boulders nor pebbles may be used, so that death is neither mercifully quick nor endlessly prolonged" (Hughes - Dictionary of Islam).

"In November 1991 a thirty year-old woman named Zahra, who managed to scramble out of the pit in which she'd been buried, had her death sentence commuted: the judiciary felt that her escape must have been the will of God. Those who have recently witnessed stonings describe all-male crowds, different from the mixed groups who attend beheadings. The mood is commonly one of rage and blood lust. Part of the ritual of the Hajj-the holy pilgrimage to Mecca-is the stoning of pillars meant to represent Satan. Witnesses say the woman being executed somehow becomes as dehumanized as those pillars-an outlet, perhaps, for the men's guilt at their own uncontrollable sexuality. Yet the stones in this case hit soft flesh. Because of the way she is buried, each impact snaps her neck backward in a series of excruciating whiplashes. Death often comes when her head is knocked completely off. It is hard to imagine a worse way to die.

Yet the punishments set down for homosexual sodomy are designed to be even more cruel. If the partners are married men, they may be burned to death or thrown to their deaths from a height. If they are unmarried, the sodomized partner, unless he is a minor, is executed, the sodomizer lashed a hundred times. The variation in the penalty reflects the Muslim loathing of the idea of a man taking the feminine role of the penetrated partner. Lesbian sex, if the women are single, draws a hundred lashes. Married lesbians may be stoned. 'Why is Islam so severe in matters of adultery, homosexuality and lesbianism?' asks Mohammed Rizvi. 'If the Islamic system had not allowed gratification of sexual urge by lawful means without associating guilt with it, then it would be alright to say Islam is very severe. But since it has allowed fulfillment of sexual instincts by lawful means, it is not prepared to tolerate any introverted behavior'."

Geraldine Brooks (R80) outlines the continuing severity of this code against women:

"For both Sunnis and Shiites, whatever license their faith allows comes walled around with ghastly penalties for sexual transgression. The limits on sexual freedom in Islam are drawn strictly around the marriage bed, be it temporary or permanent. Extramarital sex and homosexuality are prohibited, and both offenses can draw the most horrific punishments in the Islamic legal code. While the death penalty, in Islamic law, is optional for murder, it is mandatory for any convicted adulterer who could have satisfied his or her sexual urge lawfully with a spouse. The sentence is commuted to a hundred lashes if the adulterer is unmarried, or if the spouse was ill or far away when the adultery was committed. In Iran, stonings, or, as the Iranians prefer to translate the word, lapidations, are still carried out in cases of adultery. Saudi Arabia also specifies stoning as punishment for married adulterers".

"the Prophet tried hard to avoid having a woman stoned when she admitted committing adultery. Twice he turned his head to one side, so he couldn't hear her confession. It was only when she told him the third time, when she insisted on her punishment, that he ordered her to be stoned."

The key problem here is the fundamentalistic association of scripture, law and state. Although the Deuteronomic law specifies stoning for adultery, and for apostasy, even in Biblical times it was very uncommon and mitigated by many conditions, and is now never used. Even Hammurabic laws were not invoked in the inflexible way Sharia is. The Qur'anic invocations are less severe, but are combined with Sharia and interpreted literally, without any religious freedom of choice, instead of being recognized as inspired spiritual poetry.

The expression *"naqisatan 'aqlan wa dinan"* (deficient in intelligence and religion) is one of the bywords and axioms of life on the lips of the masses in Arabic countries (Rafiqul-Haqq and Newton R549). Narrated Abu Said Al-Khudri:

Once Allah's Apostle went out to the Musalla (to offer the prayer) of 'Id-al-Adha or Al-Fitr. Then he passed by the women and said, "O women! Give alms, as I have seen that the majority of the dwellers of Hell-fire were you (women)." They asked, "Why is it so, O Allah's Apostle?" He replied, "You curse frequently and are ungrateful to your husbands. I have not seen anyone more deficient in intelligence and religion than you. A cautious sensible man could be led astray by some of you." The women asked, "O Allah's Apostle! What is deficient in our intelligence and religion?" He said "Is not the evidence of two women equal to the witness of one man?" They replied in the affirmative. He said, "This is the deficiency in her intelligence. Isn't it true that a woman can neither pray nor fast during her menses?" They replied in the affirmative. He said, "This is the deficiency in her religion."

As in the Decalogue, women are equated to domesticated beasts:

Aisha: The things which annul the prayers were mentioned before me. They said, "Prayer is annulled by a dog, a donkey and a woman (if they pass in front of the praying people)." I said, "You have made us (i.e. women) dogs. I saw the Prophet praying while I used to lie in my bed between him and the Qibla. Whenever I was in need of something, I would slip away. for I disliked to face him."

Down to the present time, based on the Qur'an, a man shall have twice the inheritance of a woman and it takes the evidence of two women to equal that of one man. In Iran when a husband dies without other heirs, the state takes half the endowment that would go to the wife. Unlike some extreme forms of patriarchy, this at least provides a 'partial' inheritance:

" Allah enjoins you concerning your children:
The male shall have the equal of the portion of two females" (4.11)

"call in to witness from among your men two witnesses; but if there are not two men, then one man and two women from among those whom you choose to be witnesses" (2: 82).

A hadith narrated by Abu Said al-Khudri and Sahih Bukhari explains the connection:

"The Prophet said, 'Isn't the witness of a woman equal to half of that of a man?'
The women said, 'Yes.' He said, 'This is because of the deficiency of a woman's mind'."

al-Llah prefers men and permits women to be beaten into submission in the bed chambers:

"Men stand superior to women in that God hath preferred the one over the other ... Those whose
perverseness you fear, admonish them and remove them into bed chambers and beat them, but if they
submit to you then do not seek a way against them; surely Allah is High, Great" (4:34)

Bukhari and Imam Suyuti make clear the full significance of this in the hadith showing how far inequality goes in terms of female human worthlessness (R549):

"It is a noble sacrifice for a man to share his life with the woman; she being deficient in mind, religion, and gratitude. It is condescension on the part of the man to spend his life with her. She can not repay this favour, no matter what sacrifice she makes."

"If blood, suppuration, and pus, were to pour from the husband's nose and the wife licked it with her tongue, she would still never be able to fulfil his rights over her."

Geraldine Brooks (R80) notes in 'Nine Parts of Desire':

"When the Koran sanctions wife beating and the execution of apostates, it can't be
entirely exonerated for an epidemic of wife slayings and death sentences on authors."

Muhammad's statements in *hadith* express extreme ambivalence about women (Walther):

"I have left behind no temptation more harmful to my community
than that which women represent for men."

"The whole world is delightful, but the most delightful thing in it is a virtuous woman."

"If a man and a women are alone in one place, the third person present is the devil."

"I stood at the gates of Paradise, most of those who entered there were poor,
I stood at the gates of Hell, most of those who went in there were women".

Desire under a thin red veil.

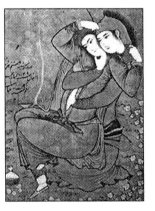

Law of Desire

If the veil is to protect women, the '*mut'a*' or temporary marriage has surprising contradictions to this. In Iran fleeting 'temporary marriages,' are endorsed by the clergy. One particular respect in which Shi'ite and Sunni branches of Islam differ is in the institution of temporary marriage: "A major difference in custom is the Shia practice of *mut'a*, or temporary marriage. An ingenious expedient created by Shiites to resolve the tension of momentary lust without resorting to either dishonor or sexual repression, *mut'a* may last only a few hours, but it legitimizes any offspring of the union. Sunnis disavow such a concept, even though their treatment of women is considerably less generous than that of the Shiites when it comes to family inheritance and participation in religious ritual" (Occhigrosso R500 432). These are marriages in name only, not least because men have the right to deny their responsibilities for any children born of the temporary liaison. This controversial law allows men to fornicate, so long as they register their intentions with a religious Sharia, court where they fill out a form specifying how long they intend to 'enjoy' their partner. Dr. Mahran Doltchahi comments: "The enjoyment marriage is nothing but a legal cover for prostitution. How can anyone in the world claim that a marriage for 10 minutes is a legal act?" The real victims of the Law of Desire are women from deprived socio-economic backgrounds.

Jan Goodwin (R246) in "Price of Honour" provides a colourful cultural vignette of mut'a:

"'You probably had your chador on the wrong way around,' my friend explained. 'That's one of the signals women use if they're looking for sigheh.' Sigheh, or mut'a agreed between a man and woman and sanctioned by a cleric, can last as little as a few minutes or as long as ninety-nine years. Usually the man pays the woman an agreed sum of money in exchange for a temporary marriage. The usual motive is sex, but some temporary marriages are agreed upon for other purposes. When sex is the motive the transaction differs from prostitution in that the couple have to go before a cleric to record their contract, and in Iran, any children born of the

union are legitimate. Otherwise, sigheh is free of the responsibilities of marriage: the couple can make any agreements they like regarding how much time they will spend together, how much money will be involved and what services, sexual or nonsexual, each will provide. Shiites believe Muhammad approved of sigheh. Sunnis, the majority branch of Islam, don't agree. Even in Shiite Iran, sigheh had fallen from favor until Rafsanjani encouraged it after the Iran-Iraq War which ended in 1988. In a 1990 sermon, he argued that the war had left a lot of young widows, many of them without hope of remarriage. Such women, he said, needed both material support and sexual satisfaction. At the same time, plenty of young men who couldn't afford to set up house for a bride were postponing marriage. Sexual tension needed healthy release, he said, and since sigheh existed for that purpose within Islam, why not use it? His remarks sparked a heated debate among Iranian women, some of whom bitterly opposed the practice as exploitative. They argued that the state should provide for war widows adequately, so that they didn't have to sell their bodies in sigheh. But others spoke out in its favor. Sigheh, they said, wasn't just a matter of money. Widows and divorcees had sexual needs and a desire for male company, and the sigheh "husband" was a welcome male presence for the children in their homes. Iran's satirical weekly magazine, Golagha, ran a cartoon lampooning the likely effects of Rafsanjani's argument. It showed two desks for marriage licenses, one for sigheh and one for permanent wedlock. The clerk at the permanent desk had no customers; the queue for sigheh stretched out the door." (Goodwin)

Shahla Haeri, authoress of "Law of Desire" (R270), says conservative clergy are behind a campaign to preserve enjoyment marriages. She cites one of Iran's leading imams, Jafar El Sadek, as declaring 'partners in enjoyment in marriages are especially blessed. When they bathe, every drop of water turns into seventy angels who will testify on their behalf on the Day of Judgment': "Khomeini was alone among senior clergy in condemning the law and the hypocrisy of those who were in favour. Still remembered on the streets of Tehran is the Persian story he once quoted on television "A religious leader said to a prostitute 'You are drunk and every moment you go and visit someone different'. She replied 'Oh Sheik! What you say about me is correct. But what you pretend about yourself, is that true too?"

"The Shi'a doctrine projects a double image of women through the contractual laws of temporary and permanent marriages. We may ask here, What is a woman from a Shi'i perspective? Is she a precious commodity that may be owned, bought, or leased? Is she a person created like a man who can be in charge of her own life, negotiate contracts, control their outcome, and exchange gifts? Is she a decision-making adult or a minor? Looking at the women's status developmentally, and through a discussion of the different forms of Shi'i marriage contracts, I have shown that at any given point in her life cycle a Shi'i Muslim woman may be perceived to be all or some of the above simultaneously. Such legal ambivalence is reflected in a variety of vastly popular binary images of women. Images of women as controller/controlled, seducer/seduced, cunning/gullible, and pious/adulterous, all hive wide currency in the Perso-Islamic literature. In one of the most fascinating literary treasures of the Middle East, the tales of A Thousand and One Nights, the superimposition of many of these binary images is elegantly portrayed. indeed, the whole story is based on one such dominant binary opposition: that of order/disorder. Through the cunning of an adulterous queen, society is brought to the brink of disorder. But the mediation of another woman, Shahrzad, restores order to society and sense to the king. The underlying ambivalence toward women is not reflected just in literature and folklore. The Qur'an itself conveys this ambivalence toward women as well. In the Holy Book women are sometimes depicted as objects to be treated kindly or harshly, and at other times as persons created of the same material as men (compare suras of Women 34 and the Cow 223 with the Private Apartment 13). Many hadiths and sayings of the Prophet, the imams, and other Muslim leaders further underscore this ambivalence. For example, the Prophet Muhammad is frequently quoted as having said: 'Women are the trappings of Satan' (cited in Burhan-i Qat' 1951 63, 2:681; Razi 1963 68, 350). In another context, however, he is alleged to have stated: 'From your world I do not like anything but women and perfume' (quoted by Ayatollah Mishkini 1974, 118). Such ambivalence finds its resonance in the following popular adage in Iran: 'Women are a pain, bala. May no house be without it.' A sigheh woman especially is a target of cultural and legal ambivalence. Personally, she might be more mature and experienced than other women (because she has married at least once and divorced), and legally, she is freer than married and virgin women to negotiate on her own behalf, choose her male partner(s), and exercise her own decision-making power. She is her own person, as it were. A divorced woman's status is the closest that a Shi'i Muslim woman can come to having legal autonomy. Autonomy, however, is not a trait socially approved of for women in Iran. Although some men may welcome it, and even be fascinated by the alluring autonomy of women, as is apparent in the 'sigheh myth,' they are at the same time fearful of the arbitrariness implied in it: just as they may be selected for a treat, they may be let go unceremoniously. Because temporary marriage is a contract of lease and its objective is sexual enjoyment, sigheh women are seen not only as objects of exchange (indeed, they are referred to as the object of lease) but also as temporary sexual partners. There is thus a close structural association with prostitution. Consequently, the custom of temporary marriage and its propriety involve cultural questioning and conflicting feelings, and women who make use of it are also perceived with moral ambivalence. Much to women's disappointment, temporary marriage often bestows them neither with the masculine protection nor with the social prestige they so earnestly seek." (Haeri)

But Khomeni also reduced the age of marriage, permitting girls as young as nine to marry. Muhammed himself married his favorite wife A'isha, the daughter of Abu Bake, one of his closest associates, when she was six years old. Muhammad was 52 and Aisha was 9 year old and still played with dolls when they sexually consummated their marriage. Muhammad followed an Arab custom in marrying a child who had had her first menstrual cycle. The legal marriage age for girls in Iran was only in 2002 increased from 9 to 13.

"Khomeini lowered the marriage age for females from eighteen to thirteen, but permitted girls as young as nine, even seven in some cases, to be married if a physician signs a certificate agreeing to their sexual maturity. 'In his book Tahrir Al' Vassilih, Khomeini writes about the legal requirement for having sex with children,' explained a woman lawyer who is concerned that child brides are dying since this ruling was instituted. 'In villages where child marriage is most common, doctors often don't even see the girl,' she told me. 'They just take the family's word that she is physically mature enough to marry. Consequently, we have had very young girls badly injured and when they have had what amounts to forced intercourse. Infection sets in and they have died.' 'Only with girls under seven did the Ayatollah say that sex was forbidden." (R246)

Contrast the severe legal punishments for women with a statement on men and mut'a:

"No one can deny that most, if not all married men have had sexual relations, legitimate or illegitimate, with other women. Is it wise then to forbid married men from having relations with other women? Is such a law just and in accordance with human nature? Of course not. Such law has not been practical and will not be so! A A Muhajir "Polygamy and Mut'a (Haeri R270 153).

This is consistent with Muhammad's approval of polygyny, including marriage to slaves:

"marry such women as seem good to you, two and three and four; but if you fear that you will not do justice (between them), then (marry) only one or what your right hands possess; this is more proper, that you may not deviate from the right course (4.3).

Islamic law requires a man to provide each of his wives with a household of her own. Thus marital polygyny was usually the privilege of the prosperous. However, in addition to their wives, men could also select any number of concubines from among their slaves (Walther).

The parties to a marriage contract are not the bride and groom, but the groom and the bride's male relative. Marriages can thus be forced (Walther R712):

The parties to the contract are the bridegroom and the bride's guardian ... her closest male relative, usually her father or brother or, if need be, even the judge himself. Two free male witnesses, or one male and two female witnesses, must be present. The Sunna recommends that the bride should not be married without her consent. However, silence is sufficient indication of agreement in the case of a virginal bride, since she is considered to be too shy or timid to speak for herself. When the girl is a minor, her guardian can also force her into marriage, but she has the right to annul this as soon as she is of age. The Maliki, Shafi'i and Hanbali [schools of Sunna] even permit an adult woman to be forced by her guardian to contract marriage.

An important part of the marriage contract is the fixing of the dowry (*mahr* or *saddq*, in Arabic), which is a form of 'bride price', not an endowment for the bride's welfare from her family. However, the *mahr* was not a purchase price, but a compensation the bridegroom had to give the parents of the bride for the loss to the tribe of the sons the woman would bear. The *mahr* was not paid when the girl married her cousin on her father's side; that is, when she remained in the tribe. This is still true among Bedouins today. The *saddq* was the wedding gift the girl received. As early as the time of Muhammed, a distinction was no longer made between these two terms (Walther R712).

Wiebke Walther (R712) notes: "In the context of divorce, the Koran says that they (women) have the same right as is exercised over them, though the men have a rank above them". In fact, husbands are given free reign in matters of separation and divorce:

"You may put off whom you please of them, and you may take to you whom you please, and whom you desire of those whom you had separated provisionally; no blame attaches to you; this is most proper, so that their eyes may be cool and they may not grieve, and that they should be pleased, all of them with what you give them" (33.51).

Under the triple talaq a husband merely has to repeat the oath of divorce three times for it to have immediate effect.Walther further notes that Islamic law permits every man in a healthy mental state to repudiate his wife (*talaq*) without having to give any reason for it and without consulting a judge. There are only a limited number of ways in which a wife can free herself from her husband. The *khul'*, or redemption, was adopted from heathen practice and consists in the wife's purchasing her freedom from her husband by the payment of a certain sum - frequently equivalent to the dowry. It is laid down in the Koran that after the divorce the husband must provide for a wife who is suckling a child until it is weaned this can extend to a period of two years. The mother has the right of custody for girls until they are of age or until they marry and for boys until puberty or the age of seven years. However, the father is the legal guardian of the children; only when they are poor he is obliged by law to maintain them. Thus the mother usually returns to her family, which maintains her, with the children she has to look after. A Muslim woman may not marry a non-Muslim, but a Muslim man is permitted to marry a Jewish or a Christian woman. After a divorce, a woman must wait three months before remarrying. Men, however, are permitted to remarry immediately. (2:234) Muhammad introduced the waiting period in order to determine whether the woman was expecting a child, so that the paternity could be established without any doubt. If the woman was pregnant, she could only re-marry after the birth of the child.

"And the divorced women should keep themselves in waiting for three courses; and it is not lawful for them that they should conceal what Allah has created in their wombs, if they believe in Allah and the last day; and their husbands have a better right to take them back in the meanwhile if they wish for reconciliation; and they have rights similar to those against them in a just manner, and the men are a degree above them, and Allah is Mighty, Wise" (2.228).

Walther notes "Here, as in later traditions in which women are defined as mothers, sisters, and daughters, their roles are defined from a man's point of view, women are seen in their family relations and in their sociability with men":

"Amongst His signs is that He hath created for you of your own species spouses that ye may find rest in them, and hath set love and compassion between you." (30.21)

However this very apparently 'merciful' sura is cited by Qortobi as a basis for a woman to have to submit to the sexual demands of the husband on call:

"When a man calls his wife to his bed, and she refuses, the One Who is in the heaven will be angry with her until he [her husband] is pleased with her" (Rafiqul-Haqq and Newton)

Such Quranic passages are reflected in hadith where sex on demand is a holy duty:

"The prophet of Allah said: When a man calls his wife to satisfy his desire, let her come to him though she is occupied at the oven." (Rafiqul-Haqq and Newton).

Muhammad imposes a taboo on women as unclean during menstruation but ordains intercourse the rest of the time under commandment of God, [as do the Jews]:

"And they ask you about menstruation. Say: It is a discomfort; therefore keep aloof from the women during the menstrual discharge and do not go near them until they have become clean; then when they have cleansed themselves, go in to them as Allah has commanded you; surely Allah loves those who turn much (to Him), and He loves those who purify themselves" (2.222).

Ever present is the role of the female as a sexual beast of burdens, light, or heavy:

"He it is Who created you from a single being, and of the same (kind) did He make his mate, that he might incline to her; so when he covers her she bears a light burden, then moves about with it; but when it grows heavy, they both call upon Allah, their Lord: If Thou givest us a good one, we shall certainly be of the grateful ones. (7.189).

To al Ghazali, woman is in this sura created as a mere plaything. She is a recalcitrant domesticated animal, valued only in her fear of her husband (Rafiqul-Haqq and Newton R549):

"In the company of women, looking at them, and playing with them, the soul is refreshed, the heart is rested, and the man is strengthened to the worship of God... this is why God said: 'That he might rest in her.' (Q. 7:189)" (Essid R195).

"If you relax the woman's bridle a tiny bit, she will take you and bolt wildly. And if you lower her cheek-piece a hand span, she will pull you an arm's length ... Their deception is awesome and their wickedness is contagious; bad character and feeble mind are their predominant traits" ...

"[A man's wife] fears him, while he fears her not, a kind word from him satisfies her, where nothing of hers has importance in his eyes, it is she who must tolerate the presence of concubines, and it is she who worries when he is ill whereas even her death would leave him indifferent."

Despite the high price of dowry settlements to wives' families in Saudi Arabia, and the shunning of divorced women, more than twenty percent of Saudi marriages end in divorce within a year. Marriages suffer from all the usual afflictions, infidelity, incompatibility, house-hold violence - but the biggest problem is polygamy. Many Saudi husbands constantly change partners, a practice that causes constant heartache (Wright L R752).

The Veil of the Shadow of Death

Hamas considers the unveiled as collaborators of a kind. It is our religious duty to execute collaborators. Hamas Graffitti, Gaza (R246)

Wiebke Walther (R712) notes: "Closely connected with the veil is the exclusion of women from public life, based on a verse in the Koran which refers only to the wives of the Prophet: 'When ye ask them (i.e. the wives of the Prophet) for any article, ask them from behind a curtain; that is purer for your hearts and for theirs" (33: 53, 55). She elaborates:

> It is reported in an Arab historical work dating from the ninth century that this revelation originated at the marriage of Muhammed to the beautiful Zaynab Bint Jahsh the former wife of his adopted son Zayd Ibn Haritha. Muhammed had once seen Zaynab in her undergarments as he was about to enter Zayd's house and had coveted her from then on. Zayd wanted to divorce her immediately so that Muhammed could marry her, but Muhammed did not want to accept Zayd's offer. But Zaynab had been married with Zayd against her will and now displayed a clear lack of affection for him. In the end, her marriage with Muhammed took place. Toward the end of the wedding feast, the guests showed no signs of departing. This shows that Zaynab's attractiveness for her guests was considered to have been very great. Muhammad impatiently left the room several times and went out into the courtyard, hoping that he would finally be left alone with his new bride. But this was not the case. It was now that the verse quoted above was revealed to him:

"O Prophet! say to your wives and your daughters and the women of the believers that they let down upon them their over-garments; this will be more proper, that they may be known, and thus they will not be given trouble; and Allah is Forgiving, Merciful" (33.59).

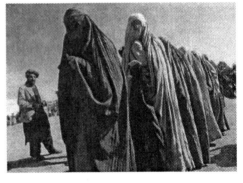

Under the Taliban, women were confined to their houses, unable to work or girls to go to school. They were beaten or imprisoned for showing any sign of make up or even clicking their shoes, in a rigid enforcement of sura 24.31 above: *"and let them not strike their feet so that what they hide of their ornaments may be known" (RAWA).*

An early Arabian historian also explains that Muhammad's wives had been bothered by his opponents in Medina when they left the house at night to 'relieve themselves', because they took unveiled women for slaves (Walther). This ties in with Assyrian traditions in which unveiling was mandatory for slaves and 'available' women and veiling was a 'privilege' of the attached (p 201). It is known that noble ladies of the trading city of Mecca wore veils even before Islam. There no specific mention of veiling the face.

Restrictions on women's modesty are far more detailed and severe than for men:

"Say to the believing men that they cast down their looks and guard their private parts; that is purer for them; surely Allah is Aware of what they do" (24.30).

"And say to the believing women that they cast down their looks and guard their private parts and do not display their ornaments except what appears thereof, and let them wear their head-coverings over their bosoms, and not display their ornaments except to their husbands or their fathers, or the fathers of their husbands, or their sons, or the sons of their husbands, or their brothers, or their brothers' sons, or their sisters' sons, or their women, or those whom their right hands possess, or the male servants not having need (of women), or the children who have not attained knowledge of what is hidden of women; and let them not strike their feet so that what they hide of their ornaments may be known; and turn to Allah all of you, O believers! so that you may be successful" (24.31).

Essentially women are regarded as sexually so provocative and sensual that unless they are completely regulated they will either entice men into fornication or they will become helpless victims of male ardour. This is confirmed by the way a woman who is no longer sexually enticing is exempt:

"And (as for) women advanced in years who do not hope for a marriage, it is no sin for them if they put off their clothes without displaying their ornaments; and if they restrain themselves it is better for them; Allah is Hearing, Knowing" (24.60).

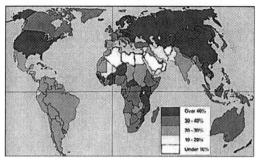

There are fewer women in the work force in many Islamic countries than any other region on Earth (1991)

Consequently women are not only hidden by the veil to varying degrees, but also confined in their movements, expected to be chaperoned in public by their husband or male relatives and limited in their educational and work opportunities.

Zaigul looked at her three daughters, their female cousins and a woman friend down the street and wept. "It is better to die than stay alive in the house. We are like birds in a cage. She had one daughter a lawyer, another studying language and literature at Kabul university and a third at school. None of them expects to study or work again, even though the Taleban say they favour women's education and will find a way for that to continue and for women to work in complete separation from men. "They always say that, but in Khandahar and Herat for a long time now the girls there don't go to school and the women don't go to work. But the Qur'an says to seek knowledge without regard for gender" (Taliban Afghanistan).

The veil is defended by some Muslim women because it protects them from harassment. This is hardly surprising given the way they will be stared at by men used only to 'black moving objects', but it is imposed in Islam from a root fear of female sexual power. It is extended to confinement of the sight of women to their partners and immediate relatives in a way which deprives women of their rights to be seen and to enter the world freely, except when accompanied by a partner or a relative: Consequently there are fewer women in the work force in Islamic countries than any other cultures.

"Women will always be the core issue that will hinder any social progress in Saudi Arabia. We limit their roles in public, ban them from public participation in decision making, we doubt them and confine them bcause we think they are the source of all seduction and evil in the world. And then we say proudly:'We are Muslims.'" - Raid Qusti Saudi journalist (Wright L. R752)

There are some parts of Saudi Arabia where a woman never unveils - her husband and children see her face only when she dies. Female education, which was introduced in 1960 was born in controversy. Although females now outnumber males at the university level, only six percent of women in the overall population are employed, a statistic that has led religious conservatives to argue that education is 'wasted on girls' (R752).

"I am worried about the next generation, They don't see any real women at all. You don't see each others wives, daughters, sisters. Everything is masculine. And yet they are bombarded by images. They can easily see porn" (A middle-aged Saudi R752).

In 2002 a fire broke out in a girl's school in Mecca of 835 students. 15 girls were trampled to death and over 50 were injured. According to the al-Eqtisadiah daily, firemen confronted police after they tried to keep the girls inside because they were not wearing the headscarves and abayas (black robes) required by the kingdom's strict interpretation of Islam:

One witness said he saw three policemen 'beating young girls to prevent them from leaving the school because they were not wearing the abaya'. The Saudi Gazette quoted witnesses as saying that the police - known as the Commission for the Promotion of Virtue and Prevention of Vice - had stopped men who tried to help the girls and warned 'it is sinful to approach them' (BBC).

Female genital mutilation, Egypt (Cohen R121).

The Sunna

Islam is the only major world religion tolerating FGM (p 283). Over a hundred million women world wide especially in the Horn of Africa suffer circumcision removing the clitoris, or infibulation the literal sewing up of the labia to prevent pregnancy. Up to 75% of Egyptian women, including Nawal el Sadaawi herself are

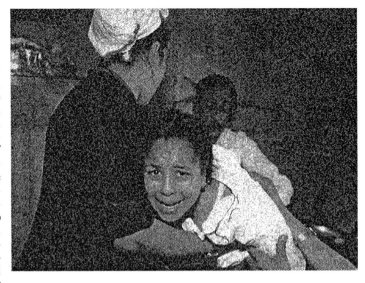

'circumcised'. Muhammad is reputed to have said "reduce but do not destroy" when faced with this practice, but this has led to the sunna cut of the female becoming as traditional as Sunni faith itself:

"The practice of circumcising girls is still a common procedure in a number of Arab countries such as Egypt, the Sudan, Yeman and some of the Gulf states. The importance given to virginity and an intact hymen in these societies is the reason why female circumcision still remains a very widespread practice despite a growing tendency, especially in urban Egypt, to do away with it as something outdated and harmful. Behind circumcision lies the belief that, by removing parts of girls' external genital organs, sexual desire is minimized. This permits a female who has reached the 'dangerous age' of puberty and adolescence to protect her virginity, and therefore her honour, with greater ease. Chastity was imposed on male attendants in the female harem by castration which turned them into inoffensive eunuchs. Similarly female circumcision is meant to preserve the chastity of young girls by reducing their desire for sexual intercourse. . Circumcision is most often performed on female children at the age of seven or eight (before the girl begins to get menstrual periods). On the scene appears the daya or local midwife. Two women members of the family grasp the child's thighs on either side and pull them apart to expose the external genital organs and to prevent her from struggling like trussing a chicken before it is slain. A sharp razor in the hand of the daya cuts off the clitoris. During my period of service as a rural physician, I was called upon many times to treat complications arising from this primitive operation, which very often jeopardized the life of young girls. The ignorant daya believed that effective circumcision necessitated a deep cut with the razor to ensure radical amputation of the clitoris, so that no part of the sexually sensitive organ would remain. Severe haemorrhage was therefore a common occurrence and sometimes led to loss of life. The dayas had not the slightest notion of asepsis, and inflammatory conditions as a result of the operation were common. Above all, the lifelong psychological shock of this cruel procedure left its imprint on the personality of the child and accompanied her into adolescence, youth and maturity. Sexual frigidity is one of the after-effects which is accentuated by other social and psychological factors that influence the personality and mental make-up of females in Arab societies. Girls are therefore exposed to a whole series of misfortunes as a result of outdated notions and values related to virginity, which still remains the fundamental. The research that I carried out on a sample of 160 Egyptian girls and women showed that 97.5% of uneducated families still insisted on maintaining the custom, but this percentage dropped to 66.2% among educated families. When I discussed the matter with these girls and women it transpired that most of them had no idea of the harm done by circumcision, and some of them even thought that it was good for one's health and conducive to cleanliness and 'purity'." (El Sadaawi R188)

"'Have you undergone circumcision?' 'Yes.' 'How old were you at the time?' 'I was a child, about seven or eight years old.' 'Do you remember the details of the operation?' 'Of course. How could I possibly forget?' 'Were you afraid?' 'Very afraid. I hid on top of the cupboard [in other cases she would say under the bed, or in the neighbour's house] , but they caught hold of me, and I felt my body tremble in their hands.' 'Did you feel any pain?' 'Very much so. It was like a burning flame and I screamed. My mother held my head so that I could not move it, my aunt caught hold of my right arm and my grandmother took charge of my left. Two strange women whom I had not seen before tried to keep me from moving my thighs by pushing them as far apart as possible. The daya sat between these two women, holding a sharp razor in her hand which she used to cut off the clitoris. I was scared and suffered such great pain that I lost consciousness at the flame that seemed to sear me through and through.' 'What happened after the operation?' 'I had severe bodily pains, and remained in bed for several days, unable to move. The pain in my external genital organs led to retention of urine. Every time I wanted to urinate the burning sensation was so unbearable that I could not bring myself to pass water. The wound continued to bleed for some time, and my mother used to change the dressing for me twice a day.' 'What did you feel on discovering that a small organ in your body had been removed?' 'I did not know anything about the operation at the time, except that it was very simple, and that it was done to all girls for purposes of cleanliness, purity and the preservation of a good reputation. It was said that a girl who did not undergo tills operation was liable to be talked about by people, her behaviour would become bad, and she would start running after men, with the result that no one would agree to marry her when the time for marriage came. My grandmother told me that the operation had only consisted in the removal of a very small piece of flesh from between my thighs, and that the continued existence of this small piece of flesh in its place would have made me unclean and impure, and would have caused the man whom I would marry to be repelled by me.' 'Did you believe what was said to you?' 'Of course I did. I was happy the day I recovered from the effects of the operation, and felt as though I was rid of something which had to be removed, and so had become clean and pure'." (El Sadaawi R188) .

Enslaving the Concubine

However, like all the ancient patriarchal cultures, slavery is explicitly permitted. Although slavery was supposed to be confined to apply to prisoners of war during a time of conflict and free people could not legally sell their children or become debt slaves.

"So when you meet in battle those who disbelieve, then smite the necks until when you have overcome them, then make (them) prisoners, and afterwards either set them free as a favor or let them ransom (themselves) until the war terminates" (47.4).

In conservative countries such as Saudi Arabia and Bahrain, slavery was ended only recently (Walther R712). The Qur'an acknowledges it as integral to the social condition:

"And marry those among you who are single and those who are fit among your male slaves and your female slaves; if they are needy, Allah will make them free from want out of His grace; and Allah is Ample-giving, Knowing. And let those who do not find the means to marry keep chaste until Allah makes them free from want out of His grace. ... " .

Slaves are allowed to become literate and slave girls should not be forced into prostitution:

"And (as for) those who ask for a writing from among those whom your right hands possess, give them the writing if you know any good in them, and give them of the wealth of Allah which He has given you; and do not compel your slave girls to prostitution, when they desire to keep chaste, in order to seek the frail good of this world's life; and whoever compels them, then surely after their compulsion Allah is Forgiving, Merciful" (24.33).

However female slaves 'whom your right hands possess' are free game as sexual concubines, as in the ancient world:

"And who guard their private parts, Except before their mates or those whom their right hands possess, for they surely are not blamable" (23.5).

Slaves are listed centrally along with the rules for cousin exogamy:

"O Prophet! surely We have made lawful to you your wives whom you have given their dowries, and those whom your right hand possesses out of those whom Allah has given to you as prisoners of war, and the daughters of your paternal uncles and the daughters of your paternal aunts, and the daughters of your maternal uncles and the daughters of your maternal aunts" (33.50).

There are several exhortations to treat slaves compassionately, along with kin:

"And serve Allah and do not associate any thing with Him and be good to the parents and to the near of kin and the orphans and the needy and the neighbor of (your) kin and the alien neighbor, and the companion in a journey and the wayfarer and those whom your right hands possess; surely Allah does not love him who is proud, boastful" (4.36).

In Algeria in a continuing 'civil jihad' which has claimed over 100,000 lives, women are young girls are taken as sex slaves on Islamic pretexts:

"They forced us to cook, wash and clean for them. Each evening, one of us was chosen for gang rape in a separate room. One night as we were eating, I noticed the men's eyes were on me. They kept asking, 'Have you finished eating?' and I would say 'No'. It was the longest dinner of my life. I thought they would get tired of waiting. When I did finish, one of them came to me and dragged me by the arm to a nearby room. There he ordered me to undress. I started crying and begged him not to harm me. I told him that adultery was forbidden by Islam, but he replied,' I am entitled to it because I am a holy warrior, a mujahid.' Before he forced me, he said he would marry me. Then he threw me to the ground - burned me with cigarette ends until I fainted. When I awoke, I was naked and bleeding. I realized I had lost my virginity."

Pregnant women were disemboweled, and children hacked to death:

"Survivors of Algeria's single most bloody massacre told in harrowing reports yesterday how terrorists blasted their way into village houses to hack to death children and women begging for their lives. Some pregnant women were disemboweled. Those fleeing were shot or axed and their bodies burned. Scores of young girls were taken away to provide sex for the attackers. At least 98 people were killed and 120 wounded during a four-hour nightmare in Sidi Rais, south of Algiers, according to official figures. The authorities blamed Muslim rebels for the killings. About 60,000 people have been killed" (Aug 1997).

A thousand people were hacked to death in one episode:

"They [the attackers] are not human ... How can you explain the head of a baby of six months being crushed and the body being trampled on?""The Islamic world should not remain indifferent towards such shocking acts, especially during the holy month of Ramadan" (Jan 1998)

We can see in all these actions as reflections of jihad - permissible in 'holy war' in which 'unbelievers' are cut at the neck and woman are taken as slave concubines noted in (47.4).

Just how central slavery is to the entire concept of Islam as submission is illustrated in the following hadith. Those with the highest rewards are Jews and Christians who convert to Islam, a slave who is faithful to their master and Allah and a master of a slave concubine who 'civilizes', frees and marries her:

Narrated Abu Burda's father: Allah's Apostle said "Three persons will have a double reward:

1. A Person from the people of the scriptures who believed in his prophet (Jesus or Moses) and then believed in the Prophet Muhammad (i.e. has embraced Islam).

2. A slave who discharges his duties to Allah and his master.

3. A master of a woman-slave who teaches her good manners and educates her in the best possible way (the religion) and manumits (frees) her and then marries her."

Defenders of Islam

There are many who claim that, despite these restrictive traditions, Muhammad was a 'radical, compassionate reformer who did much to liberate and protect women':

"Certainly the attitude of the Prophet as regards women has weighed heavily on Muslim civilization, for [his] examples and principles were forcibly warped by the natural tendency of men to seek their own advantage. He certainly improved woman's lot in the Arabia of his day. He prohibited infanticide and the prostitution of slave-women. He established the rights of women to inherit (a half-share). He proclaimed that ... married couples have reciprocal duties and rights, and that women ought to be educated. He limited the number of wives a man may lawfully have to four. He did not set himself up as a model. As it was, he hardly surprised his contemporaries; on the contrary they were inclined to admire his amatory prowess, and were accustomed, like the contemporaries of Solomon, to measure the power of a ruler by the number of his wives. Polygamy was only permitted if one was capable of being perfectly fair to all. Concubines could only be obtained from the holy war, not from the purchase of slaves. Daughters could not be married without their own consent, and this ought to have done away with the right of jabr (arranging marriages for minors). As for unilateral divorce which, more than the now rapidly disappearing polygamy, is the curse of Muslim family life, it is condemned in the famous but little observed hadith, "There is nothing created that God likes better than the freeing of slaves, and nothing that He hates more than divorce." -Emile Dermenghem - Muhammad and the Islamic Tradition" (Occhigrosso R500 404).

What is difficult to ascertain is just how true these statements are about the previous Arabic society. The strength and independence of the Nabataean queens is noted on the coinage of Aretas IV and Shaqilat II (p 221). Many of these traditions should carry over to the goddess worship of Mecca and its environs. It is said that a man pronouncing divorce by recting it three times was a reversal of the rights of women before Islam (Walker R708). The modifications Muhammad made, if we compare them with the Codex Hammurabi are not revolutionary, although they may have been a little more lenient than patrarchal tribal codes following Mesopotamian traditions. The harshest aspects of Deuteronomic law were used by Muhammad himself, including stoning. Thus the claim that the social conditions of women were improved under Islam remains specious but doubtful.

The cruel repression of the women of Daws, and the women of Hadramaut who had their hands cut off for rejoicing at Muhammad's death, the singers whose tongues were cut out and Sarah, killed the day Muhammad arrived in Mecca indicate a heavy and violent hand against any form of female independence. A master had to free a female slave to marry her and her children would then be free but he could also simply claim her as a slave concubine if she wasn't married to another. A free Muslim woman clearly did not have the right to concubinage with one of her slaves (Walther R712). By the power and force-of-arms that occurs in large social systems moral and religious imperatives and controlled domestic violence (Wright R754), men have throughout the patriarchy turned the reproductive tables against women, while claiming to 'protect their interests.' Certain writers pass some of the blame to later patriarchs who themselves had reasons to sequester and veil their women:

> "Many of the so-called cultural and ethnic habits that we see in Muslims today are not derived from the original teachings of Islam, but trace their origins back to that period of the corrupt Ummayad dynasty. Indeed dynastic rule itself was forbidden by Muhammad. The separation of men and women within the same house began in Damascus. There were men who wanted to have dancing girls in their palaces and so they created for the women of the household ladies' quarters, which had not existed in houses before. The mosque, which had been the center of the community where the general public met, and which was the center of economic, social, and political exchange as well as a place of worship, ceased to be so. The mosque became a place of ritualistic worship and lost its pivotal position in the life of the community. The caliph grew fat, often drank and did not want to leave his palace. Accordingly the palace became the center of power and governmental activities. In order not to have his debauchery openly exposed, the caliph separated the women and the children from himself, and thus the home was divided and fragmented." -Shaykh Fadhlalla Haeri, The Elements of Sufis.

Nevertheless these scriptures, if taken literally as they are in many parts of the Islamic world do not spell out freedom and protection for women, but enable men to oppress women in the name of religion and of God. Islamic women who are staunch defenders of the faith need to look a little more caregfully at the actual history of double standards that runs right back to the source events at the founding of the faith. Veiling in its history, from Assyria to Mecca, is an expression of ownership of women by men as possessions, not modesty or privacy.

Apart from the many *houris*, only *Sakina* the spirit of tranquillity, remains in Islam, as the independent expression of the concealed feminine, unsought by Muhammad, in the 'holy' peace at Hudaybiyah which is the antidote to *jihad*. Armstrong (R21 224) says: "The sakina it will also be recalled, seems to be related to the Hebrew Shekhinah, the term for God's presence in the world"(p 262). *Shekhinah* is the abstract feminine face of God, of the Kabbalah, (Scholem R609, Waite R706) the 'indwelling' spirit of matrimonial concord, which withdrew in the Fall from Eden, reflected in the ancient marital tent of Sarah, and the eagle's wings, echoed in Revelation carrying the pregnant 'queen of heaven' to the wilderness

The Sufi Martyr

Sufism is described as the 'inner garment' of Islam, but its roots lie deeper in Gnosticism. The terms comes from the rough wool of their garments. The 'drunken Sufis' exemplified by Bistami (Armstrong R22 261) desired to become one with the beloved in annihilation ('fana): "I gazed upon al-Llah with the eye of truth and said to Him: 'Who is this?' He said 'This is neither I nor other than I There is no God but I' Then he changed me out of my identity into his Selfhood. Then I communed with him with the tongue of his face, saying 'How fares it with me with Thee?' He said 'I am through Thee, there is no God but Thou'. This was taken to its visionary conclusion by al-Hallaj, the 'wool carder'

> *"I am He whom I love, and He whom I love is I: We are two spirits dwelling in one body.*
> *If thou seest me thou seest Him, And if thou seest Him thou seest us both" (Armstrong R22 263).*

However when he preached overthrow of the .Caliphate and cried *"ana al-Haqq* - I am the truth" as Jesus did, he was crucified for blasphemously claiming a name of God. When he saw the cross of nails he turned and uttered a prayer (Armstrong R22 264):

"And these Thy servants who are gathered to slay me, in zeal for Thy religion and in desire to win Thy favours, forgive them O Lord, and have mercy upon them; for verily if Thou hadst revealed to them what thou hast revealed to me, they would not have done what they have done,; and if Thou hadst hidden from me what you have hidden from them, I should not have suffered this tribulation. Glory unto Thee in whatsoever thou doest, and glory unto Thee in whatsoever Thou willest".

Even al-Ghazzali was to argue al-Hallaj had not been blasphemous but only "unwise in proclaiming an esoteric truth which could be misleading to the initiated. Because there is no reality but al-Llah, as martyrdom - *shahadah* maintains, all men are essentially divine. The Qur'an taught that God had made Adam in his own image so that he could contemplate himself in a mirror" (Armstrong R22 264). Itibari has the following to say in response:

"Mansur el-Hallaj was dismembered while still alive, and is the greatest Sufi martyr. But can you name the person who cut him up? Suhrawardi was murdered by the law, but what was the name of his executioner? Ghazali's books were thrown into the flames, but by the hand of whom? Nobody remembers these people's names, for the Sufis decline to reiterate the names of the infamous"
(Shah R622 296)

This sense of revolution against religious confinement has never ceased:

What Must Come
To those who seek truth in conventionalized religion:
Until college and minaret have crumbled
This holy work of ours will not be done.
Until faith becomes rejection
And rejection becomes belief
There will be no true believer. Abu Said (Shah R622 239)

Truth
She has confused all the learned of Islam,
Everyone who has studied the Psalms
Every Jewish Rabbi, Every Christian priest.
Ibn El-Arabi (Shah R622 86).

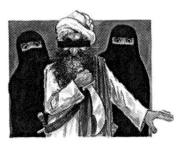 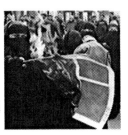

Dec 2005. Left: The Danish newspaper Jyllands-Posten is being protected by security guards and several cartoonists have gone into hiding after the newspaper published a series of twelve cartoons about the prophet Muhammad. According to Islam it is blasphemous to make images of the prophet. Unlike the Safavid (p 263) and Turkish (p 260) images, and other cartoons this one discretely covers the prophet's eyes. Muslim fundamentalists have threatened to bomb the paper's offices and kill the cartoonists. The paper's editor, said the cartoons were a test of whether the threat of Islamic terrorism had limited the freedom of expression in Denmark.. The matter has been referred to the UN Commissioner for Human Rights. The Arab League's ministers council said the cartoons were an insult to Islam. 5000 Muslims have protested in Denmark and burka-clad women have staged demonstrations as far away as Srinagar (Right). The Danish government has so far refused to become involved. The Prime Minister said "The Danish government and the Danish nation as such cannot be held responsible for what is published in independent media".

Ending Female Genital Mutilation

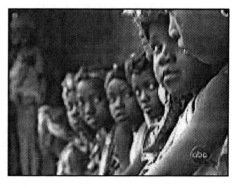

Waiting for the worst (ABC).

Today, an estimated 130 million women, averaging 6000 a day have undergone sexual mutilation. It is performed in many African countries, including Sudan, Somalia, Ethiopia, Kenya, and Chad. It is also a tradition among Muslims in Malaysia and Indonesia, and in a number of countries in the Middle East, including Egypt, the UAE, and parts of rural Saudi Arabia. Coptic Christians in Egypt and animist tribes in Africa as well as Muslims, undergo the ritual (p 278). Subincision is also practiced by some Amazonian tribes (p 170).

It appears to be driven originally by men's desire to have power over womens' sexuality to remove fear of paternity uncertainty by keeping women chaste and uninterested in love affairs, but the practice has become so old and rooted that it is now perpetuated by women upon women in many places.

Female circumcision is frequently described as an "age-old Muslim ritual," when in fact it predates Islam and is even believed to be pre-Judaic. Strabo claimed that "the Egyptians circumcised their boys and girls as do the Jews". The Virgin Mary was likewise said to have been circumcised (Briffault R75v3 324). Islamic tradition also says it was practised by Sarah on Hagar and that afterwards both Sarah and Abraham circumcised themselves by order of Allah. There is no evidence any of Muhammad's wives or daughters were circumcised. There is no mention of it in the Koran, and only a brief mention in the authentic hadiths, which states: "A woman used to perform circumcision in Medina. The Prophet said to her: 'Do not cut severely, as that is better for a woman and more desirable for a husband.' But because of this still debated hadith, some scholars of the Shari school of Islam, found mostly in East Africa, consider female circumcision obligatory. The Hanafi and most other schools maintain it is merely recommended, not essential (Goodwin R246).

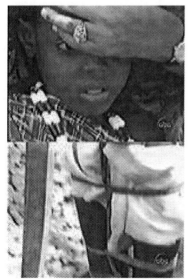

The small girl's torn genitalia are stitched with thorns and her legs tied together to reduce blood loss. Many die (ABC)

The majority of rural Egyptian women are still circumcised. Here they remove only the clitoris; they do not do the much more extensive procedure, but even so, there are many problems. Infection, bleeding, urinary tract damage, sepsis, even death.

More than 90 percent of Sudanese women undergo the most severe form of circumcision, known as "pharaonic," or infibulation, at the age of seven or eight, which removes all of the clitoris, the labia minora, and the labia majora. The sides are then sutured together, often with thorns, and only a small matchstick-diameter opening is left for urine and menstrual flow. The girl's legs are tied together and liquids are heavily rationed until the incision is healed. During this primitive yet major surgery, it is not uncommon for girls, who are held down by female relatives, to die from shock or hemorrhage of the vagina, urethra, bladder, and rectal area may also be damaged, and massive keloid scarring can obstruct walking for life.

After marriage, women who have been infibulated must be forcibly penetrated. This may

284

take up to forty days, and when men are impatient, a knife is used. Special honeymoon centers are built outside communities so that the screams of the brides will not be heard. Sometimes the husband traditionally runs through the streets with a blood-stained dagger.

Waris Dirie had to be operated on as an adult before she could have sexual relations. Dirie's mother believing she was doing the best thing for her daughter, walked her into the brush, held her down and told her to bite on a root. A gypsy woman cut at the lithe girl's genitalia, using a dirty, broken razor blade. "I heard the sound of the dug blade sawing back and forth through my skin," The woman used thorns from an acacia tree to puncture holes in her skin and sew her up, leaving a tiny hole the diameter of a matchstick, through which urine and menstrual blood could dribble. "My legs were completely numb, but the pain between them was so intense that I wished I would die." Five-year-old Waris was left in a hut to recuperate her infibulation. Two cousins died from infection. Uncircumcised girls are seen as unclean and treated as outcasts. For more than 20 years Dirie suffered health problems from her radical circumcision. Menstruation was a long, agonizing process each month, as the menstrual blood backed up in her body:

> It's when we touch on the subject of sex that Dirie becomes agitated. "Please," she implores, "lets not talk about that. Just use your imagination. I will never know the pleasures of sex that have been denied me. I feel incomplete, crippled and knowing that there's nothing I can do to change that is the most hopeless feeling of all. When I met Dana, I finally fell in love and wanted to experience the joys of sex with a man. But if you ask me today, "Do you enjoy sex?" I would say not in the traditional way. I simply enjoy being physically close to Dana because I love him. It never gets easier. It is emotionally draining to talk about something which has been locked deep for so long. The hardest part is to start somewhere. Everybody is waiting, they don't know what to do. The West are aware of the problem. But they're told to back off, it's none of your business.

The face of pain and the implements of destruction (ABC)

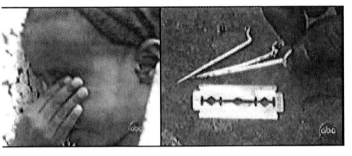

Hawa Adan Mohamed was born and raised in Somalia. At the age of 8 she underwent the most radical form of mutilation practised infibulation. Performed by her aunt in a small village, the procedure was carried out without anesthetic, using basic cutting tools and thorns. She lost an older sister who died after the operation. "In Somalia, circumcision is such a deep deep part of a girl's life. From the moment we are crawling we know about circumcision, we know that our grandmother and mother and sisters are circumcised and we look forward to it being done. Back then, no one would even dream of not being circumcised. If a mother doesn't get her daughter circumcised, her daughter will be an outcast, no one will marry her and everyone would think she is a prostitute so it is a very difficult situation we can't be angry at anyone, because the mothers' intentions are good." In 1995 she returned home, despite civil turmoil, to help her country women deal with circumcision. "I was devastated by what I saw. It seems that we have gone back 40 years. Girls were being infibulated every day with razors and thorns. Two young girls recently died following the procedure and yet still many don't question it. My dream is that in my lifetime there will be young girls living in the heart of Somalia who can run free and play without pain, without the cruel and devastating effects of circumcision. Even just a few. Even 10." (NZ Herald 25 Nov 98)

At the age of 18 Zebebu Tulu was kidnapped by her future husband, Getachew (Getu) Moneta, and taken to his brother's home. Such forced unions are not uncommon in Ethiopia, where men often have near-total control over women's lives. Tradition forbade the tearful Zenebu from returning to her parents and the pair was married after negotiations between the two families (NZ Herald).

Nawal el Sadaawi (R188) has been a prominent campaigner against female circumcision which has brought her the ire of the mullahs. The Naked Face of Eve contains several commentaries on female circumcision:

> "My blood was frozen in my veins. It looked to me as though some thieves had broken into my room and kidnapped me from my bed. They were getting ready to cut my throat which was always what happened with disobedient girls like myself in the stories that my old rural grandmother was so fond of telling me. I strained my ears trying to catch the rasp of the metallic sound. The moment it ceased, it was as though my heart stopped beating with it. I was unable to see, and somehow my breathing seemed also to have stopped. Yet I imagined the thing that was making the rasping sound coming closer and closer to me. ... At that very moment I realized that my thighs had been pulled wide apart, and that each of my lower limbs was being held as far away from the other as possible, gripped by-steel fingers that never relinquished their pressure. I felt that the rasping knife or blade was heading straight down towards my throat. Then suddenly the sharp metallic edge seemed to drop between my thighs and there cut off a piece of flesh from my body. I screamed with pain despite the tight hand held over my mouth, for the pain was not just a pain, it was like a searing flame that went through my whole body. After a few moments, I saw a red pool of blood around my hips. I did not know what they had cut off from my body, and I did not try to find out. I just wept, and called out to my mother for help. But the worst shock of all was when I looked around and found her standing by my side. Yes, it was her, I could not be mistaken, in flesh and blood, right in the midst of these strangers, talking to them and smiling at them, as though they had not participated in slaughtering her daughter just a few moments ago."

New Scientist

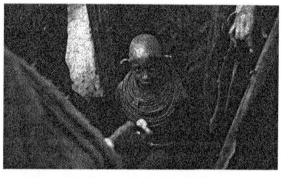

Elizabeth Lloyd (R410 36) in making a case that female orgasm is just for women to have fun with no reproductive value (p 86) has claimed that FGM has little effect on fertility:

> To date, no study has found an association between reproductive capability and FGC. While the Jones et al. study in Burkina Faso found that women who have been cut are more likely to experience obstetric complications, a 1998-1999 NHRC study found that women who were circumcised married earlier than uncircumcised women, and that circumcised women had greater total fertility than uncircumcised women (Reason 2004). Another study based on DHS surveys in the Central African Republic, Côte d'Ivoire, and Tanzania found that, when controlling for confounding socioeconomic, demographic and cultural variables, circumcised women, grouped by age at circumcision, did not have significantly different odds of infertility nor of childbearing than uncut women (emphasis added, Larsen and Yan, 2000). (Elizabeth F. Jackson, Philip B. Adongo, Ayaga A. Bawah, Ellie Feinglass, and James F. Phillips, "The Relationship between Female Genital Cutting and Fertility in Kassena-Nankana District of Northern Ghana," Paper presented at the Annual Meeting of the Population Association of America, Philadelphia, Pennsylvania, March 31-April 2, 2005, p. 4)

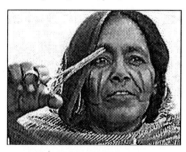

Lloyd's claims are misplaced and unhelpful. Women who have had FGM do suffer a significantly increased fertility risk (Almroth R10). It is clear that, patriarchal societies that diminish or eliminate women's capacity for orgasm, by genital cutting or any other means, also have an agenda to make women bear more children - i.e. more 'reproductively successful'. FGM occurs because men fear, not without good reason, that female arousal does influence reproductive choice. See also the Dogons (p 138), the Shipibo (p 170) and the Sunna (p 278).

2004 An international conference on female genital mutilation has ended in Kenya with a fresh call to ban the practice. Campaigners urged more countries to ratify the Protocol on the Rights of Women in Africa adopted in July 2003. It has so far been ratified by just three states, Rwanda, Libya and Comoros. Although female circumcision is banned in 14 African countries, including Ethiopia, Uganda, Ghana and Togo, the practice is still widespread.

Kedar Ghat Varanasi Feb 2000
(Chris King)

Daughters, Wives and Widows

Killing the Girl Child

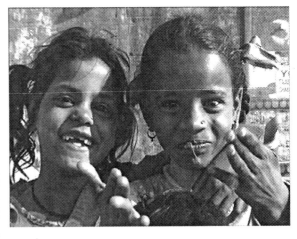

By far the most important cause of a shift in the balance of the sexes is a sexual culling, simple, brutal and carefully hidden from the eyes of seekers after the truth. Millions of girls are destroyed at or before birth, as testimony to their worthless state. In the West, young boys die at a higher rate than their sisters. In two-thirds of the less developed world, the opposite is true. Beliefs in elite male desirability permeate into the social customs of whole societies. The murder of female children is common and, in the new global economy, has become more so. Chinese, deprived of a chance to have more than one child killed more than 250,000 baby girls between 1979 and 1984. Worldwide, the average sex ratio at birth is about 105 male births to every 100 female births. In some age groups in China there are 122 boys for every 100 girls, consistent with 17% of all girls being killed at birth. In one recent study of clinics in Bombay, of 8,000 abortions, 7,997 were of female foetuses, leading to a move to ban ultra-sound for sexual differentiation. In one hospital 96% of mothers who were told they had a daughter aborted, while 100% with sons carried to term (Ridley R564).

The murder of girls is a valued Indian tradition. Rajputs, Sikhs and other warrior castes preferred to marry their daughters to a husband of higher rank which meant an expensive dowry, or the rapid disposal of the unwanted child at birth. The British became concerned when they saw the results of the first census of 1871. In some villages, the commissioners reported, not a single female child was to be found. The authorities brought in the Female Infanticide Act, which set heavy penalties on child murder, and policemen were stationed in such places but, twenty years later, some provinces still had twice as many boys as girls. For a time, the habit began to fade, but now things have changed for the worse. Dowries often take half of a poor family's disposable wealth and the death of unwanted children has become more, not less, common with India's new affluence.

Steve Jones (R340), in forthrightly decrying this situation, notes that the value of females depends on the market:

> In Kerala, a liberal society with an educated population, daughters are born unscathed. In the north and northwest of the country, in contrast, tradition rules. All over the Punjab, Haryana and the United Provinces, men want large families, and many children die young. Women move out of the household to marry, and are rarely seen in public once they have done so. The economy is based on wheat, rather than as in Kerala on rice. Wives play almost no part in the fields, and their value has been further reduced by the farm machinery brought in after the green revolution. Girls suffer as a result (the sole exception lies among the untouchables, whose poverty is such that the efforts of all children are needed to keep the family alive). In certain villages, young boys outnumber girls by three to one. Week-old girls die at twice the rate of their brothers. Often, neither the birth nor the death is recorded; but, when parents admit their child's demise, the cause is given as 'pneumonia', or that 'the baby became stiff'. Boys, the villagers tell the curious, are saved from such a fate because the correct gifts have been made to the gods. Mothers stay in hospital for several days when blessed with a son, but after the birth of a daughter leave at once. Dais, traditional birth attendants, often kill the child, for a fee of around a hundred and fifty rupees (about two pounds sterling). They can, they claim, assess a baby's gender even before birth, and stand ready to do their duty. In some places, each admits to a murder a week. The relatives may do the job themselves by forcing the mother to place tobacco under her child's tongue. If she refuses, she is herself killed or thrown out of the house.

The practice was once limited to the higher castes, but a desire to copy their betters, combined with economic pressure, has spread it even to Sikhs and Christians. As the Indian economy has evolved, so have the reproductive rules. The Kahar community in southern India was branded a criminal tribe in the days of the Raj' and many of its members were imprisoned for banditry. Their women were assertive, worked hard and supported their kin while their husbands were out of circulation. Their villages were poverty-stricken, but both dowries and infanticide were unknown. In 1958 a dam was built. A few communities could grow cash crops and became wealthy, but most stayed poor. At once a dowry system began as parents became desperate to marry their daughters into a richer household. Now the incidence of child murder is among the highest in India. In one recent year, five hundred and seventy of the six hundred girls born were dead within days. So scandalous were the figures that the law at last became involved. For the first time in India, somebody was found guilty of child murder and went to prison. She was, needless to say, a woman, but who was really responsible? No man was charged with any crime.

Nowadays a husband's relatives ask not for clothes, but for televisions. In the slums of Bombay, a dowry may represent five years' worth of household expenses. The Dowry Prohibition Act of 1961 has had no effect. Twenty years on, only the rural northwest had much of an excess of boys soon after birth. Ten years later child-killing had spread, and for the first time in history, India's cities now as a whole have a masculine bias. A dreadful recent development involves dowry murder young brides whose families have not come up with the goods are burned alive, often with the pretext of an accident with a kerosene stove. At least 2000 wives a year are the victims of such crimes, which did not become common until the 1970s.

Prenatal sex tests e.g. with ultra-sound were forbidden in 1996, because they lead to selective abortion, with a three-year sentence and a heavy fine, but the law applied only to government health centres and not to private clinics. Bombay alone has two hundred clinics that offer such abortions, with almost all the procedures aimed at daughters. Now, the job has got easier, with portable scanners taken from village to village to check whether a fetus passes its prenatal examination. Up to a million unborn girls are destroyed in India each year. To check whether his wife is pregnant with the wrong kind of child costs an unskilled worker two months' wages, but the fiscal balance makes it worthwhile. For the middle class, private clinics have begun to provide test-tube fertilisation followed by selection of the desired type; and, of the few dozen who have so far used them, every one has asked for a boy.

The murder of children which so shocked the British in 1871 led to a ratio of 972 women to a thousand men. In 1991 modern science had shifted the figure to 929 females to each thousand males. Gandhis goal of a nation in which, intellectually, mentally and spiritually, women would be equivalent to men has not been realised.

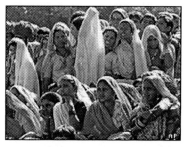

Indian women (AP)

India has an unusual gender balance. In most countries, women slightly outnumber men, but in the year 2001, for every 1,000 male babies born in India, there were just 933 girls. This has often been explained by the fact that some Indian mothers abort their female offspring because they regard them less favourably than boys. But the latest research suggests that discrimination may persist into childhood. The researchers analyzed autopsy reports of babies in three socially deprived parts of Delhi over a five-year period and discovered that the overall death rate for girls was almost one-third higher than that for boys. This was particularly the case for sudden, unexplained deaths - three out of four cases were girls. The researchers suggest some of these deaths may be cases of parents actually killing their female babies. Where death occurred because of a severe and non-preventable disease, there was no gender gap, but deaths due to diarrhoea - which is treatable - were twice as likely to happen to girls as to boys. Again, the researchers suggest that this could be due to discrimination, with parents seeking medical help more urgently for male than for female offspring.

Medical research in India suggests that baby girls are much more likely to die than infant boys, even from illnesses that can be treated. The research, published in the British Medical Journal, was carried out at St Stephen's Hospital in Delhi. The report concludes that the imbalance in the proportion of deaths may be due to the fact that baby girls are less welcome and are treated less favourably by parents (*Indian girls 'more likely to die'* BBC 18 July, 2003)

More than 10m female births in India may have been lost to abortion and sex selection in the past 20 years, according to medical research. Researchers Prabhat Jha of St Michael's Hospital at the University of Toronto, Canada, and Rajesh Kumar of the Postgraduate Institute of Medical Research in Chandigarh, India writing in Lancet said prenatal selection and selective abortion was causing the loss of 500,000 girls a year, based on a national survey of 1.1m households in 1998. The 'girl deficit' was more common among educated women but did not vary according to religion. In most countries, women slightly outnumber men, but separate research for the year 2001 showed that for every 1,000 male babies born in India, there were just 933 girls. They found that there was an increasing tendency to select boys when previous children had been girls. In cases where the preceding child was a girl, the ratio of girls to boys in the next birth was 759 to 1,000. This fell even further when the two preceding children were both girls to 719 girls to 1,000 boys. However, for a child following the birth of a male child, the gender ratio was roughly equal (*India 'loses 10m female births'* BBC 9 Jan 2006).

Indian authorities have been ordered to enforce laws designed to stop the abortion of female foetuses. The Supreme Court ruled that clinics must be punished for using womb scans to determine the sex of a fetus. The case was brought by a children's charity which said many Indians have abortions after ultrasound scans tell them to expect a baby girl (*"India confronts fetal sex checks"* BBC10 Sep 2003).

This pattern of girl slaying is an overblown response under the pressures of a changing developing capitalist consumer society to pressures on the dowry from higher technological expectations and a desire on the part of more people in lower classes to adopt the life style including the practices of girl killing of those in 'higher strata': Nevertheless, its basis is firmly rooted in the Trivers-Willard hypothesis discussed in context of the prisoners' dilemma: as elaborated by Sarah Hrdy (R323 331):

"No research on biased sex ratios in birds or mammals had been done when anthropologist Mildred Dickemann first encountered the logic laid out by Trivers and Willard in their 1973 paper. Social scientists at that time paid scant attention to the idea that there might be innate human predispositions that enhanced inclusive fitness and the long-term survival of family lines. Devaluation of daughters was viewed as a purely cultural construct. It was assumed to be the outcome of free-floating minds spinning infinitely variable webs of meaning out of locally received traditions. As far as cultural anthropologists were concerned, the ideology of son preference along with the custom of paying dowries to marry off daughters sufficed to explain female infanticide. What other reasons could there be? Yet Dickemann was struck by how well the patterning of son preference in the north Indian case conformed to predictions of an evolutionary model that applied to animals generally. Trivers and Willard proposed that parents in good condition should prefer sons, those that were disadvantaged, daughters. They even specified that this logic would be found in socially stratified human societies, where women marry up the social scale, whenever the 'reproductive success of a male at the upper end of the scale exceeds his sister's, while that of a female at the lower end of the scale exceeds her brother's. A tendency for the female to marry a male whose socioeconomic status is higher than hers will, other things being equal, tend to bring about such a correlation.' Trivers and Willard's logic even explained the most puzzling feature of daughter slaying in the Rajput case - why the most elite families were the most likely to kill half of their offspring. By contrast, sub-elites were left paying exorbitant dowries to place daughters in one of these elite households, impoverishing their sons in the process. The poorest subcastes, who really did not have enough resources to feed their children, were the ones who welcomed daughters and did not kill them. None of this made sense unless one accepted the assumption that parents were not counting offspring but looking further down the line, toward grandchildren and beyond, toward the survival of a family line."

"Eliminating daughters at the top of the hierarchy produces a vacuum sucking up marriageable girls from below, and creating a shortage at the bottom. Families don't pay dowries to place daughters in families with the same or lower status than their own. They demand payment for them instead. At the bottom of the heap, sons whose families cannot cough up the required bride price remain celibate. Far from calamities, daughters are the most valuable commodity low-status families possess. Referring to a daughter as a commodity will strike many as extraordinarily callous. But we are not talking about post-industrial Western populations that for generations have lived in an unprecedented state of ecological release, freed from concern about famines. Continued survival of such parents and their children rarely depends on choices mothers make about how much food to allocate to one child versus another. But not all mothers are so fortunate. Daughters not only offered the only prospect for upward mobility, in many cases they provided the only possibility at all of continued survival of a family line. In parts of the world where drought and famine are recurring hazards, the landless and dispossessed invariably have the worst chance of making it through. Under such harsh circumstances the likeliest survivors will be offspring of mothers who marry into families with access to resources, like arable land. Hypergamy (girls marrying up) is not a fluke. It was a long-standing necessity for lineage survival. Nor can it be denied that decisions leading to it have genetic outcomes. Centuries of hypergamous mating have left a trail of genetic markers, like bread crumbs through the forest of the Indian caste system, documenting the different paths followed by the two sexes as they married and produced offspring. An examination of genetic traits carried in mitochondrial DNA (found in somatic and egg cells but not preserved from sperm), which is transmitted only from mother to offspring, showed that these mother-transmitted traits are spread widely beyond traditional caste boundaries. For centuries, they have been carried by brides and concubines moving up in the world by marrying into higher-caste families. By contrast, paternally transmitted markers, traits passed from father to son on the Y-chromosome, are less mobile. Father-transmitted traits remain localized, rarely spreading beyond the caste where they originated. This may be one reason why male traits are more vulnerable to extinction than those carried by mothers. Thus do customs previously viewed as purely cultural have profound demographic and genetic consequences, as well as deep roots in human motivations and their decision rules regarding children".

The earliest evidence for sex-biased infanticide derives from the DNA of baby skeletons-all less than two days old and without apparent defect excavated from the sewer of an ancient brothel in Roman Ashkelon on the southern coast of modern Israel. Fourteen of the nineteen victims of what archaeologists suspected were male consistent with coming from prostitutes in lower class society where daughters would be more valuable.

Whatever the social pressures to get rid of one sex, the simple laws of reproduction will, in the end, always make their presence felt. To interfere with them can lead to painful and expensive consequences. In China girls are still sometimes called 'Too Many' or 'Little Mistake' to reflect their value, but once they were worth even less. In the nineteenth century the province of Huai-Pei suffered a series of famines which led to civil war. Daughters were despised as another mouth to feed and, quite soon, their numbers began to plunge. As their brothers grew up, they found nobody to marry. Great gangs of disaffected youths grew into a horde of a hundred thousand rebels, the Nian. They almost overthrew the Imperial dynasty before they were crushed. The problem of the friendless and discontented Chinese youth has returned. Even official statistics (which understate the problem) suggest a ratio of 117 male births for each 100 females which gives the nation eighty million young men with no hope of marriage. The age gap between groom and bride has increased as older men take teenage wives (which makes life even worse for the next generation), and bachelor villages have appeared in distant provinces. The residents of such places ('bare branches', as they are known) once became monks, or soldiers, or eunuchs in the royal household. Now they move to the cities and add to social unrest. There has been an outbreak of abduction of girls, who are sold into families in search of a daughter-in-law or as prostitutes in the male-filled cities. The government sees the problem. Selective abortion of daughters has been banned, and posters proclaim that 'Girls are fine descendants too'. It will, alas, take more than slogans to remove a habit built so deep into the nation's fabric.

A principal effect of the one-child policy was to cause children after the first to be skewed. Later births in families with more than one existing daughter were extremely male-biased, those with several sons were somewhat female-biased (R416).

Bobbi Low (R416 173) notes the effects of this process of families biased towards sons:

"In the early 1980s, the government of China instituted its "one child" policy in an attempt to slow China's population growth rate. Couples were restricted to one child per family, with some exemptions. The cultural history of son preference has interacted with the limits on family size, and possibly with marriage preferences. The proportion of families with only one child did increase, and the birth sex

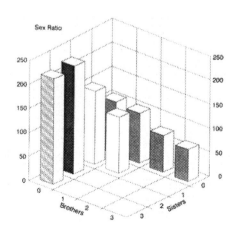

ratio became more male-biased. In one or two provinces the sex ratio. of children in single-child families to soared to over 129.

But it was primarily in later births that the sex ratio became most pronounced. In a nation-wide study in 1989-90, the sex ratio of first births was 105.6, right at the worldwide average, but the sex ratio of later-born children depended on how many older brothers and sisters already existed. The sex ratio of third-borns when there were two older sisters was 224.9 males per 100 females, and the sex ratio for third-borns with two older brothers was 74.1. Some daughter preference did exist when several older brothers were already born".

"China acts to protect baby girls" BBC 15 July, 2004:

> China says it will intensify its efforts to protect girls and address the gender imbalance of new-born babies. A senior government official said that trafficking and abandonment of girls would be severely punished, and a ban on selective abortion reinforced. Government figures show that 117 boys are born for every 100 girls. The imbalance is widely believed to be a result of China's strict one-child policy. Many parents abort baby girls, hoping to try again for a boy. "Illegal sex determination and sex-selective abortion must be strictly banned," said Zhao Baige, the deputy director of China's National Population Commission. "China has set the goal of lowering the sex ratio to a normal level by 2010."

In Korea there is a similar imbalance in the sex ration caused by selective abortion:

> "One son is worth ten daughters,'" exclaimed the exultant south Korean mother of a newborn boy. It's a harsh assessment, but one often heard. in male-dominated Asian societies. In South, Korea, however, the preference for boys has taken a disturbing turn. There are at least 113 men for every 100 women in Korea, one of the highest gender imbalances in the world which, according to sociologists has profound social implications. A shortage of wives perhaps is the most obvious of these, but more alarming is the willingness of many Korean women to abort female fetuses in pursuit of a son. About 30,000 female fetuses each year or one in every 12 girl births after tests to confirm their gender. The high rate of abortion is partially explained by the aborting of female foetuses,' Professor Cho says in her paper. She notes that in a national survey in 1991, nearly one-third of respondents approved of abortion of female foetuses. The abortion rate is extremely high in Korea. One survey says that half of women aged between 15 and 44 have had abortions, a rate that has stayed steady since the late 1970s. Abortions are a major factor behind the sex imbalance, particularly among third and, fourth-born children where there are more than 200 boys for every 100 girls. Most women pray for their first born to be a boy, consuming such bizarre folk medicines as raw rooker's testicles and holding religious services to boost their chances. They become increasingly desperate if they produce only girls, leading to more sex-tests and abortions. "When I felt that the fetus was a girl, I aborted my pregnancy,' said one woman interviewed for a recent paper in the Asia Journal of Women's Studies published by Ewha Women's University. "I almost decided to abort my third pregnancy because my dreams and the shape of my belly told [me] it was a girl." In 1990 doctors were banned from telling parents the sex of their unborn child after ultra-sound tests or amniocentesis. The Government's aggressive campaign to convince to convince Koreans that a well-raised daughter is worth ten sons has seen the imbalance dip since 1990 But, despite new moves to revoke the licences of offending doctors, a high number still take money to tell parents their child's sex, and the practice is almost impossible for the authorities to trace.

In recent years ethnic Korean women from China have been imported by marriage agencies for rural men unable to find wives. The match often ends badly as many of the women are already married and agree to the match solely to support their families back home. "Nowadays the age of the girl children subject to sexual abuse is getting lower. The problem of sexual violence is high anyway and many people think it is due to the sex imbalance." The signs are encouraging that the imbalance will gradually correct itself, but its consequences will linger for - years as the pressure on women to bear sons is still immense. The so-called 'son-preference' is rooted in South Korea's Confucian philosophy, which stresses the role of the son in carrying on the family's bloodline, and in various ancestral rituals. Bearing a son is regarded as a woman's most important role. Girls are secondary since they become part of their husband's family after marriage. But these traditions have been modified to suit South Korea's embrace of capitalism. It is a chauvinistic society where women have little prospect of a well-paid job. Boys, simply, are a better bet for parents wanting financial support in their dotage. "Boys are seen, as a guarantee against economic upheaval," says Professor Cho. But she points out that South Korea's modernisation is slowly changing the attitudes of some young women: "Many young women don't want to live like their mothers."

Authorities in Vietnam are preparing a law which will stop doctors from performing tests on pregnant women which will tell them whether they will have a son or daughter - aimed at stopping the abortion of females in a society where many parents prefer to have sons:

Senior officials are concerned that Vietnam's current population imbalance, where there are more men than women, could get worse. Vietnam has one of the world's highest rates of abortion. It is used as a contraceptive and, the authorities fear, as a way of ensuring that pregnancy results in sons, not daughters. Two-child policy The new law to ban gender testing is being prepared with the support of the National Committee for Population and Family Planning. It has warned that having an imbalance of men to women could lead to violence as men compete for partners. Vietnam's rulers urge people to control the size of their families as part of their economic and social responsibilities to the country, where the population has reached about 80 million. Women are encouraged to delay having children until their early twenties and there is a two-child policy. In the most extreme cases, parents can be penalised for having a third child. They can be expelled from the Communist Party or have their land confiscated. But Vietnam has decided against a one-child policy after looking across the border to China where the policy has led to a massive gender imbalance. There is also concern about the rate of abortions in Vietnam. The average is for a women to have two abortions in her lifetime. The high rate is attributed to the use of terminations as contraception and also to the trend for urban living and, among the young, more liberal attitudes to sex (Vietnam to ban gender testing BBC 18 Nov 2001).

Low (R416 171) also notes that highly biased sex ratios can also occur from some customary practices without necessarily implying infant mortality or abortion:

"Among orthodox Jews, marital intercourse is prohibited during menstruation and for seven days thereafter, and the husband is not to masturbate or seek other sexual outlets. At the end of the seven days, the wife takes a ritual bath, and the couple is directed to have intercourse at that time, and twice' a week during the rest of the month, with the exception of men in unusual occupations. There is additional advice if the couple wishes to conceive a son: intercourse should take place twice in succession. It is difficult to obtain birth sex ratios for orthodox Jews independent of nonorthodox Jews, and conception biases are certainly difficult to measure, for the obvious reason that important parameters are difficult to control. Nonetheless several things are true. Y-bearing sperm, which combine with the egg to make an XY (male) fetus, are slightly pointier-headed (hydrodynamically better) than X-bearing sperm; they are also smaller, with fewer resources to stay alive if the egg is not immediately ready. As a result, in humans as in most mammals, conceptions close to time of ovulation tend to be male- biased. The orthodox cultural practice of abstinence for about twelve days per month, combined with frequent intercourse near the time of ovulation, appears to interact with biological biases in conception probabilities: sex ratios for Jews in a number of traditionally orthodox locations historically average 137 males/ 100 females, while for nonorthodox Jewish populations, and nearby secular populations, they average 105, the worldwide average".

The developed world, less bound by economic pressure, is not much concerned with gender balance. Parents with two boys, or two girls, choose to have a third child more often than do those whose first pair were of different gender. This affects their own household, but has no effect on the overall balance. In the United States a third of counsellors would allow a pregnancy termination for a couple who want a child of a particular gender even if no medical issue is involved. The figure for Israel is twice as high. Britain has so far been strict, except to avoid inborn disease.

Plenty of couples try to subvert the rules of nature in a less drastic way and are happy to pay for the privilege. The author of 'How to Choose the Sex of Your Baby' retired to Las Vegas on the proceeds. The FACS machine, used to sort cattle sperm, has now been turned to our own ends. The businesses who shift the ratio for cows have been joined by the MicroSort Company, which does the same for humans. So far its services are restricted to couples who already have two or more children of the same sex and who are happy to be counselled to ensure that they do not reject a child of the unwanted variety should the device fall. At two thousand dollars a try the procedure is not cheap, but already five hundred or so American pregnancies have come from sorted sperm.

In stark contrast to parents in the developing world, Americans who make such choices much prefer girls. Three-quarters ask for a daughter rather than a son. The global shortage of a hundred million of their fellows is a reminder that in other places the economic sums add up in a different way. Remorseless as such calculations may be, human evolution follows the rules of other creatures and the laws of nature are likely to win in the end.

The Indian government says it will reward girls from single child families with free education and other benefits. The move is intended to bolster India's dwindling female population and help promote population control. India, with a population of over one billion, has only 933 women per thousand men according to the 2001 census.(*Free school for one-girl families Jyotsna Singh BBC 22-9-2005*).

Girl's less than half the value: Shanghai police are investigating a scheme to sell newborn babies on a popular auction Website, according to eBay officials. The starting bid for a baby was 1 yuan, like most items sold on eBay. If a bidder agreed to pay 28,000 yuan (US$3,457) for a boy or 13,000 yuan for a girl, the person would win the auction immediately (ShanghaiDaily.com 20-10-2005).

Till Death us do Part

There is a more sinister patriarchal logic to the burning of wives for their dowries. A new study (Swami R663), the first of its kind, provides appalling proof of what many in India already acknowledge - that many of the unusually large number of kitchen burning 'accidents' affecting young married women are in fact dowry-related murders, or forced suicides, acts of unimaginable violence against wives who can't meet their husbands' and in-laws' demands for yet more money. The study suggests that in spite of India's strict anti-dowry laws and long-running campaigns by women's groups, incidents like these are on the rise across India. Worse still, the guilty nearly always go unpunished either because police and forensic pathologists fail to investigate the cases, or because rampant corruption scuttles them at a later stage.

Hindu practices in India cause the death of more females than any other social or religious system, when infanticide of up to 15% of girl children, plus up to 25,000 wife burnings annually are taken into account. Although the dowry is illegal, social customs persist (Swami)

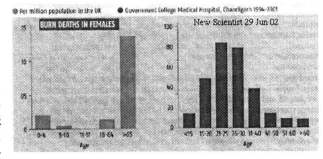

The study carried out by Baldev Raj Sharma and his colleagues shows that of 385 burn deaths at his hospital between 1994 and 2001, most of the 292 women who died were not victims of kitchen accidents (Burns, 28, p 250). What's more, the numbers are rising. In 1994, burns accounted for 12 per cent of postmortems at the hospital. In 2001, the figure had jumped to nearly 30 per cent. However, the police reports Sharma examined concluded that 97 per cent of the women, usually young women within five years of their marriage, were burnt in accidents in the kitchen, usually due to a burst kerosene stove. Yet in some of their homes, kerosene wasn't even used in the kitchens. And while most kitchen accidents cause burns on the arms, chest and abdomen, many of these women suffered 80 to 90 per cent burns.

In traditional Indian homes, girls learn to cook when they are around 13, which is when most accidents would be expected to occur. Most burns victims in the West are children and the elderly. In stark contrast, only 4 per cent of the deaths studied by Sharma were among girls younger than 15. The number jumps to 16 per cent for women aged 16 to 20 - the age at which most women marry - and to 28 per cent for those aged 21 to 25. The most damning statistic is that every one of the married women was burned in her in-laws' home. "That speaks for itself," says Sharma.

Why then, in the face of seemingly overwhelming evidence, do the guilty nearly always go free? The problem is not with the anti-dowry laws. "The villain of the piece is the investigation," says NR Menon. And the problem starts with the woman's dying declaration. "There is a belief that the dying will not lie. Invariably, the victim is brought to hospital by her husband and her in-laws, the very people who may have tried to kill her or forced her to attempt suicide (the law treats those responsible as guilty in both cases). The woman is told that her own parents will be hurt if she doesn't say it was an accident, or is beseeched to consider the fate of her children if she dies and her husband goes to jail, or warned that she will have to come back home if she survives. "Even if I send the in-laws outside, she'll invariably lie".

In fact, Sharma found that fewer than 4 per cent of the women died within an hour because of shock, while more than half survived for anywhere from three days to over a week before succumbing to infections. Sometimes, in the hours or days before her death, the woman reveals that she tried to commit suicide after being unbearably tormented at home, or even accuses her husband and in-laws of trying to kill her. In such cases, the courts are forced to consider an her statements and look at other evidence. Some evidence comes from the post-mortem, which must be performed on the body of any woman who died an unnatural death within seven years of marriage. And experienced forensic pathologists can usually tell whether burns are accidental from their nature and extent. Yet even then the system fails. The problem is that such evidence is not enough in itself. Because the police invariably do not start investigations until the woman dies, supporting evidence from the scene is usually lost. It should be completely obligatory on the part of the police to take the help of the forensic scientists and forensic pathologists. Until two years ago, Victoria Hospital's burns ward was like a railway station, she says. People wandered in and out as they pleased, and staff had to be bribed to change sheets or give injections. 'It was a hell-hole,' says Fernandes. And this remains the state of many hospitals across the country.

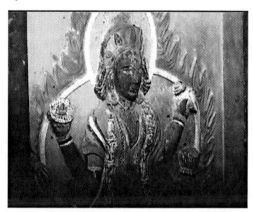

Kali in the flames Katmandu (Chris King)

"According to the reported deaths - and they are all under-reported - almost 100 women die every month in Bangalore [of unnatural causes such as hanging, poisoning or burns]. And 70 to 800 per cent of these deaths are deemed accidental", says Fernandes. "The interest and commitment to find out the truth are not there." As a consequence, official figures on dowry-deaths don't mean much. The National Crime Records Bureau in Delhi reported about 6000 dowry deaths a year in the 1990s. Unofficial estimates are much higher. Himendra Thakur of the US-based International Society against Dowry and Bride-Burning in India estimated in 1999 that nearly 25,000 women are murdered or forced to commit suicide every year. Aside from sheer negligence, corruption at all levels is sabotaging efforts to crack down on the culprits. "When they don't succeed with the police and the doctor, they get hold of the prosecutor," says Saldanha. "And he'll very cleverly sabotage the case." The problem is so bad that in Karnataka state an astounding 97 per cent of the accused in dowry death cases are acquitted. And after appeals to the High Court, the acquittal, reach nearly 99 per cent. This problem affects the entire country, creating a climate in which some men feel they can get away with murder. Saldanha adds that one section of India's anti-dowry law states that if a woman dies, any property or wealth given as a dowry should be returned to her own family, regardless of whether her husband was convicted or acquitted. "Judges in India had totally overlooked [that] section As a result, when the case fails, the husband and in-laws are left with the loot. And that gives them a tremendous appetite to do it again. Society will have to take a leading role and revolt against this, and see that the system is taken to its logical end."

Most killing of women for non-payment of 'promised' dowry have so far occurred in the urban affluent upper-caste Hindu communities, in spite of its rapid escalation and migration into traditionally incidence-free areas and non-Hindu communities of India as well as Bangladesh and Pakistan (where death of newly married women due to 'stove bursting' has often featured the news media in recent years). In places where traditionally there is an absence of caste- or dowry-based marriage system (such as the tribal communities of the far-east Indian states or predominantly caste-free Muslim, Christian, or Buddhist majority areas), dowry deaths are still not rampant (Partha Banerjee). This evidence reasserts that the problems of dowry death, bride burning, and other forms of dowry-related violence on women is a Hindu phenomenon that is now almost out-of-control. Reasons cited by one author are: (1) retention of the caste system, (2) undermining of the woman by the religious orthodox and social patriarch making herself and her family vulnerable to socio-economic pressure and extortion, (3) ever-increasing greed of the bridegroom and his family, (4) an economically strangled hyper-populated society non-supportive of unmarried women, (5) a morally depraved political system run by the pro-status quo conservatives.

(6) Apathy from the educated Indian middle-class.

The epicenter of the problem of bride burning and other forms of dowry-related violence on women is Delhi (the Indian capital), western and central Uttar Pradesh (cities such as Kanpur, Lucknow and Agra have witnessed the highest number of deaths), and places adjoining Delhi (Haryana, northeastern Rajasthan, northern Madhya Pradesh, and southern Punjab), and the problem has largely been concentrated among the upper caste above-average Hindu communities. Now the problem has spread rapidly to other traditionally incidence-free areas and classes -- south Indian states such as Andhra Pradesh, Tamil Nadu, and Karnataka, western states such as Maharashtra and Gujarat, and eastern states such as Bihar and West Bengal (the latter having been one of the bastions of leftist politics of India) have witnessed rapid surge of incidents in recent years.Incredibly, in some cases, the convicted husband will be requested by the parents of his previous bride to marry her sister. The latter is an example of the severity of the problem. The sister and her parents have no place else to go but the abuser/killer man. The death of the woman has left a permanent mark of misfortune on her family resulting outcasting/abhorrence by other prospective bridegrooms. The surviving sister can't remain unmarried: the patriarch society and the upper caste rulers would not permit that. But the incidence of the 'untimely death' of her older sister prevents her parents to find a "clean" groom for her. Now, here comes the widower willing to remarry with an batch of dowry probably a little less than the first time. And, he will now probably be more 'forgiving' to the bride's family he already so much knows. So, who should the family turn to but the 'closely related'?

Cerbera odollam, which grows across India and south-east Asia, is used by more people to commit suicide than any other plant, but doctors, pathologists and coroners are failing to detect how often it is used to murder people. Three-quarters of Cerbera victims are women. The team says this may mean the plant is being used to kill young wives who do not meet the exacting standards of some Indian families (J. Ethnopharmacology 95 123)

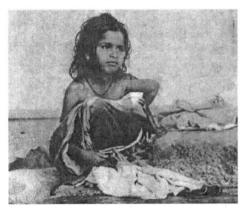

NZ Herald

Untouchable Sacred Whores

Untouchability is practised everywhere in India—until it comes to sex. Ten-year-old Yellamma perches on a stone slab in the dying light, absent-mindedly fiddling with her hair. She doesn't realise it but her hair has condemned her to a life of sexual slavery. Yellamma was born a Dalit (or untouchable) and lives in Pagidimar village in Andhra Pradesh. She has a wild mane of hair matted into dreadlocks. Her father has been told by the village chief it is a sign that she must be dedicated to the goddess Ellammal. His only daughter will become a Jogini woman - a role performed - only by Dalits - and will have to have sex with any man that wants her. She will not be permitted to marry and the men need not pay nor bear any responsibility for any children. Her father says, "We have worshipped Ellammal for many years. She gives us protection and guides us. I don't want to disobey the sign because she will punish us. Look at her hair. It means she must be dedicated." In fact her hair is so tangled because her mother died from tuberculosis when Yellamma was only six and she had no one to care for her or look after her appearance.

Her dedication as a Jogini has little to do with religion and more to do with economics. Her father is a day labourer, paid only in rice. He cannot afford meat or vegetables. Yellamma is a pretty girl and a Dalit— which is why her father has come under pressure from higher caste men to have her dedicated. She hasn't reached puberty yet but already the vultures are beginning to circle. More than 10,000 Dalit women across Andhra Pradesh are forced to work as temple prostitutes. The practice was outlawed in 1984, yet the use of

Jogini women is still extensive in rural areas. There is little will to help these women, especially as the local police also make use of them. Many temple prostitutes are bonded to their work through fear of punishment from the goddess, but Dappu employs former Jogini women to show change is possible. Ex-jogini Hajamma was brave enough to leave her profession and has married. She now travels from village to village to persuade elders and parents to abandon the custom. So far Hajamma has saved more than 1130 girls from a life of misery and sexual servitude. She is slowly trying to win the confidence of Yellamma's father, who has finally agreed to take her to the barbers to shave off her hair. If it grows back straight she will not be dedicated to the goddess. With constant support from Dappu, Yellamma may have a fighting chance. - India is the world's largest democracy, a nuclear power and at the forefront of the "' revolution. (Georgina Newman CCF NZ Herald 26 June 2004).

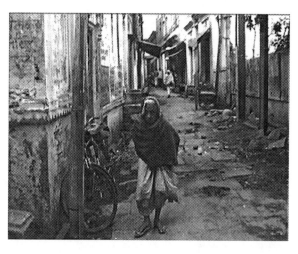

Varanasi February 2000 (Chris King)

Widows in Charnel Houses

In "Fire" Deepa Mehta had done a searing portrayal of a wife burning. In February 2000 agitated Hindu extremists, threatening violence, forced the authorities in a northern Indian state to halt her from shooting her subsequent feature film "Water" after a Hindu activist tried to commit suicide by jumping into the Ganges in protest. The film was to be about impoverished Hindu widows and their inter-caste love affairs in the holy Hindu town of Varanasi on the banks of the holy Ganges River - Mehta was requested to leave Varanasi as the authorities feared more trouble from extremists objecting to the Indian-born Canadian director 'sullying' their culture by portraying penurious Hindu widows in sexually exploitative situations (Feb 2000 NZ Herald).

Varanasi Feb 2000 (Chris King)

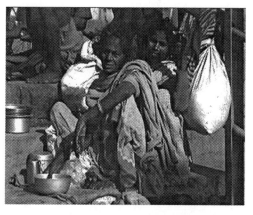

The subject of countless tragic Indian novels and stories, the hapless widows of Varanasi, mainly from eastern Bengal state have for centuries been banished by their children to this filthy and over-crowded city. Over 6000 widows live wretched lives in Varanasi today, cast aside by their sons or other male relatives within weeks of their bereavement. Many are beggars while others are forced into prostitution. Some even belong to rich Bengali families, whose sons were successful overseas businessmen. "To live and die in Varanasi can no longer be the end-all for widows today," said former Justice Dalip Basu of Bengal's High Court, who recently upheld the rights of banished Bengali widows to sue their children for depriving them of a "decent and honourable life." The widows, he declared, must be recognised as "helpless victims of family tragedies and a degenerate value system" (India's neglected widows BBC 2 Feb 2002 Jill McGivering).

India alone has almost 40 million widows. Traditionally Hinduism frowns on widows remarrying and many have their social and economic power eroded too - although in recent years many widows have benefited from moves to enhance their status. Vrindavan is a pilgrimage town now home to thousands of destitute widows. Ashtabala Mundo is one of thousands of widows who have been driven by poverty to the holy town. She was married off when she was still a baby and widowed when she was still a child. "We have to come and sing here morning, noon and night and for all that I only get is $10 a month," she said. "By the time I've paid the rent, I can't afford to buy cooking oil. So I often go all day without a The women line up, after singing for several hours, to receive a cup of rice and a few teaspoons of lentils. It isn't much. In India, widows are an invisible community. Meera Khanna, one of the conference organisers, says although many widows are treated less harshly nowadays, they still face discrimination and neglect. "We treat widowhood not as a natural stage in the life cycle of a woman, we treat it as some kind of an aberration. We accept death but we don't accept widowhood," she said. "Because somewhere in the Indian psyche, the woman's identity is with the man and the minute he's not there, it's something that cannot be accepted."

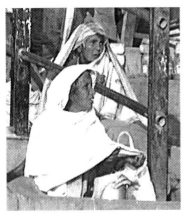

Varanasi Feb 2000 (Chris King)

Mr Madhav of Vrindavan's Shri Bhagwan Bhajan Ashram temple society says more than a thousand widows a day come to his temple alone. "Most are very poor and once their husbands die, they have to come here. We can at least give them food and clothes". Outside, loudspeakers play songs honouring Lord Krishna, in the town associated with the Hindu God. Many of the widows who flock here have nowhere else to go. Hindu widows are not supposed to remarry. With little social or economic status, many become destitute. We met Nirmala Dasi, a frail 85-year-old, begging at the temple gate. When she spoke, she dissolved into tears. "I've been too ill to sing at the temple for the last three days so I haven't had a thing to eat. You don't get anything unless you go there." We were soon surrounded by widows with sad stories to tell. "I spend almost everything I get on a room I share with four others. I've no relatives, or I wouldn't be here," said Mithila. "It's so cold here, I'm always freezing." Widows have been a marginalised and deprived group for generations.

Suttee: Ultimate Immolation

Ram Mohun Ray fought against and brought down the barbaric custom of *suttee* ('voluntary' immolation of the widow along with her dead husband -- in most cases, she would be coerced to die -- again, the custom was practised upon distortion of Hindu scriptures where the covert purpose was to surreptitiously gobble up the property of the deceased). Ram Mohun Ray, using his sharp progressive mind, thorough knowledge of the Hindu scripture, and social status as a rich landlord with connections with a few compassionate British officers and civilians, openly challenged and defeated Hindu orthodox pundits in scholarly debates on the issue of 'sutee'. At the same time, on the streets of Calcutta, he fought thugs and criminals hired by the zealots.

Sati, Shiva's wife is said to have immolated herself in shame at her lord's exclusion from the Vedic sacrificial rites of her father Daksha. She is reincarnated as Parvati Shiva's long-suffering wife who tries to introduce the wrathful and ascetic god of death and destruction to family life. In his wrath at the sacrifice, Shiva dropped a bead of sweat which became disease. The gods begged Shiva to limit the damage so he divided disease into its many forms. Like the celibate man, *sati* the chaste 'virtuous woman' became worthy of worship. She was equated to a goddess. The Ramayana drives the concept of female chastity to an extreme, where a slur against a woman's reputation becomes unforgivable. In keeping with her wifely duty Sita followed her husband Rama to the forest and endured hardships for fourteen years. In the final year of her exile she was abducted by the rakshasa king Ravana. Rama rescued her, but before accepting her back he demanded proof of her chastity. Sita jumped onto a pile of burning wood. The flames did not touch her, so pure was she. But despite this the people of Ayodhya were unwilling to accept a woman associated with another man as their queen. So Rama abandoned his wife, despite knowing that she was virtuous; he did not want his family name to be soiled in any way.

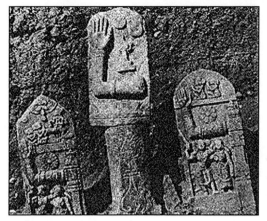

Memorial stellae on a former widow-burning ground at Kiken near Mysore, India. The symbolic rosette and lifted hand carry into the modern period motifs originally associated with Inanna and her descent into the underworld to witness the funeral rites of the bull of heaven, the star Taurus, where she hung on a nail as a rotting corpse, before ascending into heaven. They are also echoed in the Royal Tombs at Ur where whole kingly courts were buried alive (Campbell R104).

Devutt Pattanaik (R518 177) notes that widows who chose not to follow their dead husbands were not allowed to remarry and were forced to live a life of extreme austerity. They were prevented from wearing colored clothes, cosmetics, and ornaments and even had to shave their heads. While the living widow was considered inauspicious, the widow who leapt onto her husband's funeral pyre was deified. Her love and chastity, according to popular belief, prevented the flames from hurting her. Such fidelity was not demanded of husbands":

"Even today during marriage ceremonies the bride is reminded of women who obeyed their husbands no matter what: Sita, who followed her husband to the forest; Mandodari, who remained faithful even though her husband, Ravana, was a rapist; Kunti, who, instructed by her husband, slept with gods to bear him children; Gandhari, who blindfolded herself to share her blind husband's handicap; Draupadi, who obeyed her husband, Arjuna, and married his brothers; Anasuya and Arundhati, who even the gods could not seduce. Strategic narratives that glorify female chastity have contributed in many ways to the internment of Hindu women within the household, bound by marriage and maternity. In medieval India the idea of the sati, a chaste wife sharing the death of her husband, became immensely popular, a practice that aroused, and continues to arouse, outrage among Hindu social reformers. The practice had roots in the Brahmanical idea of absolute submission of female personality to that of her husband. Some scholars argue that the reason was economic - a way to prevent a childless widow from claiming her late husband's property."

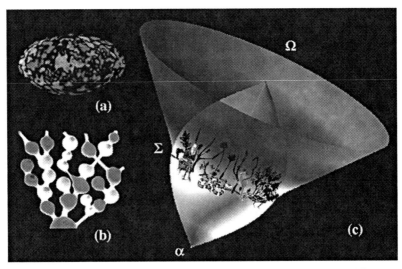

(a) The cosmic background - a red-shifted primal fireball. This radiation separated from matter, as charged plasma condensed to atoms. The fluctuations are smoothed in a manner consistent with subsequent inflation. (b) Fractal inflation model leaves behind mature universes while inflation continues. (c) Darwin in Eden: "Paradise on the cosmic equator." - life is an interactive complexity catastrophe resulting from force differentiation (Scientific American, King).

Sexual Paradox in Quantum Cosmology

To understand how sexual paradox may lie at the foundation of cosmology, it is necessary for us to digress into the spooky world of quantum reality. We exist in a quantum universe, not a classical one. We thus need to set aside the ideas of mechanism, determinism and the mathematical notions of sets made out of discrete points and come to terms with ultimate paradoxes of space-time and complementarities so deep that it may be impossible to determine which are the fundamental constituents and which are composites. To fully understand the cosmoloigcal implications of sexual paradox we need to examine all aspects of the universe in detail from the smallest particles to the universe as a whole and only then to come to a synthesis of the role sexual paradox may play at the cosmological level.

The Quantum Universe

The universe appears to have had an explosive beginning, sometimes called the big bang, in which space and time as well as the material leading to the galaxies were created. The evidence is pervasive, from the increasing red-shift of recession of the galaxy clusters, like the deepening sound of a train horn as the train recedes, to the existence of cosmic background radiation, the phenomenally stretched and cooled remnants of the original fireball. The cosmic background shows irregularities of the early universe at the time radiation separated from matter when the first atoms formed from the flux of charged particles. From a very regular symmetrical 'isotropic' beginning for such an explosion, these fluctuations, which may be of a quantum nature, have become phenomenally expanded and smoothed to the scale of galaxies consistent with a theory called inflation. Our view of the distant parts of the universe, which we see long ago because of the time light has taken to reach us, likewise confirm a different more energetic galactic early life. We can look out to the limits of the observable universe and because of the long delay which light takes to cross such a vast region, witness quasars and early energetic galaxies, which are quite different from mature galaxies such as our own milky way.

The ultimate fate of the universe is less certain, because it's rate of expansion brings it very close to the limiting condition between the gravitational attraction of the mass energy it contains ultimately reversing the expansion, causing an eventual collapse, and continued expansion forever. The evidence is now in favour of a perpetual and possibly accelerating expansion and astronomers are seeking an explanation for this apparent lack of mass in dark matter and a dark energy sometimes called quintessence, promoting accelerating expansion. The missing mass is clearly evident in close galaxies, which spin so rapidly they would fly apart if the only matter present was the luminous matter of stars black holes and gaseous nebulae. WMAP data now suggests the universe's rate of expansion has increased part way through its lifetime and that its large-scale dynamics are governed mostly by dark energy (73%), with successively smaller contributions from dark matter (23%) and ordinary galactic matter and radiation (4%).

The inflationary model explains the big bang neatly in terms of the same process of symmetry-breaking which caused the four forces of nature, gravity, electromagnetism and the weak and strong nuclear forces to become so different from one another. The large-scale cosmic structure is thus related to the quantum scale in one logical puzzle. In this symmetry-breaking the universe adopted its very complex 'twisted' form which made hierarchical interaction of the particles to form protons and neutrons, and then atoms and finally molecules and complex molecular life possible. We can see this twisted nature in the fact that all the charges in the nucleus are positive or neutral protons and neutrons while the electrons orbiting an atom are all negatively charged. Symmetry-breaking is a classic example of engendering at work. Cosmic inflation explains why the universe seems to have just about enough energy to fly apart into space and no more, and why disparate regions of the universe which seemingly couldn't have communicated since the big-bang at the speed of light, seem to be so regular. Inflation ties together the differentiation of the fundamental forces and an exponential expansion of the universe based on a form of anti-gravity which exists only until the forces break their symmetry (p 311). Inflation explains galactic clusters as phenomenally inflated quantum fluctuations and suggests that our entire universe may have emerged from its own wave function in a quantum fluctuation.

Our quantum world is very subtle and much more mysterious than a mechanical 'building blocks' view of the universe with simple separate classical particles interacting in empty space. Many people lead their lives at the macroscopic level as if quantum reality didn't exist, but quantum reality runs from the very foundations of physics to the ways we perceive. Our senses of sight, hearing, touch and taste/smell are all distinct quantum modes of interaction with the environment. Senses aren't just biological adaptions but fundamental quantum modes of information transfer, by photons, phonons, solitons and orbital interactions. Quantum processes such as tunnelling are central to the function of our enzymes and to the ion channels and synapses that support our excitable neurons (Walker R711).

The 'correspondence principle' by which the quantum world is supposed to fade into classical 'reality' is never fully realized. Many phenomena in the everyday world involve chance events which themselves are often sensitively related to uncertainties at the quantum level. Chaotic, self-critical and certain other processes may 'inflate' quantum effects into global fluctuations. Conscious interaction with the physical world may likewise depend both on quantum excitations and the loophole of uncertainty in expressing 'free-will'. We need to understand how quantum reality interacts with conscious experience, however in doing so we immediately find the most challenging examples of sexual paradox that lie at the core of the cosmological puzzle. This is the paradox of wave-particle complementarity. A quantum manifests in two complementary ways as a non-local flowing 'wave' which has a frequency and as a localized 'particle' which is created or destroyed in a single step. It can manifest as either but not both at the same time - a kind of Janus transvestite hermaphrodite - dyadic sexual complementarity in monadic primal form. All the weird quantum paradoxes of non-locality, entanglement and collapse emerge from this complementary relationship. To understand the full dimensions of this mystery we need to do a little fairly simple maths.

Wave-Particle Complementarity and the Cat Paradox

Supposing we try to imagine how we would calculate the frequency of a wave if we had no means to examine it except by using another similar wave and counting the number of beats that the 'strange wave' makes against the standard wave we have generated. This is exactly the situation we face in quantum physics, because all our tools are ultimately made up of the same kinds of wave-particle quanta we are trying to investigate. If we can't measure the amplitude of the wave at a given time, but only how many beats occur in a given period, we can then only determine the frequency with any accuracy by letting several beats pass. We then however have let a considerable time elapse, so we don't know exactly when the frequency was at this value. The relationship between frequencies and the beats is: $\Delta\upsilon\Delta t \geq 1$.

The closer we choose our frequency to get a given accuracy, the longer the beats take to occur. We thus cannot know the time and the frequency simultaneously. The more precisely we try to define the frequency, the greater the time is smeared out.

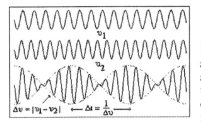

Measuring a wave frequency with beats has intrinsic uncertainty as to the time, which becomes a smeared-out interval.

Despite gaining his fame for discovering relativity, and the doom equation $E = mc^2$ which made the atom bomb possible, Einstein, possibly in cooperation with with his wife (p 496), also made a critical discovery about the quantum. Einstein's law connects to every energetic particle a frequency

$$E = h\upsilon .$$

Energy is thus intimately related to frequency - in a sense it IS frequency. Measuring one is necessarily measuring the other. If we apply the above together, we immediately get:

$$\Delta E\Delta t = h\Delta\upsilon\Delta t \geq h$$

This is the famous Heisenberg uncertainty relation. It tells us something is happening which is impossible in the classical world. We can't know the energy of a quantum interaction and the time it happened simultaneously. Energy and time have entered into a primal type of prisoners' dilemma catch 22. The closer we try to tie down the energy, the less precisely we know the time. This peculiar relationship places a specific taboo on knowing all the features of a situation and means we cannot predict precise outcomes, only probabilities. The same goes for momentum and position in each of the three spatial dimensions. Notice also that this links energy and momentum, time and space, and frequency and wavelength as three manifestations of one another. The way in which this happens is illuminating.

Each quantum can be conceived as a particle or as a wave but not both at the same time. Depending on how we are interacting with it or describing it, it may appear as either. We are all familiar with the fact that CDs have a rainbow appearance on their underside. This comes from the circular tracks spaced a distance similar to the wavelength of visible light. If we used light of a single wavelength we would see light and dark bands. We can visualize this process more simply with just two slits as in the figure below. When many photons pass through, their waves interfere as shown and the photographic plate gets dark and light interfernce bands where the waves from the two slits reinforce or cancel, because the photons are more likely to end up where their superimposed wave amplitude is large. The experiment confirms the wave nature of light, since the size of the bands is determined by the distance between the slits in relation to the wavelength where c is the velocity of light:

$$\lambda = \frac{\upsilon}{c}$$

We know each photon passes through both slits, because we can slow the experiment down so much that only one photon is released at a time and we still eventually get the interference pattern over time. Each photon released from the light bulb is emitted as a particle from a single hot atom, whose excited electron is jumping down from a hight energy orbit to a lower one. It is thus released locally and as a single 'particle' created by a single transition between two stable electron orbitals, but it spreads and passes through both slits as a wave. After this the two sets of waves interfere as shown in the figure to make bands on the photographic plate or the rainbows we see on a CD.

The evolution of the wave is described by an equation involving rates of change of a wave function φ with respect to space and time. For example for a massive particle in free space, we have a 1-D differential equation: $\left(\dfrac{\partial^2}{\partial t^2} - \dfrac{\partial^2}{\partial x^2} + m^2\right)\varphi = 0$.

This equation emphasizes the relativistic relationship between space and time. The relationship between Schrödinger's wave equation and Heisenbergs matrix mechanics (p 493) highlights a deeper complementarity in mathematics between the discrete operations of algebra and the continuous properties of calculus which may be expressed in the brain (p 367).

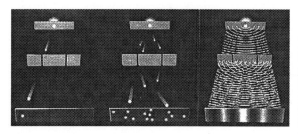

Two-slit interference experiment
(Sci. Am. Jul 92)

For the bands to appear in the interference experiment, each single photon has to travel through both slits as a wave. If you try to put any form of transparent detector in the slits to tell if it went through one or both you will always find only one particle but now the interference pattern will be destroyed. This happens even if you use the gentlest forms of detection possible such as an empty resonant maser chamber (a maser is a microwave laser). Any measurement sensitive enough to detect a particle alters its momentum enough to smear the interference pattern into the same picture you would get if the particle just went through one slit. Knowing one aspect destroys the other.

Now another confounding twist to the catch 22. The photon has to be absorbed again as a particle by an atom on the photographic plate, or somewhere else, before or after, if it doesn't career forever through empty space, something we shall deal with shortly. Where exactly does it go? The rules of quantum mechanics are only statistical. They tell us only that the particle is more likely to end up where the amplitude of the wave is large, not where it will actually go on any one occasion. The probability is precisely the complex square of the wave's amplitude at any point: $P = \varphi^*\varphi$

Hence the probability is spread throughout the extent of the wave function, extending throughout the universe at very low probabilities. Quantum theory thus describes all future (and past) states as probabilities. Unlike classical probabilities, we cannot find out more about the situation and reduce the probability to a certainty by deeper investigation, because of the limits imposed by quantum uncertainty. The photon could end up anywhere the wave is non-zero. Nobody can tell exactly where, for a single photon. Each individual photon really does seem to end up being absorbed as a particle somewhere, because we will get a scattered pattern of individual dark crystals on the film at very low light intensities, which slowly build up to make the bands again. This is the mysterious phenomenon called reduction of the wave packet. Effectively the photon was in a superposition of states represented by all the possible locations within the wave, but suddenly became one of those possible states, now absorbed into a single localized atom where we can see its evidence as a silver mark on the film. Only when there are many photons does the behaviour average out to the wave distribution. Thus each photon seems to make its own mind up about where it is going to end up, with the proviso that on average many do this according to the wave amplitude's probability distribution. So is this quantum free-will? It may be.

This situation is the subject of a famous thought experiment by Schrödinger, who invented the wave equation. In Schrödinger's cat paradox, we use an interference experiment with about one photon a second and we detect whether the photon hits one of the bright bands

302

to the left. If it does then a cat is killed by smashing a cyanide flask. Now when the experimenter opens the box, they find the cat is either alive or dead, but quantum theory simply tells us that the cat is both alive and dead, each with differing probabilities - superimposed alive and dead states. This is counterintuitive, but fundamental to quantum reality.

Cat paradox experiment (King)

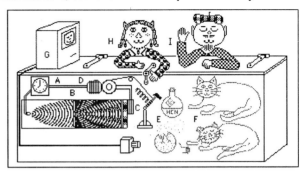

In the cat paradox experiment, the wave function remains uncollapsed at least until the experimenter I opens the box. Heisenberg suggested representing the collapse as occurring when the system enters the domain of thermodynamic irreversibility, i.e. at C. Schrödinger suggested the formation of a permanent record e.g. classical physical events D, E or computer data G. However even these classical outcomes could be superpositions at least until a conscious observer experiences them, as the many-worlds theory below suggests. Wigner's friend is a version of the cat paradox in which an assistant G reports on the result, establishing that unless the first conscious observer collapses the wave function, there will be a conscious observer in a multiplicity of alternative states, which is an omnipresent drawback of the many worlds view. In a macabre version the conscious assistant is of course the cat. According to the Copenhagen interpretation, it its not the system which collapses, but only our knowledge of its behavior. The superimposed state within the wave function is then not regarded as a real physical entity at all, but only a means of describing our knowledge of the quantum system, and calculating probabilities.

This clash between subjective experience and quantum theory has lead to much soul-searching. The Copenhagen interpretation says quantum theory just describes our state of knowledge of the system and is essentially incomplete. This effectively passes the problem back from physics to the observer. Some physicists think all the possibilities happen and there is a probability universe for each case. This is called the *many-worlds* interpretation of Hugh Everett III. The universe becomes a superabundant superimposed set of all possible probability futures and indeed all pasts as well in a smeared out 'holographic' multiverse in which everything happens. It suffers from a key difficulty. All the experience we have suggests just one possibility is chosen in each situation - the one we actually experience. Some scientists thus think collapse depends on a conscious observer. Many worlds defenders claim an observer wouldn't see the probability branching because they too would be split but this leaves us either with infinite split consciousness, or all we lose all forms of decision-making process, all forms of *historicity* in which there is a distinct line of history, in which watershed events do actually occur, and the role of memory in representing it.

Zurek (R768) describes decoherence as an inevitable result of interactions with other particles. Penrose in 'objective reduction' singles out gravity as the key unifying force and suggests that interaction with gravitons splits the wave function, causing reduction. Others try to discover hidden laws which might provide the sub-quantum process, for example a particle piloted within a wave as suggested by David Bohm (R68). This has difficulties defining positions when new particles with new quantum degrees of freedom are created. Another approach we will explore, is the transactional interpretation, which has features of all these ideas and seeks to explain this process in terms of a hand-shaking relationship between the past and the future, in which space-time itself becomes sexual. Key here is the fact that reduction is not like any other physical process. One cannot tell when or where it happens again suggesting it is part of the 'spooky' interface between quantum and consciousness.

In many situations people try to pass the intrinsic problems of uncertainty away on the basis that in the large real processes we witness, individual quantum uncertainties cancel in the law of averages of large numbers of particles. They will suggest for example that neurons are huge in terms of quantum phenomena and that the 'law of mass action' engulfs quantum effects. However brain processes are notoriously sensitive. Moreover history itself is a unique process out of many such 'unstable' possibilities at each stage of the process. Critical decisions we make become watersheds. History and evolution are both processes littered with unique idiosyncratic acts in a counterpoint to the major forces shaping the environment and landscape. Chaotic processes are potentially able to inflate arbitrarily small fluctuations, so molecular chaos may 'inflate' the fluctuations associated with quantum uncertainty.

The Two-timing Nature of Special Relativity

We also live in a paradoxical relationship with space and time. While space is to all purposes symmetric and multidimensional, and not polarized in any particular direction, time is singular in the present and polarized between past and future. We talk about the arrow of time as a mystery related to the increasing disorder or entropy of the universe. We imagine space-time as a four dimensional manifold but we live out a strange sequential reality in which the present is evanescent. In the words of the song "time keeps slipping, slipping, slipping ... into the future". There is also a polarized gulf between a past we can remember, the living present and a shadowy future of nascent potentialities and foreboding uncertainty. In a sense, space and time are complementary dimensionalities, which behave rather like real and imaginary complex variables, as we shall see below.

A second fundamentally important discovery in twentieth century physics, complementing quantum theory, which transformed our notions of time and space, was the special theory of relativity. In Maxwell's classical equations for transmission for light, light always has the same velocity, c regardless of the movement of the observer, or the source. Einstein realized that Maxwell's equations and the properties of physics could be preserved under all intertial systems - the principle of special relativity - only if the properties of space and time changed according to the Lorenz transformations as a particle approaches the velocity of light c :

$$x' = \frac{x - vt}{\sqrt{1 - v^2/c^2}}, y' = y, z' = z, t' = \frac{t - (v/c^2)x}{\sqrt{1 - v^2/c^2}}$$

Space becomes shortened along the line of movement and time becomes dilated. Effectively space and time are each being rotated towards one-another like a pair of closing scissors. Consequently the mass and energy of any particle with non-zero rest mass tend to infinity at the velocity of light: $m = \dfrac{m_0}{\sqrt{1 - v^2/c^2}}$

By integrating this equation, Einstein (p 496) was able to deduce that the rest mass must also correspond to a huge energy $E_o = m_o c^2$ which could be released for example in a nuclear explosion, as the mass of the radioactive products is less than the mass of the uranium that produces them, thus becoming the doom equation of the atom bomb. General relativity goes beyond this to associate gravity with the curvature of space-time caused by mass-energy.

In special relativity, space and time become related entities which form a composite four dimensional space-time, in which points are related by light-cones - signals travelling at the speed of light from a given origin. In space-time, time behaves differently to space. When time is squared it has a negative sign just like the imaginary complex number $i = \sqrt{-1}$ does.

Hence the negative sign in the formula for space-time distance $\Delta S^2 = x^2 + y^2 + z^2 - c^2 t^2$ and the scissor-like reversed rotations of time and space into one another expressed in the Lorenz transformations. Stephen Hawking has noted that, if we treat time as an imaginary variable, the space-time universe could become a closed 'manifold' rather like a 4-D sphere, in which the cosmic origin is rather like the north pole of Earth, because imaginary time will reverse the above negative sign and give us the usual Pythagorean distance formula in 4D.

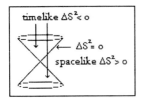

Space-time light cone permits linkage of 'time-like' points connected by slower-then-light communication. In the 'space-like' region, temporal order of events and causality depends on the observer.

A significant feature of special relativity is the fact that the relativistic energy-momentum equation $E^2 = p^2 + m^2$ has dual energy solutions: $E = \pm(\sqrt{p^2 + m^2})$

The negative energy solution has reversed temporal direction. Effectively a negative energy anti-particle travelling backwards in time is exactly the same as a positive energy particle travelling forwards in time in the usual manner. The solution which travels in the normal direction (subsequent points are reached later) is called the *retarded* solution. The one which travels backwards in time is called the *advanced* solution. A photon is its own anti-particle so in this case we just have an advanced or retarded photon.

Reality and Virtuality: Quantum fields and Seething Uncertainty

We have learned about waves and particles, but what about fields? What about the strange action-at-a-distance of electromagnetism and gravity? Special relativity and quantum theory combine to provide succinct explanations of electromagnetism, in fact they are the most succinct theories ever invented by the human mind, accurate to at least seven decimal places when describing the magnetic moment of an electron in terms of the hidden virtual photons which the electron emits and then almost immediately absorbs again.

Richard Feynman and others discovered the answer to this riddle by using uncertainty itself to do the job (p 495). The field is generated by particles propagated by a rule based on wave spreading. These particles are called *virtual* because they have no net positive energy and appear and disappear entirely within the window of quantum uncertainty, so we never see them except as expressed in the force itself. This seething tumult of virtual particles exactly produces the familiar effects of the electromagnetic field, and other fields as well. We can find the force between two electrons by integrating the effects of every virtual photon which could be exchanged within the limits of uncertainty and of every other possible virtual particle system, including pairs of electrons and positrons coming into a fleeting existence. However, note that we can't really eliminate the wave description because the amplitudes with which the particles are propagated from point to point are the hidden wave amplitudes. Uncertainty not only can create indefiniteness but it can actively create every conceivable particle out of the vacuum, and does so *sine qua non*. Special relativity and the advanced and retarded solutions that arise are also essential to enable the interactions that make the fabric of the quantum field. The advanced solutions are required to have negative energy and retarded solutions positive energy thus giving the correct reults for both scattering and electron-positron interactions within the field so that electron scattering is the same as electron positron creation and annihilation.

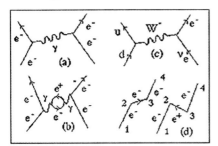

Quantum electrodynamics: (a,b) Two Feynman diagrams in the electromagnetic repulsion of two electrons. In the first a single virtual photon is exchanged between two electrons, in the second the photon becomes a virtual electron-positron pair during its transit. All such diagrams are integrated together to calculate the strength of the electromagnetic force. (c) A similar diagram shows how neutron decay occurs via the W- particle of the weak nuclear force, which itself is a heavy charged photon as a result of symmetry-breaking. (d) Time-reversed electron scattering is the same as positron creation and annihilation.

Each more complex interaction involving one more particle vertex is smaller by a factor $\frac{e^2}{hc} \sim \frac{1}{137}$ where e is the electron charge and h and c are as above, called the 'fine structure constant'. This allows the contribution of all the diagrams to sum to a finite interaction, unlike many unified theories, which are plagued by infinities, as we shall see. The electromagnetic force is generated by virtual photons exchanged between charged particles existing only for a time and energy permitted by the uncertainty relation. The closer the two electrons, the larger the energy fluctuation possible over the shorter time taken to travel between them and hence the greater the force upon them. Even in the vacuum, where we think there is nothing at all, there is actually a sea of all possible particles being created and destroyed by the rules of uncertainty.

The virtual particles of a force field and the *real* particles we experience as radiation such as light are one and the same. If we pump energy into the field, for example by oscillating it in a radio transmitter, the virtual photons composing the electromagnetic field become the real positive energy photons in radio waves entering the receiver as a coherent stream of real photons, encoding the music we hear. Relativistic quantum field theories always have both advanced and retarded solutions, one with positive and the other with negative energy, because of the two square roots of special relativity. They are often described by Feynman space-time diagrams. When the Feynman diagram for electron scattering becomes time-reversed, it then becomes precisely the diagram for creation and annihilation of the electron's anti-particle, the positron, as shown above. This hints at a fundamental role for the exotic time-reversed advanced solutions.

The weak and strong nuclear forces can be explained in a similar way, but gravity holds out further serious catch-22s. Gravity is associated with the curvature of space-time, but this introduces fundamental contradictions with quantum field theory. To date there remains no fully consistent way to reconcile quantum field theory and gravitation as we shall see.

The Spooky Nature of Quantum Entanglement

We have already seen how the photon wave passing through two slits ends up being absorbed by a single atom. But how does the wave avoid two particles accidentally being absorbed in far flung parts of its wave function out of direct communication?

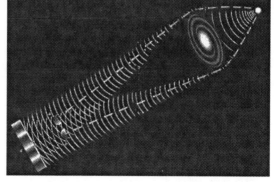

Wheeler delayed choice experiment: A very distant quasar is gravitationally lensed by an intervening galaxy. We can sample photons either by an interference pattern, verifying they went around both sides of the galaxy, or place separate directional detectors which will detect they went one way around only as particles (which will destroy the interference pattern. Moreover, we can decide which to perform after the photon has passed the galaxy, at the end of its path. Thus the configuration of the latter parts of the wave appear to be able to alter the earlier history (Sci. American).

Just how large such waves can become can be appreciated if we glance out at a distant galaxy, whose light has had to traverse the universe to reach us, perhaps taking as long as the history of Earth to get here. The ultimate size is as big as the universe. Only one photon is ever absorbed for each such wave, so once we detect it, the probability of finding the photon anywhere else, and hence the amplitude of the wave, must immediately become zero everywhere. How can this happen, if information cannot travel faster than the speed of light? For a large wave, such as light from a galaxy, (and in principle for any wave) this collapse process has to cover the universe. When I shine my torch against the window, the amplitude of each photon is both reflected, so I can see it, and transmitted, escaping into the night sky. Although the wave may spread far and wide, if the particle is absorbed anywhere, the probability across vast tracks of space has to suddenly become zero. Moreover collapse may involve the situation at the end of the path influencing the earlier history, as in the Wheeler delayed choice experiment (p 305). In this experiment we can determine whether a photon went both ways round a lensing galaxy, focusing the light from a very distant quasar long after the light has passed across the universe, by either measuring the interference between the paths as in the double slit experiment or by detecting photons from one direction or another.

Because we can't sample two different points of a single-particle wave, it is impossible to devise an experiment which can test how a wave might collapse. One way to learn more about this situation is to try to find situations in which two or more correlated particles will be released coherently in a single wave. This happens with many particles in a laser and in the holograms made by coherent laser light and in Bose-Einstein condensates. It also happens in other situations where two particles of opposite spin or complementary polarization become created together. Many years ago Einstein, Rosen and Podolsky (EPR) suggested we might be able to break through the veil of quantum uncertainty this way, indirectly finding out more about a single particle than it is usually prepared to let on.

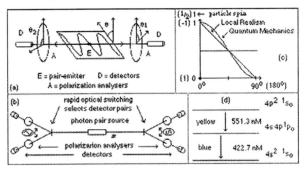

(a) Pair-splitting experiment for photons. (b) Time-varying analysers are added driven by an optical switch to fast for light to cross the apparatus. (c) The results are consistent with quantum mechanics but inconsistent with Bell's inequalities for a locally causal system. (d) The calcium transition (Aspect).

For example a calcium atom's electron excited into a higher orbital sometimes cannot fall back to its original orbital in one step because a photon always turns out to have spin 1 and the spins don't match. For example you can't go between two orbits of equal spin and radiate a spin-1 photon or the spins don't tally. The atom however can radiate two photons thereby cancelling one another's spins, to transit to its ground state, via an intermediate spin-1 orbit. This releases a blue and a yellow photon, each of which travel off in opposite directions, with complementary polarizations.

When we perform the experiment, it turns out that the polarization of neither photon is defined until we measure one of them. When we measure the polarization of one photon, the other immediately - instantaneously - has complementary polarization. The nature of the angular correlations between the detectors is inconsistent with any locally-causal theory - that is no theory based on information exchanged between the detectors by particles at the speed of light can do the trick, as proved in a famous result by John Bell (R54) and subsequent experiments. The correlation persists even if the detectors' configurations are changed so fast that there is no time for information to be exchanged between them at the speed of light as demonstrated by Alain Aspect (R25). This phenomenon has been called quantum non-locality and in its various forms quantum 'entanglement', a name itself very suggestive of the throes of a sexual 'affair'. The situation is subtly different from any kind of classical causality we can imagine. The information at either detector looks random until we compare the two. When we do, we find the two seemingly random lists are precisely correlated in a way which implies instantaneous correlatedness but there is no way we can use the situation to send classically precise information faster than the speed of light by this means. We can see however in the correlations just how the ordinary one-particle wave function can be instantaneously auto-correlated and hence not slip up in its accounting during collapse.

Since this result in the 1980s there have been a veritable conjurer's collection of experiments, all of which verify the predictions of quantum mechanics in every case and confirm all the general principles of the pair-splitting experiment. Even if we clone photons to form quartets of correlated particles, any attempt to gain information about one of such a multiple collection collapses the correlations between the related twins. Furthermore these effects can be retrospective, leading photons to be able to be superpositions of states which were created at different times. It is also possible to 'uncollapse' or erase such losses of correlation by re-interfering the wave functions so we can no longer tell the difference. This successfully recreates the lost correlations, inducing information about one of the particles and then erase it again by re-interfering it back into the wave function provided we use none of its information - the quantum eraser. In such situations the interference, which would be destroyed had we looked at the information, is reintegrated undiminished.

Quantum erasure (Scientifi American)

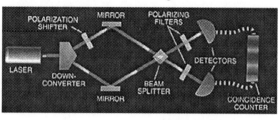

Erasing information about the path of a photon restores wavelike correlated behavior. Pairs of identically polarized correlated photons produced by a 'down-converter', bounce off mirrors, converge again at a beam splitter and pass into two detectors. A coincidence counter observes an interference pattern in the rate of simultaneous detections by the two detectors, indicating that each photon has gone both ways at the beam splitter, as a wave. Adding a polarization shifter to one path destroys the pattern, by making it possible to distinguish the photons' paths. Placing two polarizing filters in front of the detectors makes the photons identical again, erasing the distinction, restoring the interference pattern.

Quantum teleportation, in which information creating a quantum in a given state is 'teleported' by another has also become an experimental reality. These experiments give us a broad intuition of quantum reality.

Vlatko Vedral, who showed that entanglement is involved in superconductivity claims it can explain the Meissner effect, in which a magnet levitates above superconducting material. The magnetic field induces a current in the surface of the superconductor, and this current effectively excludes the magnetic field from the interior of the material, causing the magnet to hover. The current halts the photons of the magnetic field after they have travelled only a short distance through the superconductor. For the normally massless photons it is as if they have suddenly entered treacle, effectively giving them a mass. Vedral also claims a similar mechanism may be behind the mass of all particles. The source of this mass is believed to be the Higgs field mediated by the Higgs boson (p 311), thought to exist in a "condensed" state that excludes mediator particles such as gluons in the same way that a superconductor's entangled electrons exclude the photons of a magnetic field (Quantum quirk may give objects mass   New Scientist 24 October 2004).

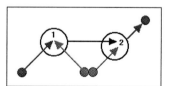

Quantum teleportation: A quantum (blue left) is combined in an interference measurement with one of an entangled pair (pink left) by experimenter 1, who then sends the result of the measurement as classical information to 2 who applies this to transform the other entangled particle, causing it to enter the same quantum state as the original blue one.

Classical computation suffers from the potentially unlimited time it takes to check out every one of the possibilities. To crack a code we need to check all the combinations, whose numbers can increase more than exponentially with the size of the code numbers and possibly taking as long as the history of the universe to compute. Factorizing a large number composed of two primes is known to be computationally intractable enough to provide the basis for public key encryption by which banks records and passwords are kept safe. Although the brain ingeniously uses massively parallel computation, there is as yet no systematic way to boot strap an arbitrary number of parallel computations together in a coherent manner.

However quantum reality is a superposition of all the possible states in a single wave function, so if we can arrange a wave function to represent all the possibilities in such a computation, superposition might give us the answer by a form of parallel quantum computation. A large number could in principle be factorized in a few superimposed steps, which would otherwise require vast time-consuming classical computer power to check all the possible factors one by one. Suppose we know an atom is excited by a certain quantum of energy, but only provide it a part of the energy required. The atom then enters a superposition of the ground state and the excited state, suspended between the two like Schrödinger's cat. If we then collapse the wave function, squaring it to its probability, as in $P=\varphi*\varphi$, it will be found to be in either the ground state or excited state with equal probability. This superimposed state is sometimes called the 'square root of not' when it is used to partially excite a system which flips between 0 and 1 corresponding to a logical negation.

To factorize a large number, we could devise a quantum system in two parts. The left part is excited to a superposition. Suppose we have a small array of atoms which effectively form the 0s and 1s of a binary number - 0 in the ground state and 1 in the excited state. If we then partially excite them all they represent a superposition of all the binary numbers - e.g. 00, 01, 10 and 11. The right half of the system is designed to give the factorization remainder of a test number taken to the power of each of the possible numbers in the left. These turn out to be periodic, so if we measure the right we get one of the values. This in turn collapses the left side into a superposition of only those numbers with this particular value in the right. We can then recombine the reduced state on the left to find its frequency spectrum and decode the answer. As a simple example, you are trying to factorise 15. Take the test number $x = 2$. The powers of 2 give you 2, 4. 8, 16, 32, 64, 128, 256 ... Now divide by 15, and if the number won't go, keep the remainder. That produces a repeating sequence 2, 4, 8, 1, 2, 4, 8, 1 ... with period $n = 4$ we can use this to figure $x^{n/2} - 1 = 2^{4/2} - 1 = 3$ is a factor of 15. The quantum parallelism solves all the computations simultaneously.

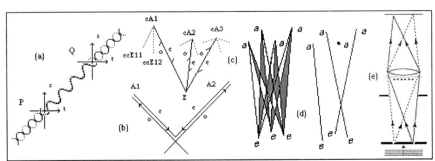

In the transactional interpretation, a single photon exchanged between emitter and absorber is formed by constructive interference between a retarded offer wave (solid) and an advanced confirmation wave (dotted). (b) The transactional interpretation of pair-splitting. Confirmation waves intersect at the emission point. (c) Contingent absorbers of an emitter in a single passage of a photon. (d) Collapse of contingent emitters and absorbers in a transactional match-making (King R355). (e) Experiment by Shahri Afshar (see Chown R118). A grid is placed at the interference minima of the wave fronts coming from two slits just below a lens designed to focus the light from each slit into a separate detector. Measurements by detectors (top) test whether a photon (particle) passed through the left or right slit (bottom). There is no reduction in intensity when the grid is placed below the lens at the interference minima of the offer waves from the two slits. The grid does however cause a loss of detector intensity when the dashed left-hand slit is covered and the negative wave interference between the offer waves at the grid is removed, so that the non-interfered wave from the right slit now hits the grid, causing scattering. This suggests both that we can measure wave and particle aspects simultaneously, and that the transactional interpretation is valid in a way which neither many worlds (which predicts a splitting into histories where a photon from the source goes through one slit or other) or the Copenhagen interpretation of complementarity (where detecting a particle forbids the photon manifesting as a wave).

Quantum Match-making: Transactional Supercausality and Reality

For reasons which immediately become apparent, the collapse in the pair-splitting experiment has to not only be immediate, but also to reconcile information looking backwards in time. The two photons we are trying to detect are linked through the common calcium atom. Their absorptions are thus actually connected via a path travelling back in space-time from one detector to the calcium atom and forward again to the other detector. Trying to connect the detectors directly, for example by hypothetical faster-than-light tachyons, leads to contradictions. Tachyons transform by the rules of special relativity, so a tachyon which appears to be travelling at an infinite speed according to one observer, is travelling only at a little more than the speed of light according to another. One travelling in one direction to one observer may be travelling in the opposite direction to another. They can also cause causality violations (King R355). There is thus no consistent way of knitting together all parts of a wave or the detector responses using tachyons. Even in a single-particle wave, the wave function in regions it has already traversed (and those it would subsequently pass through in future) also have to collapse retrospectively (and prospectively) so that no inconsistencies can occur, in which a particle is created in two locations in space-time from the same wave function, as the Wheeler delayed choice experiment makes clear.

In the transactional interpretation (Cramer R135), such a 'backward travelling' wave in time gives a neat explanation, not only for the above effect, but also for the probability aspect of the quantum in every quantum experiment. Instead of one photon travelling between the emitter and absorber, there are two shadow waves, which superimposed make up the complete photon. The emitter transmits an *offer* wave both forwards and backwards in time, declaring its capacity to emit a photon. All the potential absorbers of this photon transmit a corresponding *confirmation* wave. The confirmation waves travelling backwards in time send a hand-shaking signal back to the emitter. In the extension transactional approach to supercausality, a non-linearity now reduces the set of possibilities to one offer and confirmation wave, which superimpose constructively to form a real photon only on the space-time path connecting the emitter to the absorber as shown in the figure. This always connects an emitter at an earlier time to an absorber at later time because a real positive energy photon is a *retarded* particle which travels in the usual direction in time.

A negative energy photon travelling backwards in time is precisely the anti-particle of the positive energy photon and has just the same effect. The two are identifiable in the transactional interpretation, as in quantum electrodynamics (p 304), where time-reversed electron scattering is the same as positron creation and annihilation. The transactional relationship is in effect a match-making process. Before collapse of the wave function we have many potential emitters interacting with many potential absorbers. After all the collapses have taken place, each emitter is paired with an absorber in a kind of marriage dance. One emitter cannot connect with two absorbers without violating the quantum rules, so there is a frustration between the possibilities which can only be fully resolved if emitters and absorbers can be linked in pairs. The number of contingent emitters and absorbers are not necessarily equal, but the number of matched pairs is equal to the number of real particles exchanged.

In the pair-splitting experiment you can now see that the calcium atom emits in response to the advanced confirmation waves reaching it from both the detectors simultaneously right at the time it is emitting the photon pair. Thus the faster than light linkage is neatly explained by the combined retarded and advanced aspects of the photon having a net forwards and backwards connection which is instantaneous at the detectors. One can also explain the arrow of time if the cosmic origin is a reflecting boundary that causes all the positive energy real particles in our universe to move in the retarded direction we all experience in the arrow of time. This in turn gives the sign for increasing disorder or entropy and the time direction for the second law of thermodynamics to manifest. The equivalence of real and virtual particles raises the possibility that all particles have an emitter and absorber and arose, like virtual particles, through mutual interaction when the universe first emerged. However even if dark-energy, 'quintessence' causes an increasing expansion, or fractal inflation leads to an open universe model in which some photons may never find an absorber, the excitations of brain oscillations, because they are both emitted and absorbed by past and future brain states could still be universally subject to transactional supercausal coupling.

The hand-shaking space-time relation implied by transactions makes it possible that the apparent randomness of quantum events masks a vast interconnectivity at the quantum level, which has been termed the 'implicate order' by David Bohm (R69). This might not itself be a random process, but because it connects past and future events in a time-symmetric way, it cannot be reduced to predictive determinism, because the initial conditions are insufficient to describe the transaction, which also includes quantum 'information' coming from the future. However this future is also unformed in real terms at the early point in time emission takes place. My eye didn't even exist, when the quasar emitted its photon, except as a profoundly unlikely branch of the combined probability 'waves' of all the events throughout the history of the universe between the ancient time the quasar released its photon and my eye developing and me being in the right place at the right time to see it. Transactional supercausality thus involves a huge catch 22 about space, time and prediction, uncertainty and destiny. It doesn't suggest the future is determined, but that the contingent futures do superimpose to create a space-time paradox in collapsing the wave function.

Roger Penrose (R523, R524), has suggested that the one-graviton limit of interaction is an objective trigger for wave packet reduction, because of the bifurcation in space-times induced, leading to theories in which the random or pseudo-random manifestations of the particle within the wave are non-linear consequences of gravity. *Objective orchestrated reduction* or OOR is then cited as a basis which intentional consciousness uses to follow collapse rather than participating in it, as the transactional model makes possible. The OOR model unlike transactional anticipation thus leaves free-will with a kind of orphan status, following, but not participating in, the collapse process itself.

By reducing the energy of a transaction to a superposition of ground and excited states, the transactional approach may combine with quantum computation to produce a space-time anticipating quantum entangled system which may be pivotal in how the conscious brain does its computation. The brain is not a marvelous computer in any classical sense. We can barely repeat seven digits. But it is a phenomenally sensitive anticipator of environmental and behavioral change. Subjective consciousness has its survival value in enabling us to jump out of the way when the tiger is about to strike, not so much in computing which path the tiger might be on, because this is an intractable problem and the tiger can also take it into account in avoiding the places we would expect it to most likely be, but by intuitive conscious anticipation. What is critical here is that in the usual quantum description which considers only the emitter, we have only the probability function because the initial conditions are insufficient to determine the outcome. There is thus no useful way quantum uncertainty can be linked to conscious free-will. Only by completing the sexual paradox of time by including the advanced absorber waves can we see how anticipation might be achieved.

Engendering Nature: Cosmic Symmetry-Breaking and Inflation

The basis of the cosmic inflation concept is symmetry-breaking, in which the fundamental forces of nature, which make up the matter and radiation we relate to in the everyday world gained the very different properties they have today. There are four quite different forces. The first two are well known - electromagnetism and gravity - both long-range forces we can witness as we look out at distant galaxies. The others are two short-range nuclear forces. The colour force holds together the three quarks in any neutron or proton and indirectly binds the nucleus together by the strong force, generating the energy of stars and atom bombs. The weak radioactive force is responsible for balancing the protons and neutrons in the nucleus by interconverting the flavours of quarks and leptons (p 311).

There is a fundamental sexual division among the wave-particles. Particles come in two types, *fermions*, of half-integral spin, which can only clump in complementary pairs in a single wave function and thus, being incompressible, make up matter, and *bosons* of integral spin which can become coherent and can all enter the same wave function in unlimited numbers, as in a laser, and hence form radiation and as virtual particles appearing and disappearing through quantum uncertainty, the forces which act between the particles. We thus have another fundamental sexual complementarity manifesting as the relationship between matter and radiation. The half integral spin of electrons was first discovered in the splitting of the spectral lines of electorns in atomic orbitals into pairs whose spin angular momentum corresponded to $\pm 1/2$ rather than the 0, 1 , 2 etc. of atomic s, p - orbitals (p 318). As spin states have to differ by a multiple of Planck's constant h a particle of spin s has $2s+1$ components. A glance at the known wave-particles (p 311), indicates that the bosons and fermions we know are very different from one another in their properties and patterns of arrangement. There is no obvious way to pair off the known bosons and fermions, however there are reasons why there may be a hidden underlying symmetry, which pairs each boson with a fermion of one-half less spin, called super-symmetry, because in super-symmetric theories the infinities that plague quantum field theories cancel and vanish, the negative contributions of the fermions exactly balancing the positive contributions of the bosons. This would mean that there must be undiscovered particles. For example corresponding to the spin-2 graviton would be a spin-3/2 gravitino, a spin-1 graviphoton a spin-1/2 gravifermion and a spin-0 graviscalar.

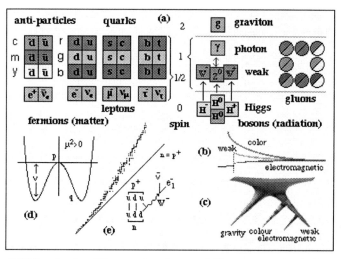

(a) Sexual paradox in the standard model of the four fundamental forces: The wave-particles are divided into two disparate groups of bosons and fermions. The fermions, which make matter are divided between quarks which experience all the forces including colour and leptons which experience only the electroweak and gravity. The bosons, which mediate the forces have integer spin and freely superimpose, as in lasers and hence also make radiation. Half-integer spin fermions only superimpose in pairs of opposite spin and hence resist compression into one space, thus making solid matter. Each quark comes in three colours(RGB) and pairs of flavours (up, down etc.) Electromagnetism is first united with the weak force ostensibly through the spin-0 Higgs boson, then with the colour force gluons and finally with gravity. (b) The forces converge at high energies. (c) Force differentiation tree, in which the four forces differentiate from a single super-force, with gravity displaying a more fundamental divergence. (d) the scalar Higgs field has lowest energy in the polarized state, (e) the stable atomic nuclei with their increasing preponderance of neutrons are equilibrated by the weak force. This force is chiral, engaging left-handed interactions, for example in neutron decay, as shown. Weak interactions may explain the chirality of RNA and proteins (King).

The four fundamental forces appear to converge at very great energies and to have been in a state of symmetry at the cosmic origin as a common super-force. A key process mediating the differentiation of the fundamental forces is cosmic symmetry-breaking. The short-range weak force behaves in many ways as if it is the same as electromagnetism, except the charged $W^{+,-}$ and neutral Z_0 carrier particles corresponding to the electromagnetic photon are very massive. One can of course consider this division of a common super-force into distinct complementary forces as a nd of sexual division, just as the division into male and female is a primary division. In this respect gravity stands apart from the other three forces which share a common medium of spin-1 bosons and broke symmetry first.

A key explanation for this symmetry-breaking is that originally all the particles had zero rest mass like the photon, but some of the boson force carriers like the W changed to mediate a short-range force by becoming massive and gaining an extra degree of freedom (the freedom to change speed) by picking up an additional spin-0 particle called a Higgs boson. The elusive Higgs may also explain why the universe flew apart. The universe begins at a temperature a little below the unification temperature - slightly supercooled, possibly even a result of a quantum fluctuation. In the early symmetric universe empty space is forced into a higher-energy arrangement than its temperature can support called the false vacuum. The result is a tremendous energy of the Higgs field which behaves as exponential anti-gravity, inflating the universe in 10^{-35} of a second to something already close to its present size. This inflationary phase becomes broken once the Higgs field collapses, breaking symmetry to a lower energy polarized state, rather like a ferromagnet. does, to create the asymmetric force arrangement we experience to form the true vacuum. In this process the Higgs particles, which are zero spin and have one wave function component, unite with some of the particles, such as $W^{+/-}$ and Z_0 to give them non-zero rest mass by adding their extra component , allowing the additional longitudinal component of the wave function associated with a varying velocity. Because the true vacuum is at a lower energy than the false one it grows to engulf it releasing the latent heat of this energy difference as a shower of hot particles, the hot fireball we associate with the big bang. Gravity has now reversed to become the attractive force we are familiar with. Two energies which cancelled now became two which add - an insignificant universe - almost nothing became one of almost incalculable proportions. The end result is a universe flying apart at almost exactly its own escape velocity whose kinetic energy almost balances the potential energy of gravitation. Symmetry-breaking can leave behind defects if the true vacuum emerges in a series of local bubbles which join. Depending on whether the symmetries which are broken are discrete, circular, or spherical, corresponding anomalies in the form of domain walls, cosmic strings or magnetic monopoles may form. In addition other weakly-interacting particles may emerge such as the axions which some researchers associate with cold dark matter.

In some models, inflation is a fractal branched structure like a snowflake which is perpetually leaving behind mature universes like ours (p 298). Recently it has become clearer that, even with additional dark matter, possibly comprising neutrinos and other exotic particles, there may not be enough mass to stop the expansion, which may even be accelerating. Various hyperbolic forms of inflation and an additional repulsion called quintessence involving a long-range repulsive dark energy have both been invoked to address this problem.

Rehabilitating Duality: Quantum Gravity and Space-time Structure

Quantum theory is formulated within space-time, but mass-energy, through gravitation in general relativity alters the structure of space-time by curving it. This has made a comprehensive integration of gravity with the other forces of nature difficult to achieve and may indicate a fundamental complementarity between the theories. Something of this paradox can be understood in graphic terms if we consider the implications of quantum uncertainty over very small time intervals, small enough to allow a virtual black hole to form. In this case a quantum fluctuation could give rise to a wormhole in the very space-time in which it is conceived raising all manner of paradoxes of connected universes and time loops into the bargain. This leads to a fundamental conceptual paradox in which space-time is flat or slightly curved on large scales but a seething topological foam of worm-holes on very small scales. These problems lead to fundamental difficulties in describing any form of quantum field in the presence of gravity.

The unification of gravity with the other forces brings new and deeper mysteries into play. Theories which treat particles as points are plagued with infinities the very points themselves imply as infinite concentrations of energy. Point particles may thus on very small scales become string, loop or membrane excitations. The theories broadly called 'superstring' explain the infinite self-energies associated with a point particle, and the different particles themselves as different excitation on a closed or open loop or string. However none have been found so far which correspond to our own peculiar asymmetric set of particles.

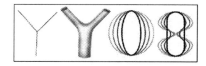

Left: Point particles have infinite self-energies and precise vertices of interaction, strings smooth these. Right: Strings have characteristic harmonic excitations (Wolfson, Sci. Am. Jan 96). They can be regarded either as open strings or loops. The different excitations being different particles.

Central to such theories is supersymmetry - a pairing between bosons and fermions of adjacent spin. The idea behind this is based on ground state zero-point fluctuations - the energies that arise through uncertainty when a quantum is considered in its lowest (ground) energy state. Only a perfect balancing of the negative zero-point energies of the fermions against the corresponding positive zero-point energies of the bosons implied by supersymmetry would cancel the potential infinities arising from the arbitrarily short wavelengths that result from the electromagnetic field when quantum gravitation is included in the unification scheme. These would effectively curl space-time to a point (Hawking 2001 46, 50). It is possible however that it is the collective contribution of the two groups which balance so that there is not an individual set of boson-fermion pairings but two symmetry-broken groups - bosons and fermions which collectively blanace one another - reflecting the standard model.

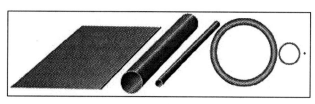

.Compactification of the 12 or so unseen dimensions leave only our 4 of space-time on large scales (Sci. Am. Jan 96). Compactification of one dimension to form a tube is a way 11-D M-theory can be linked to 10-D superstrings which are on smaller scales, string-like tubes.

Supersymmetric theories generally require over 10 dimensions to converge, all but four of which are 'compactified' - curled up on sub-particulate scales, leaving only our four dimensions of space-time as global dimensions. Such 'theories of everything' or TOEs have not yet fully explained how the particular arrangements of particles and forces in our universe are chosen out of the millions of possibilities for compactification these higher dimensional theories permit when supersymmetry is broken to produce the particles and forces we experience at low energies.

The internal symmetry dimensions of existing particles come close to the additional number required, suggesting the key can be found in the known particles. If we take 1 for the Higgs, 1 for the neutrino, 2 for the electroweak, 3 for colour, and 4 for space-time we have 11. Four-dimensional space-time is optimal mathematically for complexity. In some unification theories, one of the compactified dimensions might be much larger. Duality, in which fundamental particles in one description may become composite in another and vice versa may also enable apparently divergent theories to be understood through a convergent dual.

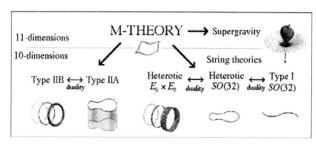

Relation between M-theory and dualities between string theories (ex Hawking R297, Duff R174).

Recently a possible unification of several theories including 10 dimensional superstring theories and 11 dimensional supergravity have been proposed in the form of M-theory -for membrane, or according to its proponents, magic. The essential idea is that 11-dimensional membrane theory looks like 10-dimensional string theory if one of the two membrane dimensions are rolled up into a tiny tube along with one of the 11-dimensions. In this point of view several of these theories are actually complementary mathematical formulations of the same object. This brings in a second mysterious concept - the 'holographic principle', in which a theory in a multidimensional region can be equivalent to a theory on the boundary of the region, one dimension lower (Duff R174).

A possible key to the higher dimensional theories is the 8-dimensional number system called the octonians. Just as complex numbers form a two dimensional plane, for which the second component is a multiple of i, the square root of -1, octonians form a system of 8-components. Associated with the octonians are the exceptional symmetry groups such as G_4 and E_8. Internal symmetries such as that of colour, and of charge, as well as the well-know Lorentz transformations of special relativity are already the basis for explaining the standard model.

Another key to a possible unraveling of the Gordian knot of the theory of everything comes from dualities. Electromagnetism is renormalizable because by adjusting for the infinite self energy of a charge we arrive at a theory like quantum electrodynamics where each more complicated diagram with more vertices makes a contribution 137 times smaller to the interaction and it is then possible to correctly deduce the combined effects without infinities creeping in. Essentially the idea is as follows:

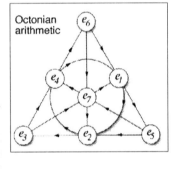

Octonians and the Fano plane: Just as complex numbers have two components $a + bi$ with $i^2 = -1$, so the octonians have eight components $1, e_1, ..., e_7$ such that $e_i^2 = -1$. Multiplication of coordinate vectors is determined by the 'Fano plane'. Any e_i, e_j, e_k connected by arrows multiply in the manner $e_i \times e_j = e_k$. Those connected in the reverse direction inherit a minus sign. Each line also loops back to the first coodinate in a cyclic manner.

Octonian arithmetic

Particles can come in two types, one vibrational states of strings (vibrating particles) and the other topological - how many times a string wraps around the compactified dimension (winding particles). The winding particles on a tube of radius R are identical to the vibrational particles on a tube of radius $1/R$. Duality is a sexually-paradoxical concept in which there is a natural relationship between theories which continue to have strong interactions and the perturbation theory fails with dual theories whose interaction strengths are the reciprocals of the originals and hence converge nicely. The nemesis comes if we end up having to deal with a TOE whose interactions are mid rage so that neither the original nor the dual can be unraveled.

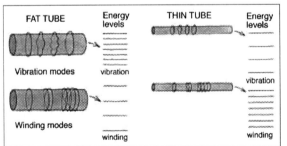

Duality between string theories. Winding particles in one have the same energetics as vibrational particles in the other and vice versa (Duff R182). The concept of duality may solve intractable infinities by finding a dual theory which is convergent. In the dual theory, particles like magnetic monopoles, which are a composite of quarks and other particles, become fundamental and electrons and quarks become composites of these. No particle is thus truly fundamental, each locked in sexual paradox with its dual.

Another dimensional issue is that the only spheres which will admit a vector field without singularities, so-called 'hairy ball's, are S^1 the circle, and S^3, S^7 the 3-D and 7-D spheres. Our two-sphere S^2 always gets places where one hair stands on end like the crown of your head. Thus the status of the unit octonians has a dual 7-D coincidence between algebra and topology, which may be essential in establishing for example a uniform time flow.

Stephen Hawking, who has been a consistent champion of the TOE quest, has lamented that although the connections implied by M-theory dualities are so convincing that to not think they are on the right track "would be a bit like believing that God put fossils into the rocks in order to mislead Darwin about the evolution of life" (Hawking R297 57), he now worries (R298) that the search for a consistent theory may remain beyond reach in a single theory because of the implications of Gödel's theorem (p 491), which proves that any logical system containing finite arithmetic admits formally undecidable propositions. If the search for a TOE runs up against this nemesis, the description of the universe may become undecidable. An indication of the possible complexity of a TOE uniting gravity and quantum field theories comes from superfluid helium 3. At close to absolute zero, helium 3 remains superfluid, and as the temperature rises fractionally a number of bound quantum excitations rather like quasi-molecules, form in the medium. Many of the known properties of unified field theories can be modeled using superfluidity and these bound structures as equivalents of gravitational and the other quantum fields. This indicates that the theory sought may not just be a limit of gravitation and quantum fields, but a deeper theory in which both of these are merely stability states hinting again at the implications of Gödel's theorem.

The possibilities remain open between our universe having unique laws derived from fundamental symmetries or being one of many types of universe whose laws happen to support complexity and life - a 'many-universes' perspective. Some theories (Smolin R636) even suggest the laws of nature might be capable of evolution from universe to universe, resulting in one containing observers. The anthropic principle asserts that the existence of (conscious) observers is a constraint delimiting what laws of nature are possible. Anthropic arguments (Barrow and Tipler R44) may enable a form of self-selection in the sense that simple universe which could not sustain life or observers would never be observed, guaranteeing our universe has dimensionalities, symmetry-breakings giving rise to fundamental constants consistent with the interactive fractal complexity (p 317). Regardless of these uncertainties in the final TOE, the general features of force unification, symmetry-breaking and inflation are likely to remain part of our understanding of the cosmic origin.

The Sexually-Complex Quantum World

We have seen that all phenomena in the quantum universe present as a succession of fundamental complementarities in a shifting vacuum ground-swell of uncertainty, out of which the super-abundance of quantum diversity emerges. In this process we have discovered a multiple overlapping series of divisions: (i) wave-particle complementarity fundamental to the quantum, (ii) the roles of emitters and absorbers, (iii) the advanced and retarded solutions of special relativity, (iv) the fermions comprising matter complementaing the bosons mediating radiation, (v) virtual and real particles distinguishing force fields from positive energy matter and radiation, and the engendered symmetry-breakings between (vi) space and time (reflecting that between momentum and energy) and (vii) between the four fundamental forces of nature, which in turn cause the quantum architecture of atoms and molecules to be asymmetric and capable of complexity of interaction to form living systems (p 317) and finally (viii) duality, which makes it difficult or impossible to determine what is a fundamental particle and what is composite in a sexual paradox between dual descriptions. Sexual paradox may also be manifest in the difficulty of separating the forces from the seething quantum 'ground' of vaccum uncertainty, which is generative of all types of quantum. To understand conscious anticipation, or free-will, may require the inclusion of advanced waves, forming a paradoxical complement to the positive energy arrow of time.

All these complementarities possess attributes of sexual paradox and are pivotal to generating the complexity and diversity of the universe as we know it. There is no way to validly mount a single description based on only one of these complementary aspects alone. All attempts to define a theory based only on one aspect implicitly involves the other as a fundamental component, just as the propagators of the particles in quantum field theory are based on wave-spreading. Classical mechanistic notions of a whole made out of clearly defined parts, as well as temporal determinism fail. The mathematical idea of a reality made out sets of points or point particle becomes replaced by the excitations of strings, again with wave-based harmonic energies. Just as we have an irreducible complementarity between subjective expereince and the objective world, so all the features of the quantum universe present in sexually paradoxical complementarities. It is thus hardly surprising that these fundamental and irreducible complementarities may come to be expressed as fundamental themes in biological complexity, thus making sexuality a cumulative expression of a sexual paradox which lies at the foundation of the cosmos itself.

Although both the Taoist and Tantric views of cosmology are based on a complementation between female and male generative principles, many people, including a good proportion of scientists still adhere to a mechanistic view of the universe as a Newtonian machine. In this view biological sexuality seems to be barred from having any fundamental cosmological basis, being an end product of an idiosyncratic process of chance and selection, in a biological evolution which has no apparent relation with or capacity to influence the vast energies and forces which shape the cosmological process. The origins of life remain mysterious and potentially accidental rather than cosmological in nature and evolution an erratic series of accidents preserved by natural selection.

However if we reverse this logic and begin with a sexually paradoxical cosmology, the phenomenon of biological sexuality then becomes a natural cumulative expression of physical sexual paradox operating in a new evolutionary paradigm in the biological world, rich with new feedback processes which give it the central role in genetics and organismic reproduction we regard as the signature and raison d'etre of reproductive sexuality.

Tissues (right) have a fractal structure (p 499) as a consequence of charge non-linearity in chemical bonding: (a) molecular level (b) cellular organelles (c) organs (skin). This fractal structure is similar to that arising from the non-linear quadratic dynamics of the Mandelbrot set (left) (King, Campbell R105).

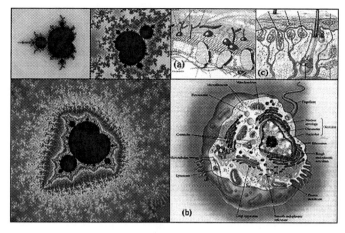

Sexual Paradox and the Tree of Life

Life is the ultimate cosmological consequence of the four forces of nature acting in hierarchical sequence, the colour and weak forces binding the quarks to form protons and neutrons, then atomic nuclei, then atoms, and finally the electromagnetic force becomes dominant in forming molecules. Complex molecular matter organized in the fractal form we find in tissues is the ultimate expression of the interaction of all the forces which emerged in the symmetry-breaking at the cosmic origin. As a precursor to looking at the reproductive nature of living sexuality we examine its genesis in the sexual paradox of physics.

Life's Emergence as Symmetry-broken Interaction

It is the twisted nature of cosmic symmetry-breaking (p 310), which makes the makes the combined action of the nuclear and electromagnetic forces capable of forming around a hundred different types of stable nuclei. The fact that the stable nucleons are neutral and positively charged polarizes the entire electromagnetic make up of atoms. The positive charges of the protons clumped together in the nucleus give atoms their unique highly polarized structure of orbital negatively charged electrons. Without this uniquely polarized situation which is itself a direct consequence of cosmic symmetry-breaking complex molecular life would be impossible.

Moreover the non-linear interaction does not stop at the major bonding types, for molecules admit a whole cascade of non-linear bonding interactions from covalent and ionic through the hydrophobic and hydrogen bond interactions that shape nucleic acid and protein structure, to the long-range cooperative weak polar and van der Waal interactions that together make the global cooperativity of enzyme action and cellular organelles including the excitable membrane possible. Symmetry-breaking has thus caused molecular matter to adopt a fractal structure, which ultimately becomes tissues and organisms on the planetary surface held together by the last force, gravity energized by the negentropic surfeit of incoming stellar radiation.

We owe to the unique twisted symmetry-breaking of the forces of nature the very capacity for molecular life and with it biological complexity and the tree of evolution to ramify. In effect biological complexity and with it the conscious brain becomes the ultimate cosmological interactive result of cosmic symmetry-breaking, the Σ at the cosmic equator, representing the fulfillment of both α and Ω, (p 298).

Chemistry is often portrayed in terms of ball and stick models as if only the particle properties of atoms are of significance in chemical bonding. Indeed the atomic nature of matter is one of the principle foundations for a reductionistic explanation of all living processes in terms of the simple actions of atoms as the "building blocks of the universe" as Isaac Asimov once put it. However wave-particle complementarity is at the very core of all chemical interactions. The periodic table of the elements has periodicity only because the wave properties of the electronic orbitals give rise to a series of s, p, d, and f orbitals of increasing spins of 0, 1, 2 etc. Thus the second row of the periodic table, after H and He, as illustrated below, consists of the second layer of one 2-*s* and three 2-*p* orbitals. Because electrons are fermions, they can only enter a given wave orbital in pairs of opposite spin, these four orbitals allow eight electrons in to complete the shell, corresponding to the eight elements in the second row, running through C, N and O - carbon, nitrogen and oxygen. In fact the energies of these orbitals equilibrate to form hybrid *sp* orbitals by wave superposition, resulting in the planar and tetradedral arrangements we find in molecules from water to diamonds.

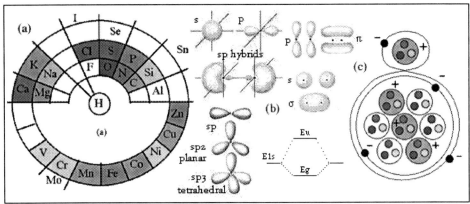

Bifurcation and wave nature in chemical emergence (a) Bifurcation diagram of the periodic table shows how the key bioelements arise from primal quantum interactions resulting from cosmic symmetry-breaking. (b) Atomic, hybrid and molecular orbitals are wave functions determining molecular geometry. Below energy diagram of the non-linear charge interactions causing molecular orbital formation. (c) The hierarchical interactive structure of a molecule (LiH) illustrating how the colour, weak and electromagnetic forces combine to form a complex polarized structure (King R353, R362).

From here the process becomes highly non-linear. Electrons are capable of forming molecular wave orbitals such as σ and π which orbit around more than one atom, often two, but sometimes in the case of conjugated single and double bonds, a whole ring. Because of non-linear charge interactions between the electrons and with the nucleus, which like gravitation obey an inverse square law in 3-D space, the lowest energy molecular orbital is lower in energy than either atomic orbital and the electron enters it binding the atoms together into a molecule such as H_2. This is the basis of the covalent bond. The ionic bond arises from a similar lowering of energy by electron transfer from one atom to another, resulting in net attraction between the resulting positively and negatively charged ions, such as Na^+ and Cl^-

These non-linearities of charge interaction are also manifest in the 'periodic' table, which is not actually periodic, because charge interactions make the properties of corresponding elements in successive rows, such as those between oxygen and sulphur or between carbon and silicon, qualitatively very different. Chemists love to describe chemical bonding as a simple ball and stick arrangement that, given appropriate energetic reagents in an artificial 'closed' system, can 'stick' almost any pair of atoms together in any arrangement we wish. This is central to the mechanistic atomic view of chemistry and biology which forms the principal alternative to the sexually paradoxical quantum view we are describing here.

This reductionist picture begins to seriously unravel, however, when we consider what happens when we ask a very different kind of question - "What will happen if we simply let the chemical elements go in the kind of situation we find in the universe at large? - What structures will emerge in the free interaction of the elements under energetic stimulation?"

We can see a first pat of this answer lies in a series of quantum bifurcations that arise from cosmic symmetry-breaking (King R353, R362). The backbone of life arises from the strongest covalent bonds of all among the elements, $-C\equiv N$ $-C\equiv C-$ and $>C=O$. Given the ubiquity of H this gives the interaction of the $1s$ orbital of H with the $2sp_3$ hybrid of carbon, nitrogen and oxygen primary status. Here we are using 'bifurcation' as a qualitative change in the interactive system caused ultimately by the underlying variables of cosmic symmetry-breaking. Despite suggested alternatives such as silicon-based life there is abundant evidence for this primary interaction being the central 'royal route' to living systems. Molecules containing chains of conjugated multiple C bonds have been detected in interstellar space. Clouds of cyanide HCN and formaldhyde HCHO have been discovered in the Orion nebula where new star and solar system formation is taking place and huge galactic gas clouds containing molecules such as the two-carbon sugar glycoaldehyde and the simplest amino acid, glycine. HCN and HCHO are also key energized intermediates in primal chemical simulations.

A second key interaction arises from the increasing electronegativity, as we move from C to O. Electronegative oxygen binds its electrons very tightly because of the larger number of positive protons in its nucleus for the same electron shell. Oxygen is actually more electronegative than corrosive chlorine. The C-H bond is covalently neutral while the N-H and O-H bonds are successively more polarized. Water H_2O has the highest melting point of any hydride because of its very strong polar and ionic interactions. This is why oily hydrocarbons don't dissolve in highly polar water, effectively separating the entire biological milieu into two distinct polar and non-polar domains, typified by the division between the fatty lipid membrane and aqueous cytoplasm, the 'micelle' or oil-droplet structure of globular protein enzymes and the stacking of nucleic acids such and RNA and DNA in their double helices. Water also has one of the highest specific heats of any substance because of its many internal quantum modes and effectively forms the quantum substrate of all living molecules.

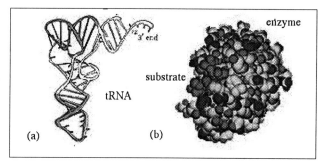

(a) (b)

tRNA substrate enzyme

Global structures of t-RNA and proteins are mediated by cooperative long-range weak bonding, in association with water structures (R396).

From here, the 'incompleteness' of the reductionistic description really begins to bite. A simple molecule like HCN, although it contains a mammoth triple bond is unstable to self-polymerization, because the triple bond's π orbitals are at a higher energy than the σ orbitals and opening them up to form only single or alternate (conjugated) double bonds as in adenine and other molecules illustrated below reduces the energy. We thus find that HCHO and its sister molecules can polymerize to form a vast array of sugars and HCN can polymerize, particularly in association with ubiquitous simple molecules like urea $(NH_2)_2$ to form the purine and pyrimidine nucleic acid bases A, G, C and U, various amino acids and polypeptides and the porphyrins we associate with chlorophyll and hemoglobin. The nucleic acid base adenine for example is simply $(HCN)_5$ and ribose is one of the forms of $(HCHO)_5$.

So where does 'incompleteness' come in? Some of the key products, such as adenine are energetically favoured, but we have a serious chicken-egg problem for the burgeoning complexity - how can a few simple molecules with only a few initial conditions give rise to an increasingly complex array of polymers with immensely varied structure and sequence? How are they guided towards those molecules, like ribose and RNA, which are biologically central? We can invoke both autocatalytic processes and random 'stochastic' interactions, but the informational paradox remains a quantum version of Gödel incompleteness (p 491).

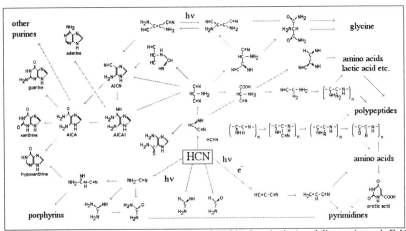

Pathways in HCN polymerization lead to many key biochemicals (ex. Mizutani et. al. R465).

Guiding further steps in this process are more bifurcations arising from cosmic symmetry breaking involving divisions between the key metal ions, $Na^+\leftrightarrow K^+$, $Ca^{++}\leftrightarrow Mg^{++}$ based partly on their ionic radii in water, as well as unique properties contributed by sulphur's relatively low energy transition between -S-H and -S-S- and the capacity of phosphorus to form dehydrated polyphosphates central to nucleic acid structure and cellular energy. Transition elements such as iron and zinc add further catalytic properties, completing a five stage quantum interactive bifurcation structure at the centre of biochemistry that has its origin right back in the force differentiation occurring in the first minuscule fractions of a second at the cosmic origin.

An indication of the recursive nature of the origin of life problem is the fact that, despite meticulous research over the last century to unearth how life began, at a time when all the details of cellular molecular interactions, from the genetic code to the ion channels of neurons, have been decoded and laid bare, the actual 'mechanics' of the origin of life remain almost as obscure as when the first primitive spark experiments were performed over fifty years ago. Although we have found galactic clouds of organic molecules, and suspect life began on Earth as early as the oceans condensed to liquid water some 3.8 billion years ago, the actual technicalities of this supposedly reductionistic process remain speculative and contentious.

There are some key pointers linking the prebiotic phase to the living epoch. The polymerizations of virtually all biopolymers including proteins and nucleic acids involve a step of dehydration by removal of a paired -OH H- to form a linking bond. Although several molecules can perform this task, one stands out, polyphosphate because it is intimately involved in the key energy molecule adenosine triphosphate or ATP, which is itself a monomer ribonucleotide, the backbone of nucleic acids and many energy processes such as glycolysis which splits sugars. A very realistic scenario which could have led directly to ribonucleotides or their analogues is the alternate drying and wetting of a shoreline enriched with precursors such as nucleotide bases, ribose and phosphates. The difficulty here is figuring out how these molecules could be selectively enriched in a manner which would avoid other similar molecules such as other sugars gumming up the works.

Certainly RNA has proven to be a molecule of potentially cosmological status. ATP is simply the stablest penta-cyanide $(HCN)_5$ (adenine) and a form of penta-formaldehyde $(HCHO)_5$ (ribose) linked together by the dehydrating power of phosphate. Syntheses have also been found, e.g. from phospho-glyceraldehyde, a 3-carbon sugar, which lead selectively to ribose. But the details of getting a viable precursor 'brew' remain muddy.

Unlike DNA which is really a genetically-engineered form of RNA designed to form only double helical data libraries, RNA can form bonds between its backbone and its bases and can thus adopt three-dimensional conformations which are able to act as active catalysts. It is thus capable in principle of both fulfilling at least some of the catalytic functions now performed by proteins and of the complementary replication characteristic of DNA.

We now meet another manifestation of 'incompleteness'. RNA is quite difficult to polymerize because it is at a higher free energy that its dissociated monomers. It has to be in unstable thermodynamic equilibrium like this or it would all polymerize once and for all, and there would be no such thing a s life, just a dead RNA crystal. So far no fully replicating spontaneous system has been devised, although RNAs attached to clays by bonding between their acid phosphate groups and the positively charged metal atoms in clay can generate short chains of up to 15 ribonucleotides. Some brilliant experimental studies on the artificial evolution of RNAs has demonstrated that simple 'random' populations of short RNA can selectively evolve to act as their own polymerases and to link amino-acids in similar was to the modern ribosomal which translates triplets of nucleotide information into protein amino-acid sequences.

On the other side of the life divide, there is abundant evidence that RNA has been a precursor to both DNA and coded protein enzymes. The eucaryotes which comprise higher organisms use extensive RNA processing within the nuclear envelope. Key structures involved in protein translation such as the ribosome are based on a core of ribosomal and transfer RNA and can function with many of the proteins removed. Retroviruses such as HIV encode RNA information back into DNA and enzymes such as telomerase essential for elongating the telomeres of chromosomes to keep the life cycle viable use enzymes with evolutionary homology to retroviral reverse transcriptases. Some nuclear processes, such as messenger RNA splicing are mediated by direct RNA catalysis.

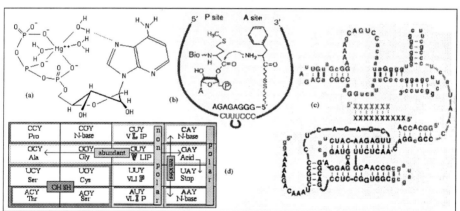

The RNA world: (a) The structure of ATP shows polyphosphate attached to adenine and ribose themselves pentamers of HCN and HCHO. (b) Trans-acting ribozyme replicates key sequence and structure of the ribosome (Zhang and Cech R762, R763). (c) The first effective ribozyme RNA polymerase - a 172 unit molecule bred by molecular selection from a ligase ribozyme through selective evolution of a pool of other intermediates. This ribo-RNA polymerase will faithfully perform complementary replication of oligo-ribonucleotides of arbitrary sequence up to 14 units long with accuracies of up to 98% per base pair (Johnston et. al .R337). (d) Origins of the genetic code in bifurcation. Centre position AU select polar (green) /non-polar (yellow) as broad groups. VLIP are Val-Leu-Ileu-Phe. First position G (cyan) determines primally abundant amino acids. Expansion: first codon C (purple) and A (blue) fix synthesis routes from Glu and Asp Subsequent bifurcations include H-bonding block and acid-base (pink). Arginine and tryptophan appear to be later additions after the evolutionary epoch has begun, possibly being only 2 billion years old as later additions to the genetic code (Cohen R122, R123).

The predominant view is that DNA-based life was thus preceded by an RNA era, but there is still a great deal of debate as to whether RNA was the first informational molecule or whether there was a more robust predecessor such as peptide nucleic acid or even replicating structured clay defects or a primitive Fe-S metabolism.

At the core of all biological function is a fundamental complementarity which is a reflection of the wave-particle complementarity at the very core of the quantum universe - the complementarity between the particulate encoded information of genetic sequences in nucleic acids and the enclosing topology of the cell membrane essential to maintain a non-equilibrium open thermodynamic system, with its wave-based excitation. All life today depends on cells, with viruses acting only as cellular parasites, although the discovery of metabloic genes in a very large mimi-virus (Peplow R553, Raoult R525) reinforces speculation that the eucaryote nucleus could have arisen from a large virus which gained processing and regulatory power over the cellular genes. Primal processes can also generate lipid molecules which have both a polar watery end and a long hydrophobic fatty tail that spontaneously stack to form the bilayer membranous films we find in the membranes of living cells.

A living cell is an open thermodynamic system able to remain far from equilibrium because the enclosure of the membrane provides a distinct internal cyto-environment aided in living cells by active transport. Various models of cooperative affinities between molecules have been advanced to explain how one might arrive at a spontaneous cellular formation. Indeed simple mixtures of cyanide and related molecules can form microcells of a similar size of eucaryote spores as shown from my own work above. Various mechanisms have been suggested for binding RNA to membranes using various intermediates to ensure cellular reproduction. Out of this membranous envelope a series of other critical wave properties emerge - chaotic electrochemical excitation and the capacity for perception and ultimately cognition.

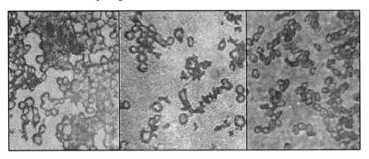

HCN microcells (left and centre) compared with psilocybe mushroom spores [right]. (King)

The emergence of the genetic code is also a process which displays strong indications of fundamental bifurcations in its genesis. As shown in the above figure (p 321) centre position A/U show selectivity for polar and non-polar amino acids. As well the most abundant amino acid glycine and alanine have specific affinity with first base G. Further divisions specify successive polar and other specializations to a four and eight member code and finally to the code we find today. Optimality arguments also can be applied to show the existing code is now close to the best possible.

There are several other biochemical aspects of cellular metabolism which are sourced in fundamental bifurcations of the chemical milieu, including the bilayer membrane, ion and electron transport, the carboxyllic acid cycle, phosphyrlation and the use of Fe-S centres. Many of the organisms at the root of the evolutionary tree of life tolerate high temperatures, suggesting life went through a high temperature phase, associated with volcanic hot pools, or hydrothermal vents. Connected with this environment are aspects of the cellular metabolism revolving around iron-sulphur Fe-S centres and reversible sulphur reactions with hydrogen which occur in volcanic processes. The electron transport process of respiration and photosynthesis in the membrane uses FeS proteins, some of which, such as ferredoxin, are very primitive, and sulphur respiration and photosynthesis occurs in a one-electron process which is a precursor of the two-electron oxygen photosynthesis. These processes are also associated with nucleotide coenzymes such as nicotene-adenine dinucleotide NAD and the flavin nucleotides, suggesting that these redox (oxidation-reduction) reactions may have begun in the RNA era, using these nucleotides as co-factors. The hot era could have occurred however, well into the RNA era, epochs after the hypothetical cooler, drying shoreline made the first self-replicating 'genetic' RNA based on phosphate metabolism.

Excitable Membrane: (a)Primitive nucleotides appear to have preceded protein enzymes, as evidenced by nucloetide coenzymes. NAD structure permits linkage of other energies to a redox bifurcation. (b) H+ and e- transport linked by H_2 in mem-

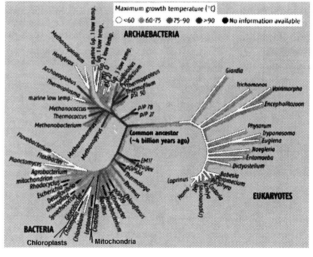

brane due to insolubility of e- and solubility of H+. (c) Prebiotic link between catecholamines and indole via quinone-type photoreduction. (d) Hypothetical form of primitive electron transport as a non-equilibrium limit cycle. (e) Acetyl-choline and phosphatidyl choline compared. Phosphatidyl choline lipid stacks tail to tail as shown in the clothes pegs (b) (King).

This brings us to the geological evidence which from the Isua deposits in Greenland and in a few other ancient strata suggest evidence of life at around 3.5 to 3.8 billion years ago almost as soon as the oceans cooled to liquid water. This raises further questions. Was life already extant in the solar system. Did it originate in space or on Mars which may have coalesced sooner? Certainly the Earth has ben peppered with cometary and other material which would have given the Earth a rich source of prebiotic organics but many questions remain and few conclusive answers are yet forthcoming.

Evolutionary root of the tree of life and its diversification into archaea, bacteria and eucaryotes may have gone through an early period of high temperature (Woese, Anathaswamy R12).

The Living Epoch: Bifurcation, Complexity and the Prisoner's Dilemma

We are now into the living epoch and can turn our attention to the base of the evolutionary tree of life, where we find three great groups, the eucaryotes, the bacteria and the more recently recognized archaea which comprise various thermophilic and methano-

genic organisms which are as closely related to higher organisms as they are to true bacteria.

The five kingdoms of plants, animals and fungi, protista and procaryotes, along with the archaea reflect major bifurcations of the thermodynamic and metabolic environment. There is a fundamental bifurcation of energy metabolism between photosynthetic fixation of incident solar energy, the principal incident energy source at the planetary surface, and all other forms of heterotrophic energy-pillaging budget, including animals as frank predators, fungi as partially symbiotic decomposers, and the highly energetic catalytic biochemical pathways of prokaryotes. The major divisions of life are thus universal in nature. Such universality also extends to the formation of excitable cells using amine-based neurotransmitters and ion channels. Some of these changes such as development of an oxygen metabolism are consequences themselves of an oxygen atmosphere induced by the biota

324

themselves.

However, as we have noted in 'The Inescapable Game of Life', the tree of living diversity and all the niches it contains are ramifications of the prisoners' dilemma game of survival, adaption and mutation. A game in which sruvival means continuing to play and the only coulmination is defeat in death or species extinction. In effect heterotrophic animals are defectors against the autotrophic photosynthetic strategy of plants, by consuming plants and other life forms as as predators. Likewise, the carnivores are defectors against the herbivores. Thus the very diversity of the tree of life is generated by the most complex prisoners' dilemma game we know of in the universe - the biological giame of life. Moreover the chaotic population dynamics and genetic Red Queen races in which predators and prey and parasites and host interact are also manifestations of this ever increasing game of climax diversity. Niches are not just adapted to, but actively created in this process. As we have seen in the chaos chapter, evolution is described as a primary instance of complexity at the edge of chaos (p 506), and indeed in a climax ecosystem, many or all of the species are in a prisoners dilemma game in which species, niches and populations are in unstable relationship including chaotic fluctuation. The 'balance of nature' is thus a misnomer - it is the imbalance of nature which sustains living diversity, albeit precariously.

Cataclysmic events have also shaped the life tree. Five great mass extinctions have irreversibly shaped the diversity of life as we know it. The most recent is the Cretaceous-Tertiary extinction caused by a massive asteroid hitting the Yucatan, also causing volcanic instability, a reduction in oxygen levels and the demise of the dinosaurs. An earlier more grave extinction of a similar kind occurred in the Permian era. The capacity of multi-celled organisms to diversify may be also a consequence of a period of almost global glaciation - the 'snowball Earth' scenario - shortly before the Ediacaran epoch that preceded the Cambrian, causing a bottleneck in the procaryote domination of the Earth and allowing multicelled eucaryotes to diversify. There have likewise been several great radiations of life into new diversity, including the Cambrian radiation of the metaphyta and the mammalian radiation.

Mutation, Selection and the Quantum Limit

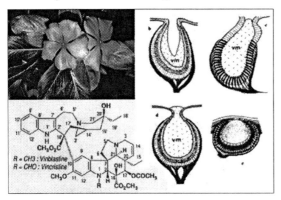

Two aspects of evolution, adventitious mutation and cumulative selection are contrasted. Left: *Cantharanthus rosea* makes the indole vincristine, unusual in structure and almost unique to the biological world. While this has been preserved through natural selection, it is an unusual molecule which appears to be the result of an initial fortuitous mutation. Right: By contrast, the development of the camera eye (Dawkins R153), is virtually inevitable by natural selection, because its formation results from a simple topological bifurcation of a photoreceptive hollow and the fact that directional photon reception is a core quantum interaction as fundamental as photosynthesis itself.

Evolution is traditionally regarded as an opportunistic drunkard's walk by occasional random mutation into a variety of rare advantageous configurations, which then become fixed by selective advantage as stunningly effective incremental historical accidents. The vast majority of mutations are deleterious and only a vanishing minority advantageous.

Evolution is thus partly a stochastic opportunistic process and partly an optimizing selective response to bifurcations in the natural, sexual and ecological landscape. The balance between the adventitious and the selectively optimized is a reflection of the deeper underlying process of quantum complementarity. In an interference experiment, the trajectories of individual photons are unpredictable through quantum uncertainty of position and momentum. The pattern of wave interference only becomes established statistically through the passage of many photons, which through their statistics of particle absorption by individual atoms demonstrate the wave amplitude variation of the interference pattern. This convergence to the probability interpretation is even more marginal in the complex macroscopic biological world than it is in the quantum world of small numbers of events.

Although their effects are large in macroscopic organisms, mutations themselves are unique kinetic events in the quantum world of molecules and molecular orbitals. Such highly specific mutational transformations are vastly rarer than the photons in a conventional interference experiment and tend to the uncertainty of a single unrepeated event which by its very fixation permanently changes the context which created it. This makes it possible for adventitious aspects of evolution to become enduring historical manifestations of the underlying nature of quantum uncertainty. Effectively adventitious mutations are single quantum events which become fixed and replicated by the genetic process. They thus never converge to the classical interpretation under the correspondence principle, becoming in effect a frozen series of cat paradox experiments piled one on top of the other.

Complementing this, selective advantage can and will over time, given sufficient mutations, explore any bifurcations or optimalities in the physical environment. Thus many of the marvels of evolution, such as the camera eye, are almost inevitable because of the capacity for bifurcational change, which incrementally enhances the immense optimality in survival of accessing the fundamental quantum mode of directional photon absorption, the most selective and discriminatory sense we have.

There is even a degree of paradox in the functioning of chaperone proteins such as heat shock protein hsp90 which inhbits protein folding instabilities and thus devlopmental changes which could precipitate phenotypic malformations in development but causes diverse potentially adaptive genetically-based phenotype changes when stress reduces the organism's capacity to repress the backlog of hidden mutations (New Scientist 28 Sep 2002, Nature, 396 336, 417 398). A similar stress-adaptive role has been attributed to prions (True et. al .R692).

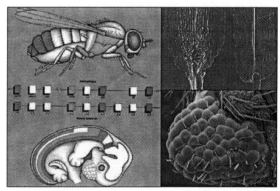

Left: Sequence of homeotic genes compared between insect and vertebrate, showing their common role in segmental organization (De Robertis et. al R158, .McGinnis et. al. R447), Top right: Knotted maize mutants have a mutation in a homeobox gene regulating differentiation. Similar homeobox genes have been found in tomatoes and rice (Homeobox Harvest Sci. Am. June 91). Lower right: Mammalian regulatory gene, pax6 elicits ectopic eyes on the leg of a fruit fly, showing the genes even have comparable action. (Dawkins R153).

Evolutionary Universality

A major quantum-leap of universality in the evolutionary realm is the ubiquitous use of homeotic genes for morphogenic organization of the multicellular organism, particularly the segmental organization from the head to the tail, common not only to all metazoa but to plants and fungi as well. The underlying mechanism of homeotic gene morphogenesis may represent a type of universal solution to developing body plans. The development of this system seems to be the key step enabling the emergence of multicelled organisms and their divergence into plants, animals and fungi, particularly in the Cambrian radiation. Although the homeobox sequence and the key proteins are too complex to be accounted for by a cosmological argument, the principles by which they evolved and the chemical morphogens may be an evolutionary universal. This is consistent with the long time from the first emergence of eucaryotes to metaphyta in the Ediacaran and Cambrian radiations about 600 million years ago. This long delay is indicative of there being only one, or a few effective solutions to this problem, giving it potential universality beyond our own metaphyta.

A second type of universality is manifest in the mammalian evolution to form an emotionally-based brain and cerebral cortex generalizing the less structured smell-brain to form a universal perceptual and cognitive organ.

The mammalian brain is functionally different from its reptilian predecessor. The elaboration of the cerebral cortex and limbic system has made possible a generalization of function which has replaced imprinted mechanisms of instinct with more generalized and flexible emotional and cognitive processes which permit complex social and strategic behavior in mammalian societies. These have had significant effects on the whole mammalian kingdom because they make for new subtleties which modify instinctual reactions supporting strict kin altruism with complex social reciprocal altruism, changing the face of the evolutionary game of survival.

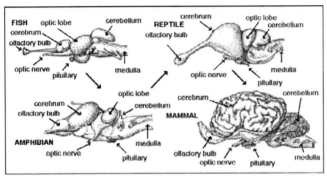

Evolution of the mammalian brain showing development of the cortex and relative reduction of the midbrain (redrawn from Keaton R346)

The architecture of the sensory cortices appears likewise in evolutionary terms to be an elaboration of a new and more generalized embryogenic scheme which can represent the dynamics of all of the quantum sense modes within the same general scheme. The generality of these neuro-embryogenic 'algorithms' is also attested to by the plasticity of the cortex in terms of the evolving function of particular areas over time after injury or learning a new skill. The result is a brain converging to the quantum and cognitive limit, both sensorily sensitive in each of the principal quantum modes of interaction and possessing generalized sensory processing capabilities arising from edge of chaotic dynamics and quantum electro-physiology, thus representing a universal and in this sense cosmological solution generated by evolution to the existential dilemma.

Overpage: Tree of Life (King).

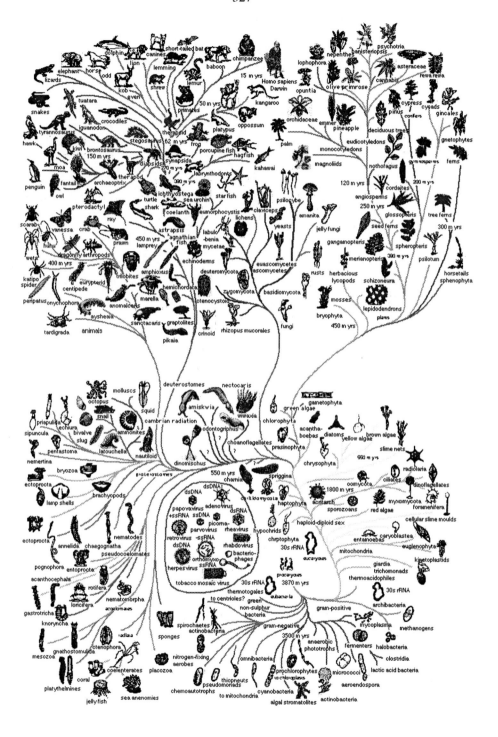

The Entanglements of Biological Sex

Human Fertilization (Porritt R537)
The symmetry-breaking of egg and sperm (see also (p 442)) emphasizes the polarization between the sexes.

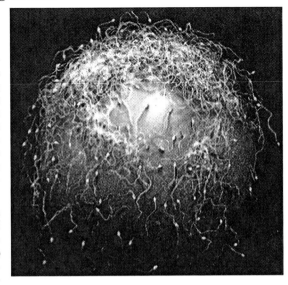

Although we perceive sex as a simple division into male and female rooted in fertilization, sexuality is a complex interwoven relationship with many forms of interaction more subtle and pervasive than the raw sexual urge. To fully understand sex we thus need to appreciate this deep relationship between sex and the warp and weft of entanglement.

Much of this entanglement comes from the long history of biological sex as a prisoners' dilemma relationship from which there is no escape but reproductive fertilization, except for brief periods of parthenogenesis, interrupted by cryptic sexual exchange and adaption.

Central to the dark nature of sexuality is the Edenic notion that sex is central to our downfall into the mortal coil and hence that our sexual desire is at the root of our fallibility, without which we could have become 'as Gods'. We need to understand the source of this fallacy in coming to terms with the redemptive nature of sexuality in the perpetuity of life.

Sex, Death, and Ecosystemic Immortality

Sex is of course the source of individual organismic mortality because, rather than reproducing clonally or parthenogenetically as bacteria do, when they are not using viral or plasmid promiscuity to exchange DNA, we share only half our genes with a partner, in conceiving new offspring, rather than transmitting all our genes and hence a complete replicon of ourselves in parthenogenesis. None our offspring will thus ever have the same genes as ourselves again in the entire history of the universe, because of sex's endless recombination. This teeming complexity, which is central to Taoistic notions of nature never repeating itself exactly, is one of the most insightful affirmations of the power of sexual exchange in creating almost endless variety from the molecular dance of the primal ooze.

Contrasting and complementing sex's tryst with death is its role in immortal life, for sex is also our salvation in the perpetual passage of the generations. For us to come into existence at all, our living germ-line, or more appropriately germ-web has had to have run in an unbroken chain of ancestors for the entire three and a half billion years back to the first beginnings of life on Earth. While sexuality gives every non-parthenogenetic organism a limited life-span, we thus owe our very existence to the immortal sexual genetic web.

Moreover, sex is the most fundamental nemesis of selfishness, for in transmitting only half our genes, we have entered into a fundamental pact with the 'other' to share our very identity and our reproductive destinies. To do this we must ultimately elicit the cooperation of the other, for defection once mutual becomes our collective nemesis. Thus the unmitigated selfishness of the parthenogenetic gene is compromised, cleaved to a break-even between selfishness and altruism, which remains the founding paradox of all sexual engagement.

Bacteria engage an even more radical form of pan-sexuality utilizing viruses and plasmids, themselves separate mobile genetic elements. This enables them to move genes around in the bacterial genome and to exchange DNA between cells, even between different species.

of bacteria. This form of sexuality is a mirror to our own form of dyadic sexuality. Sexual exchange of material can happen both through viral exchange and through a conjugation plasmid which can spool DNA from one bacterium into another, resulting in a net donation of genes from one strain to another, which ensures and exchange of genetic material.

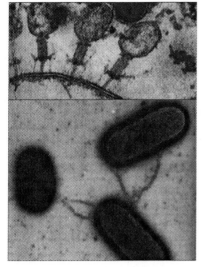

Bacterial pan-sexuality. Above: Syringe-like bacteriophages injecting their DNA are capable of transferring genes between bacteria, carrying bacterial genes with them when they multiply and are released. Some phages also integrate with the host chromosome. Below: A positive sex-strain bacterium using plasmid sexual pili to transfer DNA simultaneously to two other bacteria. Sexual plasmids also integrate with the host chromosome during sexual conjugation (Wolfe R743).

Because the genes driving this exchange are from a separate 'organism', a genetic plasmid, carrying its own genes and conferring male doning capacity on bacteria harbouring it, there are no bounds on exchange between the same species. Indeed plasmid sexuality is promiscuous between many bacterial species, resulting in sharing of genetic information on a pan-sexual basis. In addition to plasmid-mediated genetic exchange, bacteria also engage extensive genetic recombination, through viral exchange, which carries genes between bacteria, as temporary additions to a viral genome. Although some of these elements, such as the phages, are parasitic, the sexual conjugation plasmids are essential for bacterial survival and also depend on the bacteria for their existence. The overall relationship is thus a symbiotic one of mutual genetic inter-dependence amid competition. Plasmid sexuality has resulted in major aggregations of antibiotic resistance genes onto a single plasmid in infectious drug resistance.

This view of sexuality as an ecosystemic process of sharing genetic information and providing recombination into new genomic arrangements capable of new forms of survival in new ecological niches is central to the ecosystemic foundation from which sexuality gains its immense variety. It is also important in understanding the deep relationship between sexuality as an interdependent sharing of information and variety and the dyadic form of sexuality we find in higher organisms, to which we shall now return. However this ecosystemic sexual exchange has certain limitations. Notice that this form of sexuality is not directly linked to bacterial reproduction. Basically it is transferring part of a single copy genome from one cell to another. It works very well at sharing key genes among many types of bacteria. It also does well at providing new types of genome, or even new species, with new combinations of existing genes, however it doesn't provide for recombining an existing genome characteristic of a given species in a way which can make new viable varieties of individual which remain viable and interfertile within a given species. Also it is too scrambled and chaotic a process to enable the evolution of complex genomes with many chromosomes and elaborate organismic regulation which needs to be conserved.

The dyadic sex of higher organisms is the enchanted loom of emergence of all living animals, plants and fungi, because the immense genetic variety produced by sexual recombination, virtually all of whose combinations are viable genomes, is what has made evolution into complex organisms possible. If we had to rely on parthenogenetic cloning we would still be single-celled animals of unremitting genetic selfishness. The few higher species which do reproduce by parthenogenesis generally also rely on cryptic sexuality to restore variation, particularly in times of stress. If we had had to rely only on bacterial sex, we would likewise have remained at the stage of single celled single chromosome organisms. Deborah Blum (1997) notes that dyadic sex at the most basic level ensures we recombine only with a single genome of the same species and don't have to cope with the chaotic multiple agent mixing of bacterial pan-sexuality. But what is absolutely unique about higher organismic sex is that it enables specific recombination of the variants, or alleles, of a singe gene to be recombined in ways which make for almost endless variety while still preserving the overall organization of the genome.

This creative bounty comes despite sex's supposedly 'destructive' carnivorous origins (Margulis and Sagan R427). The first eucaryotes seem to have engulfed the typhus-like bacteria which became the mitochondrion, giving us our respirative energy and the cyano-bacteria which became the chloroplasts of plants which provide the energy of photosynthesis. A more controversial suggestion by Margulis has been that the kinetochores at the base of flagella which form the centrioles organizing the spindles which make both mitotic cell division of paired chromosomes and the meiotic recombinations of sex cells possibly originated from spirochaete flagella. Closer analysis may not support this idea because spirochaete flagella now appear to be rotary engines like the bacterial flagellum, rather than flexing. Lynn Margulis suggests merging of two (haploid) genomes, each containing a single copy of each of our genes, doubling our chromosome number to the diploid form, and hence fertilization itself, originates in amoeba which found 'eating one's mate alive was as good as being twins'. Diploid sexuality and possibly the separation of the nucleus and multiple chromosomes as well may thus have originated from beneficent cannibalism.

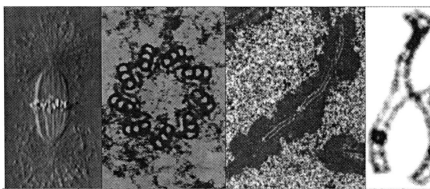

Eucaryote sexual reproduction: Both normal mitotic cell division in eucaryotes (a) and sexual meiosis involve the spindle apparatus centered on the semi-autonomous centriole (b) which must itself divide before the chromosomes can separate and is also the source of the flagellum. Crossing over requires spooling of the DNA to find homologous points of exchange, mediated by the synaptonemal complex (c) after which the crossed chiasmata can be seen in later stages (d) (R145, R743, R346).

A new form of sexuality emerges, in which there is an alternation between haploid sexual generations, each containing one copy of each gene, which fuse in fertilization to diploid generations containing two copies of every gene which can, before again forming the next sexual generation, recombine this double-headed genome to mix the genetic characteristic of 'father-sperm' and 'mother-egg' into new son and daughter sexual genomes containing a viable serially-ordered mix of each. From this elegant, stunning and still not-fully-understood process, whose evolutionary roots remain obscure, comes the immense capacity for variety we find in multi-celled organisms. Pivotal to this is the kinetochore and spindle apparatus that can pull daughter chromosomes apart after every cell division and the sifting and ordering of the genes at the crossover points during generation of sexual gametes in meiosis. The mechanism for homologous crossing-over has recently been clarified.

Eucaryotic sex has a very complex origin. Bacterial cells contain only one chromosome attached to the cell membrane. Eucaryotic cells containing many chromosomes divide mitotically, by replicating each chromosome and pulling them apart using microtubules (a) organized around the centrioles (b). The centriole itself has a cryptic origin, being partially autonomous in the sense that division of the crossed centrioles, which come in pairs at right angles, to form a new pair, precedes separation of the replicated chromosome pairs.

Centrioles are also the source of the flagellum in the sperm and other cells. Lynn Margulis has suggested that, like the mitochondrion and chloroplast, the centrioles arose from symbiosis with motile spirochaetes, which have tubulin-like proteins. However spirochaete flagella appear to be more like the rotatory bacterial flagella (Charon and Goldstein R113), so centrioles may originate internally in the apparatus linking the chromosome to the cell membrane. Studies show that at least some animal cells can generate new centrioles if their centrioles are destroyed by laser microsurgery (Khodjakov et. al. R350). These generate random multiple arrays from a cloud of microtubules, implying that mother-daughter centriole pairs serve to ensure clean bipolar spindles rather than disorganized chromosome division, which centriole-less anastral plant spindles suffer from more than animal cells (Marshall et. al. R434). Series of studies searching for independent cytoplasmic DNA or RNA in centrioles which could form a genetic symbiosis like the mitochondrion have not produced clear evidence for either (Hinchcliffe et. al. R309, Marshall et. al. R435).

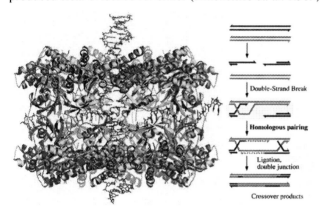

Double-Strand Break

Homologous pairing

Ligation, double junction

Crossover products

The 16-unit protein Dmc1, which shows homology with the bacterial recombinase RecA (Watson et. al. R720 319), mediates homologous recombination between DNA of maternal and paternal versions of chromosomes in meiosis, by spooling double-stranded and single stranded DNA vertically and horizontally, as shown, consistent with the scheme at right (Kinebuchi et. al. R352).

Some primitive eucaryotes still have chromosomes linked to the nuclear membrane. In a scenario in which cell fusion or cannibalism led to a doubling of a single chromosome, to a diploid cell, these could again subdivide to form haploid cells. Mitotic spindles could have begun on one diploid chromosome pair and subsequently developed to separate several chromosomes cleanly into the daughter cells. From here the double division of the tetrad of chromatids arising from replicated diploid chromosomes to regain haploid sex cells during meiosis would follow naturally. However the validity of sex depends on the variety created by sexual exchange and this requires recombination between sister chromosomes through crossing over. This is again a complex and not fully understood process mediated by the synaptonemal complex, requiring the DNA of the pair of chromosomes being crossed over to be carefully spooled to find homologous regions, so that the crossing does not interrupt a gene and retains a perfect complement of genes in each sex cell.

In addition to their selfish gene load, there are also indications of genetic symbiosis between cellular and mobile elements, which may facilitate a variety of regulatory and evolutionary processes. The incidence of genes with associated mobile elements is high. Of 12,000 human genes investigated in one study (Trends in Genetics 19 p 68) 27% were associated with transposable elements. More rapidly evolving genes, such as those in the immune system, had more transposable elements. The huge variety of antibody type in immunity is induced through many factors including large gene libraries and hyper-variable regions prone to mutation and translocation. In turn, the RAG1,2 immune system genes induce editing processes characteristic of transposon activity. 25% of human genes contain multiple promoters, including those of transposed elements, which provide an adaptive basis for complex forms of regulation. Primates have a unique capacity to regulate estrogen in the placenta independently of the gonads because of such an adaption.

This co-evolution is also fraught with the mutual antagonism we have seen between male and female sexes. In the 0.4% of genes which contain transpositional insertions into coding regions there are alternative forms of RNA splicing, which can mask and tolerate what could otherwise be a lethal mutation (for both host and endogenous element). The sexual imprinting of genes through methylation may be an adaption of a defence against genes infected by deleterious mobile elements by rendering a section of DNA inactive. In turn transposable elements may have driven sexuality itself. According to Donal Hickey (R307) transposable elements are at a two-for-one advantage to sexual genomes because they can transfect sex-cells during the reproduction cycle (as LINEs are known to do) thus ensuring all offspring of any host partner are infected, while each of the sexual partners can contribute only half their genes. It is thus possible that sexuality itself was generated as a adaptive response by transposable element evolution rather than the host genome. Species which are highly sexual have large transposable element loads. Those in between have lower loads and asexual species very few. However the transposable elements can neither be considered benign nor entirely selfish. The chromosomal and mobile genomes are in a truly sexual genetic entwinement too, with the benefits to both arising indirectly through the mutual defences each has set up to the strategic onslaught of the other (Kingsland R366). Thus the answer to the selfish gene thus turns out to be a form of sexually antagonistic coevolution (p 16).

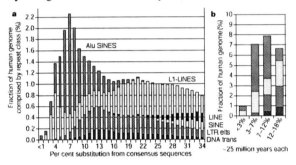

Human transposable element evolutionary history of L1-LINEs (cream), Alu elements (lt. blue), retrovirus-like LTR (long-terminal repeat) elements (green) and DNA transposons (dk. brown). Older LINEs and SINEs are in yellow and dk. blue. This history extends back over 200 million years indicating the very ancient basis of this potentially symbiotic relationship (Human Genome Consortium R329).

Coding sequences comprise less than 5% of the human genome, whereas repeat sequences account for at least 50% and probably much more. Transposable LINE or long-intermediate repeat retroelements common to vertebrates, with a history running back to the eucaryote origin are specifically activated in both sperms and eggs during meiosis (R73, R671, R685). These replicate from transcribed RNA copies of themselves thus using RNA to instruct DNA copies, indicating an origin in RNA-based life, as does the active RNA processing of our own eucaryote cells. Their RNA-based reverse transcriptase shows homologies with the telomerase essential for maintaining immortality in our germ line, indicating a common and symbiotic origin. 100,000 partially defective LINEs and their 300,000 dependent smaller fellow traveller Alu SINEs make up a significant portion of the human and mammalian genomes. These elements travel passively down the germ line with chromosomal DNA, so their specific activation during meiosis suggests they may perform a role of coordinated regulatory mutation. This suggests that the type of symbiotic sexuality embraced by bacteria and plasmids also continues to function in higher organisms in a form of sexual symbiosis between our chromosomes and transposable genetic elements. This is consistent with the 1.4% point mutation divergence between humans and chimps, being overshadowed by an additional 3.9% divergence to 5.4% overall (Britten R77), when insertions and deletions are accounted (p 97).

SINEs, such as human Alu, a free-rider on the LINE reverse transcriptase derived from the small cellular RNA used to insert nascent proteins through the membrane, are in turn implicated in active functional genes (Reynolds R561, Schmid R602) particularly some involved in cellular stress reactions, again suggesting genetic symbiosis. Humans have about 13 times as many RNA edits as non-primate species, including inosine insertions associated with Alu elements, as well as intron deletions (Holmes R318) and newly inserted exons (Ast R26), which may differentiate humans from other apes through alternative splicing of genes expressed in the brain (p 102). RNA editing is abundant in brain tissue, where editing defects have been linked to depression, epilepsy and motor neuron disease. There is a new Alu insert about every 100 births. As many as three quarters of all human genes are subject to alternative splice editing.

Although the data from the human genome project indicated that human LINEs are becoming less active as a group by comparison with the corresponding elements in the more rapidly evolving mouse genome, there remain about 60 active human LINE elements which are known to be responsible for mutations in humans. More recent investigation (Boissinot et. al. R70) shows that the most recent families are highly active. Around four million years ago shortly after the chimp-human split, a new family Ta-L1 LINE-1 emerged and is still active, with about half the Ta insertions being polymorphic, varying across human populations. Moreover 90% of Ta-1d, the most recent subfamily are polymorphic, showing highly active lines remain present. LINEs are more heavily distributed on the sex chromosomes with X chromosomes containing 3 times as many full length potentially active elements and the Y chromosome 9 times as many! This is consistent with a continuing mutational load on humans which is removed more slowly from the sex chromosomes by crossing over in proportion to the degree to which crossing over is inhibited in each (i.e. totally on the Y and largely in males in the X but not in females). We have noted (p 28) that sexual recombination is a protection from mutational error in a process called Muller's ratchet.

Evolution of reverse transcriptases from a common ancestor bearing a LINE archetype (Xiong and Eickbush R757 Nakamura et. al. R487). The root of their evolution goes back to the transfer from RNA to DNA at the beginning of life. They form a complementary evolutionary tree to that of cellular life as genetic symbionts of metazoa travelling down the germ line. Their group includes telomerases essential to the reproductive cycle.

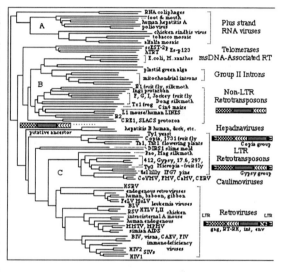

LINEs are preferentially expressed in both steriodogenic and germ-line tissues in mice (Branciforte and Martin R73, Trelogan and Martin R685), suggesting stress could interact with meiosis. L1 expression occurs in embryogenesis, at several stages of spermatogenesis including leptotene, and in the primary oocytes of females poised at prophase 1. Conversely the SRY-group male determining gene SOX has been found to regulate LINE retrotransposition (Tchénio et. al. R671). Similarly LINE elements have been proposed to be 'boosters' in the inactivation of one X chromosome that happens in female embryogenesis (Lyon R417). This could enable somatic stress to have a potential effect on translocation in the germ-line which might enable form of genetic adaption in long-lived species such as humans.

Both L1 and Alu elements may be able to self-regulate rates of replication, through the existence of stealth drivers, viable elements which maintain a low transcription rate of active elements, with little genomic impact and hence little negative selection. These occasionally seed daughter master elements, which may replicate actively to form new families when conditions permit. This picture is consistent with long periods of quiescence, punctuated by bursts of 'saltatory' replication leading to large copy numbers (Han et. al. R281).

Endogenous retroviruses, or ERVs, which also travel down the germ line as free-riders, although some may retain infectious capacity, may be essential for placental function, as every mammal tested has placental blooms of endogenous retroviruses which appear to both aid the formation of the syncytium, the super-cellular fused membrane that enables diffusion from the mother to the baby and the immunity suppression which prevents rejection of the embryo, both characteristics of retroviruses such as HIV. Mi and colleagues (R461) found a placental whose sequence was homologous to several viral envelope proteins. The sequence, now called syncytin, is identical to the envelope protein of the HERV-W retrovirus. It is expressed at high levels in the syncytiotrophoblast (and at low levels in the testes) and nowhere else. Most of the other genes of the provirus have been mutated, suggesting that the envelope glycoprotein function was specifically selected. If cultured cells are made to express syncytin, they will fuse together, and this fusion can be blocked with antibodies against syncytin. HERV-W is only found in primates, but mice have similar retroviral blooms. Our ability to form the placenta may thus depend on our harnessing a viral gene somewhere in our evolutionary lineage.

The 'lampbrush' phase of extended chromosomes during meiosis has also been suggested to enable forms of genetic re-processing. In non-mammals this extended phase involves open transcription of coding and non-coding regions and has been proposed to be a form of genetic processing (Wolfe R743), which probably occurs in a less obvious way in mammals as well. Some of the early radioactive tracer studies of diplotene 'lampbrush' chromosomes in amphibians showed apparent spooling of the DNA during maturation of the ovum, consistent with a gene comparison mechanism (Callan R99, R100). The purpose of such openly transcribing stretches of the whole chromosomes including vast regions which are not coding for any protein remains obscure (Angelier et. al. R17). All transcription units functioning in lampbrush loops synthesize RNA at a maximum rate. In situ hybridization has provided evidence for transcription of both unique coding sequences and highly repetitive sequences. For repetitive sequences, their intense transcription appears to be non-productive, in that RNAs are not translatable and might be useless products of read-through transcription, unless they have a role in genetic modulation as RNAs.

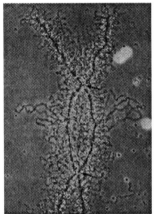

Lampbrush chromosomes in the newt (Gall, Wolfe R743).

The much longer time primary oocytes remain in meiotic stasis before eventual maturation might to give the female a tendency to express stress-induced translocational effects during adult life, 'compensating' for the up to four-fold higher base rate of male point mutation, because the continual mitotic production of sperm cells leads to more cell divisions, by contrast with quiescent immature oocytes (Ellegren R186, Nachmann and Crowell R486, McVean and Hurst R451). X-chromosomes evolve more slowly, presumably because they spend three quarters of their time in the female line.

Sex appears to become a necessity, linked to reproduction as a means of generating genetic variation when the generation to generation reproduction rate slows to the point that mutations occur at too low a rate to provide enough genetic variation for populations to fully adapt. This means a strict reliance upon sex as a means of reproduction is largely a feature of larger and relatively slowly reproducing, multicellular organisms. Many unicellular organisms have no known sexual reproduction, and can be considered to be obligate asexual. No unicellular organism is obligate sexual. Not all multicellular organisms are obligate sexual, but all the obligate sexual organisms are multicellular.

Symmetry-breaking, Gene Wars and the Ovum.

Before there was gender there was symmetrical sex. In many fungi today, and in some simple plants, like spirogyra, any two distinct strains of a species can fertilize one another by passing a nucleus through a conjugation tube. Some 'primitive' single-celled protoctists still use identical isogametes.. All multi-celled animals however depend on the cytoplasm of the egg to differentiate into the tissue layers of the developing embryo, and its organs. Egg and sperm have become symmetry-broken into complementary yin and yang genders, as wave and particle are in physics - exemplified above by a large enveloping egg membrane covered in many particulate sperm endeavouring to fertilize the ovum. This relationship with wave-particle complementarity may be more than just an analogy. It may be an expression of quantum reality at the organismic level.

Here 'sex' means the formation of haploid sexual gametes which fuse their genes again through fertilization. Each haploid sex cell contains one copy of each (non-sex) chromosome - half of the number of 'paired' chromosomes found in the diploid form of the organism, in which there are two of each. Some organisms such as mosses and coelenterates also have active haploid phases. 'Gender' is here the symmetry-breaking of sex cells, and the sexual organisms bearing them, into complementary masculine and feminine morphologies. This is the sense Kim Walen also uses it in describing 'gender predispositions' in sex as a minimum energy genetic solution breaking sexual symmetry in the simplest most efficient way - "The effect of a predisposition is essentially to open up the path of least resistance". He compares the development of gender with the way the visual nervous system responds dynamically to visual input, in stimulating development (Blum R65 18). It is clear the brain is far more complex than the 60% or so of our 30,000 genes could produce by hard wired genetic determinism. Thus the developing brain uses genetic cues to establish a dynamical process conducive to the development of a much more complex organ than the genes themselves can determine. This provides a window on a fascinating complementarity and interactivity between nature and nurture in which nature finds the simplest most efficient route in responsive relationship with the natural and social environment to give rise to engendered sexuality. In this view all the variations in transsexual development along with sexual orientation are just results of 'having enough slip' in this predisposing biological pathway.

We contrast 'gender', as symmetry-broken environmentally responsive sexuality with 'cultural engendering' - social or politically acceptable (or indeed transvestite) sex roles which a given society may impose, encourage or seek to exorcise. While acknowledging, especially in the critique of patriarchy, that imposed cultural roles can and do result in cultural variation in cultural engendering, we will argue that the health and viability of a human culture depends on a whole engagement of the 'human animal' in which culture responds to and resonates creatively with our underlying biologically 'engendered' evolutionarily sustainable nature, rather than imposing its values upon it. Thus rather than a confrontation between the conflicting influences of nature and nurture, nature in evoking complexity seeks a constructive and responsive complementation. It is this complementation that a fully abundant society gives expression to in evolutionary time.

Richard Dawkins (R150) mischievously portrays the 'engendering' of sex as the original sin of a sneaky Adam seeking to spread his reproductive investment like wild oats: "In some respects a big isogamete would have an advantage ... because it would get its embryo off to a good start. ... But there was a catch. The evolution of isogametes which were larger then were strictly necessary would have opened the door to selfish exploitation. Individuals who produced smaller than average gametes could cash in provided they could ensure that their smaller than average gametes fused with extra-big ones. ... There was a large-investment, or honest strategy. This automatically opened the way for a small-investment exploitative or 'sneaky' strategy. Each honest one would prefer to fuse with an honest one ... [but] the sneaky one's had more to lose, and they therefore won the evolutionary battle. The honest ones became eggs and the sneaky ones became sperms".

There is an irony of dramatic oversimplification here because this very differentiation may have been caused by killer genes in the female cytoplasm resulting from the selfishness of cytoplasmic genes, not the male. Isogametes frequently display cytoplasmic genetic conflict, sometimes destroying 90% of their cytoplasm in fertilization. The single celled alga *Chlamydomonas* illustrates this phenomenon. Most of its life cycle it is haploid. It is only diploid when two haploid cells fuse. Fusion can only occur between a 'plus' type and a 'minus' type (which can be regarded as distinct male and female gametes) but both types have cytoplasm and cell organelles such as mitochondria and chloroplasts. When two *Chlamydomonas* cells undergo sexual reproduction, the haploid nuclei fuse, become diploid, undergo meiosis and become haploid again. Meanwhile, however, a 'war', or better, a genetic conflict breaks out. By means of restriction endonuclease enzymes, the mitochondria of one individual 'kill' the mitochondria of the second, whilst the chloroplasts of the second 'kill' the chloroplasts of the first. The process wipes out 95% of all chloroplasts of both types illustrating how destructive the process is. This damaging cytoplasmic genetic war strongly favours one mating type digesting any cytoplasm in the other, driving the symmetry-breaking into fully-fledged gender - giant sappy egg and a lean sperm with little more than DNA. The prevailing idea has been that all sperm organelles in higher animals are digested are digested, but the story in humans is a little more subtle as we shall see.

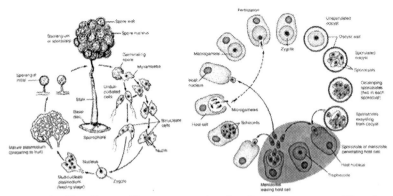

Sex becomes gender. The slime mold myxomycota has flagellated isogametes, while apicomplexa although a simple single celled protoctist already has sperms and ova (Margulis and Schwartz R428).

For this reason eucaryotes either have conjugation sex (in which case only nuclear DNA, without the symbiotic organelles are exchanged) or fusion sex, but in that case only one gamete should deliver the endosymbiont organelles. Cytoplasmic incompatibility thus neatly explains why we generally see only two sexes, one contributing the cytoplasm and one not. With conjugation sex there is really no such limitation and we find in mushrooms and ciliated protozoans there are many tens of different genders. In the ciliate hyptotrich which uses both fusion and conjugation, there are but two fusion genders but tens of conjugation ones. Some slime molds have 13 fusion sexes arranged in a hierarchy, contributing organelles strictly in order of precedence (Low R416 41, Ridley R564 97). *Physarum* has 29 variants of sex-controlling genes, dispersed among eight different types of sex cells. To ensure genetic diversity, each slime mold sex cell can only fuse with a sex cell that has completely different variants of genes than its own. The possible combinations of genes and sex cells, give *Physarum* more than 500 different sexes (Tidwell R678).

In algae, there is indication of a link between sex and stress, with different stress conditions activating related sex inducing genes. *Volvox carteri* responds to oxidative stress with a sex inducing gene related to the gene family in *Chlamydomonas reinhardtii* responsibile for sexual response to nitrogen stress (Nedelcu R488), suggesting sex evolved to spawn new genetic variants in response to stress, consistent with the Red Queen hypothesis (p 26).

Bobbi Low (R416) has a more 'dispassionate' description of the symmetry-breaking of gender based on natural selection for two fundamental traits - nurturing - that is ensuring there are sufficient cytoplasmic resources favouring large gametes, and seeking - being able to find a complementary gamete e.g. through motility favouring small ones. Natural selection thus favours a skewing of characteristics because mid-sized isogametes fail to compete at both tasks. This leads to two characteristics which continue into higher organismic behaviour - parenting investment and mating investment (p 29). Broadly speaking females invest in parenting and males in mating, though both do each to varying degrees in a given species.

We have noted the origin of sex in a Red Queen race between parasites and hosts (p 26) and that this extends to a genetic race between the sexes themselves (p 28). This extends to killer genes in one sex which affect the other. Male killer genes are found intermittently in various species because they favour the female. This can happen even with nuclear genes if they spend a selectively advantageous time in the female as is the case for male-killing 'dishonest-X' in fruit flies, but the majority are cytoplasmic in origin, since cytoplasmic organelles are transferred exclusively down the female line. Cytoplasmic genes can originate from plasmids, from DNA in our symbiotic organelles and from endoparasitic bacteria. Sometimes these stunt or kill males or render them infertile, or even incite parthenogenesis. Many hermaphroditic plants from beans to maize harbour sterilizing mitochondria which disable the male parts and promote propagation down the female line.

By far the most diverse and notorious sexual distorters are *Wolbachia* (Majerus R422). These bacteria are inherited and widespread among insects and other arthropods, infecting more than a fifth of all insect species, the most diverse among all living phyla. They may govern every facet of arthropod lives. Infection produces a catalogue of weird effects on arthropod sex and sexuality. In most cases, infected males only produce viable offspring if mated to a female infected with the same strain of *Wolbachia*. This has been demonstrated to potentially enable speciation by causing a fertility barrier between populations, so it may even contribute to insect diversity. Such fertility barriers and severe sex imbalances, which in some butterflies will result in clouds of unrequited virgins competing to pounce on the odd remaining male's advances can be cured by antibiotics. Like many parasites, Wolbachia has a small genome. Even high temperatures can cleanse *Wolbachia* infection, so there are frequent outlets from the cul-de-sac of male 'silencing'. In some crustaceans, gender-bending *Wolbachia* transforms infected males into females. In colonial insects such as bees, wasps and ants, infection abolishes males altogether, so that females reproduce clonally, without sexual reproduction, creating female-only populations. In other cases, arthropods come to depend on the presence of *Wolbachia* to perform their most basic functions. Sex determination in most creatures depends on the presence or absence of certain sex chromosomes, but in some populations of the pill wood louse, it depends on the presence or absence of *Wolbachia*. In two species of ladybirds and butterflies Wolbachia kills all males outright, only half the eggs hatching to maturity. This actually helps the ladybirds, whose hatching larvae can eat the dead males and develop more quickly. It severely distorts the sex ratio, but occasional bacteria-free males which escape vertical transmission, keep the sexual population alive. Some species, such as the parasitic round worms causing elephantiasis, depend on *Wolbachia* to survive, opening the prospect of using antibiotics to cure the human parasitic disease. Henry Gee quotes in Nature: "Long ago, some male chauvinist wag suggested that a suitable mascot for the feminist movement should be the angler-fish, in which a tiny, insignificant male is dominated by (and dependent on) a gigantic, bloated female. The work on *Wolbachia* suggests an altogether more sinister alternative."

Engendering causes a symmetry-breaking in the forms and reproductive strategies of male and female organisms, which is particularly pronounced in mammals and even more so in humans. Dawkins (R150) notes: "Sperms and eggs too contribute equal numbers of genes, but eggs contribute far more in the way of food reserves: indeed sperms make no contribution at all, and are simply concerned with transporting their genes as fast as possible to an egg. At the moment of conception therefore, the father has invested less than his fair share (i.e. 50 per cent) of resources in the offspring. Since each sperm is so tiny, a male can afford to make many millions of them every day. This means he is potentially able to beget a very large number of children in a very short period of time, using different females. This is only possible because each new embryo is endowed with adequate food by the mother in each case. This therefore places a limit on the number of children a female can have, but the number of children a male can have is virtually unlimited. Female exploitation begins here".

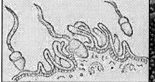 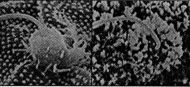

Fertilization displays amoebic engulfing by the ovum (King R353 1978 left) in the sea urchin (Sci. Am. right).

Pertinent to the issue of female reproductive choice is the question of whether it is the first sperm which fertilizes the egg by simply pushing its way in, or whether it is the ovum reacting to a sperm's presence, through a coordinated amoe-bic and electro-chemical response elicited at the time of fusion, during the complex chain-reaction ensuring only one sperm enters the egg. Sarah Hrdy (R323 70) comments "Rather than being penetrated by a sperm, the egg (or oocyte) more nearly engulfs it, quite possibly selecting which sperm to accept and producing the chemicals that are necessary for fertili-zation to take place." This speaks of fertilization itself as strategic paradox.

In mammals, an outer follicle cell glycoprotein, ZP3, binds to the sperm heads causing the release of the acrosomal cap which dissolves the eggs jelly-like outer layer. A protein in the exposed sperm head can now bind with a receptor on the egg's membrane precipitating membrane fusion. These receptors go by the names of integrin on the egg and disintegrin disintegrin on the sperm, a domain on a protein called fertilin from the ADAM family con-volutedly named after "A Disintegrin And Metalloprotease containing protein". This leads to binding and insertion of the protein into the egg's membrane, bringing the two mem-branes together; resulting in a pore. The oily membrane-fusing domain from fertilin shares features with viral integration proteins, suggesting viral membrane fusion could have played an early role in sexual fusion (White R726, Bloebel et. al. R64, Wolfsberg et. al. R744). Integration proteins evolve very rapidly in HIV and other viruses and in many spe-cies of animal in mutually antagonistic co evolution. Consequently fertilins cannot pro-mote fusion on their own in the way viral integration proteins do (White personal communication). A hair-trigger cortical response of membrane electrical depolarization ensues, as in a neuron reacting to a neurotransmitter (fast block to other sperm). A calcium ion release is set off by a G-protein, a type common to sensory transduction, certain neu-roreceptors and hormone amplification. This causes an explosive blowing off of the outer layers by the cortical granules in the sea urchin, or an outer hardening within seconds in mammals (slow block). It is also accompanied by active amoebic engulfing of the sperm by the egg. Once the sperm and egg fuse, the beating of the tail stops immediately, the sperm is drawn into the egg by elongation and fusion of egg's microvilli, forming the fer-tilization cone. Microvilli grow and surround the sperm, and via actin polymerization draw the sperm into the egg. As a result the entire contents of the sperm, including the nucleus and other organelles, are incorporated into the egg cytoplasm.

At this point the nucleus of the egg, still suspended in meiotic arrest now divides again to form the haploid egg pro-nucleus and a polar body. The condensed sperm DNA now expands and a nuclear envelope also forms. The sperm carries along with its axonene and basal bodies, centrioles, which nucleate new microtubules in the egg cytoplasm. With pushing forces, the male pronucleus migrates to the center of the egg. The female pronu-cleus uses the same microtubules as a track to meet the male pronucleus in the center of the cell. The two pronuclei fuse to form the diploid nucleus.

Recent evidence confirms another bizarre twist to this for the superficial sex war between the egg and sperm has entered into a deeper state of sexual paradox over time. The mam-malian zygote relies on the paternal gamete to provide the centrosome component essen-tial for the first mitotic division. It is the sperm centriolar apparatus that is one which survives to shepherd the chromosomes apart in the embryo. Eggs fertilized by dissected sperms which lack an intact centriolar flagellum base do not undergo correct spindle cleav-age. Electron microscope study has traced the paternal centrioles extensively. The sperm proximal centriole is introduced into the oocyte at fertilization and remains attached to the expanding sperm head during sperm nuclear decondensation, as it forms the male pronu-cleus. A sperm aster is initially formed after the centriole duplicates at the pronuclear stage. At syngamy, centrioles occupy a pivotal position on opposite spindle poles, when the first mitotic figure is formed. Centrioles were traced from fertilization to the hatching blastocyst stage. It is very likely that the paternal centriole is the ancestor of the centrioles in fetal and adult somatic cells (Sathananthan et. al. R599, Moomjy et. al. R470). There are also up to 18,000 RNA transcripts, found in sperms, not present in unfertilized ova, includ-ing genes for fertilization, the stress reaction, embryogenesis and implantation (Oster-meier et al. R509).

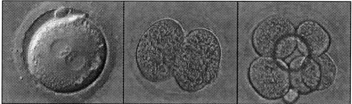

Fertilized human ovum at the point of nuclear fusion, two and eight-cell embryos (Morris).

The passage of the mitochondria is, by contrast, more of a feminine tale. Mitochondria from the sperm remain during early cleavage stages and may play a role in development. One hypothesis is that they set up the embryonic axes. 5-15% of the mitochondrial DNA in the placenta is derived from the sperm, but little or none appears in the embryo (R426). Paternal mtDNA usually comprises only 0.1% of the mtDNA in the gametes at normal conception, minimizing any chances of serious sex war of the organelles. However recombination between paternal and maternal mitochondria has recently been found to take place in a small proportion of cells (Kraytsberg et. al. R383).

Evidence has also been found for inheritance of paternal mitochondria in some organs which has implications for evolutionary genetics (p 103). A 28-year-old man had a normal heart and lungs and his muscles appeared healthy, but absorbed very little oxygen. His mitochondrial DNA had two mutations, one of which was responsible for his extreme fatigue. Muscle biopsies showed that about 90 per cent of his mitochondria came from his father. However, the mitochondria in his blood, hair roots and fibroblasts came entirely from his mother. (*Mitochondria can be inherited from both parents* 23 August 2002 New Scientist).

Up to 50% of conceptions end in miscarriage due to serious genetic errors in the developing body. Allen Enders of UC Berkeley noted we could consider God the world's greatest abortionist on this basis (Blum R65 20). Twin conceptions form a large proportion of pregnancies but in the majority of cases, one embryo fails to develop. Some researchers suggest the female can assert choice over the sex of the offspring either by her response to X and Y sperm during fertilization, or by differential reaction during or after implantation (Grant R251, King R353). Water voles are known to produce 5 times more male offspring under stress (J. of Applied Ecology, 42, 91). Variations of the sex of offspring suggest that dominant, higher testosterone women who are better fed may give birth to more boys (R251). Children of famous men also appear to be more frequently male (Jones R340). Men may also conceivably be able to modulate sex through differential activation of X and Y sperm.

Fertilization is itself a manifestation of sexual paradox through sexually antagonistic co-evolution. In the shellfish the abalone, for instance, the lysin protein that the sperm uses to bore a hole through the glycoprotein matrix of the egg is encoded by a gene that changes very rapidly (the same is probably true in us), probably because there is an arms race between the lysin and the matrix. Rapid penetration is good for sperm but bad for the egg, because it allows parasites or second sperm through (Ridley R566). The semen of flies is similarly in sexual conflict with the reproductive interests of the female forcing her to devote a disproportionate share of her reproductive energy to the siring from the ejaculate.

While it is facile to blame the male gender for what has now become a biological necessity for virtually every sexual organism, this symmetry-breaking has continued to have a significant impact on the evolution of life and reaches its 'long arm' into human sociobiology, for while the investment of the human female in the egg itself is small, her investment in the fertilized ovum is immense and pivotal to both her own survival and the survival of her offspring. It continues through pregnancy, lactation and some ten to fifteen years of child-rearing. Human pregnancy has a massive effect on the female physiology, which is unique among mammals. Although the human male often does play a significant and sometimes pivotal share of this work, being 'left holding the baby' is not a figure of speech without reason. This very ancient biological motif has become a theme we must respect in our very 'conception' of evolving human society. We fail to do so at our peril.

"One sex has a large investment to protect and looks for quality and stability. The other has little to lose and tends to be far more interested in quantity and variety. So it pays males to be aggressive, hasty, fickle and undiscriminating. They pounce, they generally make the first moves and are more ardent in them. While it is more profitable for females to be coy, to find out as much as possible in advance and to wait and see what happens. They play hard to get and play for time by flirting. All moves with a sound grounding in evolutionary psychology. Genes which allow females to be less inhibited leave fewer copies of themselves than genes which persuade them to remain highly selective. Amongst males, the best strategy is exactly the opposite one. The maximum advantage goes to those males with the fewest inhibitions. "Love 'em and leave 'em" is not so much a nasty piece of male chauvinist piggery as an accurate reflection of biological reality. In a very real sense, each sex still finds it pays to use the other as a vital resource. ... Men are a little like selfish genes, looking for convenient vehicles to carry their inheritance into the next generation. Women are more cautious, like canny investors or developers, seeing men as inconvenient sources of a seminal substance that is nevertheless necessary to realize the potential of their precious nest eggs. These bald descriptions sell both sexes short, but the two who differ so widely in interest and intent are bound to have different agendas and a conflict of interest. The fact that they manage to agree on anything at all is miraculous. Yet they do. (Watson R721).

Even this fairly obvious expression of has been challenged by social constructionists with a feminist political agenda. Anne Fausto-Sterling for example (Campbell R102 16) claimed that an association between low parental investment and promiscuity was just an argument for the male status quo, citing birds called sea snipes or phalaropes, in which it is the females which are promiscuous: "you name your animal species and you make your political point". However the species she has used to make her point confirms the evolutionary argument precisely. The non-political point which she conveniently ignores is that sea snipes are a species in which the male makes the greater parental investment. Male parental investment is also true of the midwife toad and several fish species, such as sea horses, where females inject their eggs into the males pouch through a penis-like appendage.

Sex Determination, Chromosomal Paradox and the Genius Nemesis

In lower primates, sex is often determined environmentally by the temperature of the maturing fertilized egg, as in alligators and turtles. Here the warmer the egg the larger, so alligators with larger competing males have hot eggs, becoming male whereas most turtles, which mate peaceably in the ocean have the egg-laying female the warmer sex, except for male-competing snapping turtles which follow the alligator pattern. Snails are hermaphrodites and can form sexual chains of mutual fertilization.

Halichoeres chlorocephalus
In many species of wrasse, the dominant female becomes the next male (www)

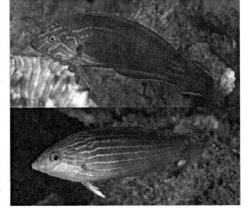

Sexual dominance is also a determinant. In several wrasse species, including the cleaner fish, the dominant female switches to the male sex when the alpha male dies or is injured, adopting the advantages of the high gain sex. Females are actually hermaphrodites as they all have small amounts of active (but walled-off) testicular material scattered through their ovaries. This again presents as an innovative solution to the sexual prisoners' dilemma, the fittest female becoming the alpha male with no loss of wasted male offspring. In a monogamous variation, the Nemo-like anemone fish *Amphiprion bicinctus* nestled like a sultan upon a bed of pink-tipped sea anemone tentacles. When a male chances on another male one transforms into a female. and invites the other fish to mate. Nobody gets hurt and in time both get to pass their genes into the next generation. "Perched upon their anemone, the two will live in prim monogamy until death do them part. At which time, the survivor may once again shift gender to secure a mate". This sex shifting goes to dynamic extremes. Hamlets (genus Hypoplectrus) are simultaneous hermaphrodites. Hamlets hold the sex-shifting record, switching from one set of gonads to the other and back in 30 seconds or less, with an average of 14 spawns in one day (Tidwell R678).

Achieving dominance in non-sex-reversing Cichlid fish also brings males to immediate maturity., . Within minutes of the dominant male being removed from an aquarium, a subordinate male turns from grey to flashy blue or yellow, cells in the anterior preoptic area swell to 8 times their previous volume with gonad-stimulating hormones, his testes grew and matured, and sperm production went into overdrive (Burmeister R94). This was due to switching on of a gene, egr-1 also found in humans, which may help us to respond to social cues.

The same sexually paradoxical logic applies again to the recently discovered whale bone worm *Osedax frankpressi* (Rouse et. al. R581), where any individual gaining a foothold on a rich whale bone becomes female and those who cannot become male. If there is no place for the larva to land except on another female, it does the next best thing and becomes a male, to provide that female with sperm. Whereas female worms are several inches in length, males are little more than microscopic threads, which act as nothing more than sperm factories.

Whether a species is protoandrous, and switches to female, or protogynous, and switches to male, depends on the payoffs in the sexual prisoners' dilemma game. Species where an individual can monopolize resources and become a large egg bearer tend to be protoandrous and have small males. Species where a large male is dominant tend to be protogynous and have small females. Sex changing species are common in highly stratified ecological societies as on reefs where niches are highly defined and mating opportunities which preserve territory are restricted. In free schooling species there is no advantage to the added cost of sex change. So Roughgarden's point about the influence of social factors gains good ground among the coral, even if it is not apparent in the open ocean or among mammals.

Hermaphroditic molluscs such as slugs and snails also ensure the payoff for eachindividual maintains a prisoners' dilemma realtionship. Sea slugs donate sperm only on the condition that they receive it, so thwarting the male desire to fertilise and run. Each slug inserts its penis into the other and one transfers a small package of sperm. The transfer of further sperm will only proceed if the partner reciprocates, transferring a pack of its sperm (Current Biology 15 92).

Chromosomal sex has become a pervasive and successful sexually defining strategy among many groups of organism, including mammals. Genetic sex determination enables early and precisely programmed sexual differentiation. Temperature sex determination is also unfeasible for warm-blooded internally-fertilizing animals. But there is a deeper reason. Externally fertilizing animals can sustain major fluctuations in the sex ratio that may result from temperature-mediated sex determination because both sexes produce a relatively large number of gametes. By contrast mammals only produce a vanishingly small number of eggs in a lifetime and cannot afford a serious imbalance in the sex ratio towards males. Following Kim Walen's energy-minimizing sexual symmetry-breaking paradigm (Blum 18), genetic sexuality provides a strongly fixed complementarity and stable sex ratio with only moderate slippage into transsexual and homosexual variations.

The pattern of uterine gestation and lactation in mammals results in great reproductive success, by passing the vast majority of the child-rearing energy and attention budget to the female. It is thus little wonder that the vast majority of mammals species are polygynous with males often contributing little to child rearing. By contrast birds, being uniquely warm-blooded while still laying eggs have an overweening need to have two partners to hatch the egg and provide sustenance, causing most bird species to become overtly monogamous.

In mammals sexuality is determined by additional X and Y chromosomes, XX being female and XY male. In fact it is the Y which contains the few genes, including SRY (sex-determining region Y) or TDF (testis determining factor) essential for switching the female mammalian form to the male path. Birds, some fishes, butterflies and moths have a reverse female-determining chromosome system with ZW being female and ZZ being male. In grasshoppers, roaches and some other insects, the presence of the diploid X is female determining with a single X male. The platypus has a bizarre variation to this with no less than five X and five Y with males being $(XY)_5$ and females $(XX)_5$ (DOI 10.1038/ nature03021). While the platypus X1 chromosome has 11 genes that are found on all mammalian X chromosomes, the X_5 carries a gene called DMRT1, also found on the Z chromosome in birds. Finally in social bees and ants, the diploid condition is female, with fertilized eggs becoming female queens and workers andunfertilized eggs becoming male drones. The queen also courts many drones thus forming several superfamilies in the hive adding adaptive resistance. Workers in the same superfamily are supersisters, sharing more genes (100% from father and 50% from mother=75%) than their own offspring (50%). Social stability is thus underpinned by the haploid-diploid sexual determination.

In another dimension to sexual antagonism and sexual selection, unlike the female ZW sex pairing of birds (male ZZ) where female selection favours male genes and hence showy sons, the XY male (XX female) mammals have female selection skewed to favour alleles advantageous in daughters, (R4) a discovery which may explain why women appear to be a step ahead of men in evolution, being more neotonous (child-like), less hairy, and explain pronounced female sexual characteristics in breasts, buttocks, concealed estrus and ecstatic clitoris.

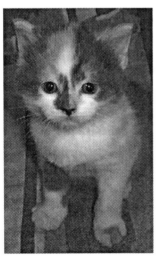

X-linked tortoise-shell gene variation demonstrates X-mosacism in a female cat (King). The confinement of this phenomenon to female felines combined with an elusive contracted genetic element in female somatic cells, the Baar body, was the trigger for Mary Lyon, the discoverer of mosaic X-inactivation to make the discovery (Jegalian and Lahn R332).

Mammals have an ingenious sexual genetic scheme to align sexual selection with the effects of the honest egg and the cheating sperm. The female XX and male XY means that the male is haploid X and the female diploid XX. The haploid state provides for maximal selective advantage, because there is just one 'pure' copy of each gene on this entire chromosome, not two interacting copies. When the female embryo begins to divide about the 10 to 20 cell stage, in each somatic cell i.e. apart from the germ-line sex cells, one or other X randomly collapses. So a female brain is single X, like the male, but with a difference - it is a mosaic of cells of two genetic X-identities, those of her father and mother, as in the picture of the tortoise-shelled cat. The male by contrast is endowed with one pure maternal X-dose. When he is good he is very very good - but when he is bad he is singularly retarded. There are at least 8 forms of X-linked male mental retardation because the X chromosome, the hemizygous 'haploid' X is carrying several key genes for brain development at the spearhead of human evolution, as noted by Gillian Turner (R696). According to one analysis, there are 221 known human genetic defects that can cause mental impairment, some 10% of which reside on the X chromosome, even though it carries less than 4% of known human genes. In our own species, where intelligence and social skills are thought to be central to success, genes on the X chromosome seem to have evolved rapidly to provide us with the necessary brain power (Check R114). Many genes on the X chromosome associated with human brain function seem to have distant relatives with different functions in other vertebrates, such as chickens and fish, posing a paradox of conservatism amid rapid change.

X-mosaicism has many other subtle effects in human females. Female monozygotic twins are often not genetically identical because X-inactivation occurs differentially between the two twins, more commonly than expected by chance, leading to the conjecture that genetic discord can also promote twinning. Specific organs may display mosaic genetic defects normally seen only in susceptible males, such as colour blindness, muscular dystrophy and autoimmune diseases, which are more common in females may result from the thymus educating t-cells only to recognize tissues with the same X-inactivation type (Bainbridge R38).

When the occasional man gets the pure benefit of a fortuitous X complementing his other good brain genes on the diploid chromosomes he may become a genius. The irony is that the male never can transmit this heritage to his sons. It is always the maternal X that goes to the son, because to be a son he must have got the paternal Y. Females are thus the progenitors of male prodigies, but the prodigies are doomed ducks. This is the sacrificial saga of the sex gene. The only hope for a male genius is to have daughters! By contrast, females can fortuitously give direct birth to male geniuses. This doesn't mean only males display creative genius. Neither does it deny the capacity of culture and education to mediate natural differences.

It is common to animal species that the reproductive potential of individual females is relatively equivalent to one another, but that of the males varies widely depending on opportunity and reproductive fitness. Females compete only for scarce resources but males directly for impregnation. Mammalian evolution has put the X with its largely haploid single dose gene expression in both males and females into the position where it can be subject to strong sexual selection by the female where the evolutionary selection can have the greatest effect. This has now become a central motif in a theory of human culture as runaway sexual selection. A revolutionary idea is that female genes encouraging female sexual selection for intelligence are strongly linked to genes for high intelligence selected for in the male (Zechner et al R759). These X-linked genes then ran away together without any limitation by natural selection, because of the adaptive advantage of intelligence, unlike the peacock's tail. Intelligence presents a unique exception to the genuine indicator of fitness having to be costly. But there is an irony to this, in the Machiavellian theory of intelligence as strategic bluffing.

The sequence of genes on the X-chromosome is almost entirely conserved across mammal species, possibly as a result of the conservatism of X-inactivation. Long sections on each arm of X are homologous to non-sex chromosomes 1 and 4 in birds, showing X and Y both originated from autosomes. Unlike the Y, the X does not contain female-determining or developmental genes and even encodes among its array of housekeeping and specific functional genes male genes for sperm production. Since the X is also expressed in males, this is logical and consistent. There is a greater probability that a recessive mutation beneficial to males will appear on the X than on an autosome (Ross R578). This may give rise to a tug of war, in which X-genes favouring one sex may be selected for, even though they impose a cost on the other sex. The fertile mother effect in homosexuality (p 384) and the skewing of X-inactivation (p 385) are provocative hints of sexually antagonistic coevolution (p 16).

The Y-chromosome (Jones R340) is a genomic enigma. It was originally an X which gained the male sex-determining SRY gene. Consequently it still contains some active and 'fossil genes' showing correspondence to genes on the X. It also contains large stretches of genetic desert as well as 78 genes (Kirsch R370) some involving maleness which have moved to the Y. The Y crosses-over with homologous areas of the X only on 5% of its meagre length, at their very tips, although it has many other relics of homologous genes in other areas, some still active. The X suffers none of this, as it recombines actively in oogenesis, while also being able to express each X gene fully in a haploid manner in males and in female somatic lines. Over time, the SRY gene, which itself cannot logically cross with female-default X, has been the nucleus for four inversions of whole sections of the Y chromosome, leaving these regions unavailable for homologous recombination. Given no serial homology to enable crossing-over, these regions have degraded to a genetic desert and many genes have been eliminated by deletions. At some point, SRY has moved to the short arm of the Y chromosome again close to the tips of the Y that are still able to recombine with the X, thus leaving open the possibility of occasional crossing-overs that cause XX-SRY$^+$ males and XY-SRY$^-$ females because an SRY has been transferred from Y to X in the father's spermatogonia.

Such non-recombining regions along with the nine times higher intermediate repeat LINE incidence and inverted repeats causes the Y to be prone to deletions which cause male reproductive deficiencies. Over time such deletions continue to reduce the size of the Y. In addition there are the effects of conflicting gene drive. Because females have two X chromosomes while males have an X and a Y, three-quarters of all sex chromosomes are Xs and only one-quarter are Ys. An X chromosome thus spends two-thirds of its time in females, and only one-third in males. Therefore, the X chromosome is three times as likely to evolve the ability to take pot shots at the Y as the Y is to evolve the ability to take pot shots at the X. Any gene on the Y chromosome is vulnerable to attack by a newly evolved driving X gene. The shrunken state of the Y indicates it is heading for oblivion. The combined processes of decay are causing the Y to disappear up the fundamental orifice of the very male-determining gene SRY which caused it to diverge in the first place. In some species, such as platypus and kangaroo, the Y is under significant risk of complete deletion being only a shadow of our shrunken size. In some mice and voles, the sex determining role of the Y has already been corrupted, resulting in XY females or a loss of Y determination.

Humans have the worst sperm count of any mammalian species, with the exception of the gorilla, possibly because of the fragile location of these sperm production genes on the Y chromosome. A recent study suggests that there has been a slight decline in human sperm counts in every year that it has been documented (p 404). Speculation on the reasons for the decline include environmental toxins, estrogen-fed beef, or even statistical bias in studies due to geographic differences in sperm production rates among different populations of men. It is very clear, however, that sperm production is genetically controlled, and that humans are in some ways 'genetically programmed' to have an unstable sperm count (Ridley R566, Jegalian and Lahn R332, Jobling and Tyler-Smith R333).

Even more bizarrely, but logically, the X inactivation that causes X-mosiaicism in female somatic cells happens principally only for the X genes which do not remain active on the Y. This explains why X inactivation occurs in the female. As Y genes became inactive as a result of loss of recombination and mutation, their dosage was firstly halved in men, who were relatively disabled by having only a half dose from the X . Evolutionary selection then tends to double the level of expression of these genes to correct for male disability, and to evolve to inactivate one copy in the XX female, to correct for overdosing her, so one equal dose occurs again in both sexes. However sequencing of the human X has shown that there is significant variability in individual women in 10% of the 'inactivated' X genes (R107), giving females a more varied genetic disposition of these X genes.

Several male fertility genes have converged on the Y, in the non-recombining region near SRY, thus making up to some degree for the relative decay overall. The Y thus harbors specific genes, and protects them from further recombination, providing these genes with a safe place in which to amplify and not be carried in the women. Compensating for the lack of homologous recombination, these genes exist in multiple copies on the Y, active versions becoming seeds of further multiplication as other copies become inactivated by mutation. Associated with this process are huge palindromic regions with reverse reflections like "Madam I'm Adam" up to 3 million bases long. There are 8 palindromes 6 of which carry male determining genes. It has now been established that these palindromic repeats are a fundamental way the Y compensates for not crossing-over by providing instead a gene conversion process in which sections of the palindromes are copied to one anther - about 600 base pairs per newborn male child.   Male-specific genes in these regions display 99.97% homology to their counterparts. Six of the palindromes were established before the human-ape divergence confirming a continuing role in maintaining human male specific genes from creeping errors (Rosen et. al. R582, Skaletsky et. al. R632).

Many of these genes, including SRY itself, lack introns, the non-coding inserts punctuating the functional sub-domains of most higher organism genes. This indicates they have been made through reverse transcription from the already processed messenger RNAs that code proteins. They may have been generated by retroviruses or the LINE type retroelements dispersed throughout the genome and in effect jumping retrogenes- mobile DNA in the classic sense of the 'selfish gene'. In a paradoxical reversal, closing the logical loop, the SRY family gene Sox-11 has been found to regulate LINE-transcription, consistent with the coupling we have seen of LINE to the meiotic cycle (Tchénio R671). SRY evolved from a Sox gene on the X - to which it is related but now has a different function (Jegalian and Lahn R333).

Moreover LINEs appear to play a key role in X chromosome inactivation (Ross et. al. R578), with the defective LINE elements resulting from the inactivation of the LINEs resulting from natural nuclear resistance to the onslaught of active disruptive mobile elements, functioning to inactivate the receptors of X genes. X-inactivation is a very unusual process in several respects. It is controlled by a gene called Xist, but this gene does not produce a translated protein. It merely produces a messenger RNA which appears to 'paint' the inactivated X chromosome from end to end. An anti-sense complementary version of this mRNA is also produced, appropriately called Tsix. In mice, the active X secretes Tsix to oppose Xist (Sado et. al. R593) however in humans Tsix does not repress Xist and is expressed on the inactive X (Migeon e. al. R462). The original central dogma of Crick and Watson is that DNA makes RNA makes protein which carries out the essential catalytic tasks. However X inactivation smacks of the ancient forms of RNA processing that may have preceded the DNA genome of eucaryote cells, which still appear to be major players in processing mRNAs from the majority of genes containing introns, non-coding inserts between functional sub-domains of genes. The key violation of the central dogma that opened up a major reconceptualization of the field was the discovery of reverse transcription from RNA to DNA, a process shared by retroviruses, LINE elements and the telomerase which adds new telomeres essential to maintaining the immortality of the germ line. There are sequencing homologies between the reverse transcriptases of all of these indicating a viral origin for telomerases. Significantly LINE elements, which are concentrated in specific regions of other chromosomes are also spread over the X-chromosome and concentrated around the inactivation centre where Xist lies (Lyon R417). This mechanism suggests a very ancient symbiotic relationship between cellular RNA processing and retroelements.

The SRY gene sequence is very strongly conserved among men: there are virtually no point mutations in the human race. It is a variation-free gene that has changed hardly at all since the last common ancestor of all people around 200,000 years ago. Yet our SRY is very different from that of a chimpanzee, and different again from that of a gorilla. There is, between species, ten times as much variation in this gene as is typical for other genes. Compared with other active genes, SRY is one of the fastest evolving. The answer appears to lie in selective sweeps. From time to time, a driving gene appears on the X chromosome that attacks the Y chromosome by recognizing the protein made by SRY. At once there is a selective advantage for any rare SRY mutant that is sufficiently different to be unrecognized. This mutant begins to spread at the expense of other males. The driving X chromosome distorts the sex ratio in favour of females but the spread of the new mutant SRY restores the balance. The end result is a new SRY gene sequence shared by all members of the species, with little variation. The effect of this sudden burst of evolution would be to produce SRYs that were very different between species, but very similar within species (Ridley R566, Jones R340).

There are several genes related to SRY in the genome, the closest neighbour of which is a gene on the X chromosome involved in early brain development (R340). A cluster of Y genes involved in sex characteristics include ones for sperm manufacture, growth rate, formation of teeth, left-handedness, aggression (in mice) and a gene for a protein active in the brain, adding to the logical entanglement of the sexuality of brain function and consciousness. Certain genetic anomalies can be explained by an aberrant crossing over between the X and the Y in the father , in regions neighbouring the SRY, transferring it to the X, resulting in an X containing SRY and a Y failing to do so. This leads to both XX individuals who may develop somatic characteristics of males and XY individuals who turn out female.

The XY signature is a source indicator of the divergence between reptiles and internally fertilizing, lactating and gestating mammals. The first of four Y inversions happens around the time of the platypus and echidna, the next close to the divergence between marsupials and true mammals, the next at the main mammalian radiation and the fourth around the time apes differentiated from other primates. The fact that birds have a mirror-complementary female-determining ZW sex-chromosome arrangement suggests this chromosomal form of sexual differentiation has specific evolutionary advantages.

Non-sex chromosomes (autosomes) are also sexually-imprinted in a way which may give the mother's genes a key developmental role in the cerebral cortex, striatum and hippocampus with the father's being more significantly expressed in the mid-brain emotional centres - the hypothalamus, amygdala and pre-optic area. (Keverne et. al. R347, R348, R306, Gibbons R234). This would mean children tend to inherit their father's personalities, but they inherit their mother's astuteness, intellect and memory. Eric Keverne sees this as being evidence of evolution of executive areas of the cortex in a context of prolonged association between female relatives, consistent with the matrilocal pattern of most mammals and primates but not apes (Hrdy R323 143). This also suggests an early arms race in which competition for a male drive for emotion was countered by a major growth of controlling factors in the cortex including the frontal areas maintaining overall integration (Campbell R102 239).

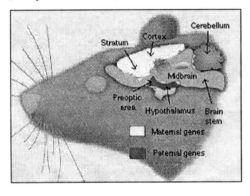

Sexually imprinted genes and their locations in the brain. Maternally-imprinted genes red in the cortex and paternally in emotional centres green (New Scientist 3 May 1997)

Chris Badcock (R32) claims the conflict between the male-imprinted limbic system and the female cortex may reflect a parallel with a paternal *id* making egocentric, infantile and constant demands on the mother while the maternally-controlled cortex represses them. This reflects Haig's (R272, R273) theory of an arms race between paternal genes favouring growth promotion in the hypothalamus and the invasive placenta and maternal genes spreading the effort among offspring. Notably the insulin growth factor IGF II is paternally expressed while the IGF IIR receptor is maternally expressed and seems to have a role in inhibiting excessive growth in the embryo. However the evolution of these genes is not accelerated as in active arms races so the process may have stratified.

Genes for telomere length and hence long-levity also appear to be peternally imprinted, correlating only with the father's pattern, rather than the mother's (Nordfjäll R494). There is evidence that telomere length in sperm increases with age, so "it is possible that children with older fathers would inherit longer telomeres", Nordfjäll says. This shows an ultimate sexual paradox at work - female reproductive choice applied to older successful men causes successful genomes to become even more long-lived.

The small minority of about 50 genes (Hrdy R323 432) which are sexually imprinted by paternal or maternal descent display some stunning examples of a genetic 'tug-of-war' between the sexes, although some are more difficult to interpret. Daughters inheriting a mutant form of a male imprinted mouse gene called Mest display, in addition to a slight reduction in body size, failure to eat the placenta on birth and deficiencies in mothering (R323 433). The key theory about 'fatherly' imprinting of genes is interpreted in a conflict model to favour the selective replication of paternal genes, by encouraging the female to devote more energy to the current offspring of the father than consistent with her overall reproductive commitment to all her potential offspring, favouring for example larger babies which consume more of the mother's resources. David Haig has suggested this sexual 'tug of war' may have become an essential feature and that disruption of the counter-balances on either side could compromise fertility (ibid). Haig's predictions have been confirmed in experiments where specific genes were modified to have only maternally imprinted versions of vice versa The female imprinted offspring were only 60% of normal size and the male imprinted 130% (R323). However paternally imprinted Mest and Peg-3, which affect mothering by affecting oxytocin-related bonding appear to equally favour maternal fortunes.

Children with Turner's syndrome are genetically neuter. They have a single X-chromosome, inherited from either their mother or their father, instead of the usual two X chromosomes of a girl or the X and Y of a boy. Since a female body plan is the default among mammals, they look and act like girls. Turners syndrome females with a single X differ in their symptoms, with the maternally-inherited X displaying more serious problems of social maladjustment and those with a paternal X being better at interpreting body language, reading emotions, recognizing faces, handling words, and getting along with other people. This is consistent with the adaptive imprinting of the maternal X for the social restiveness of males who always have a maternal X to prime them for reproductive competition (Hrdy R323 142).

Methylation of the cytosine bases on DNA is one key mechanism that leads to imprinting, permitting the independent expression of maternal and paternal genomes during early development and after. The female germ line is more highly methylated than the DNA of the male germ line. The methylation of some genes may lead to their silencing into inactive clumped regions, while others may be activated. Imprinting appears to have a sexually-polarized role in the primal development of the embryo. A tumorous uterine growth called a hydatidiform mole is caused by the lack of female imprinted genes, as a result of more than one sperm entering the egg. Either all the genes are paternally inherited, or there is one maternal and two paternal sets. The hydatidiform mole is effectively an exclusively placental pregnancy, supporting Haig's theory of an arms race in which the paternal genes promote invasive growth (p 16) in line with males ensuring the survival of their offspring in 'captive' females.

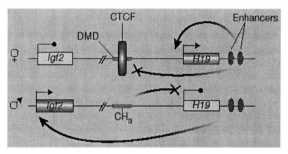

Sexual imprinting master switch: Key imprinted H19 and Igf2 genes on the same mouse chromosome are oppositely 'imprinted' in normal embryos. On the maternal chromosome, an enhancer-blocking protein CTCF, which recognizes the DNA sequence CCCTC binds to the differentially methylated domain (DMD), blocking the access of enhancers to Igf2 and instead favouring H19 expression. On the paternal chromosome, the DNA of the boundary element is methylated; the blocking protein cannot bind, and Igf2 is expressed (Loebel and Tam R411).

Recent experiments have suggested that the maternal and paternal genomes have different roles during mammalian gastrulation. Mouse zygotes can be created that have only sperm-derived chromosomes or only egg-derived chromosomes. The male-derived embryos (androgenones) die with deficiencies in the embryo proper but form well-developed chorions. Conversely, the female-derived embryos (gynogenones) die with deficiencies in their chorions, even though the actual embryo seems normal. It appears that sperm-derived genes are needed for the proper development of the chorion, while egg-derived genes are necessary for the normal development of the embryo itself (Barton et al., R47; McGrath and Solter, R448; Surani et al., R661). This has been confirmed by making allophenic mice in which blastomeres from a normal 4-cell embryo are aggregated with blastomeres from either androgenetic or gynogenetic embryos. In both cases, cells from both the normal and abnormal embryos were originally seen in all regions of the blastocyst. However, by the end of gastrulation, androgenetic cells are seen almost exclusively in the trophoblast, while gynogenetic cells are hardly ever seen in trophoblast-derived tissues (Thomson and Solter, R674). This strongly suggests that the maternal and paternal genomes serve distinct functions during early mouse embryogenesis.

In 2004 the first successful 'parthenogenetic' mouse pups have been raised by manipulating maternal imprinting to repress it in one maternal haploid genome, and introducing this into an ovum, to mimic the natural imprinting expression above, resulting in two live pups out of 598 oocytes, one of which proved fertile in adulthood (p 411). Kono et. al. (R377) comment "These results suggest that paternal imprinting prevents parthenogenesis, ensuring that the paternal contribution is obligatory for the descendant".

Varieties of sex hormones: The steroid hormones (a) are synthesized sequentially from progesterone through testosterone to estrogens. (b) Prostaglandins (c) Polypeptides oxytocin and vasopressin. (R396)

Hormonal and Pheromonal Paradoxes

The steroid sex hormones, like neurotransmitters are an ancient feature of evolution. In the turtle which determines its sex by temperature, eggs incubating at the female temperature have a rising estrogen flush which then tapers off once sex determination has taken place. At male-determining temperatures, while estrogen levels still rise, there is a pulse of testosterone at the time sex determination takes place. These patterns echo strongly the patterns of human embryogenesis even up to the time of a brief testosterone burst around the time of birth that is believed to have an engendering effect on the human brain.

The main steroid hormones are in a state of yin-yang complementation. The dominant male hormone testosterone is a metabolic intermediate sandwiched between the two female hormones, progesterone and estradiol, which have an oscillatory nature driving the menstrual cycle and ovulation. Steroids are lipid molecules which can drift through cell membranes, pass the blood brain barrier, and act directly on gene regulation in the nucleus of target cells. This makes them ideal for hormonal signalling from the gonads to the brain and other tissues. Invertebrate species also use steroids as hormone signallers. Ecdysone is the key hormone in the stages of insect molting and metamorphosis and ecdysone variants maintain ovarian function in adult mosquitoes (Hagedorn et. al. R271).

Progesterone stimulates the implantation of the fertilized embryo and the maintenance of pregnancy. Estrogen is largely secreted by the ripe ovarian follicles as they come to maturity, triggering the bursts of follicle stimulating hormone and lutenizing hormone from the pituitary that cause ovulation to occur. Then in the latter part of the cycle, progesterone from the corpus luteum, the yellow remains of the follicle prevents the endometrial lining of the uterus from sloughing of for long enough for implantation to occur.

Part of the paradox of this situation for the human female is that estrogen is supplied by the follicles of the germ-line ova rather than maternal tissues. In males testosterone is manufactured in the somatic interstitial cells of the testis, rather than the sperm-producing germ-line cells of the seminiferous tubules. This means that males continue into later life with only about a 1% decline in testosterone a year. However in females, the lioness' share of female sex hormones come directly from the oocytes. Unlike sperms, which are produced continuously from germ-cell primordia, oocytes are not generated afresh during adult life, but remain dormant, since first multiplying prenatally, When their supply runs out in mid-life, menopause occurs. Female chimps remain fertile until too aged to bear pregnancy, so it is unclear whether this is an ironic penalty of human evolution, or an adaption to provide grandmotherly support for the next generation's parents rather than competing with one's own long-lived offspring (Hrdy R323). Estrogen levels fall by about half in menopause and progestogen levels precipitously. In menopausal women, as estradiol levels fall, fat cells and to a certain extent muscle cells begin secreting estrone. A moderately well-endowed menopausal woman may circulate more estrogens than a skinny woman having normal cycles.

Although men have ten times as much circulating testosterone as estrogen and women the reverse, both sexes secrete several steroid sex hormones, including both androgens and estrogens. The formation of breasts depends rather sensitively on the balance and starving prisoners of war were known to grow breasts in their first flush of a good diet. XY males who have androgen receptor intolerance fail to develop as normal males, having no penis, but instead a shallow vagina, with only the outer labia since they also lack the estrogen required for a fully developed female anatomy. Since they appear anatomically as female many have their defunct testicles removed at birth and given estrogen replacement therapy in adolescence. Since the default condition in mammals is female, they identify as women and appear as sometimes beautiful women.

Those madly in love also have converging levels of testosterone, higher in women and lower in men, suggesting nature seeks to mediate the dissonance of differing sex strategies when love is the binding glue (Marazziti Psychoneuroendocrinology *to appear*, R13). NGF or nerve growth factor has also been cited as an albiet transient accompaniment of falling in love (*Truly, madly, deeply in love - but not for very long* NZ Herald 28 Nov 2005) Music has been found to have a similar effect, confirming it has a complex role in human bonding (Fukui R226), not only developed as a signal of courtship, as Darwin remarked, but also evolved to influence human love in a complicated way.

Storey et al. (R655, R473) have also found increased levels of prolactin and decreased levels of testosterone, consistent with findings in other paternal mammals suggests human males are hormonally modulated to promote fatherhood and reduce aggression.

However the paradox does not end there. Males have an enzyme called aromatose which converts testosterone to estradiol, just as the ova convert androgens to estrogen. In women testosterone is produced in the adrenals and ovaries as a principal estrogen precursor. In rats, estrogen is essential for masculinizing the brain. In mice, α-fetoprotein binds to estrogen stopping it from masculinizing the brain. This process is different in humans. While human 'males' with androgen receptor intolerance have both feminized external genitalia and feminine brain and behaviour, the corresponding rats have masculine brains because of these paradoxical effects of fetal estrogen. Human males with estrogen receptor intolerance, although they appear to be normal but perhaps oversized men, are infertile because estrogen receptors are essential for full fertility in the male. Rare disturbances in the aromatose pathway result in men who cannot mate. Parts of the testis have higher estrogen concentrations than the ovary and sperm are during their journey in the male subjected to higher estrogen levels than the ovum. In both men and women aromatose activity increases with age. In men, estrogen production is not confined to the brain. Estrogens are also secreted from the skin, blood and fatty tissue. A man of over 50 may have higher estrogen levels than a menopausal woman (Angier R18, Blum R65). Conversion to estrogen in men has been associated with irritability. It appears essential for maintaining important classes of brain neurons, such as those involved in Parkinson's, and in the maintenance of memory. Women suffering sudden falls in estrogen notice memory impairment. The brains of female rats fluctuate noticeably in the density of their hippocampal synapses during the estrus cycle, coming to a maximum in proestrus as the endometrium and follicles are maturing, driven by estradiol. Progesterone is also present in men, rising in the evening.

The sex hormones are also in feedback with one's sexual charisma, sense of success, libido , sexual arousal and male dominance (Mazur and Booth R440). Men, experience a noticeable rush of 100% increase in testosterone watching pornographic movies. Astrid Jutte also found (New Scientist 22 Aug 98 11) that women also have an 80% rise in testosterone under the same circumstances (albeit from a ten times lower baseline). It is thus no surprise to hear that some women find testosterone also enhances their libido if taken as a drug. Though testosterone levels in men and women do not overlap, variations in level have similar kinds of effects in the two sexes. High-testosterone women smile less often and have more extramarital affairs, a stronger social presence, and even a stronger handshake. In men testosterone is very volatile, rising in single men on the prowl, and before a contest, falling during stress and plummeting when a man is beaten, rising after success. It is also responsible for the growth of a female's genital hair just as it is in the male. However one should note that there is a hundred times more testosterone bound in the blood proteins of a male than available to receptors, so levels are smoothed out over time. Broadly speaking testosterone has a ravaging effect across many species, diverting energy from immunity and repair towards reproduction, and reducing pain sensitivity (Hau R292), suitable for a sex which has to contest risking death and is expendable in the reproductive process. Males tend to age more rapidly and often accrue more parasites. The effects are exaggerated in highly polygynous species. By contrast estradiol promotes immunity and protects women against effects of aging such as heart disease and osteoporosis, suggesting part of its function is to ensure the females of the species retain good health throughout their valuable reproductive years (Blum R65).

"The rush of a T shot is not unlike the rush of going on a first date or speaking before an audience. I feel braced. After one injection, I almost got in a public brawl for the first time in my life. There is always a lust peak-every time it takes me unaware" (Andrew Sullivan Pinker R532 348).

When estrogen levels are high, women get even better at tasks on which they typically do better than men, such as verbal fluency. When the levels are low, women get better at tasks on which men typically do better, such as mental rotation. A variety of sexual motives, including their taste in men, vary with the menstrual cycle as well, tending to more hunky male features during ovulation. Baron Cohen (R42) has found that high testosterone at birth correlates with autism, less curiosity and less eye contact. Valerie Grant (R251) suggests a link between higher testosterone, female dominance and the birth of additional sons, possibly involving selection for Y-sperm by the ovum or differential implantation, something which may be an evolutionary adaption to take advantage of the reproductive opportunities of male offspring. Blum however notes that higher testosterone women in modern society seem to be more interested in careers rather than child-rearing. There is also a correlation between more sons and the aftermath of major wars, like WW1 and WW2. A better diet is also said to favour boys. Girls with excess exposure to androgens show early preferences for male toys and 'tomboyish' behavior even when the condition is treated at birth, indicating pre-natal determination (p 386).

Men are reputed to have reduced testosterone levels around the time of the birth of their children, which may facilitate parental bonding and paternal support for the baby, but in men trying for a baby, peaks in testosterone levels coincided far more often with periods of intense sexual activity (Hirschenhauser). Rises in testosterone also trigger a hormonal pathway that increases sperm production, making conception more likely. At ovulation in the flush of high estrogen, women will naturally shift their choices in male faces from a preference for androgynous figures towards a classically 'high-testosterone' male archetype for example with thick-set jaws. These features are in turn caused by a very high testosterone peak at puberty. Why should that be attractive? Because - so the argument runs - only men with robust immune systems are able to tolerate such a surge. A firm jaw line, in other words, is an outward sign of hidden biological fitness. Gordon Gallup has also found that semen makes women happier than use of a condom (New Scientist 29 jun 2002). The results aren't a complete surprise because semen does contain several mood-altering hormones, including testosterone, estrogen, follicle-stimulating hormone, lutenizing hormone, prolactin and several different prostaglandins.

Disturbances of the sex hormones can also lead to genital and social changes. CAH or congenital adrenal hyperplasia (p 386), also called AGS or adrenogenital syndrome, is a group of conditions of similar source: a family of autosomal recessive disorders of steroid hormone production in the adrenal glands leading to a deficiency of cortisol, the stress fighting hormone. The pituitary, sensing the deficiency, secretes massive amounts of the stimulating hormone corticotropin to bring the cortisol levels up to normal. This hormone in turn causes the adrenal glands to overproduce certain intermediary hormones which have testosterone-like effects on the fetus and child, leading to so-called 'virilization.' In females, the clitoris of girls is enlarged, and may resemble the male penis to the point that the sex of the child is questioned or mistaken. Males have enlarged penile size.

Along with the steroid sex hormones are prostaglandins. These are conjugated fatty acids which have a modulating effect on the actions of steroid hormones. They were first discovered in semen, where there are over 40 different prostaglandins. Certain prostaglandins are also agents of uterine contraction. They also function in many tissues, having a role in malaise. Asprin for example inhibits cyclo-oxygenase, which elicits prostaglandin synthesis.

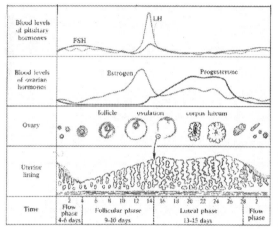

The menstrual cycle, showing variations in follicle stimulating hormone, lutenizing hormone, progesterone and estrogen (R396).

However another class of hormones, polypeptides - small strings of amino acids, and with them glycoproteins - longer strings of amino acids with sugars attached, are major hormonal feedback molecules in both vertebrate and invertebrate species. The hormones which regulate the steroid pathways fall into these categories. During development and in the menstrual cycle, secretory neurons in the hypothalamus secrete gonadotropin releasing hormone GnRH, which passes through a portal vein through the pituitary, and controls the levels of two glycoproteins, follicle-stimulating hormone FSH, and lutenizing hormone LH, named for its role in causing the follicle envelope to form the *corpus lutetum* or yellow body, after ovulation, which enables the embryo to implant, by releasing progesterone, as shown in the figure above. These two hormones are common to both male and female and also act in complementary ways on disparate testis tissues in the male, FSH directly stimulating spermatogenesis in the tubules and LH stimulating interstitial androgen production and indirectly sperm production. The cyclic behaviour of FSH and LH in the hypothalamus appears to be ablated about the time of birth by androgens in the male. Low levels of a related polypeptide hormone corticotropin-releasing hormone (CRH), is also associated both with the calm of breast feeding mammals, including humans, and with the fearless aggression a mother shows towards males or other predators who may attack her offspring (Behavioral Neuroscience DOI: 10.1037/0735-7044.118.4.000).

The Menstrual cycle starts with low level FSH stimulation of immature egg follicles which at this point are insensitive to LH. One of these becomes predominant and begins to grow, secreting small amounts of estrogen. This responds to the FSH by growing and secreting estrogen. This estrogen holds the process in check, by suppressing FSH over the two weeks that it takes for the follicle to fully ripen, and stimulates growth of the endometrial tissue in the uterine lining. Eventually rapidly rising estrogen levels in the follicle cause a hypothalamic rise of GnRH stimulating both FSH and particularly LH in the pituitary where in addition estrogen increases LH sensitivity to GnRH. By now, the mature ovum has developed LH receptors and the LH now sends the follicle toward ovulation within 48 hours. Subsequently the remains of the follicle, the corpus luteum continues to excrete estrogen and with it the progesterone necessary for maintaining the lining and permitting implantation. The precipitating factor in ending the cycle may be prostaglandins in the uterus At this point both steroid levels plummet and menstruation sets in as the uterine lining is shed. In many mammals species the uterine linings are absorbed. If implantation occurs, human chorionic gonadotropin causes the corpus lutetum to continue making progesterone. In humans the placenta also makes progesterone after the first two months. See also related primate cycles (p 76).

(New Sci. 19 Jul 2003)

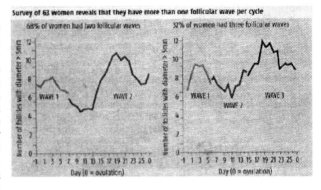

Survey of 63 women reveals that they have more than one follicular wave per cycle

Actually things are by no means as simple as this cyclic picture suggests. Many ovarian follicles mature in a given cycle although only one is released and the others atrophy and die. In recent research 68% of women were found two have two follicular flushes a month and 32% had three (Pierson et. al.R529). This is more consistent with a chaotic dynamical system than a simple periodicity. Even given progesterone masking of later flushes, in some of these cycles, two ova will be released, explaining the 10% incidence of non-identical twins, and possibly why menopause has an earlier onset in some women.

Progesterone is just one of a series of progestins which affect the cycle and maintain pregnancy. In addition estradiol is replaced by placental estriol, with some additional estrone, as well as the progestins. Estradiol is known to boost killer T-cell immune reactions so its suppression in pregnancy may help prevent rejection of the embryo (Blum R65).

Two other hormones secreted by the posterior pituitary are believed to have an important role in sex and bonding, the polypeptides: oxytocin, sometimes romantically called the 'love molecule', and vasopressin. Oxytocin is involved in both uterine contractions in childbirth and, along with another pituitary polypeptide prolactin, in lactation, where it triggers the let down reflex that releases milk for breast feeding and may help both mothers and fathers bond closely to protect young offspring. It also has other effects increasing insulin and the effective assimilation of food. In an experiment with masturbating women, oxytocin levels were found to rise, albeit slightly on orgasm, and to correlate to some degree with the pleasure experienced (Fisher R209 257). Oxytocin was released also in massage in women but not in erotic fantasy (Campbell R102 241). The fact that oxytocin functions in overcoming avoidance behavior and establishing a trusting bond in men, despite the apparent circumstances has been established in an experiment, where men sniffing oxytocin were unknowingly much more likely to give their money to a trustee in a trustee investment game (p 51).

Oxytocin effects of hugs hugs can be particularly good for women's hearts. In a study, hugs between partners were found to both increase oxytocin levels and reduce blood pressure, particularly if the relationship was loving, but the effects were highest in women, accompanied by a reduction in cortisol (*How hugs can aid women's hearts* BBC 8 Aug 2005).

Vasopressin is essential in water regulation through the kidneys. Those lacking it flush so much urine that they lose glucose and become victims of diabetes insipidus. The relatively neutral comments of humans given vasopressin as a drug which is claimed to have beneficial effects on memory retention give vasopressin a similarly ambiguous status as a bonding agent in humans.

However there is evidence these two chemicals function as female and male bonding neurotransmitters in some species. Experiments injecting them into the nervous systems of voles and sampling the natural secretion of them in rats and simian monkeys suggest that oxytocin functions to elicit maternal child-grooming behaviour, even in animals which have never given birth. Prairie voles (p 34), (p 375) are socially monogamous and there is a strong association between oxytocin in females and vasopressin in males generated by conjugal love-making up to 30 times a day, acting on dopamine pathways in maintaining bonding (Campbell R102 240) through the 'addiction' of partnership. Aragona et al. (R19) have mapped out two domapine recptors D-1 and D-2 which can unravel or enhance prairie vole fidelity. Aragona's team discovered the D-2 receptors are activated during the first mating encounter, which results in pair-bond formation. After extended cohabitation with the female, however, there was a significant increase in stimulation of D-1 receptors, which led to aggressive behaviour towards other females. Blocking D-1 at this point prevented the aggression. A virgin male adult injected with a D-2 activating chemical formed an instant and lasting pair bond with the nearest female, even if she were not sexually active and no mating took place. The injection also triggered aggressive behaviour towards other females, even ones that offered sex. D-1 activation in virgin males, conversely, prevented them from committing to a female in the first place. Non-monogamous montaine and meadow voles do not show this pair-bonding relationship. However they can be induced to do so simply by altering the promoter region of the V1aR vasopressin receptor gene to that of the prairie vole (Lim et al R408). Prairie voles with variants containing 19 more micorsatellites than other strains show greater monogamous attention and better parenting (Hammock and Young R280).

The key region contains micro-satellites which are highly variable and provide for rapid evolutionary adaption. Humans possess a corresponding region, with polymorphisms in the population. The corresponding human region is not as long as that of the prairie vole, and among the polymorphisms have been found promoters of 17 different lengths, suggesting that the population contains individuals with a wide variety of genetic responses to fidelity. Divorce rates in fact show a degree of heritability. We have also noted that a paternally-imprinted gene which affects oxytocin neurons disrupts mothering in mice (p 346). In plain fin midshipman fish, which like some other species have two types of male, courting males which sing and sneakers which don't (p 33). Sneakers, like the females can only grunt, and vasopressin and oxytocin seem to be associated with singing and grunting in this species, rather than male or female behavior per se. (Campbell R102 241). These differential reactions are characteristic of polypeptides, which may act quite differently as a neurotransmitter to their effect in the blood, since they do not easily cross cell membranes and the blood-brain barrier like steroids do. Interestingly testosterone has been found to stimulate the growth of oxytocin receptors in the brain hinting at a neuronal feedback between reproduction, arousal and bonding (Blum R65).

Here we flow into the complex question of how neurotransmitters as well as hormones facilitate love and sexual and parental bonding. Falling in love affects not only our hormone levels but neurotransmitters such as serotonin which affect the relaxation and elevation of our mood. Love is by its nature addictive and has to be so in the most healthy of ways for sexual reproduction to remain the mainstay of an increasingly intelligent autonomous organs like humanity. We know opiates, and the dopamine and serotonin affecting drugs exhibit tolerance and severe withdrawal symptoms. 'Falling in love' is by its very name a partially involuntary process beyond our rational control whose energies are wild and completely addictive, with in some ways the most severe withdrawal reactions of all the source of all love's tragedies. The ecstasy and fulfillment of love clearly involves all these neurotransmitters and hormones interacting in a symphonic manner.

This carries us finally to the most subtle and pervasive molecular dance of all, that of the pheromones. The term pheromone means 'excitement bearer' a term appropriate to their 'galvanizing' sexual role. The first to be discovered was the sexual pheromone which attracts a male moth to the female, discovered to be a volatile alcohol, even one molecule of which is said to be capable of eliciting a response from the male. Research on human pheromones has been slower to mature and it is only recently that science has acknowledged that we have specialized pheromonal organs and that human pheromones may play a major part in our hormonal cycles and in our mate choice.

Folk wisdom tells not only that the menstrual rhythm is subtly coupled to the phases of the moon (Cutler et. al. R140), but that women together often become 'mode locked' into phased cycles. This was confirmed experimentally by Martha McClintock in the dormitories of a women's college. Synchronized ovarian cycles have been found to be common to humans, non-human primates, rodents and oppossums (R442, R443). The airborne nature of such phasing indicates it is mediated through a pheromone. This has been confirmed in a series of experiments by Winnifred Cutler (R140) and George Preti and co-workers (R539) who dabbed under arm sweat from males and females on the upper lips of test women. Female pheromones, possibly volatile fatty acids, called copulins, apparently 'caused' test women to enter phase synchrony with the pheromonal donor, and male pheromones, possibly the steroid androstenone, which is a female sex attractant in pigs, tended to bring long and short cycles towards the optimally fertile 29.5 day length. The result has been an explosion of interest in human pheromone attractants which has seen Cutler and Preti part company on critical terms, with Preti questioning the scientific validity of her findings, when Cutler began marketing the supposed 'attractants' for $600 and ounce, becoming overnight a scientist millionairess with advertisements in Esquire.

Astrid Jutte (New Scientist 7 sep 1996) has found that men's testosterone levels increase by half when they inhaled synthetic copulins linked to ovulation however from the study it is not clear they were more attracted. One should be warned that all is not necessarily wine and roses for male pheromones. Many studies show no consistent effects or even a filtering one promoting female choice but not mindless attraction, although in one study it seemed to make women feel 'submissive' (Benton R57). In a rating study, 289 women rated the smell of androstenone (Grammer R250). Subjects rated the main component of male body odor 'unattractive'. This changed only to a 'neutral' emotional response at the conceptive optimum around ovulation. Karl Grammer notes: "The finding has direct consequences for hypotheses concerning the evolutionary loss of estrus. The cyclic-dependent emotional rating of androstenone might facilitate active female choice of sex partners and may be a proximate cue for female mate-choice". There is a natural logic to ovarian synchrony. It provides a way to ensure the costly investments of reproduction are coordinated with an appropriate social and physical environment. Although this is common to many mammalian species, Chris Knight (R373) has suggested lunar and pheromonal ovarian synchrony may have favoured female reproductive choice in a monthly 'sex strike' to motivate the men to hunt for meat (p 77). Mild coupling to the lunar cycle may occur through the light-responsive melatonin cycle in the pineal (p 76).

Mammals have been discovered to have not one nasal organ of smell, but two - the usual one for the smells we experience in the everyday world and the other for a variety of body chemicals which affect our feelings of intimacy, not because of their particular smell, but rather the people and connotations they invoke. Like the G-spot, the human vomero-nasal organ or VNO is only a recent item on the list of accepted human discoveries, but it plays a pivotal role, not only in influencing who we feel has the 'right body chemistry' but the entire sexual development of the male. A defective X-linked gene called KAL-1 encoding the cell-adhesion protein anosmin, causes lack of smell because olfactory axons from the nose fail to receive the correct signals to fan out in the olfactory bulb. But it also has another bizarre effect in men who, having only one X are more exposed to this defect. In males, cells in the embryonic VNO actually migrate into the brain along the fascicles - the rail-like paths made by the olfactory axons taking up residence in the brain to become gonadotropin releasing hormone secretors. Hence lutenizing hormone is not released, testosterone is suppressed and the resulting males with Kalman's syndrome have small gonads and penis and no sexual attraction to women. Thus we find an organ we didn't know about may not only be governing our sexual bonding but the entire maturation of male sexuality (Ridley R567 138-9).

Vertebrates, with the aid of sexual recombination, have built up comprehensive libraries, not only of immune genes, but of histocompatibility genes, which define compatible tissue types. The major histocompatibility MHC proteins produced by these gene libraries vary

significantly between individuals and play a part in giving the person their natural pheromonal body odour, in combination with other glandular substances which give the stimulated vagina and semen their subtly attractive fragrances, referred to in the song of songs as
mountains of spices. These contribute to the intrinsically exogamous nature of sexual
health - breeding with someone whose genes are different enough to be complementary.
Even in cousin marriages the sharing of 1/8 of our genes constitutes a significant load of
inbreeding homozygosity, reducing our genetic variety and hence our fitness even when it
doesn't result in outright genetic disease, as indicated in research by Lucas Keller (R166).

Evolution has served us well in our innate reactions to these molecules. A woman responds
to ovulation by finding the exotic allure of men with complementary histocompatibility
particularly attractive. Men likewise find women of complementary type most attractive.
This makes evolutionary sense because the offspring from such liaisons will have
increased immunity and natural resistance. With even more focus on reproductively successful genes, ovulating women in long-term relationships found the odor of socially-dom-
inant men more alluring (R293). These factors appear to be moderated by other visual and
sensory impressions that mediate towards having partners not too different to ourselves.
By contrast, when a woman becomes pregnant, she becomes more responsive to the smells
of her immediate kin in what would appear to be a protective reaction to seek the safety of
kin not inconsistent with a matrilineal scenario. This swing of olfactory affinity is consistent with incest avoidance, suggesting the 'incest taboo' has a biological basis. The contraceptive hormone pill appears to mimic the pregnant state, running a potential risk of
altering long-term mating patterns to favour people of the same compatibility type with
lower natural viability. Klaus Wedekind has found that in exclusive religious groups with
increased inbreeding and lowered MHC complementarity, pregnancy rates drop and miscarriages increase (Blum R65). Protecting against self-fertilization is a major issue in hermaphroditic plants, where for example, broccoli has no less than 50 genes involved in the
process. Human pheromones are coming to be marketed as if they are sure-fire way to a
quick sexual fix in ways which are almost certainly fallacious. However there are a whole
spectrum of new viagra-like sexual arousal potentiators being developed which are rapidly
effective by nasal inhalation, attesting to the power of pheromonal attractants.

Pheromones can also have unpredictable effects. Ironically although male pheromones
ususaly turn off males, men under the influence of androstenol - a pheromone found in
men's underarm sweat - find men's lifestyle magazines to be more attractive and are more
likely to purchase them than those not exposed to the pheromone. Women appeared to be
completely unaffected by the pheromone. (Kirk-Smith et. al. R369).

Sex Cells: Mystery, migration, tragedy and fulfillment

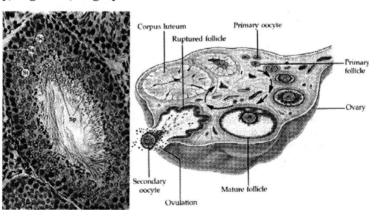

Testis with semin-
iferous tubules
generating sperm
from primordial
spermatogonia
near the edge,
with interstitial
spaces lower left
(Keaton) and
Ovary with devel-
oping follicles and
ovulation (Camp-
bell R105)

The origin of the
sex cells is a
tortuous tale of
migration,
enticement and
complementarity, of tragedy and success, despite extra-ordinary odds. It is also the immortal story of the single cells which literally pass from generation to generation between diploid primary germ cells to haploid egg and sperm, alongside which the organism is just a

multicelled offshoot the germ-line, spawned to ensure fertilization takes place. This is a story of this giddy dance, taking place alongside the doomed organism (p 356), the very cells which tricked us into sexual mortality and yet escape from us to regain immortality.

Human primordial germ cells first appear in the epiblast which will form the first ectodermal and endodermal layers of the embryo, in the region that will become the extraembryonic mesoderm. While in simpler animals such as insects, a region of the ovum cytoplasm continuing specific RNAs acts an organizing centre, in mammals the determination is more gradual. In the mouse the germ cell lineage only becomes defined during gastrulation, not during oogenesis or early cleavage as it does in lower animals. Grafting experiments have shown that many regions of the mouse embryo are capable of forming germ cells when they are transplanted to the extraembryonic mesoderm region of the epiblast prior to gastrulation.

Germ cells are proto-stem cells. Like stem cells they are totipotent, and have the capacity to generate embryonic stem cells, although this totipotentiality is only expressed after meiosis and fertilization. Consistent with this, stem cell factor is expressed throughout the stages of development of the germ line and is coupled to a specific receptor on the germ cells called ckit. Mutations disabling either of these cause infertility. Some germ determining genes particularly the anti-Mullerian male determining hormone AMH are, like the homeotic developmental genes, universal to arthropods and vertebrates. AMH, along with BMP, is a member of the transforming growth factor TGF-β family, highly conserved among animals having members common to humans, frog, fruit-fly and nematodes. These belong to the major class of high-mobility group HMG-box proteins which bind to four-way junctions that arise when self-complimentary single strands of DNA loop out to form twisted hairpins in the regulatory regions 'heading' active genes. SRY is also an HMG-box protein. HMG-box genes are involved in fundamental speciation events. Another universal sex-determining gene is Daz, 'deleted in azoospermia', first discovered in fruit flies which has a human homologue whose mutants also result in male infertility, showing it plays a key factor also in human spermatogenesis. This is one of the several male fertility genes that has moved from the autosomes (chromosome 3) to the Y chromosome around when the great apes began to develop. Oct, a nuclear transcription factor is also critical for the origin of primordial germ cells. It is expressed in cell lineages that give rise to them as well as in the germ cells and oocytes but not in sperm once they are in the testes.

Primordial germ cells temporarily migrate to the yolk-sac stalk (www)

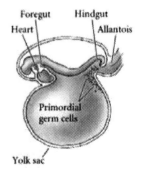

While they cannot properly be called any of the three layers ectoderm, mesoderm nor endoderm, since all these are doomed to become the somatic layers of the organism, primordial germ cells do display certain endodermal characteristics. They produce rich enough amounts of alkaline phosphatase, a key enzyme in bone, to become a key means in their detection. They also appear to use forms of bone morphogenic protein BMP, as mutant mice without this gene lack primordial germ cells. The primordial germ cells move from the epiblast to extra-embryonic mesoderm, then about two weeks after fertilization they migrate into the yolk sac stalk. The reason for this remains obscure, but may be to ensure they do not become imprinted as somatic cells. This does not seem to be to avoid X-inactivation which begins in humans almost immediately after fertilization. Both the tortoise-shell cat's large blotches and the genetic analysis of human blood cells indicates this switch happens at about the 10-20 cell stage and may even appear as soon as the first division (Montiero et. al. R468 , Puck et. al .R544 , Brown R83).

At about four weeks, the primordial germ cells migrate again through the hindgut endoderm, up the dorsal mesentery to the genital ridge where the indifferent gonad, a mesodermal structure forms near the embryonic kidneys. They proliferate during the migration, starting with 50-80 cells and becoming 30,000 by the time they reach the ridge. They move by extending filopodia (fine pseudopods), developing long processes, linked to each other in a stream-like fashion. They can pass between cells in tissues. There is evidence the genital ridges secrete a chemo-attractant that guides the primordial germ cells towards them. In addition, they may follow extracellular matrix "roadways" leading to the genital ridges, lined with a protein called fibronectin.

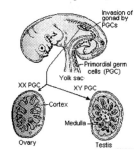

Migration of primordial germ cells into the gonads (www).

Integrins, which act as fibronectin receptors, are involved in the migration. In mutants lacking integrins, primordial germ cells fail to migrate into the gonads. If they do not successfully migrate to the gonad they can become the source of totipotent tumorous growths called teratomas which differentiate as they grow onto organs such as teeth, ears, and bones. The primordial germ cells now enter the gonads and elicit a series of interactive changes with these tissues. Female XX primordial germ cells proliferate in the cortex, the outer layer of the gonad and male XY germ cells proliferate in the medulla or core. Their presence now sets off a series of reactions in the somatic tissue of the indifferent gonad. At about 6 weeks of gestation in humans, a difference in the sexes becomes apparent: in females the genital ridge remains unchanged in morphology, whereas the male gonad develops sex cords. A series of genetic and hormone switches also occur which lead to the sex-determining pathways.

If SRY is present, cells of the medullary sex cords will differentiate into Sertoli cells. Once Sertoli cells form, the gonad is committed to becoming a testis. Sertoli cells secrete a glycoprotein called anti-Mullerian hormone or AMH also called MIS. These involve a simple dimeric signalling cell-surface receptor which activates a nuclear transcription factor. AMH is a major switch which represses the female Mullerian developmental pathway. It also stimulates intermediate mesoderm to differentiate into Leydig cells, which secrete testosterone. The medullary sex cords also form the testis cords.

Development of the indifferent gonad into testis and ovary involves development of either the Mullerian or Wolffian ducts (Sarawer www).

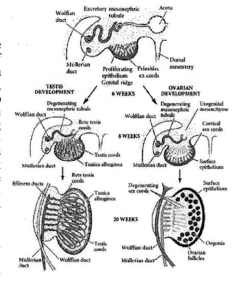

In males, the primordial germ cells become diploid spermatogonia. In the genital ridges of the male, mitosis of the diploid spermatogonia continue until puberty. Cell death is minimal, however AMH causes the germ cells to remain in meiotic arrest until puberty, when they undergo spermatogenesis, developing from spermatogonia into spermatozoa. Simultaneously, testosterone induces the testis cords to become the seminiferous tubules. At puberty some of the spermatogonia become committed to meiosis. However, diploid spermatogonia persist throughout life and serve as a continuous stem cell population. The spermatogonia committed to meiosis become primary spermatocytes, and it is in these cells that genetic crossing over occurs. After completion of meiosis, the diploid spermatids develop a tail and a condensed head. During spermiogenesis, the spermatids move toward the lumen of the testicular seminiferous tubule and are released into the lumen. Around 200 million sperm are produced a day, vastly more than the number of eggs a female produces in a lifetime.

The testis develops several weeks sooner than the ovary and is larger. Because the right side of the body also tends to develop sooner, this makes it possible for true hermaphrodites to exist who have an ovary on the left side and a testis on the right. Such individuals generally have some Y-related activity on a non-sexual chromosome, although they are generally XX and may have ovarian cycles at puberty and some even bear children.

In females, the pattern of differentiation is markedly different. In the genital ridges of the female, cell death of the primordial germ cells will begin and continue; mitosis does not continue. The primordial germ cells associate with the cortical region of the sex cords undergo a few further mitotic divisions. Shortly after arrival in the genital ridge, the female primordial germ cells cease dividing and become primary oocytes or oogonia. Sex cord cells become the granulosa cells supporting and nutrifying the ovum and the medulla gives rise to the layer of thecal cells secreting the androgens which are precursors of the estrogen generated by the follicles. In the absence of SRY and AMH, the medullary sex cords atrophy. Ovaries develop in the presence of the germ cells and the activation of both X chromosomes during gonadal differentiation, so that the germ-line again has a fully active XX complement. The primary oocyte together with a surrounding layer of flat epithelial cells is known as the primordial follicle. These cells replicate their DNA for the first meiotic division and then undergo crossing over. While still in the prophase of the first meiotic division with the points of chromosome synapsis still visible, these cells then become arrested. While eggs may remain in this state until puberty when menarche occurs, the majority resume meiosis I at varying times (in utero, infancy, prepuberty) only to be lost short of ovulation in atresia.

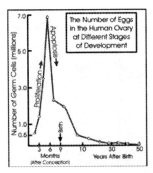

By the fifth month of prenatal development, the total number of germ cells in the ovary is estimated at around 7 million. By the seventh month, many of the oogonia and primary oocytes have atrophied in a programmed cell-death or apostosis. Surviving primary oocytes enter prophase of the first meiotic division, where they arrest until puberty.

A tragic mass extinction of oocytes has taken place, with their numbers falling precipitously to about 500,000 by the time puberty begins, leaving the woman throughout her reproductive life with only around 70,000, a mere shadow of her founding endowment, only some 400 of which will ever become ovulated. However recent research chemically destroying ova in pre-pubic in mice suggests ovarian stem cells persist which can regenerate viable oocytes. It remains to be seen whether it is possible to activate germ-line stem cells in human ovaries (BBC 'Female fertility extension hope' 11 Mar 2004). For a while, it was believed that the female pathway was the default, since in the absence of SRY the gonad becomes an ovary. Recently, genes have been discovered that challenge this view.

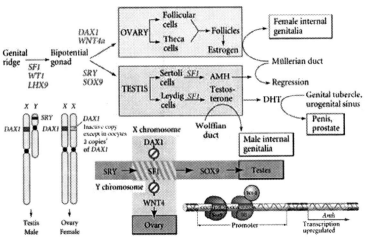

The principal genes and their related hormones and effects in the sex-determination pathway (www).

The gene Dax-1, when duplicated in the XY individual, results in sex reversal to form an XY female. It is located on the X chromosome and one copy is typically expressed in both males and females, where only one X chromosome is active in somatic lines. In some XY females, Dax-1 is duplicated on the X. Having 2 copies antagonizes SRY, leading to sex reversal to female type despite the presence of Y and SRY. Dax-1 appears to be involved in induction of the ovary and female sex-determination through Wnt-4. This antagonistic relationship between Dax-1 and SRY is a classic case of interlocus contest in sexually-antagonistic co-evolution - so sexual determination is founded on genetic warfare as manifested also in the 'fitful' evolutionary jumps of SRY.

Sex Organs: Homology in Complementarity

Originally the female sex organs were believed to be just an inverted version of the male, turned inside out from a lack of the 'heat' ascribed to male generative 'lust' (Jones, Friedman). This 'inverted shadow' of the female perpetuated from another older fallacy - that the female was simply a ripe garden for the planting of the male seed (MacElvaine R446), a complete male sperminal homunculus, which Nicholas Hartsoeker claimed to have actually perceived under the microscope in 1694, and which persisted until the discovery of the ovum by von Baer in 1827.

It is in many ways a fitting epitaph to the patriarchal dominion of the last four millennia that a process which obviously involves both sexes and was at least intuitively understood in animal husbandry and which is predominantly the 'issue' of the female in all externally fertilizing animals, from insects' to fishes and frogs, from whose ova we have quintessential delights such as caviar, were so neglected and repressed in human culture. Of course these ideas were fallacious also in the male, whose penis was believed to become erect by air pressure rather than blood, but it is nevertheless a commentary on the grim confines of sexually antagonistic coevolution that such fantasies could prevail along with dire punishments for women found in adultery or lacking the tokens of virginity. This sets a fertile stage for a discovery process in which the development of the external sex organs is found to be in many ways a homologous inversion, albeit in a context in which the female form is in many ways the default and the male an inversion of the female, via the SRY gene and its sequellae.

The mechanism appears to involve SRY blocking the inhibition of the Dax-1 pair on SF1 which then teams up with Sox-9 and Wt-1 to upregulate AMH production. In the female Dax-1 stimulates the formation of the ovary via Wnt-4. Interestingly some genes in the female pathway, such as Daz, are conserved between human and insects. The system has many more emerging components. TGF-β and LIF regulate further mitosis of PGCs in the gonad. In the male, these are primarily inhibited. Bone morphogenic protein Bmp-8 also seems to be involved in sperm development.

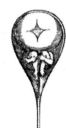

Homunculus in the sperm - Hartsoeker (Welcome library, London)

At the end of the seventh week, the gonads have differentiated to either male or female. However, the rest of the reproductive tract is still bipotential. The mesonephros begins to degenerate, but the mesonephric tubules and mesonephric (Wolffian) ducts remain, connected to each other. A second duct system, the paramesonephric (or Mullerian) ducts form as an invagination of the coelomic epithelium on the lateral side of the gonadal ridge. At the end of the eighth week, there are thus two sets of ducts. In males, with the presence of testosterone, the Wolffian ducts and the mesonephric tubules are maintained. The Wolffian ducts eventually become efferent ductules and the vas deferens. The Mullerian ducts degenerate in the presence of AMH. In females, in the absence of testosterone, the mesonephric tubules and Wolffian ducts degenerate. In the absence of AMH, the Mullerian ducts are retained. These eventually become the uterus, oviducts, and two-thirds of the vagina. These organs are missing in males with androgen insensitivity, resulting in a shortened vagina in an otherwise apparently female external anatomy. A similar condition can arise from hypoplasia of the Leydig cells caused by a failure of pituitary hormones.

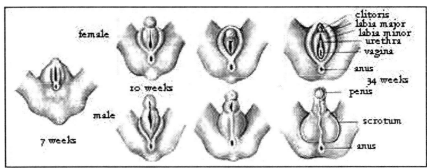

Developmental homology between the external sex organs (Keaton R346).

If the ovaries are removed, before the ducts differentiate, Wolffian ducts degenerate, but the Mullerian ducts are retained. When the testes are removed, again the Wolffian ducts degenerate, and the Mullerian ducts are retained. This is due to the absence of testosterone and AMH. Again, the female pathway appears to be the default.

Testosterone is converted to dihydrotestosterone (DHT) by the enzyme 5-alpha reductase during fetal life. DHT is the active hormonal key to the differentiation of external genitalia into a penis and scrotum. It also induces prostate formation. If the enzyme is mutated so that it is completely nonfunctional, an apparently female pattern of external genitalia develops. 'With undescended testes and a penis so short and stubby it resembles an oversized clitoris'. However at puberty something very unusual happens. The flush of androgen appears to trigger a late onset maturation of male penis and scrotum. Where these mutations are concentrated in the Dominican Republic, such people are called *guevedoces* meaning "eggs (testes) at 12." The girl has become a man, who now dates girls in a natural 'sex change'. (Blum R65 34).

Human Reproductive
Tracts (Keaton R346)

In the fifth week, cloacal folds develop on both sides of the cloacal membrane (which breaks down to form the anus). Elongation of the cloacal folds and fusion with the urorectal folds gives rise to the labioscrotal folds, urogenital folds, and genital tubercle. In the male, the urogenital folds

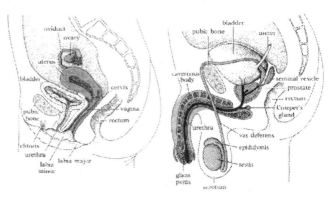

becomes the penis shaft, the labioscrotal folds become the scrotum, and the genital tubercle becomes the head of the penis. At the end of the third month, urogenital folds on the caudal end of the cloacal folds fuse to form the penile urethra. In the female, the urogenital folds become the labia minora, the labioscrotal folds the labia majora, and the genital tubercle the clitoris.

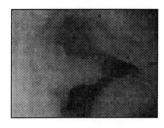

Homologous origins of the penis and clitoris: The external sex organs in a human embryo begin a generic androgynous state. In the 12-week old fetus it is difficult to distinguish male penis from female clitoris. (The Human Body BBC)

The sex organs are thus intimately entwined, both homologous in many parts such as the indifferent gonad, the penis and clitoris, labia and scrotum, and complimentary in others such as the Mullerian and Wolffian ducts, cortex and medulla which in turn give rise to inverted paradigms, the testes full of internal tubing and the ovaries externally ovulating to be enveloped by Fallopian motions of the fully developed Mullerian duct. This is an internal inversion of the sex organs as profound as the inversion of the sex organs in the fully developed penis and vagina, despite their homologous origin.

Orgasmic Physiology

Associated with each sex are differing and complementary types of orgasm. A man has a well defined pattern of spontaneous or stimulated excitement, erection, plateau, and ejaculation necessary to the act of fertilization. A female has a more complex and diverse sexual response. Firstly the female body and tactile sense is very sensually endowed, (e.g. breasts, buttocks and sexual areas), and secondly female orgasm serves a more mysterious function which is not directly connected with fertilization, but appears to be an evolutionary adaption of great significance to the female (p 85). Sexual excitation happens in more than one area. The vagina and/or cervix is a claimed source of major convulsive muscular orgasms which can become multiple, repeated or continual. It is these that some people suggest could cause deferential upsuck of sperm from the desired partner although confirmation is elusive. At another extreme, the clitoris although small carries up to twice as many merge endings as the entire penis. It is thus sensitive sexually in a way not dissimilar to the fovea of the retina - a very focussed organ with knife edge energetics. Somewhere in between the two between the bladder and the vagina is the G-spot, which includes Skein's glands, the female equivalent of the prostate, and an area of erectile tissue on the front of the vagina which uses nitric oxide in the same way as the penis. These seem to vary extensively in size in different women. The breasts are also directly sexual. Female orgasm is not linked directly to ejaculation which causes a refractory period so, although strong clitoral orgasms may result in a short period of quiescence, female orgasm is much more like surfing the great wave.

Geoffrey Miller (R464) notes that the penis and vagina are in an evolutionary race, with the clitoris coquettishly evolving to demand more and more pleasure to be 'satisfied' and the penis evolving to try to deliver it in the paradigm of evolution by female sexual selection. The clitoris is thus not attuned to the monotony of monogamy so much as the thrill of the chase and the novelty and abandon of falling in love.

The G-spot, associated Skeine's glands and erectile tissue (New Scientist 6 Jul 2002)

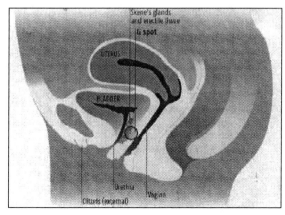

Sarah Hrdy (R323) suggests that female sexual ecstasy is to aid the survival of offspring and the degree of resourcing from males, but not exclusively to one. In most species, including humans, female sexuality acts to both to seek 'choice' genes and more disquietingly for the males, to reduce paternity certainty. There are extremely valid reasons for this. By inviting 'many possible fathers', females significantly reduce the risk of infanticide by any given male and at the same time encourage one or more of them to act in a broadly supportive manner - thus reducing paternity certainty. In socially monogamous species, females invest both in a resourceful partner and an insurance in good genes in some 'time on the side'. Human society is no exception. In DNA tests, over 10% of children in many Western societies are not sired by their ostensible father. Pair bonding has increased paternity uncertainty by comparison with chimps, from around 50% to about 80%, although in some matrilineal societies it could be lower than 33%, the point where investing in the children of your sister is more worthwhile than those of your partner, which is a common motif in such societies.

Are the Biological Sexes just Cultural Genders?

The gender feminist Anne Fausto-Sterling argues that all sex differences, other than the anatomical ones, come from the expectations of parents, playmates, and society:

"The key biological fact is that boys and girls have different genitalia, and it is this biological difference that leads adults to interact differently with different babies whom we conveniently color-code in pink or blue to make it unnecessary to go peering into their diapers for information about gender."

Pinker (R532 345) notes that the pink-and-blue theory is becoming less and less credible, listing a dozen kinds of evidence that the difference between men and women is more than genitalia-deep.

1. In all human cultures, men and women are seen as having different natures, divide their labor by sex, with more responsibility for childrearing by women and more control of the public and political realms by men. Men are more aggressive, more prone to stealing, more prone to lethal violence and war, and more likely to woo, seduce, and trade favors for sex. And in all cultures one finds rape, as well as proscriptions against rape .

2. Many of the psychological differences between the sexes are exactly what an evolutionary biologist who knew only their sexual differences would predict, in particular the greater parental investment of women and the greater mating investment of men. Other physical traits of men, such as later puberty, greater adult strength, and shorter lives, also indicate a history of selection for high-stakes competition, male polygyny.

3. Many of the sex differences are found widely in other primates, indeed, throughout the mammalian class. Including the above sex differences and the male having a greater range, reflected in men's advantage in using mental maps and performing 3-D mental rotation may not be a coincidence.

4. Geneticists have found that the diversity of the mitochondrial DNA (which men and women inherit from their mothers) is far greater than the diversity of the DNA in Y chromosomes (which men inherit from their fathers), implying men have had greater variation in their reproductive success than women.

5. The human body contains a mechanism that causes the brains of boys and the brains of girls to diverge during development. The Y chromosome triggers the growth of testes in a male fetus, which secrete androgens, the characteristically male hormones (including testosterone). Estrogens, the characteristically female sex hormones, also affect the brain throughout life. Receptors for the sex hormones are found in many parts of the brain, as well as in the cerebral cortex.

6. The brains of men differ visibly from the brains of women in several ways, size (men), proportion of grey matter (women), cerebral commisures and hypothalamic nuclei involved in arousal.

7. Variation of testosterone levels among different men, and in the same man in different seasons or at different times of day, correlates with libido, self-confidence, and the drive for dominance.

8. Women's cognitive strengths and weaknesses vary with the phase of their menstrual cycle.

9. Androgens have permanent effects on the developing brain, not just transient effects on the adult brain. Girls with congenital adrenal hyperplasia, though their hormone levels are brought to normal soon after birth, grow into tomboys.

10. Attempts to surgically feminize boys with a damaged penis such as that of John Money, below, fail and the individuals though reared as a girl insist on identifying as males and even marrying.

11. The evidence from girls with Turner's syndrome indicates that the X-chromosomes are differently imprinted from fathers and mothers in ways which have long-lasting effects in adult life.

12. Contrary to popular belief, parents in contemporary America do not treat their sons and daughters very differently. Nor do differences between boys and girls depend on their observing mas-

culine behavior in their fathers and feminine behavior in their mothers, even when they have two 'mothers' and no father.

Two key predictions of the social construction theory - that boys treated as girls will grow up with girls' minds, and that differences between boys and girls can be traced to differences in how their parents treat them - have gone down in flames.

As to the first Pinker illustrates a poignant example of attempted sex reversal at birth.

"The ultimate fantasy experiment to separate biology from socialization would be to take a baby boy, give him a sex-change operation, and have his parents raise him as a girl and other people treat him as one. If gender is socially constructed, the child should have the mind of a normal girl; if it depends on prenatal hormones, the child should feel like a boy trapped in a girl's body. Remarkably, the experiment has been done in real life-not out of scientific curiosity, of course, but as a result of disease and accidents. One study looked at twenty-five boys who were born without a penis (a birth defect known as cloacal exstrophy) and who were then castrated and raised as girls. All of them showed male patterns of rough-and tumble play and had typically male attitudes and interests. More than half of them spontaneously declared they were boys, one when he was just five years old. .In a famous case study, an eight-month-old boy lost his penis in a botched circumcision (not by a mohel, I was relieved to learn, but by a bungling doctor). His parents consulted the famous sex researcher John Money, who had maintained that "Nature is a political strategy of those committed to maintaining the status quo of sex differences." He advised them to let the doctors castrate the baby and build him an artificial vaginal and they raised him as a girl without telling him what had happened. I learned about the case as an undergraduate in the 1970s, when it was offered as proof that babies are born neuter and acquire a gender the way they are raised. A New York Times article from the era reported that Brenda (née Bruce) "has been sailing contentedly through childhood as a genuine girl." The facts were suppressed until 1997, when it was revealed that from a young age Brenda felt she was a boy trapped in a girl's body and gender role. She ripped off frilly dresses, rejected dolls in favor of guns, preferred to play with boys, and even insisted on urinating standing up. At fourteen she was so miserable that she decided either to live her life as a mate or to end it, and her father finally told her the truth. She underwent a new set of operations, assumed a male identity, and today is happily married to a woman".

In 2004 David Reimer committed suicide after the departure of his wife and the suicide of his twin brother, cementing this misadventure in history:

As to the second prediction, Pinker quotes the following summary:

"A recent assessment of 172 studies involving 28,000 children found that boys and girls [in the US] are given similar amounts of encouragement, warmth, nurturance, restrictiveness, discipline, and clarity of communication. The only substantial difference was that about two-thirds of the boys were discouraged from playing with dolls, especially by their fathers, out of a fear that they would become gay. (Boys who prefer girls' toys often do turn out gay, but forbidding them the toys does not change the outcome.) Nor do differences between boys and girls depend on their observing masculine behavior in their fathers and feminine behavior in their mothers. When Hunter has two mommies, he acts just as much like a boy as if he had a mommy and a daddy."

Anne Campbell (R102) notes that many sex differences are universal, extend to primates and the developmental onset of behavioural differences in young children predates the ability to name the sex of others, to name one's own sex, to appreciate gender constancy and knowledge of gender stereotypes.

Principal areas in the human brain (Redrawn from Scientific American). Although the brain does not display overt sexual polarization, there are a host of subtle differences from the cellular to the neurosystems level.

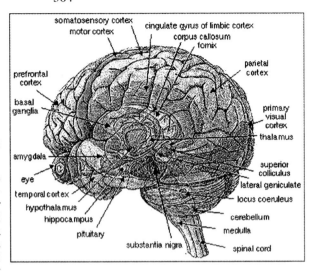

Sexual Paradox in the Conscious Brain

The Enigmatic Three Pound Universe

The brain is the gateway to the deepest enigma of modern science - the biological basis for subjective consciousness and the paradox of free will in a physical universe. It thus holds all the trump cards in the final frontier of scientific discovery whose surface has only so far barely been scratched. Although many people in the reductionistic paradigm from artificial intelligence and other areas have sought to see the brain as simply a glorified computer, there is little about the brain which in any way resembles the sort of digital device we have invented to carry out our computational tasks. For a start, the brain is a very bad computer. We have a memorizable digit span of only about seven figures and find even simple arithmetic calculations difficult without the aid of a pencil and paper. By contrast, we are able to remember whether or not almost a million different scenes are familiar or have been seen before, hinting at an almost unlimited 'environmental' memory capacity.

This kind of contrast is reflected in everything we know about the anatomy and physiology of the brain. Although the first nervous system to be studied, the giant axon potential of the squid, does have an apparently discrete response, it is in fact a pulse coded analogue signal which is being transferred, whose rate of discharge is proportional to the continuous depolarization at the cell body. When we come to examine even the simplest nervous systems such as the ganglia of the sea slug *aplysia* we find that it is the 'silent' analogue cells with continuous potential changes which act as the organizing centres for behavior, with the pulse coded cells merely acting as long distance relays.

Similarly when we look at brain waves in the cortical electroencephalogram or EEG, we find so-called 'brain waves' such as the α, β, and γ rhythms, which are not only continuous changes but broad spectrum vibrations more characteristic of chaos or edge of chaos dynamics, than the exact resonances of an ordered dynamical system. In complete contrast to the essentially serial nature of the digital computer despite attempts to introduce some relatively trivial parallel architecture, the overweening paradigm for the central nervous system is 'parallel distributed processing'. Generally there are as little as 10 synapses between input and output despite there being between 10^{10} and 10^{11} neurons and around 10^{15} synapses in the cerebral cortex. Central nervous networks are also intrinsically fractal in architecture because of the many-to-many nature of connections arising from the tree structure of a neuron's dendrites and axons. The combination of this many-to-many fractal architecture and the wavelike nature of neuronal transmissions is a key concept in Karl Pribram's description of the 'holographic brain' (Pribram R540). Phase-locking can mark out populations of cells sharing a common 'experience' or process from other randomly related stimuli. This 'holographic' view is supported by much physiological evidence. EEGs, particularly in the gamma band 40-60 Hz (cycles/sec), and their averaged event-related potentials, display phase coherence in a situation when a given perception is recognized, and out-of-phase chaotic 'hunting', when we are trying to orient to an unfamiliar experience. Phase beats are the basis of the quantum uncertainty relationship (p 299) implying a potential connection. The complementarity between continuous wave coherence and the discrete local information carried to a given neuron or synapse is deeply similar to wave-particle complementarity.

Another important complementarity is provided by the reliance many neuronal connections make on highly non-linear and diverse chemical neurotransmitters to transduce information across the synaptic junction. These neurotransmitters come in a variety of types both excitatory and inhibitory and also of temporary short-term effect or of long-term potentially permanent effect in the long-term potentiation or LTP involved in memorization.

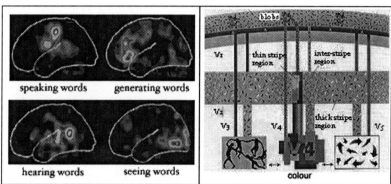

Despite the development of sophisticated techniques for visualizing brain activity such as those for speech (left), and ingenious work tracing connectivity of activity between neurons in the cortex such as that establishing distinct parallel processing regions for colour and movement in vision (right, Zeki R761), no objective brain state is equivalent to a subjective conscious experience. The difficulty of bridging this abyss is called the hard problem in consciousness research (Chalmers R111)

If we consider what brains actually have to do to ensure our survival we can see at once why this might be the case. Many problems which simulate environmental decision-making are computationally intractable. A good example is the travelling salesman problem - finding the shortest distance around n cities, which to be computed classically requires tracing every possible route which grows super-exponentially as $(n-1)!/2$ To calculate a route around some 30 cities would take a modern serial computer the entire history of the universe to complete.

Thus if a gazelle is standing at a forking in the paths to the water hole it would become stranded and eaten by the tiger if it had to resort to classical computation. Moreover many of these problems are prisoners' dilemma problems in which the 'opponent' is forever changing their strategy, making computation historically out-of-date. The tiger may for example choose the safest looking path, or switch unpredictably. Finally there is no single answer to many of these decisions, most of which have many possible outcomes rather than one computational solution, which is why we have evolved to have free choice in the first place.

The way the brain appears to have evolved to solve this problem is to engage a kind of Darwinistic internal ecosystem of resonating excitations which are chaotic in time and enable holographic wave processing in 'space' across the cortex. In a dynamic brain, phases of chaos are essential, both to provide the sensitivity on initial conditions of chaos which is essential to respond acutely sensitively to the outside world, and to provide the unpredictable, seemingly random, variation required to prevent the system getting caught in the rut of one overwhelming 'attractor' - the nemesis of all ordered systems.

The overall architecture of the mammalian brain consists of an overarching cortex acting as a modifier of resonant excitations ascending from mid-brain centres in the thalamus and deeper basal brain centres driving phases of alertness, sleep and dreaming. The cortex has a modular parallel architecture with sensory and cognitive processing for different modes occurring in parallel in distinct centres. For example upward of 24 centres have been identified for vision, handling colour and motion in separate parallel processing units. These parallel differentiations extend to specific types of feature such as separate regions for recognition of different human faces and of human facial emotional expressions. Each of these modular regions is in turn organized into a series of columns on a scale of about 1mm which act as feature detectors for example of lines with a specific orientation. Processing occurs in three to five distinct cellular layers comprising a mix of excitatory and inhibitory cells forming feedback loops enabling processing such as contrast enhancement.

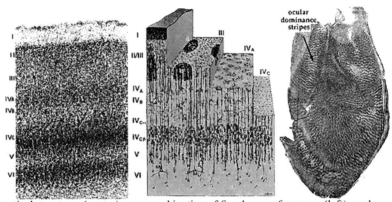

Typical cortical structures (centre) are a combination of five-layers of neurons (left), each composed into columnar modules about 1mm on the cortical surface. Such modules are sensitive to stimuli such as a line of a given orientation. Blob centres in layer II are also shown (p 365). Although specific sensory area have functional and anatomical specializations neural plasticity can enable changes of functional assignment indicating common principles throughout the cortex. Ocular dominance columns (right) for left or right eye illustrate functional columnar architecture (www).

Given only some 30,000 protein-producing structural genes in the human genome, there are far too few to genetically determine exact details of brain structure on a cell-to-cell basis in a hard-wired manner. The best specificity that can be managed consists of general rules of synaptic growth between specific cell types in different areas, which is what we see in cell migration and synaptic contact during development. In the visual system, the developing retina first begins to manifest chaotic excitation. Only then does differentiation in the lateral geniculate become evident and in turn from its dynamical excitation the visual cortex becomes differentiated for pattern recognition. Thus while genes may be able to encode interconnections between specific excitatory and inhibitory cell types and to promote growth of axons between cell types in different regions, the central nervous system depends on dynamical excitation to establish the developed architecture of its connections. Genetic determinism is thus a myth. Genes create developmental potentialities, which are shaped by excitation in both development and the environment. Nature thus utilizes nurture.

This dynamical basis for development is reflected in cortical plasticity, where emerging changes in function can result in regions previously assigned to one function taking over another. Examples are changes in binocular optical dominance when one or other eye is covered, through to the phenomenon of the phantom limb, where regions assigned to a removed limb become invaded by other functional areas, resulting in sensory confusion, and the illusion that the limb is still present, perhaps even painful. Changes also take place during higher learning such as becoming fluent in a new language. These kinds of specialization and development are reflected in the modular organization of the cortex we see in positron emission tomography (PET) and functional magnetic resonance imaging (fMRI) studies of the language and perceptual areas of the cortex.

The cerebral cortex is divided between front and rear broadly into motor and perception areas by the Sylvian fissure, which divides frontal regions and the motor cortex from the somatosensory (touch) and other sensory areas, including vision and hearing. The broadly sensory 'input' and associated areas of the parietal and temporal cortices are complemented by frontal and pre-frontal areas which deal with 'output' in the form of action rather than perception and with forming anticipatory models of our strategic and living futures. These active roles of decision-making and 'working memory', which interact from pre-frontal cortical areas complement the largely sensory-processing of the temporal, parietal and occipital lobes with a space-time representation of our 'sense of future' and of our will or intent.

Another motif with undertones of sexual complementarity (p 388) is the fact that we possess two left and right hemispheres which are to all purposes separate cortices linked only by massive underlying parallel circuitry in the corpus callosum. Although much has been romanticized about our left and right brains in terms of the contrast between intuition and structured reasoning, and some people almost banish the sub-dominant hemisphere to inarticulate zombie-like status, there is abundant evidence for a degree of complementarity between foci in the two hemispheres, for example analytic language versus creative expression, linguistic versus musical perception, and holistic versus mechanical modes of thought.

Such lateralization has also been associated with the complementarity between different types of mathematical reasoning, the continuous ideas of topology (p 492) and calculus being associated with the right hemisphere by contrast with the discrete operations of algebra (p 301) hypothetically assigned, like language to the left. The two key language areas, Broca's frontal area for verbal speech fluency and Wernicke's temporal area for semantic resolution are traditionally on the left. However one should note that lateralization is more prominent in males and that females have generally greater facility with language, despite their language processing being less lateralized (p 390). The cortex itself is relatively inert in electrodynamical terms and may actually form a complex boundary constraint on the activity of more active underlying areas such as the thalamus, which contains a number of centers with ordered projections to and from corresponding areas of the cortex.

Characteristic of the mammalian brain is also the peripheral 'limbic' system forming a loop around the periphery of the cortex, connecting primary frontal regions mediating integrated decision-making in action and the emotional centres of the cingulate cortex with the flight and fight centre of the amygdala, the long-term sequential memory of the hippocampus and basic bodily and sexual functions of the hypothalamus in great feedback loops whose dynamics are characteristic of changes in emotional mood and its influence on our outlook and strategic direction. The limbic system lies at the core of mammalian emotionality from fear and anger to love and our capacity to transcend immediate genetic determinacies.

The overall dynamical organization of the mammalian brain is also evident in the major ascending distributed pathways from the basal brain using specific neurotransmitters such as dopamine, noradrenaline and serotonin, which modify alertness and light and dreaming sleep (see New Scientist 28 Jun 2003 29) and are also modulated by psychedelics such as psilocin and mescaline. These fan out from basal brain centres into wide areas of the cortex connecting into specific cortical layers where processing is taking place. The large pyramidal cells which coordinate output thus have several different types of neurotransmitter modulating their excitation, both in an excitatory and an inhibitory manner.

Walter Freeman's model of chaos in sensory perception (Skarda and Freeman R633, Freeman R224) gives a good feeling for how dynamical chaos (p 498) could play a key role in sensory recognition, for example, when a rabbit sniffs the air for a strange smell. The olfactory cortex enters high energy chaotic excitation forming a spatially correlated wave across the cortex, causing the cortex to travel through its space of possibilities without becoming stuck in any mode. As the sniff ends, the energy parameter reduces, carrying the dynamic down towards basins in the potential energy landscape. If the smell is recognized the dynamic ends in an existing basin, a recognized smell, but if it is a new smell, a bifurcation eventually occurs to form a new basin (a new symbol is created) constituting the

368

learning process. The same logic can be applied to cognition and problem solving in which the unresolved aspects of a problem undergo chaotic evolution until a bifurcation from chaos to order arrives at the solution in the form of a flash of insight - "eureka!".

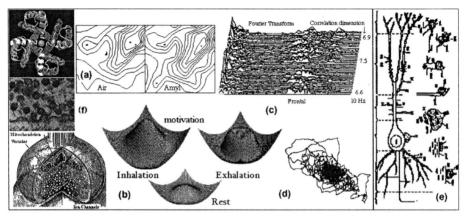

Chaos in perception: Freeman's model of olfaction is represented (a) by differing distributed excitations on the cortex. (b) A state of high energy chaos during inhalation gives rise to a lower energy attractor under recognition or learning. (c) Electroencephalogram shows broad spectrum waves with a finite correlation dimension, consistent with chaotic excitation. (d) A chaotic orbit generated by an EEG. (e) Neurons are fractal trees, potentially enabling inter-relationship between global instability and molecular or quantum uncertainty if the system is critically poised. (f) Top to bottom, ion channel is a single molecule which may display non-linear (quadratic dynamics) being turned on by two neurotransmitter molecules; synaptic vesicles budding at the membrane; a synaptic bulb containing vesicles and their recipient ion channels across the cleft. Eddington pointed out that the uncertainty of position of a vesicle is approximately the width of the membrane. Ion channels display stochastic activation (Liljenström R407) and have been modelled using fractal kinetics (Liebovitch R404).

Indicators of the use of chaos in neurodynamics come also from measurements of the fractal dimension (p 499) of a variety of brain states, from pathology through sleep to restful wakefulness. Recordings from single neurons, and from other cells such as the insulin-releasing cells of the pancreas confirm their capacity for chaotic excitation. The organizers of neural systems are also frequently non-pulse coded 'silent' cells capable of continuous non-linear dynamics. Despite the approximate linearity of the axonal discharge rate with depolarization, virtually all aspects of synaptic transmission and excitation have non-linear characteristics capable of chaos and bifurcation. For example the acetyl-choline ion channel has quadratic concentration dynamics, requiring two molecules to activate. Many cells have sigmoidal responses providing non-linear hyper-sensitivity and are tuned to this threshold. The electroencephalogram itself although nominally described as having brain rhythms such as alpha, beta, gamma and theta actually consists of broad band frequencies, rather than harmonic resonances, consistent with a ground-swell of chaotic excitation (King R357, R359, R360, R363). Broadly speaking neurodynamics is "edge of chaos" (p 506) in the time domain and parallel distributed in a coherent 'holographic' manner (Pribram) spatially. Phase coherence (e.g. in the 40 Hz band) has been associated with binding between related parts of the brain supporting an integrated perceptual experience, providing a mathematical parallel with quantum wave coherence. While artificial neural nets invoke thermodynamic 'randomness' in annealing to ensure the system doesn't get caught in a sub-optimal local minimum, biological systems appear to exploit chaos to free up their dynamics to explore the 'phase space' of possibilities available, without becoming locked in a local energy valley which keeps it far from a global optimum.

Into this picture of global and cellular chaos comes another scale-linking property, the fractal (p 499) nature of neuronal architecture and brain processes and their capacity for self-organized criticality at a microscopic level. The many-to-many connectivity of synaptic connection, the tuning of responsiveness to an arbitrarily sensitive 'sigmoidal' threshold, and the fractal architecture of individual neurons combine with the sensitive dependence of chaotic dynamics (p 500) and self-organized criticality (p 501) of global dynamics to provide a rich conduit for instabilities at the level of the synaptic vesicle or ion channel to become amplified into a global change. The above description of chaotic transitions in perception and cognition leads naturally to critical states in a situation of choice between conflicting outcomes and this is exactly where the global dynamic would become critically poised and thus sensitive to microscopic or even quantum instabilities.

Evidence for complex system coupling between the molecular and global levels. Stochastic activation of single ion channels in hippocampal cells (a) leads to activation of the cells (c). Activation of such individual cells can in turn lead to formation of global excitations as a result of stochastic resonance (d). Individual cells are capable of issuing action potentials in synchronization with EEG peaks (e) (Liljenström R407).

From the synaptic vesicle, we converge to the ion channel, which in the case of the K^+ voltage-mediated ion channel with its fractal kinetics (Liebovitch R404), and further to the structure and conformational dynamics of proteins, both of which operate on non-linear fractal protocols. The brain is thus capable of supersensitivity to the instabilities of the quantum milieu (Eccles R180).

Chaotic excitability may be one of the founding features of eucaryote cells (King R353, R356). The Piezo-electric nature and high voltage gradient of the excitable membrane provides an excitable single cell with a generalized quantum sense organ. Sensitive dependence would enable such a cell to gain feedback about its external environment, rather than becoming locked in a particular oscillatory mode. Excitation could be perturbed mechanically and chemically through acoustic or molecular interaction, and electromagnetically through photon absorption and the perturbations of the fluctuating fields generated by the excitations themselves. Such excitability in the single cell would predate the computational function of neural nets, making chaos fundamental to the evolution of neuronal computing rather than vice versa. The chemical modifiers may have been precursors of the amine-based neurotransmitters which span acetyl-choline, serotonin, catecholamines and the amino acids such as glutamate and GABA, several of which have a potentially primal status chemically. Positively charged amines may have complemented the negatively charged phosphate-based lipids in modulating membrane excitability in primitive cells without requiring complex proteins. It is possible that chaotic excitation dates from as early a period as the genetic code itself and that the first eucaryote cells may have been excitable via direct electrochemical transfer from light energy, before enzyme-based metabolic pathways developed.

It is thus natural to postulate that, far from being an epiphenomenon, consciousness is a feature which has been elaborated and conserved by nervous systems because it has had unique survival value for the organism. We are thus led to an examination of how chaotic excitation may have evolved from single-celled animals through the early stages represented by Hydra, which, despite having an unstructured neural net, has no less than 12 modes of locomotion, to the complex nervous systems of metazoa. We have seen how chaotic excitation provides for exploration of phase space and sensitivity to internal and external fluctuations. However the conservation of consciousness may also involve features expressed only by chaotic systems which are fractal to the quantum level.

It is a logical conclusion that the conscious brain has been selected by evolution because its biophysical properties provide access to an additional principle of predictivity not possessed by formal computational systems. One of the key strategies of survival is anticipation and prediction of events (King R355, Llinás R409). Computational systems achieve this by a combination of deductive logic and heuristic calculation of contingent probabilities. However quantum non-locality may also provide another avenue for anticipation which might be effective even across the membrane of a single cell, if wave reductions are correlated in a non-local manner in space-time.

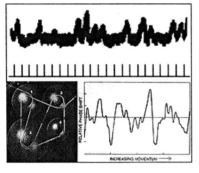

Above: Output from a frog retinal rod cell displays sensitivity to single quanta (Blakemore). Below: Phase shift in an electron traversing an open molecular medium shows chaotic phase shift (Gutzwiller R269) supporting a quantum chaotic model at the molecular level despite quantum suppresion of chaos in closed systems (p 501). Enzymes also depend on quantum tunneling to lower their transition energies, supporting a variety of quantum effects at the molecular level in brain function.

The limits to the sensitivity of nervous systems are constrained only by the physics of quanta (p 298) rather than biological limits. This is exemplified by the capacity of retinal cells to record single quanta, and by the fact that membranes of cochlear cells oscillate by only about one H atom radius at the threshold of hearing, well below the scale of thermodynamic fluctuations. Moth pheromones are similarly effective at concentrations consistent with one molecule being active, as are the sensitivities of some olfactory mammals. The sense modes we experience are not merely biological. They encompass the basic qualitative modes of quantum interaction with the physical universe - giving sensory consciousness plausible cosmological status. Vision deals with interaction between orbitals and photons, hearing with the harmonic excitations of molecules and potentially with membrane solitons as well. Smell is the avenue of orbital-orbital interaction, as is taste. Touch is a hybrid sense involving a mixture of these.

The very distinct qualitative differences between vision, hearing, touch and smell do not appear to be paralleled in the very similar patterns of electrical excitation evoked in their cortical areas. If all these excitations can occur simultaneously in the excitable cell, its quantum-chaotic excitation could represent a form of cellular synaesthesia, which is specialized in representing each individual sense mode. Thus in the evolution of the cortical senses from the most diffuse, olfaction, the mammalian brain may be using an ultimate universality, returning to the original quantum modes of physics in a way which can readily be expressed in differential organization of the visual, auditory, and somatosensory cortices according to a single common theme of quantum excitability. This is consistent with cortical plasticity which enables a blind person to use their visual areas for other sensory modes. Chaotic excitation thus leads naturally to a cellular multi-quantum-mode sense organ responding to external perturbations of the environment by sensitive dependence.

Can Transactions explain Conscious Intentional Will?

Supposing this chaotic sense organ found that these quantum properties also aided not just the perception of the world around it, but the anticipation of situations in the world critical to survival, through a novel form of physics which forms the basis of subjective consciousness. This is the critical function of any nervous system. A form of quantum anticipation of its own immediate future may be possible using the inner relationships of quantum entanglement - **transactional handshaking** with future states (p 308). This anticipation would have critical selective advantage for the organism and thus became fixed in evolution. This may explain directly why the brain is sentiently conscious rather than just being a computer. Computational capacity could be complemented with transactional anticipation through the chaotically fractal central nervous system. The work of Libet (R402) suggests the brain engages such time referrals. The transactional process is also compatible with quantum computation (Brown R85) using a superposition of states. The use by the brain of complex excitons may make it sensitive to an envelope of states spanning immediate past, present and future - the anticipatory 'quantum of the conscious present'. Such excitons might have restricted interactions which would isolate them from quantum decoherence effects (Zurek R768) as illustrated by quantum coherence imaging (Samuel R595, Warren R714). Hameroff and Penrose (R278) suggest that the brain may be able to function as a quantum computer and have speculated that neuronal microtubular protein units may function as quantum cellular automata in such computations, however their OOR model lacks the anticipatory properties and thus the *raison d'etre* for subjective consciousness described here (p 310).

What is interesting here is that the 'binding problem' - how sensory experiences being processed in parallel in different parts of the cortex are bound together to give the conscious expression we associate with our integrated perception of the world - has no direct solution in terms of being hard-wired to some collection point - the ultimate seat of consciousness. Every indication is that consciousness is distributed and bound together by non-linear resonances in the brain, such as gamma band phase coherence. This is very similar to the problem of quantum measurement (p 300) and exactly what we would expect if self-resonances were being used as part of a quantum transactional (p 308) solution to the perception-cognition dilemma. Just as with phase coherence, transactional interactions involve wave components interfering - the usual retarded ones and advanced ones travelling backwards in time, superimposing to form the real waves occurring in phase coherence. In the transactional model of conscious intention, subjective consciousness enters into the picture as the inner complement of the quantum space-time hand-shaking process. This violates the classical causality of initial states determining future states, which we associate with the Newtonian universe and temporal determinism. This is a consequence of special relativity and the fact that the boundary conditions of collapse include future contingent absorbing states (p 308). Since quantum transactions are general to all quantum interaction, their manifestation in resolving the fundamental questions of intentional action in the physical world gains a cosmological dimension. The conscious brain may thus be a key avenue for the expression of quantum non-locality in space time - a consummation of cosmology, not in the alpha of the big-bang, nor in the omega of finality but in the sigma of interactive complexity (p 298).

The brain has at the same time been evolving towards a type of universality (p 325) expressed in flexible processes for multi-sense processing and modeling. The qualitative differences between the sense modes are not matched by qualitative differences of cortical structure and electrochemical activity. Experiencers of synaesthesia witness multi-sense perception, suggesting conscious neural activity is potentially multisensory. A cosmological question is now raised. Is evolution simply accident, or is it part of the way the quantum universe explores its own space of possibilities, in reaching towards a universal expression of the entangled physical universe? If so what is the status of sensory consciousness?

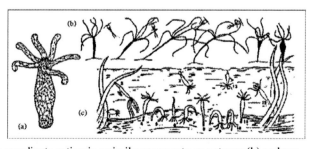

Hydra poses a dilemma for theories of cognitive development based on neural net organization rather than the complex adaptability of individual neurons. Hydra can reassemble ectoderm and endoderm if turned inside out and has a disseminated neural net (a) with no global structure, except for a slight focus around the mouth. Nevertheless it can coordinate eating in a similar manner to an octopus (b) and possesses more diverse types of locomotion than animals such as molluscs and arthropods which have structured ganglia. These include snail-like sliding, tumbling, inch-worm motion and use of bubbles and surface films.

In a quantum universe we have the many-universes dilemma, inspiring the Schrödinger cat paradox (p 302). In the real world, if we wire a cat to a Geiger counter with possibly lethal consequence, when we open the box, the cat is either alive or dead, not in a superposition of both. Transactional supercausality (p 308) explains this paradox as follows - the many probability multiverses solve a problem of super-abundance by hand-shaking across space-time to reduce the packet of all possible emitter-absorber connections to one 'happy marriage' . The universe, thus becomes experientially historical. Napoleon meets his Waterloo, but Britain wins Trafalgar, despite the feigned uncertainty of Nelson's blind eye. The same goes for all the hopeful monsters of evolution when mutations become success-ful. Quantum non-locality appears to have a method, through space-time hand-shaking, to determine which of the multi-verses hovering in the virtual continuum will actually become manifest. The role of consciousness as a cosmological process appears to mediate effectively between the world of the cosmic subjective, represented in physics as quantum non-locality, with the uniqueness of historicity, which never fully converges to the statisti-cal interpretation of the cosmic wave function, because each change leads to another, throughout cosmic epochs.

This leads to a deep question, shared by all human cultural traditions, from the dawning of shamanism, through Vedanta to the Tao and even in the Judeo-Christian prophetic tradi-tion, that mental states of awareness and subsequent happenings are interrelated. If histo-ricity is interactive with both the quantum realm and the existential condition, what are the consequences for science, society and cosmology itself? Our description of reality here suggests that the physical universe has a complement - the subjectively conscious existen-tial condition. Such a view both of the cosmological role of evolution to sentience and the brain as an interface between the cosmic subjective and the physical universe puts us right back into the centre of the cosmic cyclone in a way which Copernicus, Galileo, Descartes, Leonardo and Albert Einstein would have all appreciated. Consciousness may then not just be a globally-modulated functional monitor of attention, subject helplessly to the physical states of the brain, but a complementary aspect to physical reality, interacting with space-time through uncertainty and quantum entanglement in a manner anticipated by Jungian synchronicity.

Although subjective consciousness, by necessity, reflects the constructive model of reality the brain adopts in its sensory processing and associative areas, this does not fully explain the subjective aspect of conscious experience. Conscious experience is our only direct ave-nue to existence. It underlies and is a necessary foundation for all our access to the physi-cal world. Without the consensuality of our collective subjective conscious experiences as observers, it remains uncertain that the physical world would have an actual existence. It is only through stabilities of subjective conscious experience that we come to infer the objec-tive physical world model of science as an indirect consequence. For this reason, despite its seemingly ephemeral basis in a sappy organismic brain at the 'apex' of evolution, sub-jective consciousness may be too fundamental a property to be explained, except in terms of fundamental physical principles, as a complementary manifestation to quantum non-locality, which directly manifests the principle of choice in free-will in generating history.

This cosmology is intrinsically sexual. Subject-object complementarity is different from either panpsychism or Cartesian duality. The subjective aspect is described as complimen-tary to the physical loophole of quantum uncertainty and entanglement, just as the wave and particle aspects of the quantum universe are complementary. Subjective and objective are interdependent upon one another with neither fully described in terms of the other. Furthermore, the transactional interpretation is intrinsically sexual in the sense that all exchanges are mediated through entangled relationship between an emitter and an absorber in which reduction of the wave function is a match-making sequence of mar-riages. This sexual paradigm is not simply an analogy, but is a deep expression of the mutual complementarity and intrinsic relationship manifest in the existential realm, physi-cally and subjectively.

Furthermore, the theory suggests the evolution of sexuality, as it is found in metaphyta, is not simply an analogy with quantum complementarity, but is an emergent expression of the same complementarity principle. The single ovum, by necessity, is driven to seek fer-tilization through a solotonic wave of excitation which extends across the membrane. The multiple sperm, by contrast, are particulate packets of molecular DNA, without a cellular cytoplasmic contribution. Thus biological sexuality is utilizing quantum complementarity in the symmetry-breaking of gender.

The pivotal role of complementarity is reflected in both the Tantric (p 459) and Taoist (p 452) cosmologies. In Tantra, the subject-object relation is an intimate sexual union, which, in its retreat from complete intimacy, spawns all the complexity of the existential realm. In the Taoist view the same two dyadic principles are the creative and receptive forces which in their sequential transformation in the I Ching (p 457) give rise to all the dynamic states of existence. In Taoist thought, the cosmological principle is manifest in three phenomena, chance, life and consciousness, the very same phenomena appearing here in quantum physics, evolution and brain dynamics. The transactional principle clearly establishes the marital dance of emitter and absorber as the foundation of historicity - the collapse of the infinite shadow worlds of multiverses into the one line of history we experience in life, evolution, consciousness and social and natural history.

Randomness remains a scientific mystery, explained ultimately by quantum entanglement. The source of the scientific concept of randomness lies in theories, such as probability theory, statistical mechanics, and the Copenhagen interpretation of quantum mechanics which draw generalities from an incomplete knowledge of the system. However the source of supposedly random events in the real world lies either in highly unstable systems, which themselves may draw their uncertainty from the quantum level, or directly from the phenomena of reduction of the wave function under the probability interpretation. The transactional approach seeks to explain the sub-stratum of entanglement in a deeper interaction. This could provide an ultimate explanation for the origin of randomness in the underlying sexual weave of transactions.

The diversity of wave-particles resulting from cosmic symmetry-breaking (p 310) finds its final interactional complexity, in which all forces have a common asymmetric mode of expression, in complex molecular systems. It is thus natural that fundamental principles of their quantum interaction may be ultimately realized in the most delicate, complex and globally interconnected molecular systems known - those involved in brain dynamics. In this sense the brain is the culmination of a fractal interaction induced by' alpha limit' of cosmic symmetry-breaking - the cosmic sigma limit just as the heat death is an omega limit (p 298).

What is the relationship between the existential observer and the universe at large? What is the relation between conscious subjectivity and the objective physical world? This is a question which has plagued philosophers and scientists from the early Greeks through Bishop Berkeley and Descartes to modern researchers, from Francis Crick (Crick and Koch R136), who believes consciousness to be a product specific brain oscillations and their neural mechanisms, to David Chalmers (R111), who sees the 'hard problem in consciousness research' as a fundamental philosophical chasm, which can only be crossed through a greater description of reality.

Despite the advances of modern scanning techniques, a chasm still remains between the brain states under a researcher's probe and the subjective experiences of reality we depend on for our awareness of the physical world. This comes on top of a fundamental complementarity upon which we depend for our existence. Although we live as biological organisms, raise families, navigate our lives and perform our science on the assumption of the existence of the physical world, we access physical reality only through our subjective sensory experiences. Without the direct veridical access we have to subjective experience, there would be no conscious 'observers'. It remains unclear under these circumstances that one could establish that the physical universe would exist in any objective 'sense'. Ironically, a purely objective physical world description considers only brain states, leaving subjective consciousness to the perilously ephemeral status of an epiphenomenon, or not existent at all. However the physical world is really a consensual stability property of our conscious experiences, despite the fact that we are physical organisms whose consciousness appears to depend on our remaining alive. We can both consciously agree that the table is a table or that we will bleed if cut, so the subjective aspect is capable of representing the objective. The objective is capable in turn of 'incorporating' the subjective in terms of uncertainty in the physical. A fully cosmological theory would thus have to encompass both

This access to the subjective is profoundly augmented by a variety of subjective states, some of which have no direct correlate in the physical world, yet can be commandingly real to the observer. Firstly consciousness is constructive, and fills in details to generate a subjective description of reality which can often lead to peculiar results as illustrated by visual illusions). More significantly we have a spectrum of subjective states, from meditative trance, through psychedelic hallucination, the intense phases of dreaming, to near death experience. Although various tests can be made by the astute subject to distinguish dreaming from waking reality, the very fact of dreaming as an alternative veridical reality raises a deep question about the nature of the everyday world we perceive. Is it nothing but an internal dream state anchored by additional stability constraints provided by sensory input? If we are actually witnessing exclusively and only our internal model of reality, what then, if at all, is the manifest nature of the physical world? And what IS the existential status of this 'internal model' we ALL appear to share subjectively even if in somewhat differing ways? If this is the only reality we actually do experience, isn't subjective reality in some sense a universal?

The brain may be one of the few places where the supercausal aspect of wave-packet reduction can be fully manifest, as a result of its unique capacity to utilize entanglement in its dynamic resonances. It is difficult to conceive of a physical system which could in any way match the brain as a potential detector of correlations and interrelationships within the domain of quantum mechanics. Cosmology is not simply a matter of vast energies, but also quantum rules. In these rules of engagement more fundamental even than symmetry-breaking, the stage appears to be set for the emergence of sentient organism as the culminating manifestation in complexity of quantum interaction. In this sense the conscious brain may be the ultimate inheritor and interactive culmination of the quantum process at the foundation of the universe itself.

Understanding the Sexual Brain

The human brain, by comparison with that of any other species shows extreme adaptable generality - the hallmark of humanity as a metaspecies, defining its own ecosystemic niches in an environment now determined in significant measure by the interactions between humans and the varied social strategies they adopt to ensure survival in a human society.

This picture extends well back into our gatherer-hunter emergence where, despite the occasional ravages of large carnivores, humanity has been a resourceful long-lived species with a life expectancy not dissimilar to our current span amid long periods of leisure and socio-sexual activity. By comparison with other species, which are often primed by chemical or other overt cues of estrus of a specific programmed nature which drives reproductive opportunity, humans have a subtle and complex set of cues for sexual attraction. Women remain sexually attractive throughout most of the ovarian cycle (all if you count Tantric practices) and pheromonal influences are so subtle, given concealed ovulation, that neither sex is fully aware of these cues, even when they are conscious of their existence.

Nevertheless love and sex are both highly addictive, central drives whose energy and vitality are absolutely essential for our survival so we would hardly expect them to have evolved to be a matter of whim. As we shall find, they are woven into the deepest and most ancient parts of our brains as well as being expressed in an elegant and complex way in the cortex.

If the development of the visual system is any clue to sexual differentiation, we would expect to see differentiation emerging dynamically in the same way vision does. On the other hand, the effects of hormonal modifiers such as steroids are pervasive. Given that development occurs under markedly different hormonal regimes in male and female embryos, this provides a rich opportunity for evolution over time to adapt to specific enhancements of the nervous system in each sex that prove favourable to survival. We would thus expect sexual differences to be pervasive and subtle at all levels, from neuro-systems down to cellular and synaptic, and for these to vary in a variety of ways which reflect the ongoing dynamic process of adaption in individual species.

Consistent with this picture, the mid-brain centers, which researchers seek to identify with specific sexual behaviors, such as sexual orientation, are less clearly defined in humans than in rats and other mammals with clearly defined mating patterns. Moreover the most interesting sexual differences so far discovered revolve around major differences in emphasis of skills relevant to the gatherer-hunter way of life in a variety of ways which extend far beyond issues of simple sexual orientation. It is these differences and their con-sequences that are of profound interest to human society in reaching for a fertile social paradigm which takes best advantage of our complementary faculties. Again, consistent with maximum adaptability of the human CNS, individual differences in many of these skills are greater than the overall differences between the genders.

This all occurs in a context that paternal imprinting in mammals (p 346) appears to specif-ically favour development of mid-brain emotional systems while the maternally imprinted genes favour the development of cortical structures. The entire development of the cortex and its relationship to the emotional centres may thus be a product of a genetic arms race between the male and the female.

Some trends which have been regarded as a hallmark of human 'superiority' such as later-alization and cerebral lobe dominance turn out to be more a characteristic of male mam-mals generally, extending to testosterone-promoted cortical asymmetry in rats, shared by men in language and other development in a way which makes for intriguing contrast with women. However even some of these features, such as the differences in size and shape of the corpus callosum connecting the two cerebral hemispheres remain ambiguous to vary-ing degrees in humans. One should note that handedness appears to operate with a distinct, although related basis, to cerebral lobe dominance. Most left-handed people, have the same cerebral lateralization as right-handed people.

Love's Addictive Hunger, Empathy, Cooperation and Revenge

Nisa's penetrating comment (p 102), "Sex is food: ...hunger for sex can cause people to die" shows that the idea of sex and sexual lust as 'gratification' and a hunger and thirst abound. Falling in love is particularly 'driven' by sentiments like "I can't get enough of you".

Love, sex and addiction are associated in the popular mind, by addicts and lovers alike, and also now, by scientists. Stimulants like cocaine act on the brain's dopamine system, and so mimic the thrill of desire and anticipation. Depressant drugs like heroin, on the other hand, produce the opposite kind of pleasure - a dreamy satiation and freedom from pain, caused by their action .on the brain's opioid system. A speedball, a cocktail of cocaine and heroin, can be likened to a rapid, hyped-up sex simulation, moving rapidly from desire to climax. According to neuro-scientist Annarose Childress, what those sys-tems usually do is control our sexual behaviour : "This circuitry has been well preserved throughout evolution to enable animals to eat and reproduce. Those functions have been around long before cocaine and opiates" (Szalavitz R667).

Whether nicotine, cocaine, heroin or alcohol, the more directly or profoundly a drug affects the dopamine system, the more craving and pleasure it produces. Dopamine responses to sex are known to vary between male and female rats. In male rats, she says, dopamine levels go up when they smell a female, see her or have sex. Anything to do with being introduced to a female, dopamine goes up, but female rats only get a 'hit' of dopam-ine when they can control sex". In the wild, females normally allow the male near, then flee, returning a few times, before they will eventually accept his advances. This 'pacing' ensures the rat is optimally primed for pregnancy. A release of estrogen sensitizes the dopamine system, so it will give her a 'kick', and simultaneously maximizes the odds of successful conception.

High levels of the receptor VlaR in the ventral pallidum are associated with monogamous behaviour in the prairie vole, a species specifically associated with oxytocin and vaso-pressin bonding (p 352). Other voles with fewer of these receptors seek multiple partners. It seems as though the monogamous voles get more pleasure from their partners, or become more addicted to them, while the promiscuous voles get more joy from novelty. Intriguingly oxytocin seems to reduce both the extreme effects of cocaine and opiates and their withdrawal symptoms, indicating that bonding may also heal the cravings of love.

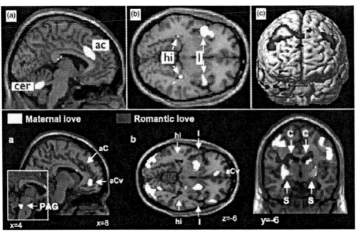

Top: (a,b) regions with higher activity in romantic love (c) lat-eralized lower activ-ity. Bottom: Romantic and Mater-nal love compared. (Bartels and Zeki R45, R46)

Bartels and Zeki (R45) used func-tional magnetic res-onance imaging fMRI to scan the brains of 17 volun-teers who described themselves as 'truly and madly' in love. During the scans, each was shown pictures of their loved one, or a friend of the same sex as their part-ner. Seeing a lover prompted activity in four brain regions that were not active when look-ing at pictures of a friend, and caused a significant reduction in the activity of another area. Two active areas lay deep in the cortex, the medial insula which may be responsible for 'gut' feelings, and a part of the anterior cingulate, which is known to respond to euphoria-inducing drugs and believed to be involved in emotional experience. Two lie in a deeper region known as the striatum, which is active when we find experiences rewarding. Deac-tivations were observed in the posterior cingulate gyrus and in the amygdala (regulating flight and fight) and were right-lateralized in the prefrontal, (a region that is overactive in depressed patients), the parietal and middle temporal cortices. This suggests that the cor-tex is functionally specialized for 'love'. The combination of these sites differs from those in previous studies of emotion, suggesting that a unique network of areas is responsible for evoking the most overwhelming of all affective states, that of romantic love. The authors note that "given the complexity of the sentiment of romantic love, it was not surprising to find that the activity was within regions of the brain found to be active in other emotional states, even if the pattern of activity evoked here is unique".

Bartels and Zeki (R46) have extended this work to compare romantic and maternal love and find some interesting parallels and differences. In particular, aspects of female roman-tic love fall closer to the patterns seen with maternal love than those in men. Romantic and maternal love are highly rewarding experiences, both linked to the perpetuation of the spe-cies and therefore have a closely linked biological function of crucial evolutionary impor-tance. The authors used fMRI to measure brain activity in mothers while they viewed pictures of their own and of acquainted children, and of their best friend and of acquainted adults as additional controls. The activity specific to maternal attachment was compared to that associated to romantic love. The authors conclude that: "Both types of attachment activated regions specific to each, as well as overlapping regions in the brain's reward sys-tem that coincide with areas rich in oxytocin and vasopressin receptors. Both deactivated a common set of regions associated with negative emotions, social judgment and 'mentaliz-ing', that is, the assessment of other people's intentions and emotions. We conclude that human attachment employs a push − pull mechanism that overcomes social distance by deactivating networks used for critical social assessment and negative emotions, while it bonds individuals through the involvement of the reward circuitry, explaining the power of love to motivate and exhilarate". Those madly in love also have converging levels of test-osterone (p 349).

In a study of the process of falling in love, Helen Fisher, Arthur Aron and Lucy Brown (Fisher R210) asked 7 male and 10 female volunteers who claimed to be 'madly in love' to look at pictures of either their loved one or another familiar person. Their fMRI scans show that, early on in a romantic relationship, dopamine-rich brain regions associated with motivation and reward become overactive when people see pictures of their sweetheart. The more intense the relationship, the greater the activity. Yet although love feels like an intense emotion, the researchers were surprised to see no extra activity in the emotional parts of the brain, such as the insula and parts of the anterior cingulate cortex. These regions are not activated until the later, more mature phases of a relationship. The findings suggest that romantic love is merely a motivation or drive, like hunger or thirst. Fisher explains: "Early on in a relationship, the brain seems to be very focused on planning and pursuit of pleasurable reward. This drive is mediated by the right caudate nucleus and right ventral tegmentum - the same brain regions that become active when you eat chocolate" (Szalavitz 2003).

The team saw patterns of brain activity in the anterior cingulate cortex that resembles those in obsessive-compulsive disorder. The activity is correlated with the length of a rela-tionship, lasting just into the emotional stage, by which time we overcome our obsession and form a more lasting bond, or not as the case maybe. An Italian team has reported that serotonin levels in the blood plummet in people who fall in love (New Scientist, 31 July 1999 42). People who suffer from OCD as well as those with depression, also have low levels of serotonin, however the cingulate area is very sensitive to serotonin levels, so tak-ing antidepressants could wreck a person's chances of falling in love.

There are also noticeable sexual differences. Women in love show more emotional activity earlier on in a relationship. Their memory regions are more active as they look at pictures of their partner, perhaps paying more attention to past experience. In men ,love looks more like lust, with extra activity in visual areas that mediate sexual arousal and the regions associated with penile erection. Despite all this, the region responsible for making aes-thetic judgements rates attractiveness in a very honest way, agreeing well with the ratings of independent observers. Fisher comments: "We say beauty is in the eye of the beholder, but part of the brain keeps track of the objective view" (ibid).

A PET study shows that many areas of the brain switch off during female orgasm. "

At the moment of orgasm, women do not have any emotional feelings," says Gert Holstege of the University of Groningen in the Netherlands. His team compared the brain activity of 13 heterosexual women in four states: simply resting, faking an orgasm, having their clitoris stim-ulated by their partner's fingers, and clitoral stimulation to the point of orgasm. As the women were stimulated, activity rose in the primary somatosensory cortex, but fell in the amygdala and hippocampus, involved in alertness and anxiety, confirming that women cannot enjoy sex unless they are relaxed and free from worries and distractions. However, during orgasm, activ-ity fell in many more areas of the brain, including the prefrontal cortex, compared with the resting state. From an evolutionary point of view, the brain may switch off emotions during sex because the chance to produce offspring becomes more important than the survival risk to the individual. Only one small part of the brain, in the cerebellum, was more active during female orgasm. The cerebellum is normally associated with coordinating movement, though there is also some evidence that it helps regulate emotions. When women were faking an orgasm areas of the brain involved in controlling conscious movement lit up, and there was none of the extreme deactivation (*Orgasms: a real 'turn-off' for women* New Scientist 20 June 2005 Michael Le Page).

Hypothalamic differences in activity when men and women watch erotic images consistent with the activity of dimorphic centres in the hypothalamus. Left: male and female responses subtracted show a unique male activation centre. This has a close relationship to a region (right) differentially illuminated when males find erotic scenes particularly exciting (Karama et. al. R345).

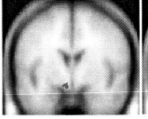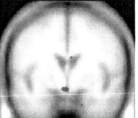

Mario Beauregard (Karama et. al. R345) uses fMRI to explore which brain areas become activated when men and women view erotic films. Not surprisingly, the visual areas are busy; but so too are many evolutionarily ancient circuits associated with emotion - the limbic system, anterior temporal pole and amygdala, and a region of the orbito-frontal cortex (OFC). Previous research found that these areas are important in prioritizing, decision making and giving emotional colour to an experience, and may subconsciously trigger physiological responses and desire. Pornographic images have been found to make men briefly blind to the orientation of immediately following neutral images (Sexy images cause temporary blindness New Scientist 20 August 2005).

Such response mechanisms extend further than sexual love into cooperation, defection and all the dimensions of the prisoners dilemma. De Quervain et. al. (R157) asked whether choosing to punish a defector would recruit brain circuits implicated in reward processing. They found that when subjects administered a monetary punishment to defectors, a the striatum was activated, indicating that punishing a defector activates brain regions related to feeling good about revenge rather than feeling bad about having been violated (Knutson R374). Indeed, these striatal foci lie near brain areas that rats will work furiously to stimulate electrically. They then asked whether the striatum would be activated even when administering the punishment carried a personal cost. They found that the striatum was still activated, as was a region in the medial prefrontal cortex, implicated in balancing costs and benefits. Effective punishment, as compared with symbolic punishment, activated the dorsal striatum, which has been implicated in the processing of rewards that accrue as a result of goal-directed actions. Subjects with stronger activations in the dorsal striatum were willing to incur greater costs in order to punish. The degree of striatal activation during no-cost punishment predicted the extent to which subjects chose to punish at a personal cost (that is, under less satisfying conditions). This finding suggested to the investigators that striatal activation indexed subjects' *anticipation* of satisfaction, rather than satisfaction *per se*.

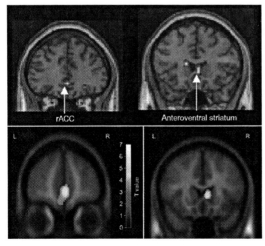

rACC

Anteroventral striatum

Above activation of areas by cooperative playing of the prisoners' dilemma game among women (Rilling R570). Below Left frontal and right striatal areas activated by 'sweet revenge' (de Quervain R157). The similarity of the areas suggests anticipated social rewards motivate both these contrasting behaviors.

Ironically, punishment of defectors in this study activated the same regions (that is, striatum and MPFC) that were activated when people rewarded cooperators in a recent functional magnetic resonance imaging (fMRI) study (Rilling et. al. R570). The monetary awards were apportioned after each round. If one player defected and the other cooperated, the defector earned $3 and the cooperator nothing. If both chose to cooperate, each earned $2. If both opted to defect, each earned $1. Mutually cooperative social interactions in the prisoner's dilemma game were associated with activations in anteroventral striatum, rostral ACC, and OFC that were not observed in response to monetary reinforcement in a nonsocial control condition. OFC activation but not the other areas was also observed for mutual cooperation with a computer partner, suggesting that the ACC and striatal activations may relate specifically to cooperative social interactions with human partners.

A pattern of neural activation is thus identified that may be involved in sustaining cooperative social relationships, perhaps by labeling cooperative social interactions as rewarding, and/or by inhibiting the selfish impulse to accept but not reciprocate an act of altruism. These seemingly diametrically opposite social behaviors are united by a common psychological experience - both involve the *anticipation* of a satisfying social outcome. While the former study of defectors included male subjects, the f MRI study of cooperators included only females. Future research will undoubtedly need to explore which social interactions most powerfully motivate men compared with women (as well as members of different social groups).

Activation of left frontal and right parietal areas involving mirror neuron activity (Iacoboni R328).

Another set of brain areas to do with both empathy and one's reactions and behavior in relation to others associated with 'reading the minds' of others (Motluk R480) has been dis-

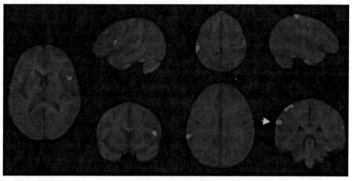

covered in the form of so-called 'mirror neurons' which although they may be in areas we usually associate with motor function intentional action and even the expression of language, contain a population of neurons which react in the same way when the same action is being performed by another individual (or even another species). Monkeys were found to have neurons in a frontal area (Di Pellegrino R167, Rizzolatti and Craighero R573) that discharge both when the monkey does a particular action and when it observes another individual (monkey or human) doing a similar action. Imitation may be based on a mechanism directly matching the observed action onto an internal motor representation of that action.

To test this hypothesis (Iacoboni et. al. R328), normal human participants were asked to observe and imitate a finger movement and to perform the same movement after spatial or symbolic cues. Brain activity was measured with functional magnetic resonance imaging. If the direct matching hypothesis is correct, there should be areas that become active during finger movement, regardless of how it is evoked, and their activation should increase when the same movement is elicited by the observation of an identical movement made by another individual. Two areas with these properties were found in the left inferior frontal cortex and right superior parietal. Rizzolatti and Arbib (R572) have commented that such mirroring, occurring in 'motor' areas such as Broca's area associated with language expression would give a basis for a transition to language, based on mirroring of actions gestures, cries and facial expressions. Such mirroring is also central to the empathy we associate with the way emotions transcend simple barriers of genetic determinism through imprinted instinct as well as the capacity to assess complex social situations of deceit and betrayal.

Sex, Brain and Steroids

One of the most outstanding examples of sexual dimorphism is in the brains of song birds where a whole sexually-typed brain region grows in the male only, waxing each spring and waning in the autumn. In mammals, timed bursts of hormones such as testosterone are believed to play critical roles in gender-typing certain key areas of the hypothalamus involved in female and male reproductive behavior around the time of birth, particularly in species such as rats and voles. Roger Gorski and his colleagues at the University of California at Los Angeles have shown that a region of the pre-optic area of the hypothalamus is visibly larger in male rats than in females. The size increment in males is promoted by the presence of androgens in the immediate postnatal, and to some extent prenatal, period. Laura Allen in Gorski's lab has found a similar sex difference in humans.

While rats have a very marked difference in their sexually dimorphic nuclei, humans vary only moderately between males and females. This is exemplified by the spinal bulbocavernosus centre which exists only in rat males, but is merely 28% different in human males and females because the muscles it controls work both in the base of the penis, promoting ejaculation and in the muscles constricting the vagina (Blum R65 30). To make matters worse, excision of such nuclei in rats causes only transient disturbance to sexual behavior and in monogamous prairie voles, the sexually dimorphic nuclei, whose differences between adolescent males and females are evident, become difficult to differentiate in parentally engaged bonded male and female pairs (Blum). This suggests that these centres may be dynamic consequences of activity rather than simply genetic differences determining sexual orientation. Each case of sexual dimorphism seems to be part of a distributed network of sexually dimorphic neuronal populations which normally interact with each other.

There are also marked differences in hormonal specificity in the development of brain and behaviour across mammalian species. Paradoxically in rats for example, testosterone aromatized to estradiol plays a major role in sexual determination in the male brain, preventing programmed apostosis (cell-death) the sexually dimorphic centres. This flood of estrogen is apparently quenched in females by binding to excess α-fetoprotein (Kandell et. al. R344). In prairie voles oxytocin in females and vasopressin in males are linked to parental care of the newborn (Angier, Blum) ((p 352), (p 34)). Neither of these clear-cut processes can be demonstrated to work in the same way in primates and in particular in humans. Even the role of testosterone in imprinting the human brain around the time of birth is debated. The review by Marc Breedlove's team (Cooke et. al. R130) notes "there is ample evidence of sexual dimorphism in the human brain, as sex differences in behavior would require, but there has not yet been any definitive proof that steroids acting early in development directly masculinize the human brain". Many studies link testosterone to dominance in men (Mazur and Booth R440) and women (Grant R251).

Because the nervous system is plastic, any sexual dimorphism seen in the adult brain could be the result of differences in experience, either during development or in adulthood, rather than as a direct result of fetal steroid action. Obviously a sexual dimorphism present at birth could not be due to sex differences in experience or social stimulation. One dimorphism present at birth is the sex difference of some 15% in the weight of the human brain, an issue trumpeted by some male scientists with political agendas. Deborah Blum (R65 38) notes: "More than any other gender comparison in biology, it's fair to say feminist scholars hate this one the most. Brown University geneticist Anne Fausto-Sterling argues this work is biased from the start. Male scientists consistently find male scientists have bigger brains. Since we tend to assume bigger is better the implications are obvious." Bente Pakkenberg claims there is a corresponding slightly higher number of brain cells in a man, 23 billion as against 19 billion. However Raquel and Reuben Gur have found that the male human brain loses neurons at almost three times the rate of women, probably due to the influence of androgens, so in mid life the male frontal lobe ends up the same size as in women (Blum 52). Similar results apply to the hippocampus involved in sequential memory. Sandra Wittelson has also found that women have about 15% more neurons in layers four and five, packed more tightly than in men - 35,000 in women in each sample and 30,000 in men (Blum 60). Because it is mirrored by the sex difference in body weight, brain size may be the indirect result of steroid hormone action. Most likely, testicular androgens masculinize the secretion of factors such as growth hormone or its companion factors to give males a larger body and brain. But the effect does not seem to be specific to the nervous system, so it is unlikely that it can account for sex differences in human behavior.

The brain structure that has been best studied in humans is the sexually dimorphic nucleus of the pre-optic area (POA) also called INAH-1. Swaab and Fliers (R662) found that males had a larger nucleus, with more neurons, than females, but this sex difference in neuronal number is not detectable in children younger than 6–10 years of age. Allen and Gorski (R9) and Le Vay (R399) could not replicate this sex difference but both did find dimorphism in INAH-3. However no one has examined its size in human development, so we do not know whether dimorphism is present at birth (and likely to be engendered by fetal steroids) or arises later in life (and could alternatively be due to social influences). The conflicting reports concerning sexual dimorphism in the human brain indicate sexual dimorphism is more subtle in the brains of humans than of other animals (Cooke et. al. R130). It may also be a consequence rather than a cause of sexual orientation.

Another strategy for asking whether fetal steroids affect the human brain is to find whether inadvertent exposure to fetal hormones alters sexually dimorphic behaviors. Unfortunately, the results of such studies are contradictory. Females with androgen overproduction from congenital adrenal hyperplasia (CAH) do behave more like boys, showing more rough and tumble play and tomboy behaviors than other girls. As women, CAH patients usually are sexually attracted to men, but are also more likely to be attracted to women than are other women (p 386). However it is hard to eliminate cultural factors here. CAH females have slightly masculinized genitalia and this effect could also be due to differences in their social experience, because of family or personal gender confusion.

Androgen insensitive XY individuals, who look like normal females externally, display feminine spatial learning behavior and verbal behavior, and are sexually attracted to men. But this might be due to their unambiguous upbringing as girls. If, as in rodents, the estrogens coming from aromatized testosterone masculinized the developing human brain, then we would expect these people to display masculine behaviors despite their feminine exterior. Androgen insensitive rats present feminine exterior, but a masculine SDN-POA, and a refusal to display feminine 'lordosis'. The feminine behavior of androgen insensitive humans indicates that aromatized metabolites of androgen cannot be playing a major role in masculinizing the human brain, either because steroids have no effect on the developing human brain, or because steroids act through androgen receptors themselves to exert such an effect. It is also possible that in humans, androgen receptors must be functional for estrogen receptor activation to be effective or to occur at all.

Contrasting this, Melissa Hines (R311) found that women who had been exposed to the estrogen diethylstilbestrol (DES) in utero showed greater evidence of cognitive lateralization (for a dichotic listening task and a visual search task) than their non-DES-treated 'sisters'. We shall see that this is a characteristic of males. However the effect is small and cannot be readily related to most human sex differences in behavior, so estrogen may be making only a small contribution to human neural sex differences. On the other hand a twin boy who had had a surgical mishap at 8 months and was given a sex change operation and reared as a girl decided at puberty to identify as a male and successfully became married with step children, suggesting masculinization had occurred (p 362).

Sexual differences in specialized abilities also fluctuate with hormone levels in both women during the ovarian cycle and in men, suggesting hormones continue to have a dynamical influence on gender difference in brain function (p 348).

Despite the fact that there is not yet any conclusive proof that fetal steroids directly masculinize the human brain, the rampant masculinizing effect of androgen during early brain development of other vertebrates makes it seem likely that at least some such influences remain in our species. There is however no doubt that adult steroid

382

manipulations do alter human behavior and both the behavior and the neural structure of other species.

Gay Genes and Cultural Brains

The saga of the 'gay gene' is probably one of the most sensational and hotly disputed genetic discoveries. Bailey and Pillard (R34) made the first of two twin studies in which a genetic basis for sexual orientation was found in both human males and subsequently females. The same year Simon Le Vay (R399) found an area in the hypothalamus (INAH-3) which was larger in men than women but more intermediate in gay males. Homosexual men are also claimed to have a larger suprachiasmatic nucleus and a larger anterior commissure than heterosexual men. Moreover another dimorphic nucleus the so-called 'bed nucleus' of the stria terminalis BNST or BSTc, which is larger in human males than females is even larger in homosexual men (Zhou. et. al. R765) suggesting hyper-masculinization rather than 'feminization'. However these measures, made in adulthood, cannot tell us whether the brain caused, or are a result of the differences in sexual orientation. As few of these orientation dimorphisms have been replicated, their status remains uncertain.

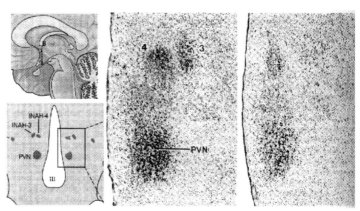

Interstitial nuclei of the anterior hypothalamus INAH-3,4 display sexual differences (Kandel et. al. R344). Section of the hypothalamus showing differences between male (left) and female (right). It is this centre that Le Vay claimed was closer to the female profile in homosexual men. Because these are adult structures and the brain adapts to behavior, it is difficult to distinguish fetal cause from cultural effect..

In adult rodents, the BNST, is 75% larger and contains many more cells in males and the anteroventral periventricular nucleus, or AVPV, is both larger and richer in cells in females. If a male rat is castrated shortly after birth, its BNST and AVPV will develop in the female pattern. Conversely, if a female rat pup is treated with testosterone its adult brain will be indistinguishable from a male's. A single gene Bax, from the Bcl2 family shaping neuron growth and death, has been found to govern the pruning of neurons. In the Bax-"knockout" mice used by Forger and her colleagues (R215), both the BNST and AVPV had many more cells than are seen in mice and the number of cells was equal in males and females.

Pathways linking odor to reproductive activity include the vomeral nasal organ (VMO) olfactory bulb (AOB) medial amygdala (MeA) bed nucleus (BST) and preoptic area (mPOA) (Cooke et.

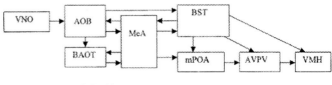

al. R130).

In 1993 Dean Hamer announced (R277) that he had found a gene on the X-chromosome that had a powerful influence on sexual orientation. Homosexuality is highly heritable, as twin studies show. Among 54 gay men who were fraternal twins, there were 12 whose twin was also gay. Among 56 gay men who were identical twins, there were 29 whose twin was also gay. Since twins share the same environment, whether fraternal or identical, such a result implies that a gene or genes accounts for about half of the tendency for a man to be gay. A dozen other studies came to a similar conclusion. Hamer's team interviewed

110 families with gay male members and noticed that homosexuality seemed to run in the female line. If a man was gay, the most likely other member of the previous generation to be gay was not his father but his mother's brother. That suggested the gene might be on the X-chromosome, the only set of nuclear genes a man inherits exclusively from his mother.

By comparing a set of genetic markers between gay men and straight men in the families in his sample, he found a candidate region in Xq28, the tip of the long arm of the chromosome. Gay men shared the same version of this marker seventy-five per cent of the time; straight men shared a different version of the marker seventy-five per cent of the time.

Consistent with this discovery, Trivers noted that, because an X-chromosome spends twice as much time in women as it does in men, a sexually antagonistic gene that benefited female fertility could survive even if it had twice as large a deleterious effect on male fertility. However Michael Bailey's research on homosexual pedigrees has failed to find a maternal bias to be a general feature. Other scientists, too, have failed to find Hamer's link with Xq28. However the discovery of the fertile mother effect in about 14% of gay men (p 384) may clarify these contradictions.

Table 57-5 Concordance for Homosexuality in Twins

	Males[a]	Females[b]
Monozygotic twins	(29/56) 52%	(34/71) 48%
Dizygotic twins	(12/54) 22%	(6/37) 16%
Adopted same-sex siblings	(6/57) 11%	(2/35) 6%
	Males[c]	Females[c]
Monozygotic twins	(22/34) 65%	(3/4) 75%
Dizygotic twins		
Male/male	(4/14) 29%	
Male/female	(3/9) 33%	

[a]Bailey and Pillard 1991.
[b]Bailey et al. 1993.
[c]Whitman, Diamond, and Martin, 1993.

Homosexual orientation shows heritability in both sexes. By comparing identical and dizygotic twins we can estimate how much genes (~30%), family and siblings (~20) and environment and culture (~50%) affect sexual orientation. Even given the strong genetic influence, culture is still the major determining factor. Nature is more than complemented by 'nurture' here (Kandel et. al. R344).

There have been reports of several physiological differences between homosexual and heterosexual men that could reflect nervous system involvement. Homosexual men are, on average, shorter than heterosexual men, will have undergone puberty at an earlier age than heterosexual men and will have more symmetrical left-versus-right fingerprint patterns than heterosexual men.

The proportion of gay people is also a matter of debate. Michael Bailey estimates that 2-3% of US men are exclusive homosexuals and 1.5% of women. Occasional bisexuals double the number and the idly curious swell it to perhaps 8.7% of men and 11.1% of women - considerably less than the 20% some political proponents would claim. Masters, Johnson and Kolodny (R438 373) report even lower figures from a specturm of international studies, around 1.4% of men and 0.4% of women reporting same sex contact in the previous year in a typical French study, with similar figures from Britain, Japan, Philippines, Thailand, Denmark and Holland with no study reporting figures as high as 10% when bisexuality is included. Gwen Broude (R82) points out the higher incidene of male homosexuality is consistent with the shotgun male reproductive strategy of trying to have sex with everything in sight. There is little evidence for a biological pattern of exclusive homosexual orientation in ape societies (p 66) nor in world societies in which male homosexuality is part of the social norm, from Greece (p 203) through Amazonia (p 149) to New Guinea (p 171), where Sambia males go through a period of obligate homosexual activity before entering marriage.

Deborah Blum in 'Sex on the Brain' (R65) devotes a chapter to differences in sexual orientation, aptly entitled 'the second date' for its quotable quote, attributed to Daryl Bem:

> *"There's a joke in the gay community that goes like this -*
> *'What does a lesbian bring on her second date?' - 'A U-Haul'.*
> *'And what does a gay man bring on his second date?' - "What second date?'*

Don Symons elaborated this into the theory that male gay behavior, rather than mimicking female behavior, is an extreme of where biology leads men without women - i.e. to sew male wild oats to oblivion. By contrast lesbian women display extreme nesting.

384

Left: Percentage of partners who were strangers. Right: Lifetime number of homosexual partners (R438).

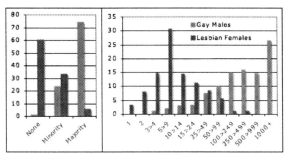

In studies, gay males and lesbian females do show diametrically opposite sexual behaviors, which conform strongly to the reproductive strategies of their own sex, rather than the implied gender reversal of their same-sex orientation. Gay men display a runaway-male pattern of sex with many strangers, while lesbians bond with established partners. This belies claims of gay men to be more 'feminine' sexually than heterosexual men. These sexual strategies of males and females are confirmed in heterosexual dating experiments, where women consistently refuse casual offers of sex from male strangers, conforming to the careful, choosy strategy, while almost all men offer to accept a sexual advance from a strange woman (R438 433). There is however a large difference between married heterosexual and homosexuals on whether love is central to a sexual relationship. 41% of married women and 27% of married men do not approve of sex without love, but only 19% of lesbians and 7% of gay men do so (R438 320).

Blum (R65) claims women seem to be more flexible sexually and more tolerant of sexual orientation. She reports that many lesbian women experience attraction to men but simply don't act on it. By contrast men tend to subdivide more into homophobic males and freely flaunting gays. Bem also considers the gay genetic influence may be about another personality trait than sexual orientation, which may cause social factors which predispose to sexual orientation, such as sex differences in play interest between classic childhood sex role play such as dolls and making house versus action games and sports, which themselves seem to be partially inherited. Edward O. Wilson also suggested gay men might favour survival of their relatives by helping with children and in cementing family ties. There is some evidence for this in ancient American Indian cultures and it might apply in matrilineal societies, where mother's brothers figure strongly in parenting without having to reproduce, but it is far from established generally.

Roughgarden (R580) suggests same-sex orientation is too frequent to be a genetic 'error' and proposes that social selection in the form of both same-sex and heterosexual bonding acts as a major filter to reproductive opportunity (p 55). However, only a few species use social sex profligately and often have purely non-sexual forms of grooming and amatory behaviour, so it remains unclear that a 'rainbow' of sexual orientations plays a significant role in reproductive advantage. Even in bonobos where socio-sexual bonding is abundant (p 66), it is only female socio-sexuality which is a significant selector of reproductive fitness.

	Incidence		Fecundity
	Maternal	Paternal	
Hetero (100)	0.000	0.013	2.3
Gay (98)	0.056	0.020	2.7

In 2004 Camperio-Ciani and co-workers (R133) discovered the 'fertile mother effect' - that female relatives of gay men had more children on average than the female relatives of straight men. But the effect was only seen on their mother's side of the family. Mothers of gay men produced an average of 2.7 babies compared with 2.3 born to mothers of straight men. And maternal aunts of gay men had 2.0 babies compared with 1.5 born to the maternal aunts of straight men. The effect accounts for about 14% of the incidence of gay individuals. This provides a resolution of the sexual paradox implied by the reduced heterosexual fertility of gay men - in Camperio-Ciani's words: "The same factor that influences sexual orientation in males promotes higher fecundity in females." Simon LeVay puts a genetically determinist spin on the idea this is a gene for overweening attraction to males: "This is a novel finding. We think of it as genes for 'male homosexuality', but it might really be genes for sexual attraction to men. These could predispose men towards homosexuality and women towards 'hyper-heterosexuality', causing women to have more sex with men and thus have more offspring." However the evidence doesn't necessarily indicate that this is a gene causing genetically deterministic sexual orientation but merely female fecundity. "There is no single gene accounting for these observations. It's a combination of something on the X chromosome with other genetic factors on the non-sex chromosomes," Camperio-Ciani says. He estimates that about 20% of the predisposition to being gay is caused by genetic factors, including the following birth order effect, to which he attributes 7%.

A male with one or more elder brothers is also more likely to be gay than a man with no siblings, only younger siblings, or with one or more elder sisters. Each additional older brother increases the probability of homosexuality by roughly 1/3. Since the most important variable is how many sons their mother carried before them (rather than how many older brothers grew up in their household), these data suggest a maternal effect on the developing fetus. The effect has now been reported in Britain, the Netherlands, Canada and the United States, and in many different samples of people. Ray Blanchard (Blanchard and Cantor R63), who has pioneered studies on the 'fraternal birth order effect' estimates that 1 out of 7 gay men can attribute their sexual orientation to this cause (see "The big brother effect New Scientist 29 Mar 2003 44-8). The best explanation concerns a set of three active genes on the Y chromosome called the H-Y minor histocompatibility antigens. One of these genes encodes AMH. What the other two genes do is not certain. They are not essential for the masculinization of the genitals, which is achieved by testosterone and anti-Mullerian hormone alone.

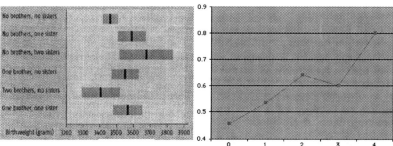
Effects of successive older brothers on birth weight and the probability of being gay from an equal population of heterosexual and homosexual men (New Scientist 29 Mar 2003 44-8).

These gene products are called antigens because they provoke a reaction from the immune system of the mother. As a result, the immune reaction is likely to be stronger in successive male pregnancies. Ray Blanchard, one of those who studies the birth-order effect, argues that the H-Y antigens' job is to switch on other genes in certain tissues, in particular in the brain and indeed there is good evidence that this is true in mice. If so, the effect of a strong immune reaction against these proteins from the mother would be partly to prevent the masculinization of the brain, but not that of the genitals. That in turn might cause them to be attracted to other males, or at least not attracted to females. Baby mice immunized against H-Y antigens grow up to be largely incapable of successful mating, consistent with this idea. Paradoxically, data from John Manning and Marc Breedlove with both gay men and those with older brothers suggests there is an increase in testosterone consistent with the idea that later male offspring may be primed to be more competitively physical.

Researchers have also noticed skewing in the usually random X-chromosome inactivation (p 342) when investigating 97 mothers of gay men with 103 mothers of heterosexuals. They found this in 23% of mothers with two gays sons, 14% of mothers with one but only 4% of those with none, although there appears to be no skewing in their daughters (New Scientist 6 Nov 2004 14). The article notes that such skewing is usually associated with genetic disorder but the mothers all appear to be healthy.

Whether of biological or socio-dynamic, origin, gay men and straight women appear to share stimulation of sexual centres when sniffing a male pheromone AND, by contrast with estrogenic EST, lavender, cedar oil, eugenol or butanol. PET and MRI scans revealed that the ordinary odours activated parts of the brain associated with smelling in all test subjects. But AND also excited the anterior hypothalamus and medial preoptic area of gay men and straight women alike, brain areas associated with sexual behaviour, as did EST for straight men. However the brain scans revealed no anatomical differences between any of the participant's brains (Savic et. al. R601). In a second study by Dr. Charles Wysocki due to appear in Psychological Science, gay men preferred the odours of other gay men and heterosexual women, but the smell of gay men were least liked by heterosexual men and women and lesbians, suggesting sexual orientation affects both pheromone production and responses.

In women, testosterone comes predominantly from the adrenals. Congenital adrenal hyperplasia, or CAH, and another associated condition, polycystic ovarian syndrome PCOS, in which ovulation fails to complete, result in increased testosterone levels in females. Mild 'symptomless' forms of the polycystic condition are 2-3 times as common in lesbian women, in whom a high proportion - up to 80% in one study (BBC) - display mild signs of the condition, suggesting a linkage between hormones and female sexual orientation. Otoacoustic emissions (faint clicks emitted from the tympanic membrane either spontaneously or in response to click presentation) are also more masculine (i.e., quieter) in lesbians compared to heterosexual women. A similar, effect is seen in the female twins of boys, a slight freemartin-like effect echoing the sterile androgenized twins of male calves which Frank Lillie correctly observed in a classic 1917 publication was due to male hormones altering a genetic female (Fausto-Sterling R201 163).

CAH is caused indirectly by a failure of 21-hydroxylase which the adrenal cortex uses to produce other steroids such as cortisol, causing an overflow of precursors to testosterone (p 351). With CAH as well, some researchers note changes of play in girls to more traditionally rough and tumble 'tomboyish' interests, forsaking "clothing, cosmetics, doll-play and infant care", even when the condition is hormonally corrected shortly after birth. These trends were found to continue in adolescence in "modeling, football, working with engines" as opposed to admittedly contrived 'feminine' traits such as "fashion magazines, cheer-leading or keeping a diary" (Campbell A R102 126). Those who are treated with hormones only later in childhood show male patterns of sexuality when they become young adults, including quick arousal by pornographic images, an autonomous sex drive centered on genital stimulation, and the equivalent of wet dreams.

Anne Fausto-Sterling (R201 75) critiques such studies as imposing expectations of gender biased behavior, questioning the lack of doll play because there was more interest in pets, stating that: "All in all, the results provide little support for a role for prenatal hormones in the production of gender differences". She extends this however to a professedly political position, working from an avowedly cultural constructionist feminist attitude toward sexual orientation, and lesbianism in particular, as if 'gender' itself is simply a social construct and there are as many 'genders' as human cultural 'morality' or transsexual and individual gender orientation will embrace. Simply equating the democracy of human equality with a genderless social construction fails to understand the critical issue about biological gender. Since we do have two sexes, evolution is likely to select for biological traits which, in their complementarity achieve a greater prospect of survival than any genderless social construction. Just as there is a danger in jumping overboard with political correctness in assuming male homosexuality is 'born in the genes', so assuming a political rejection of biology may commit cultural feminists to exactly the fate committed by patriarchs throughout history, who, in rejecting the completion of sexuality, while seeking paternity certainty, repressed woman and nature alike, by refusing to accept the healing power of natural sexuality on the human condition. Neither is it clear such 'political science' is good biological science.

Fausto-Sterling (R201 26) openly admits such a highly political position in regard to the gay gene research so avidly pursued by gay male scientists.

"A few years ago, when the neuroscientist Simon Le Vay reported that the brain structures of gay and heterosexual men differed (and that this mirrored a more general sex difference between straight men and women) he became the centre of a fire storm. Although an instant hero among many gay males, he was at odds with a rather mixed group. On the one hand, feminists such as myself disliked his unquestioning use of gender dichotomies, which have in the past never worked to further the equality of women. On the other, members of the Christian right hated his work because they believe that homosexuality is a sin that individuals can choose to reject."

Fausto-Sterling then pinpoints the issue central to her:

"politically the nature/nurture framework holds immense dangers ... In most public and scientific discussions, sex and nature are thought to be real, while gender and culture are seen as constructed. But these are false dichotomies".

She then cites trans-gender individuals, female genital mutilation, and sex-change operations, (while opposing some of these practices), as instances of the shaping of 'sex' by culture, as if this avowedly political position can be realized by 'affirmative' action.

Anne Campbell (R102 22) criticizes this political approach as deceptive:

"Many feminists have objected that the very questions posed by scientists are laden with tacit political agendas and that the scientific method can never be value-free. The solution they offer is for researchers to announce their politics at the same time as their results ... this has the side effect of allowing the reader to pick and choose in terms of the author's politics and to be prejudicially positive to articles that gel with their own agendas. Fausto-sterling for example writes of the difficulty she experiences in distinguishing between 'science that is well done and science that is feminine'. She is also surprisingly honest about the double standard that she employs in evaluating data which are not congenial to her ideological position: 'I impose the highest standards of proof for example on the claims about biological inequality, my high standards stemming directly from my philosophical and political beliefs in equality'. Theories that are not consistent with a feminist viewpoint usually fail to achieve this higher standard. Feminists are keen to promote high-quality research - but this claim is made difficult by their inability to distinguish between feminist science and good science. many feminist journals will refuse to publish data that are unacceptable to their ideological position. This state of affairs has already inhibited open debate among those who fear that they will incur feminist wrath, and if it continues, it will seriously jeopardize academic freedom."

Campbell goes on to note a fundamental issue about the pursuit of knowledge. "The postmodern rejection of grand theory (feminist theory excepted) which emphasizes close qualitative description of experiences and discourse which are contextually and historically bound. This effectively replaces theory with subjectively interpreted description. Since there are multiple possible descriptions of any event and no objective criterion for deciding between them the best one is the one that resonates with the feminist readers own experience and intuition" - but this invalidates any notion of validity outside one's own personal perspective, hence also any historical truth of men's oppression of women as well.

We have mentioned that biological gender may be a minimum energy solution which allows for natural slippage in transsexual and homosexual behavior. Orientation to the same sex is noted in many species besides humans. Certain male sheep seem to display a rigid orientation to other males, suggestive of a genetically imprinted effect. However one of our closest species, the bonobo uses frank homosexual engagement in sexual socialization. Females will engage sexual rubbing to orgasm and males sexually massage one another's genitals. The female clitoris has even evolved to facilitate mutual female-female 'coitus' called 'hoka-hoka' for its ecstatic cries. However here the context of sexual activity is manifestly psycho-social and not just reproductive. An entire troop may engage a sexual spree on sight of food and many of these homosexual encounters appear to be appeasement to reduce tension rather than driven by sexual appetite. Moreover this behavior fits naturally without conflict into the reproductive behavior of bonobo colonies. Although bonobos are genetically adapted to such behavior it is flexible bisexuality with a motive of reconciling tensions rather than committed exclusive attachment to the same sex.

In studies of human sexual orientation, a gulf separates culturally constructionist ideas of sexual orientation advanced in particular by some schools of lesbian feminist thought which see sexual orientation as a social choice and the professed enthusiasm the male gay community has for each discovery that suggests a 'born to be gay' genetic basis for exclusive homosexuality either in genetic or neuroscience discoveries. There is some justification to both these points of view. Twin studies of Bailey and Pillard show that a genetic component may explain 30% of both male and female homosexual orientation, familial influences another 20%. Bailey himself worried that the statistics might have been inflated by the fact that the respondents had been found through gay activist newspapers (Blum R65133). However the remaining cultural influence of some 50% is still the major factor and even though genetic influences may play an early formative role, we need to keep in mind the hallmark capacity of human adaptability is over and above all other species to retain a personal autonomy over our choices and fates. The evidence both from bonobos and our own physiology suggests this remains true for sexual orientation, despite genetic influences.

The Gatherer-hunter Cortex

Although women's brains are slightly smaller on average than men, Jill M. Goldstein and co-workers have found that certain areas in the frontal cortex and emotional limbic system, including the hippocampus, are relatively larger in women, while parietal regions dealing with spatial orientation and the amygdala dealing with emotional impulses are relatively larger in men. Moreover Sandra Witelson and colleagues have found that language areas in the temporal lobe and in the frontal lobes have a greater density of neurons in women (Cahill R98). Such variations are likely connected with steroids in development as they contain some of the highest levels of sex hormone receptors.

Doreen Kimura (R351), studying sex differences in the human brain notes broad differences in activities, contrasting spatial and linguistic ability, as well as mathematical reasoning.

Differences in incidence of aphasia after stroke are significantly different between men and women (Kimura R351).

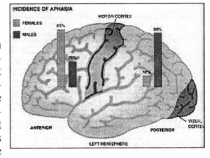

Women have on the mean, comparable (and often superior) intelligence to men. Females are generally more accomplished in language development and social maturity, particularly during adolescence, although men tend to have the edge in the mechanics of mathematical manipulation and spatial map reading (R351). In all of these, except mathematical manipulation individual differences are much greater than gender differences. These differences also reflect, to a degree, gatherer-hunter specializations of the two sexes.

Major sex differences in intellectual function seem to lie in differing patterns of ability rather than in overall level of intelligence. Men, on average, perform better than women on certain spatial tasks. Men have an advantage in certain spatial tasks, such as tests that require the subject to imagine rotating an object or manipulating it in some other way. They outperform women in navigating their way through a route. Map reading has become a cliché of gender difference. Further, men are more accurate in tests of target-directed motor skills-that is, in guiding or intercepting projectiles. They do better on disembedding tests, in which they have to find a simple shape, once it is hidden within a more complex figure and men tend to do better than women on tests of mathematical reasoning (R351). Deborah Blum jokingly comments "my favorite part of this is that the wonders of human math/spatial skills are based on sexual promiscuity" noting that map reading is not just for hunting but for keeping track of one's sexual partners. See also Geary (R231).

These maths skills differences appear to be real. The most comprehensive study published in Science in 1995 found that in maths and science in the top ten percent, boys outnumbered girls three to one. In the top one percent there were seven boys to each girl. By contrast in language skills there were twice as many boys at the bottom and twice as many girls at the top. In writing skills girls were so much better, boys were considered 'at a rather profound disadvantage' (Blum R65 58). This tallies with the less lateralized distribution of language in females, as the creative use of language may occur in the subdominant right hemisphere.

Women tend to be better than men at rapidly identifying matching items, a skill called perceptual speed. They have greater verbal fluency, including the ability to find words that begin with a specific letter or fulfill some other constraint. Women also out perform men in arithmetic calculation and in recalling landmarks from a route. Moreover, women are faster at certain precision manual tasks, such as placing pegs in designated holes on a board. In addition, women remember whether an object, or a series of objects, has been displaced. On some tests of ideational fluency, those in which subjects must list objects that are the same color, and on tests of verbal fluency, in which participants must list words that begin with the same letter, women also outperform men. And women do better than men on mathematical calculation tests (Kimura R351).

Deborah Blum (R65 56), following the research of Thomas Beaver, notes that there are two ways of following a route, using landmarks or calculating distances travelled and that women tend to navigate by landmarks 'the gas station past the furniture store' as opposed to 'turn left on 69 for 15 miles then right for a mile and left'. Beaver has found that, in both rats and humans, although males did better on featureless mazes; in tests where the distances were changed, but the landmarks were correct, females performed better than males. This difference in approach may be reflected in the larger hippocampus in women. There is some evidence gay men make more use of landmarks than heterosexual men (R550), although they also use male distance and direction strategies, but no evidence for a difference between lesbian and heterosexual women. The only measure on which they appear to shift is on language production or verbal fluency. Like straight men, lesbians tend to be more sparing with words than straight women. Gay men, however, are inclined to speak as much as straight women.

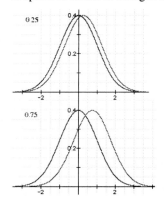

Effect sizes of 0.25 and 0.75
illustrated for a normal distribution

To compare the magnitude of a difference across several distinct tasks, the difference between groups is divided by the standard deviation. The resulting number is called the effect size. Effect sizes below 0.5 are generally considered small. There are typically no differences between the sexes on tests of vocabulary (effect size 0.02), nonverbal reasoning (0.03) and verbal reasoning (0.17). On tests in which subjects match pictures, find words that begin with similar letters or show ideational fluency such as naming objects that are white or red-the effect sizes are somewhat larger: 0.25, 0.22 and 0.38, respectively. Women tend to outperform men on these tasks. Researchers have reported the largest effect sizes for certain tests measuring spatial rotation (effect size 0.7) and targeting accuracy (0.75). The large effect size in these tests means there are many more men at the high end of the score distribution.

We have noted that women also have slightly smaller brains with slightly fewer cells on average, but all these features are in relation to the relative body size of women, and do not indicate any significant differences in mental capacity. There are also significantly different types of functional organization in the cerebral cortex between men and women. These are strongly illustrated in the differences in the aphasias which result from strokes in the frontal and parietal regions of the cortex (p 388).

One of the most outstanding studies of language is that of the Sally and Bennett Shaywitz, in which a series of language tasks were examined under functional magnetic resonance imaging. The tasks were subtracted to highlight language activity over other functional activity. They show the less lateralized language function in women very clearly. The

Gurs' studies on the resting brain (Blum R65 61) found male activity occurred more from the amygdala and women from the cingulate gyrus, two parts of the limbic emotional system, one ancient and reptilian and the other of more recent evolution, suggesting men are primed to react physically and women verbally. Contradicting these studies, Steven Petersen found little or no differences in region, although the male brains worked a little harder (R65 62). This increased activity may be correlated with the higher rate of cell death in males.

Sexual dimorphisms in language under letter recognition, rhyming and semantic category tasks, with a visual task as control, averaged over 19 males left and 19 females right, all right handed. By subtracting task fMRIs one can test for semantics or phonology alone (Shaywitz et. al. R623).

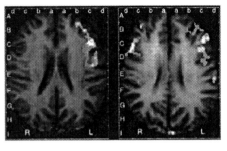

It is assumed by many researchers studying sex differences that the two hemispheres are more asymmetrically organized for speech and spatial functions in men than in women. Parts of the corpus callosum, a major set of axons connecting the two hemispheres, may be more extensive in women. Perceptual techniques that probe brain asymmetry in normal-functioning people sometimes show smaller asymmetries in women than in men, and damage to one brain hemisphere sometimes has a lesser effect in women than the comparable injury has in men. In 1982 it was reported that the back part of the corpus callosum, an area called the splenium, was larger in women than in men. This finding has subsequently been both refuted and confirmed. The view that a male brain is functionally more asymmetric than a female brain is long-standing. Androgens have been claimed to increase the functional potency of the right hemisphere.

In 1981 Marian Diamond found that the right cortex is thicker than the left in male rats but not in females. Jane Stewart, and Bryan E. Ko lb (R98), pinpointed early hormonal influences on this asymmetry: androgens appear to suppress left cortex growth. In the 1990s Marie-Christine de Lacoste and her colleagues reported a similar pattern in human fetuses (Kimura R351). They found the right cortex was thicker than the left in males. Thus, there appear to be some anatomic reasons for believing that the two hemispheres might not be equally asymmetric in men and women. Despite this expectation, the evidence in favor of it is meager and conflicting, which suggests that the most striking sex differences in brain organization may not be related to asymmetry.

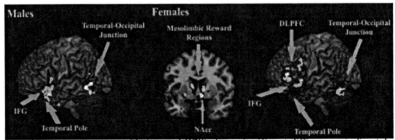

Responses to humourous cartoons (Azim et al.R29) show significant differences in frontal processing and a more decisive response in emotional centres when women appreciated the joke.

There are also significant differences in the way the two sexes respond to and process humour (Azim et al. R29) Males and females share an extensive humor-response strategy as indicated by recruitment of similar brain regions: both activate the temporal– occipital junction and temporal pole, structures implicated in semantic knowledge and juxtaposition, and the inferior frontal gyrus, likely to be involved in language processing. Females, however, activate the left prefrontal cortex more than males, suggesting a greater degree of executive processing and language-based decoding. Females also exhibit greater activation of mesolimbic regions, including the nucleus accumbens, implying greater reward network response and possibly less reward expectation. Women were more analytical in their response, and felt more pleasure when they decided something really was funny. "Women appeared to have less expectation of a reward, which in this case was the punch line of the cartoon, so when they got to the joke's punch line, they were more pleased about it." Women were subjecting humor to more analysis with the aim of determining if it was indeed funny. Men were prepared to laugh along with slapstick.

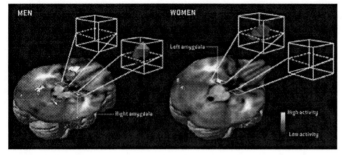

Response to an unpleasant experience, in the amygdala, differs between men, who respond in the right amygdala and are drawn to central features, and women who respond in the left amygdala and remember more of the context (R98).

There are significant limbic differences which reflect these trends. Males hippocampi appear to thrive on short-term stress but to succumb to long-term stress while females have the reverse pattern (Cahill R98). Emotionally stressful experiences also fire up the right amygdala in men but the left in women. This tends to make men acutely aware of central aspects of the situation while women are made more aware of the surrounding details and ambience. Men also tend to have significantly higher serotonin levels making them less liable to depression.

Tania Singer et al. (R631) analysed the brain activity of 32 volunteers after their participation in the Prisoners' Dilemma, which we know allows players to cooperate or double-cross one another, and so fosters camaraderie or enmity between them. Following the game, participants were placed inside an fMRI imager and saw their fellow players zapped with electricity. The scans revealed changes in activity as players who had cooperated got zapped, compared with those who had double-crossed them in the game. The results suggest that men get a much bigger kick than women from seeing revenge physically exacted on someone perceived to have wronged them.

Baron-Cohen (R42, R43) suggests the female brain is adapted to 'empathy' while the male brain is adapted for understanding and building systems. These differences are at least partly innate. Even at 24 hours after birth sex differences emerge with girls looking longer at faces and boys longer at inanimate mobiles. This appears to relate to pre-natal testosterone with higher levels correlating with less eye contact and slower vocabulary development at 12 and 18 months respectively. Of course parents tend to reinforce such gender stereotypes in their boys and girls often claiming male maths skill is 'a whizz' while female achievement is 'hard work', but the innate differences still appear to exist. Similarly the preference of boys for action toys and girls for dolls is reflected in similar choices made by monkeys (R98).

Serotonin levels are often higher in men, consistent with women suffering more from depression (R98).

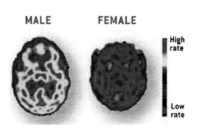

MALE   FEMALE

High rate

Low rate

The empathic factor also appears to relate to networking. In "The First Sex", Helen Fisher (R209) contrasts step-by-step analytic thinking, which discounts extraneous data to get at the essential principles, with a web-based associative networking mentality that gathers together disparate facts and nuances and integrates them into a coherent social process. Although both sexes do both, she claims from a host of studies that across disparate cultures, men more naturally assume the former and women the latter.

Many of the sexual differences found between women and men may be adaptions to gatherer hunter life. Good map reading is important for hunting in the wild. By contrast women are better at classifying a large number of similar objects in a space consistent with recognizing plants and tubers. These factors also relate to differing styles of social grouping between the male hierarchies and coalitions of females we find in ape societies, although here again both sexes can and do use both strategies. For example, although male chimps form hierarchies, and female chimps and bonobos form coalitions, female competition can also give rise to hierarchies, and male coalitions play an important role in dominance and competition. Women also often show a much more developed sense of place, developing a sustaining 'home' environment, while single men tend towards a more shiftless existence.

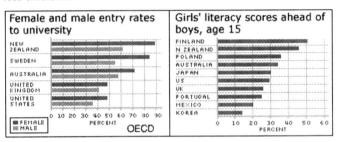

(a) Changes of educational trends from male preferential patterns have seen girls leap ahead in university admission rates. Compare figure (p 49) (b) Female adolescent literacy surpasses that of males (BBC 16 Sep 2003).

It seems clear that the sex differences in cognitive patterns arose because they proved evolutionarily advantageous. And their adaptive significance probably rests in the entire period of say 100,000 years during which Homo sapiens has emerged, and not just the cultural phase of the last 10,000 years, although this too will be having a cumulative effect. The organization of the human brain was determined over many generations by natural selection. As studies of fossil skulls have shown, our brains are essentially like those of our ancestors of 50,000 or more years ago. For these longer epochs during which our brain characteristics evolved, humans lived in relatively small groups of gatherer-hunters (p 83). The division of labor between the sexes in such a society probably was quite marked, as it is in existing hunter-gatherer societies (p 106). Men were responsible for hunting large game, which often required long-distance travel. They were also responsible for defending the group against predators and enemies and for the shaping and use of weapons. Women most probably gathered food near the camp, tended the home, prepared food and clothing and cared for children. Such specializations would put different selection pressures on men and women. Men would require long-distance route-finding ability so they could recognize a geographic array from varying orientations. They would also need targeting skills. Women would require short-range navigation, perhaps using landmarks, fine-motor capabilities carried on within a circumscribed space, and perceptual discrimination sensitive to small changes in the environment or in children's appearance or behavior. Men's hunting is often silent vigil, while women's gathering is frequently talkative and full of gossip which could explain some of the linguistic differences. Nevertheless both sexes and particularly men who are uncertain of their offspring depended on the grapevine and their intuitive senses of fidelity and betrayal to ensure their genes were passed on into the selective process.

In an ironic reflection of these differences, a study by the Pew Internet Project found that as of late 2005 roughly the same percentage of men and women in the US are serious internet users, but use it differently. Men value the net for the freedom it gives them to try new ways of doing things. By contrast women like the opportunities the net gives them to make and maintain human connections (*Gender gap alive and well online BBC 29-12-05*). "This moment in internet history will be gone in a blink," said Deborah Fallows, senior research fellow at Pew who wrote the report."We may soon look back on it as a charming, even quaint moment, when men reached for the farthest corners of the internet, trying and experimenting with whatever came along, and when women held the internet closer and tried to keep it a bit more under control." Yet these differences are older than culture itself.

Reproductive Technology: Utopia or Nemesis?

The future of human evolution and how it will be effected, both by the relationship between the sexes and new emerging technologies is a key question overshadowing all our reproductive futures. Major changes have happened to our entire reproductive profile as a result of effective contraception, choices in sex roles and careers, and increasing use of highly technological medical science, in fertility treatments, genetic testing, in-vitro fertilization and emerging new techniques such as germ-line engineering. These are issues that effect everyone, their hopes for a reproductive future for their progeny and the whole nature of what it is to be human. Changes in genetic technology are overtaking us so rapidly that there is a large risk of watersheds being crossed before we have even begun to consider their potential future implications. This chapter asseses these and their impact on our reproductive futures.

Human Evolution: Accelerated, Inverted or Extinguished?

Attitudes to the question of the current status of human evolution are varied. Some researchers have taken the position that we are still pretty much the same as the gatherer-hunters of 50,000 years ago. We have already discussed the differing time scales on which factors influencing human genetic makeup occurs, from the very long term trends in use of molecules such as prolactin, through gatherer-hunter traits in perception and sexuality to very rapid changes in allele frequency over cultural time scales. Simon Conway Morris for example considers effective weapons removed most of the threat of predators, and agricultural development beat back starvation, noting that the technological innovations that took place during the cultural period have been astounding with no sign that this was due to genetic changes. And that while we still haven't banished human hunger or disease from the planet, we are cushioning ourselves from many of the forces that shaped our biology for aeons.

Steve Jones says that culture and technology spelled the beginning of the end for evolution in its classic sense - natural selection of genes better suited to their environment. In the developed world, child mortality has declined drastically and family size tends to be small. Put simply, natural selection doesn't take place if everyone, regardless of the genes they carry, has two children who survive to reproduce. Jones also cites the low variation in human genomes. There is only about a 0.1 per cent difference between your DNA and that of any passerby, but among chimpanzees, the variation is at least five times that. Jones believes that modern life continues to chip away at the few remaining differences. For instance, mutations in the chromosomes of eggs or sperm become more common as parents age, but this source of genetic variation is disappearing because parental age is decreasing as couples tend to stop at two kids. What's more, in the past, some human mutations were preserved because they provided protection from disease. But as public health measures eliminate deaths from these diseases, the number of people who carry the mutation decreases. There is now also a great deal of mixing across the entire human gene pool, something which prevents the genetic isolation which makes species barriers able to emerge. With mutational fuel running low and the engine of natural selection idling, Jones concludes that our evolution is, at most, coasting slowly to a standstill. However, our genetic variability is still high enough to pose significant medical problems.

It is clear that genetic factors mean that new drugs often prove ineffective on a significant chunk of the population. Others such as Lynn Jorde consider that evolution is not slowing, but simply changing direction as new selective factors particularly associated with culture become the principal drivers. Agricultural developments may have made famine less frequent, he points out, but they have also caused people to live in larger, more densely populated areas, increasing the likelihood and impact of epidemics such as cholera and HIV. In addition, our frequent globe trotting has allowed disease organisms to hitch rides into even the most remote communities, presenting our immune systems with greater challenges. Science may have spawned medicine, but it has also unleashed an industrial and technological revolution that spews out radioactivity and chemicals that can contribute to an increase in our mutation rate-or act directly as selective forces.

Christopher Wills (R735) believes that as the deadly blows of past selective pressures disappeared, we began to be shaped by more subtle but equally persuasive forces and that rather than slowing us down, our culture has probably propelled us into developing at unprecedented speeds. Culture itself shapes our genes. In those societies where milk drinking is an ancient practice, for example, people have genes that allow them to digest the milk sugar lactose. People whose ancestors were not milk-drinkers tend to lack these mutations. Wills argues that today's globalisation increases the potential diversity of the human gene pool by bringing together such specialised versions of genes that had been separated through much of history to make new combinations that may never have been seen before. Wills argues that the major evolutionary influence of culture is to create new environments and select for human genetic diversity. Fine motor skills, for instance, may have been of less use when our ancestors were doing little more than smashing rocks. But in a more modern society you can benefit from both big muscles, and the delicate manipulations of a watchmaker. One talent of the human animal is to devise ever more exacting mental and physical challenges. Diversity itself can be selected for. Outside our species, for example, researchers have found that trees that are rare in forests reproduce more often than more common varieties. The thinking is that a sparse population gives species-specific parasites less of a chance to breed. Similarly rare traits are rewarded in our culture. Musical geniuses for example thrive precisely because they are exceptional talents and it is in intellectual and psychological areas that our culture generates the greatest advancement and diversity. Pivotal to this is evolution of the brain and the some third of our genes which are involved in this. Some genes also overlap the brain and other areas The dystrophin muscle gene, for example, which causes muscular dystrophy when faulty, is also expressed in the brain. So too are XRCC4 and Lig IV, which are involved in immunity. As a result, genetic changes that have improved muscle tone or our ability to fight disease could have had psychological or intellectual repercussions.

The influence of culture and particularly cultural attitudes to reproduction in an age of contraception bring us to the precipice of some searching questions. The decision not to have children, for example, has exactly the same evolutionary impact as losing a child through predation or disease. Do increases in the use of birth control select for better parents, because only those that really want children tend to have them? Or does it mean that a great many more children are born to parents who mess up their use of pills or condoms, selecting for parents who are less than careful, socially incompetent or maladjusted or less able to cope? On the other hand, selection against having children given choice might also be triggered by our genetic constitution. People who cope badly with stress in their lives often choose not to have children, so the effect may be a bloodless coup where those genes that allow us to deal with the stresses of modem life emerge victorious.

This brings us to a critical issue involving women and reproduction and the effects of culture. There has been a major trend in Western societies for women to seek careers and reduce or postpone their reproduction. This is partly associated with feminist rejection of the 'essentialist' role of mothering and partly to do with general attitudes to emancipation, equal opportunity and the unique skills women bring to the workplace. Such changes are certainly helping alleviate the population explosion as women in developing countries take the cue partly through television and seek smaller families, but it is also causing almost catastrophic declines in reproduction below replacement levels in countries from Italy to Japan, and here in New Zealand among middle class Europeans.

A study of 2710 female twins in a contemporary Western population in Australia by Ian Owens and others (Kirk et. al. R368) has elucidated several key heritable and cultural factors affecting female reproductive fitness. Cultural factors had a big impact on the women's fitness - 50 to 60 per cent of fitness is environmentally determined, but 40 to 50 per cent is genetic. Prominent among the cultural factors are education and religion. University-educated women have 35% lower fitness than those with less than seven years education, and Roman Catholic women have about 20% higher fitness than those of other religions. We can see here a striking negative relationship between educated women and reproduction and a positive one between religions advocating unrestrained reproduction and its incidence.

This leads to some dangerous conclusions - that both education, which also to some degree reflects genetic factors involved in intelligence (about 50% genetic 15% uterine, and the rest divided between family, peers and culture) and freedom from religious conformity are being selectively bred out of the human population. Such trends carry over to other major religions which actively encourage reproduction, such as Islam, as reflected in the high birth rates and large adolescent populations in Iran, Palestine, Saudi Arabia and other countries.

When the cultural factors of choice are taken aside and we turn to heritability, the conclusions are also striking. There is substantial heritable variation in fitness itself, with approximately 39% of the variance attributable to additive genetic effects, the remainder consisting of unique environmental effects and small effects from education and religion. The strongest genetic factor is a tendency of some women to begin reproducing earlier. Structural modeling, reveals significant genetic influences for all three life-history traits, age at menarche, age at first reproduction, and age at menopause, with heritability estimates of 0.50, 0.23, and 0.45, respectively. Strong genetic covariation with reproductive fitness was demonstrated for age at first reproduction. In later work they found that extroversion and neuroticism affected the 'fitness' score of women. And some 'social attitude dimensions' such as family values and militarism boosted fitness. These personality traits are about 50 per cent heritable and could contribute quite a lot of the genetic variance in fitness. It remains to be seen whether the family values were conservative or the shorter term reproductive investment strategy of sexually precocious girls growing up in single parent families.

Natural selection of this sort could have worrying implications. "If our results are correct, one would predict steady selective pressure toward earlier reproduction," says co-researcher Nick Martin, "and selection against women who delay childbearing, and the traits that currently drive women to professional success". So as society encourages women to have children later, the biological urge to have kids early could discourage them from having careers. "The genes are pushing in the other direction," says Owens. "There's a fierce conflict between a career and wanting to reproduce" (New Scientist 5 May 2001).

Part of the solution to this problem has to lie in a better recognition both by those in the business community, in government, feminists, and mothers themselves that Western society needs to find better ways of acknowledging and integrating careers with mothering. The two have remained in opposition party because of intransigence in the work place aided by cultural attitudes to sex roles which do not respect the importance of biological mothering. A social revolution is needed here towards an intelligent matricentric society if we are going to enhance, let alone retain our qualities of intelligence, astuteness and non-militaristic freedom of choice.

Another technological innovation, genetic testing, has the capacity to strip bare all our subtle evolutionary characteristics of female reproductive inscrutability and male philandering. Paternity testing, in one step, places a searing spotlight on female infidelity, as well as men who sew wild oats who are being sought by women or governments for compensation. The penalties for women in many countries are dire. If female reproductive choice has been a paramount catalyst for human cultural and intellectual emergence, we need to respect it, perhaps even safeguard it with the same aura of sacredness that patriarchal religions have given to male paternity certainty. Males need to develop a culture of tolerance towards female reproductive choice and a preparedness to support children who may not be their own in the interests of our reproductive future, as well as the welfare of their partners.

There is a rising tide of expectation that human assisted reproduction will bring in techniques of germ-line engineering for all sufferers of genetic disabilities that will remove defective genes and replace them with 'healthy' ones. This leads to a new form of utopian social eugenics in which virtually any trait, from the sex of a child, to their teeth, sexual orientation, extroversion, or love of sports, will be sought by prospective parents to enhance features they find desirable, resulting in frank destabilization of the human gene pool at the behest of human whim. They could also be used to eliminate counter-cultural traits. Genes in development and brain function are profoundly interactive. This leads to another dangerous scenario where our entire natural evolutionary paradigm - as an evolutionarily stable strategy will be replaced by an auto-creationist technological life-expectancy in which human survival becomes totally subject to the brittle instabilities of advanced technology.

Contraception, Abortion and the Divorce of Social Sexuality from Reproduction

Human fertility has throughout our evolutionary emergence been naturally regulated by the inhibition caused by lactation and regular demand feeding, which as we have noted in the !Kung (p 107) markedly reduces the number of children a woman will bear in her lifetime. The release of prolactin in turn suppresses progesterone production provided in is very regular. Societies have often also practiced forms of infanticide to avoid a new offspring becoming too burdensome on existing children to protect the overall parental investment in children who can survive and fend for themselves.

The Greeks, for all their patriarchal fetishism, were intimately familiar with female hormonal feedback mechanisms: Hippocratic aphorism V50 says "to restrain a woman's menstruation, apply the largest possible cupping glass to the nipples". V39 also: "If a woman who is neither pregnant nor has given birth produces milk, her menstruation has stopped. Caustic or blocking vaginal pessaries were known and used in the ancient world. The Egyptian Kahun gynaecological papyrus (1900 BC) prescribes hydrated sodium carbonate mixed with crocodile droppings. The Ebers papyrus mentions acacia gum. Many herbal abortifacients were also used in earlier times, such as penny royal or Queen Anne's lace, mentioned by Hippocrates and later by Aristophanes, as well as species of fennel, myrrh, Artemisia and rue. Eight out of ten plants mentioned by Soranus in the 2nd century AD for either contraception or abortion are now known to have distinct effects. Dioscorides also mentions a male contraceptive herb. Ayurvedic medicine mentions 28 plants useful in this respect (Taylor R670 86). Knowledge of medicinal plants appears to go back 40,000 to 100,000 years where plum stones and borage seeds have been found by the hearth (R670 108).

However now with the advent of modern 'scientific' forms of contraception, from the pill, through condoms, intra-uterine devices, to male or female tubal ligations, for the first time social sex between reproductively fertile partners has become functionally divorced from the reproductive quest (p 100). This is continuing to have far-reaching consequences and leads to deep evolutionary contradictions. At the same time the various techniques of abortion from the morning-after pill to late term partial birth terminations have created a near continuum, from contraception to infanticide which raises a host of new ethical questions that wrack society. While no one wants to see dehumanization of the value of life, the debate pits the rights of a mother against those of the child and patriarchal religious attitudes against the rights of a woman to make choices over her own reproductive life. Although there are obvious exceptions, particularly in an alienated society, mothers don't generally abort for fun or evil intent. Every woman in history who has aborted has risked her life and limb for a child a male has causally impregnated her with, at no risk to himself.

Not only has Christianity adamantly opposed abortion throughout its history, but contraception as well. Up to the Lambeth Conference of 1936, Christian churches, following the fecund pronunciation of Genesis 1 'be fruitful and multiply' have opposed all forms of contraception (O'Grady R502). Catholics, citing also the 'natural law' theory of Aristotle, Augustine and Aquinas vehemently oppose contraception to the present day, despite a world in population crisis which can't or won't look after all the children well that we are bringing forth. Although birth rates in traditional Muslim societies remain some of the highest in the world (p 421), most Muslim traditions permit the use of birth control, although the emphasis remains on procreation within the family.

In several developed countries, the reproduction rate, especially of successful career women, who by any sociobiological measure would normally be at a reproductive advantage, has fallen to catastrophic lows, so that many of the more socially successful genetic traits which would support the creative viability of future generations are likely to be lost. At the same time members of cultural sectors who have religious or social attitudes against contraception advocate unrestricted reproduction. Those who are too dysfunctional or incompetent to contraceive, now also tend to reproduce disproportionately. Against this trend, several societies from China, through India to Peru have embarked on mass campaigns to restrict human population, often discriminating against certain classes of people, including ethnic minorities.

These factors combine with the preservation of potentially non-naturally viable genes through IVF and other treatments to raise serious questions about the future viability of the human genetic resources of the human species. Thus one can speculate that all the beneficent factors leading to sexual selection of humanity as a species are rapidly being replaced by detrimental or disruptive factors likely to undermine our future viability.

Into the centre of this debate has also come an assault on the very link between social sexuality and human regeneration which has seen social sexuality take centre stage in moves to make any form of sexual connection between consenting adults of either sex on the same footing as reproductive 'marriage'. We are thus seeing a heightened polarization between religious traditionalists who see marriage and the reproductive family as central and social libertarians who see any form of discrimination even between social and reproductive sex as reprehensible. Just as all of us who read this book were born as humans, so the reproductive process is the foundation of human 'relationship' and of human society in its widest and deepest sense. The implications of sexual union, extend from passion and infatuation, to belonging, loving empathy, then to parental commitment and finally to the whole genealogical fabric of a people in time and space. Without this fabric the institutions of society become a corrupt exercise in personal gratification to no meaningful end.

Although we may make love some ten thousand times in a lifetime and have fewer than ten offspring, so more than 99.9% of our sexual connections are social, this doesn't mean social sex is simply sensual recreation for gratification or adult bonding alone. To define relationship simply in these terms, whether heterosexual or homosexual, is perilous. There is an urgent need to for humanity to redefine its values to take into account and respect the evolutionary paradigm and how sexual complementarity and the deep connection between social sexuality and the reproductive passage of the generations gives us the full dimensions of what human 'relationship' means in terms of the entire social fabric and why and how we continue to engage as a society of living biological beings into the future.

Caesarian deliveries are beginning to
overtake natural births

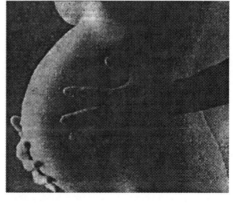

Surviving by Caesarian and IVF

Entering into such questions come a host of questions in reproductive technology and medical science which are transforming the very nature of the reproductive process and even our viability as a species. The first of these is the ancient art of the Caesarian section which goes back at least to Roman times. Although many of these ancient operations may have been lethal to the mother, Caesarians are now becoming so routinely common that they threaten to undermine the natural viability of human birth. The rates of Caesarian births are rising to epidemic levels partly for social or cosmetic 'designer deliveries'.

Gynecologists have predicted rates of over half live births within ten years, although other authorities seek to reduce current levels around a quarter of all births to the WHO guideline of 10-15%. This raises a huge issue of balancing individual needs against the future viability of the human race, if a majority of the population come to be delivered by unnatural means. The human delivery is already at the threshold of difficulty with head size. Human evolution has progressively delayed brain development to keep natural delivery viable as head size has increased. Caesarian delivery also leads to increased risks of complications in future pregnancies rather than the realtively greater ease with natural childbirth, as well as an increase of the still birth rate from 1.4 to 2.4 per 10,000.

More than half women having babies will opt for Caesarian deliveries by 2010 a leading British doctor predicts. Patient choice is all important to maternity care and given this "I believe efforts to reduce Caesarian deliveries are doomed" Professor Nicholas Fisk said the risks were finely balanced between Caesarian and vaginal birth. It was wrong to deny women the choice when research indicated attempting a vaginal birth could be riskier for the mother or the baby. But New Zealand health leaders sound warnings over the risks of a Caesarian delivery which they emphasized was a minor operation. There are still serious risks including a woman have a subsequent caesarian haemorrhaging so badly her uterus would have to be removed. Caesarians still carry a risk nine times higher than births. New Zealand's Caesarian rate has soared - in 1989 it was 12% but in 2000 it was 27% at National Women's Hospital, Australasia's largest, and in 1999 it was 45.8% at St. George's Hospital, Christchurch (Untimely from the Womb NZ Listener 25 Jan 2003). In the UK it is 25% (BBC Huge rise in Caesarian births Friday, 26 Oct 2001) and in some countries it is now up to 35%. The World Heath Organization recommends a rate no higher than 15% (*Caesarians Normal by 2010* NZ Herald 16 Mar 2000).

However, overall fertility is reduced in those who deliver by Caesarian section. A study of 25,371 women from 1980 to 1997 found that just 66.9% of mothers undergoing Caesarean section went on to have another pregnancy, compared with 73.9% of women who had spontaneous deliveries. They then took an average of 36.3 months to conceive a second child, compared with the 30.4 months taken by women who gave birth naturally. And they were more likely to suffer an ectopic pregnancy next time around, with 9.5 per 1000 pregnancies, than women with spontaneous delivery, who suffered 5.7 per 1000 pregnancies (Bhattacharya R61).

Women opting for a Caesarean also face a small chance that it will jeopardise later natural births. They face a slightly higher risk of serious medical problems, including tearing of the womb, Ohio State University researchers conclude based on a study of 46,000 women. Of the 46,000 women included in the study, about 16,000 chose to undergo a repeat Caesarean delivery, 12,000 had to have a Caesarean for medical reasons and 18,000 attempted a vaginal birth - 73% successfully. In the UK about a third of Caesarians are elective rather than because of a medical emergency (*Caesarean 'low birth risk link'* BBC 15 Dec 2004).

Rates of in-Vitro Fertilization, or IVF birth are rising precipitously. This process directly introduces into the human gene-pool genetic defects which will multiply and continue to plague future generations, resulting in perpetuated infertility and developmental abnormalities. This raises again a very serious question of balancing future human viability against individual rights and needs. Multiple births as a result are coming to dominate the population, with a huge increase of medical costs and genetic defects. Estimates of triplet births as high as 350,000 a year are conceived of in the US as a result, costing billions of dollars.

The developed world is facing a disastrous 'epidemic' of twin and triplet births. Changes to fertility treatments are being called for to prevent a huge increase in problem pregnancies and birth defects. Increased use of IVF is one reason for the rise in multiple births. "The incidence of multiple pregnancy after IVF in Britain is about 25 per cent. That is a real concern" says Robert Winston. Multiple births often occur after IVF because doctors transplant more than one embryo to make a successful pregnancy more likely. Another problem is that the drugs used to induce ovulation often make ovaries release several eggs at once. Multiple pregnancies are a problem for health services because they're plagued by complications. Babies are often premature, underweight and need expensive intensive treatment, and their mothers need more prenatal and antenatal care. Multiple births can also lead to neurological disorders, with triplets being 20 times more likely than singletons to have cerebral palsy. The epidemic of multiple births arising from fertility treatments escalated swiftly, experts warn. Between 1980 and 1997, the twin birth rate in the US increased by 42 per cent. Triplet and higher multiple births increased by 370 per cent. If current trends for triplet births continue, almost a third of all people born will be a triplet in some countries within a decade or so. In the US, triplet births could rise to around 350,000 each year. The figure for the health care costs is into billions and billions of dollars a year, not even counting the psychosocial costs for the families and for the triplets themselves (*Two's a crowd* New Scientist 14 jul 2001).

Benefits and Risks of IVF

Current techniques of IVF are causing concern because of the much higher fetal abnormality rates between two and three times ("IVF babies at risk of defects" NZ Herald 2002) as high as natural conceptions. Some of the reason for this is the frequency of multiple births which themselves lead to complications.

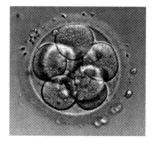

> One of the most comprehensive studies to date suggests that babies conceived by IVF are more than twice as likely to suffer major birth defects as babies conceived naturally. The controversial findings, which are the first to suggest such a high rate of malformations, come amid concern about the aggressive marketing and growing use of IVF in countries such as the US. No one knows whether the defects are linked to the factors that make couples infertile in the first place, or to aspects of IVF, or to both. But even with the increased risk, a couple who conceive after IVF or intracytoplasmic sperm injection (ICSI) still have over a 90% chance of having a healthy baby. Of the 837 IVF babies, 9% had major defects, such as a hole in the heart or a cleft palate. For the 301 babies conceived by ICSI, the figure was 8.6 %. By contrast, only 4.2% of the 4000 naturally conceived babies had major defects (*Test tube trauma* New Scientist 16 mar 02).

In a development which is rewriting text books, young healthy women donating eggs have been found to have chromosomal abnormalities including incorrect numbers of chromosomes (aneuploidy) in 42% of their eggs, leading to a recommendation that people undergoing IVF should have preimplantation genetic screening (PGS). Experts believe it might be that the drugs used for IVF that stimulate a woman's ovaries to produce eggs add to the risk of genetic damage. It could also be that defective eggs are common among the general population but are rejected early on by the body if they are fertilised as up to a third of conceptions are believed to misscarry early term (*IVF defects higher than expected* BBC 19 Oct 2005).

However ICSI babies appear to fare as well as the naturally born in development:

> The first study of ICSI children at age eight suggests children conceived this way are slightly more intelligent than normal, allaying fears that the technique is not as safe as standard IVF. Lize Leunens' team at the Free University of Brussels (VUB) in Belgium has compared the intelligence and motor skills of 151 ICSI children at age eight with those of 153 naturally conceived children. There was no difference in motor skills, and the ICSI children scored slightly higher on intelligence tests than those conceived naturally. There was no difference in the education levels of the mothers, which is known to influence children's intelligence, so Leunens thinks the most likely explanation for the finding is that mothers of ICSI children provide more stimulation (*ICSI kids become smarter than average* New Scientist 21 June 2005 Michael Le Page).

Further technical advances may take ICSI further towards chromosomal manipulation:

> Removing the tiny cap of potent enzymes from human sperm prior to the common assisted-fertility treatment, ICSI, could boost the efficiency of this reproductive technology, new research suggests (Stripped sperm may boost ICSI success rate Anna Gosline NewScientist 19 Sept 2005).

IVF babies are three times more likely to develop neurological disorders among the 50,000 babies currently born by IVF a year worldwide.

> Babies born after in vitro fertilisation (IVF) are three times more likely to develop neurological disorders including cerebral palsy than children conceived naturally, a study has found. Scientists believe the findings could be explained by the complications that often arise when two or more IVF embryos share the same womb, rather than because of the IVF techniques themselves. Dr Bo Stromberg, said the findings supported the view that only one IVF embryo should be implanted into a woman rather than the two or more routinely used in many countries. "We think that IVF is a good treatment and a vital option for couples who can't have babies naturally, but we have to think of a baby's life, and not just that of the couple" The study compared 5680 IVF children aged between 18 months and 14 years with 11,360 youngsters of the same age who were conceived naturally. Stromberg also compared twin births with single births. IVF in Sweden produces a relatively high number of twins because two embryos are routinely implanted into patients to raise the chances of a successful pregnancy. Worldwide,

there are about 50,000 IVF children born a year, yet next to nothing is known of any possible long-term effects on their health (*IVF babies at risk of defects* NZ Herald 2002).

A major survey in 2004 has focussed more on premature death and prematurity:

Children conceived by IVF are at greater risk of certain health problems, the first comprehensive analysis of medical data has found. Around 1% of babies in the US are conceived in vitro. Babies born after IVF are at least twice as likely to die at or soon after birth, or to be born prematurely or with a clinically low birth weight. Premature and low-birth-weight babies are thought to suffer more health and developmental problems later in life. The evidence also suggested that IVF children are at greater risk of some rare genetic abnormalities. Twins born after IVF were at no greater health risk than twins born conventionally. However, doctors know that bearing twins or triplets is itself linked to a range of long-term health problems, and that IVF boosts the risk of multiple births tenfold. The evidence does not show any increase in major birth malformations, cancer or psychological development. However, the cause remains unknown. One possibility is that the technique of fertilizing and growing young embryos in the lab somehow disrupts their normal development, resulting in problems later on. But it is also possible that infertile couples themselves are the source of the problem, perhaps because they pass on detrimental genetic sequences to their babies (*IVF health risks pinpointed* Helen Pearson Nature 20 October 2004 doi:10.1038/news041018-9).

Multiple implantation has been found to be unnecessary as well as potentially harmful:

Pia Saldeen and her colleagues at IVF Klinken CURA in Malmö, Sweden, examined the pregnancy rate in Swedish fertility clinics. In January 2003, health authorities in the country banned the transfer or more than one embryo at a time except in exceptional circumstances. Saldeen found that the rate of pregnancies after the legislation was just as high as it was before (around one-third were successful). [The pregnancy rate among those given single embryos and saving a second frozen embryo was 39.7%, compared to 43.5% in the double embryo group *IVF 'should use one embryo'* BBC 29 June, 2004,]. However, the frequency of twin pregnancies fell from 23% to less than 6%. Transferring a single embryo can still result in twins if one embryo splits naturally into two. Two studies from US fertility clinics mirrored the Swedish results. When otherwise healthy women were offered the choice of having one embryo implanted instead of two, pregnancy rates remained just as high (over 70%). The high rate of twins, triplets or higher multiple births is one of the most pressing problems in fertility treatment. Multiple births are associated with health problems for the mother such as high blood pressure, and increase the risk that their babies will be born prematurely or with low birth weight. The high rate occurs because doctors routinely place several embryos into the womb during treatment. This practice continues because both doctors and patients widely believe that it boosts the chances of pregnancy. "The challenge is to get people to accept it" (Big success for single embryos in IVF Helen Pearson Nature 22 October 2004 doi:10.1038/news041018-15).

PGD or pre-implantation genetic diagnosis has itself been found to present no problems:

Carrying out tests on embryos to screen for genetic disorders, does not harm their health, a large scale review of the procedure has found. The Reproductive Institute of Chicago study looked at 754 babies born after IVF pregnancies where preimplantation genetic diagnosis was used. It found they were no more likely to suffer birth defects than babies born after natural pregnancies (*Embryo screening 'no health risk'* BBC Wednesday, 18 August, 2004).

Advertisements for egg donors have been published on the internet and in several American college newspapers. The specifications include: height, 5 foot 10 inches, athletic build, high score on the test given to all college applicants, and no major family medical problems. The reward for the lucky winner, $50 000! 'Egg donation' has been banned in the UK because of the strain on a mother's health.

IVF watchdogs have ruled out a scheme that would allow women to have cheap treatment if they are prepared to do it twice and donate half their eggs. The Human Fertilisation and Embryology Authority (HFEA) says that 'egg giving' means a woman risks her health by having extra treatment for financial reasons (*Ban imposed on IVF egg 'giving'* 29 Nov 2003).

Pre-implantation Genetic Diagnosis

While finding an egg or sperm donor with certain characteristics might give prospective parents an edge in designing their children, a more predictable way to 'intervene' comes with genetic diagnosis before implanting an embryo produced through IVF.

[Robert] Winston, developed the technique of "pre-implantation genetic diagnosis" (PGD) in the mid-1980s using sex selection as a proxy for genetic testing for diseases, such as haemophilia, most of which are carried by women and affect only their sons. The technique has since been developed to detect a range of genetic defects. One or two cells are removed from an embryo at the eight-cell stage, amplified and then biopsied. Only embryos that are found to be healthy are then implanted in the uterus. Great expectations New Scientist 1 May 99 Arlene Judith Klotzko. A recent study has found the technique does not increase the risk of fetal abnormalities (*Embryo screening 'no health risk'* BBC18 August, 2004).

All IVF embryos should be checked for genetic abnormalities before the pregnancy is allowed to go ahead, say international genetic experts. A London conference on preimplantation genetic diagnosis (PGD) heard how this technique greatly increases the chance that a healthy child will be born. IVF pioneer "By selecting to transfer only a normal embryo, we fulfil our dreams to have a healthy child" Dr Verlinsky. Robert Edwards and PGD leader Yury Verlinsky also said couples should be allowed to choose a child's sex for "family balance". Critics strongly opposed these ideas. Both Life and Comment on Reproductive Ethics (CORE) said these approaches were unethical and discriminatory. At the Sixth International Symposium on PGD, Dr Verlinksy, famed for selecting a test-tube baby whose tissue matched that of a sick sibling, presented new results showing PGD increased the take home baby rate seven-fold. His team at the Reproductive Genetics Institute in Chicago looked at the pregnancy outcomes of 709 women undergoing IVF.Overall, PGD increased the chance that a woman would take home a baby from 11% to about 80%, due to fewer miscarriages and better foetal implantation rates. Dr Verlinsky said: "It should be implemented to all IVF cases. (*'Make IVF genetic screen routine'* BBC 19 May, 2005.)

New Scientist

IVF is blossoming into a potential central technique of choice rendering natural conception obsolete. A new technique of routine IVF by 'chip' combined with genetic testing for a battery of genetic defects could become so inviting for parents that its attraction could lead to it becoming standard for all births. Another reason potentially driving such a process is the extraction of a few cells to be kept as a clone for stem cell transplants or organ replacement clones with perfect genetic matching. Couples are flocking to use the technique simply to chooose the sex of their child, despite the risks to the woman of ovarian hyperstimulation, because it has higher reliability than sperm sorting (Westphal R726). Routine IVF and genetic selection could have a major irreversible effect on the gene pool, whose implications we have not begun to research. It will also render all conceptions potentially inviable naturally, through loss of the genes supporting natural conception over time as a result of lack of natural selection.

Children in future may be conceived and spend their first few days of development on a computer-controlled chip. In a move recalling Aldous Huxley's famous production lines in Brave New World, researchers David Beebe and Matthew Wheeler are building a 'chip' that can automatically carry out all the steps involved in IVF, from fertilising eggs to preparing embryos for implantation. Ultimately, such devices which amount to artificial reproductive tracts - may even be able to sort and test embryos for genetic flaws. Far more mouse embryos develop successfully on these devices than by traditional IVF methods. The work could be the first step towards a future in which IVF becomes the norm, says George Seidel "Fifty or 100 years from now, our in vitro procedures for parts or even all of pregnancy may end up being safer than dealing with the various things that occur in the body-in terms of viruses that the mother comes across, toxins, and so on." In conventional IVF, sperm and eggs are dumped into a Petri dish where the fertilised eggs grow until they're ready to be implanted. As embryos need different culture media at different stages, embryologists transfer them from one dish to another via a pipette. "In 48 hours, in the traditional Petri dish, none of them made it to the blastocyst stage. In our channels, about 75 per cent made it" says Beebe. "The embryos were transplanted into hosts and live pups were born. So there doesn't appear to be any detrimental effect" (*Brave New Babies: An automated IVF chip could lead to production-line embryos* New Scientist 26 May 2001).

Complementing this the procedures for whole genome genetic testing for signs of abnormality are advancing rapidly:

Within a few years it could be possible to boost the success of IVF by checking for major chromosomal abnormalities before embryos are transferred to the womb. "Potentially, this is a major advance," says Mark Johnson of Imperial College, London. At present, it is only possible to check a handful of chromosomes. But by adapting existing techniques, Joy Delhanty and

Dagan Wells of University College London were able to check all the chromosomes in 12 three-day-old embryos. Abnormalities were surprisingly common, Delhanty says. Only three of the 12 embryos had the right number of chromosomes in all their cells. The researchers used a technique called comparative genomic hybridisation (CGH). They compared the chromosomes from the embryos with ones from normal cells by staining them with different dyes. Any departures from the normal number of chromosomes, or any large deletions or insertions, show up as differences in the amount of fluorescence. Large amounts of DNA are needed for CGH, so Delhanty and Wells had to make many copies of a cell's DNA by improving on a second method known as whole genome amplification. At present the test takes three or four days- far too long for pre-implantation screening, says Delhanty. The time will have to be reduced to around 24 hours to make it practical, she says. "It'll be a year or two before it might be applied." (*Only the best* New Scientist 29 Oct 2000 13).

PGD is to become a tool of choice for avoiding genetically-inherited forms of cancer:

The Human Fertilisation and Embryology Authority UK approved the screening following a request from couples for IVF treatment. The watchdog said there was a strong chance of bowel cancer being passed from parent to child. One of the couples to win the right to have their IVF embryos screened said they were delighted with the decision. "We are overjoyed to have been given this chance, not only to do as much as possible to make sure our children don't have the gene, but to stop them passing it on." The technique is already used in screening for other disorders such as cystic fibrosis. But this is thought to be the first time it has been used for a disease that does not affect the sufferer until early adulthood.Dr Mohammed Tarannisi, director of the Assisted Reproduction and Gynaecology Centre in London, said the latest decision should have been 'put to a wider audience'. "We are still talking here about medical conditions that have serious implications, but we are talking about conditions that are not going to be there at the time of birth. These are conditions that may or may not develop 20, 30, 40 years down the line. Is this the right thing to do?" Dr Tarannisi has an application for a licence to test for breast cancer genes being considered by the HFEA. Josephine Quintavalle of Comment on Reproductive Ethics said: "It's a very big ethical step forward. "The HFEA has yet again taken a big ethical decision without consulting the public." She said it was moving down a slippery slope from what had started as intervention for only disease that threatened the viability of the embryo to diseases that might appear in adulthood. "We should be looking for medicines that cure not medicines that kill".

The combination of IVF and genetic testing makes it possible for couples who know they have a defect or who have a child with a potentially lethal defect which could be repaired using gene therapy from a healthy sibling's genes, to raise 'designer babies' either to escape a genetic flaw or as therapy for an existing child:

Six more couples plan to apply for permission to have a designer baby to save a sibling's life. The Human Fertilisation and Embryology Authority Britain's fertility watchdog insisted it had not opened the floodgates after Raj and Shahana Hashmi got the go ahead for embryo selection last weekend. The couple at the centre of the medical row say they are not 'playing God' by creating a child to save the life of their terminally ill son. Dr Simon Fishel, who is treating the Hashmis, said he had six other patients who were eager to -go ahead. (*Couples queue for Designer Babies* NZ Herald 2002).

A woman has chosen to have a genetically selected baby to ensure it does not develop early onset Alzheimer's disease which runs in the family. The child is now 18 months old and genetically 'safe'. The woman, who is 30 and has not been identified, may be unable to recognise or care for her daughter within 10 years. She and her family carry a mutation which causes the onset of Alzheimer's disease before the age of 40. However, the child, who is now about 18 months old, did not inherit the tendency to develop the disease. Researchers said the baby's birth marked the first time pre-implantation genetic diagnosis, as the technique is called, has been used to weed out embryos carrying the defect that causes early onset Alzheimer's (*Screening creates 'disease free' baby* BBC 27 Feb, 2002).

It also makes possible some very unusual forms of 'incestuous' parenting between brother and sister without genetic inbreeding:

A 62-year woman who this month became France's oldest mother has revealed that her brother was the biological father of the baby. The woman said she got pregnant using her brother's sperm and a donor egg, and that a second baby fathered by her brother a girl was born to a surrogate mother. The 62-year-old woman, identified in the media only as Jeanine, said she underwent treatment at a Los Angeles clinic and gave birth on May 14 in southern France. The woman told Le Parisian newspaper that her child was conceived from her brother's sperm and an egg donated by an American woman. The woman also said her 52-year old brother's sperm was used to conceive a second baby born in May with the same egg donor, who acted as a surrogate. Both babies live in Frejus with the woman and her brother, who share their house with their 80-year-old mother. Jeanine, a retired teacher, said she told the clinic that her brother was her husband. "We are both healthy in mind and body," she told the paper. "I couldn't pass on my genes because of my age, so I wanted to pass on his and give life so our line could continue." The woman and her brother are both single and had been childless. According to a 1994 French law., only couples can have 'medically -assisted procreation,' and the techniques are forbidden for menopausal women (*Mum at 62, pregnant by brother* NZ Herald June 2001).

Sex Determination and Sexual Imbalance

Humans across the planet have practised infanticide, particularly of girl children. The advent of abortion has drawn the lines of this battle right through the uterus. Female choice and its antithesis the right to life. Selective abortion has in turn become a battle-ground in which girl children become the overwhelming targets in countries from Saudi Arabia through India to China, Vietnam and Korea.

Now new technologies are making it possible for people to have selective conception and take the battle out of the ovary and into the IVF apparatus. The impact of such techniques in the West leads to planning of balanced families, but can lead to runaway selection for boys, just as abortion in turn has.

The first of these two techniques is a high quality version of sperm sorting:

> Hundreds of couples are using a medical technique to choose the sex of their children, many for social reasons. The 'sperm sorting' procedure, which allows gender selection before conception, is particularly valuable in avoiding passing on genetic illnesses that usually affect only boys, such as haemophilia and muscular dystrophy. But Dr Harvey Stern, of the Genetics and IVF Institute in Fairfax, Virginia, said that of 200 couples who had used the procedure, 40 per cent had done so for non-medical reasons. Many of his patients, who paid E1400 ($4625), were seeking to 'balance out' families. 'There are concerns that some parts of the world would use it only to have boys ... We only do this for balancing families, not for a first child.' The Human Fertilisation and Embryology Authority, which regulates IVF and sperm donation in Britain, said the technique was legal, but it opposed using it for nonmedical reasons. Sperm are sent through a sorting machine one by one and stained with dye. A laser is then shone on each sperm to measure its fluorescence and the larger ones are separated out. Because "female" sperm are slightly larger, carrying 2.8 per cent more DNA, it is possible to sort them out before conception (*Sperm sorting and gender choice* NZ Herald July 2001).

The second is much more expensive and has close to 100% reliability, but involves IVF to select and then implant a single fertilized embryo known to be of the desired sex (p 401).

> Launching what he claims is the "world's first 100 per cent guaranteed baby sex selection project," British gynaeoologist Paul Rainsbury is unbothered by criticism that he is playing God. Dr Rainsbury offers parents the chance to choose the sex of their unborn child by embryo selection for the equivalent of about $25,000. Using existing in-vitro fertilization (IM technology, his clinics in Riyadh, Saudi Arabia and Naples, Italy, will take eggs and sperm from the couple, fertilise the eggs in a laboratory, then choose an embryo with the preferred sex to implant in the womb. Dr Rainsbury said the sex of the fertilised egg is evident after about 48 hours. The rate of live births will be the same as those for IVF. The difference is that the sex of any foetus that is born is '100 per cent guaranteed.' In Saudi Arabia, they love it." Dr Rainsbury said his clinics have a place in a world where sex selection is already commonly practised but in cruel and inhumane way, the result of pressure to produce a male heir in many parts of the Middle and Far East and Africa. 'Around the world tens of thousands of babies, whose only crime was being born of the 'wrong' sex, are deliberately abandoned to starve and die.' (*Doctor's happy playing God* NZ Herald 19 Mar 1997).

PGD confirms a run of one sex does not arise from a genetic predisposition (p 96) although hormones, social ranking and stability of relationships do bias the sex ratio (p 95).

IVF and Heritable Defects

Most studies of IVF suggest there is no increased risk of birth defects compared with natural conception although a rare defect Beckwith-Wiederman syndrome is increased 9-fold to 1 in 4000 (Holding R317 2004). Some techniques of IVF such as intra-cytoplasmic sperm injection ICSI appear to cause higher rates of malformations (New Scientist 12 July 2003 18) including Angelmans syndrome . ICSI is specifically prone to generating infertility which is passed down the generations, resulting in the dissemination of defective genes and unstable chromosomes, which undermine natural human viability. In some cases these are already known to create deleterious effects in future generations, but are still used because parents assume their offspring can also rely on the technology.

Since its introduction in the early 1990s, controversy has dogged the IVF technique called intra-cytoplasmic sperm injection. ICSI involves injecting a single sperm into an egg and is used mainly when men cannot fertilise an egg because their sperm count is too low or their sperm abnormal. A series of recent studies has associated ICSI with infertility in children, chromosomal abnormalities, birth defects and delays in mental development. The latest research suggests that children created by ICSI have a raised risk of being born with Turner's syndrome or ambiguous genitalia. For roughly 5 per cent of men seeking fertility treatment because they have few or no sperm, the cause is a tiny mutation in the Y chromosome called a microdeletion. As long as the man still produces a few sperm, however, it is sometimes possible to inject one directly into the egg. One of the reasons ICSI is controversial is that if there's a genetic reason for the man's infertility, it will be passed on to his sons. Many couples are prepared to use ICSI anyway, arguing that it will also be available to their children. But evidence suggests that microdeletions on the Y chromosome are a precursor to more serious genetic faults. Ken McElreavey found that in eight men with microdeletions, Y chromosomes were missing in about 10 per cent of the cells in their bodies. In the three who had enough sperm to test, up to 18 per cent of the sperm lacked a Y chromosome. These findings suggest that the microdeletion is a sign of a chromosomal instability that causes some cells to lose the entire Y chromosome, The loss of the Y chromosome in some of a baby's cells-called genetic mosaicism can cause either ambiguous genitalia or Turner's syndrome, or both. Women with Turner's have normal female genitals, but they are unusually short and do not go through puberty. Men with Y chromosome microdeletions make up just a small fraction of those using ICSI, but they might be largely responsible for offspring with Y chromosome losses. If so, then the technique may be too risky to use on them. David Page from MIT reports (NS 22 jun 02) the results of treating 26 men who were infertile because of a deletion in their Y chromosome. Of these, 11 were able to have children thanks to ICSI, but all 10 sons inherited their father's deletion-which probably means they will be infertile when they grow up, Page says (*Genetic roulette: A small problem for a man can become a disaster for his children* New Scientist 15 dec 2001).

A warning has also been issued over heritable failures of correct imprinting in men with a low sperm count who use IVF (Lancet 363 1700):

In a study led by Mario Souza, one in four of 96 men with low sperm count had imprinting faults in H19 a gene which switches on the growth factor IGF2 important for placental growth. Imprinting conditions include Beckwith-Wiedemann syndrome, which causes too much growth and is linked with an increased chance of tumours, and Angelman's syndrome, which affects the development of the brain. No such errors were found in 27 men with normal sperm.

There are some notable exceptions to the heritability of ICSI. Men with an extra X-chromosome can father normal children from selected sperm:

Several men with a serious genetic fault have been able to father normal children thanks to the controversial IVF technique known as ICSI. Men with Klinefelter's syndrome have an extra X chromosome. While many don't know about the condition until they discover they're infertile, others have symptoms such as mental retardation. Since the men cannot produce viable sperm, for the past few years Zev Rosenwaks's team has been retrieving immature sperm directly from their testicles. The best-looking ones are used to fertilise eggs from their partners using ICSI, or intracytoplasmic sperm injection, in which a sperm is injected into the egg. Rosenwaks told a conference in Montreal last month that 9 of the 15 patients with Klinefelter's treated this way have managed to have children. All 14 babies have a normal number of chromosomes, even though some parents refused pre-implantation genetic diagnosis to ensure that this was the case. The result is surprising because there's concern that ICSI allows genetic abnormalities to be passed on to the next generation. His team is also using the method of retrieving sperm directly from the testicles to help men unable to father children after chemotherapy (*Men with extra X chromosome father normal children* New Scientist 22 jun 2002).

Declining Fertility, Feminization of Nature and Ephemeral Males

Such techniques exist in a context where there are fears that male fertility is declining, even without the intervention of such processes. Some have attributed this to the 'feminization of nature' associated with environmental pollution with estrogenic industrial chemicals (Cadbury R97, Colborn et. al. R126) with widespread effects on wildlife, from fish to frogs.

A study of 7,500 men attending the Aberdeen Fertility Centre suggests average sperm counts have dropped by 29% in 14 years. While the fall may be a result of more men coming forward for treatment, doctors are concerned by the findings. The results of the study were presented at a British Fertility Society meeting in Liverpool. In one of the biggest studies of its kind, researchers analysed nearly 16,000 semen samples taken from men attending the clinic between 1989 and 2002. They found that the average sperm count of men attending the clinic had dropped sharply. "The drop in sperm counts must cause concern": Dr Siladitya Bhattacharya In 1989, the average sperm count of men with "normal" amounts of sperm in their semen was 87 million sperm per millilitre. By 2002, that had dropped to just over 62 million sperm per millilitre (*Fresh fears over men's fertility* BBC 5 Jan 2004).

There are several other features of this picture causing concern, including fewer men with healthy sperm, smaller testicles with more fibrous tissue, increasing testicular cancer. Many agents from tobacco to marijuana, and physical activities like riding a racing bike can also cause damage to sperm and the sperminal apparatus. At the same time there is confirmation that chemical pollutants thought harmless destroy male fertility in mice:

> Pressure to control the pollution of drinking water by oestrogen and compounds that mimic the female sex hormone is growing following two worrying discoveries. Last week, Finnish scientists published the most convincing evidence yet that sperm production by men in industrialised countries is declining. Among the men who died in 1981, 56.4 per cent had normal, healthy sperm production. By 1991, however, this figure had dropped dramatically to 26.9 per cent. The average weight of the men's testes decreased over the decade, while the proportion of useless, fibrous tissue increased. The incidence of testicular cancer is increasing every year, and in Denmark now affects 1 per cent of young men. Meanwhile, an American team has found that octylphenol, an oestrogen mimic which is a breakdown product of a detergent used in the manufacture of paper, textiles and plastics, that pollutes many rivers, but which was thought to be relatively benign, can render male rats infertile within two months (*Fresh Alarm over Threatened Sperm* New Scientist 11th Jan 1997).

Difficulties over measuring sperm counts and regional and seasonal fluctuations add to the dilemma of gaining an accurate picture. In a 1996 study sperm counts in the US appeared to have increased and there was a trend following overall fertility rates as well. However regional differences may confirm environmental effects.

American men are not suffering from declining sperm counts. What's more, sperm counts are closely correlated with birth rates. Fisch's findings contradict those of European researchers, who have been amassing evidence for a worldwide decline in sperm counts. Fisch renewed sperm counts of 1283 men who banked sperm between 1970 and 1994 before they had a vasectomy, in Los Angeles, Roseville in Minnesota, and New York City. He found a statistically significant increase in New York and Minnesota and a slight but not statistically significant increase in California. The average sperm count rose from 77 million per millilitre

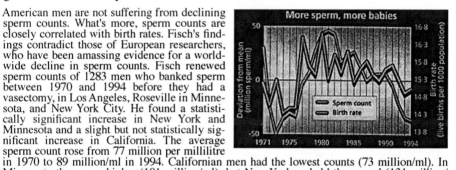

in 1970 to 89 million/ml in 1994. Californian men had the lowest counts (73 million/ml). In Minnesota they were higher (101 million/ml), but New Yorkers held the record (131 million/ml). But Fisch also points out that variation from one year to the next could be greater than the variation over 25 years. The study that first put men on alert was Skakkebaek's huge multi-study analysis, in which he looked at the data from 61 sperm count studies in the medical literature since 1930, covering 14 947 men. He found that between 1940 and 1990, sperm counts fell by 60 per cent on average, and he concluded there was 'a genuine decline in semen quality' (*Panic Over Sperm Counts May be Premature* New Scientist 11 May 1996).

The effects on male fertility also appear to be reflected in a small but noticeable decline in male birth rates, which may also be related to pollution as the Seveso dioxin disaster caused a profound shift to only daughters in the most contaminated couples.

> Male fetuses are generally less likely than females to come to term: although 125 males are conceived for every 100 females, only about 105 boys are born for every 100 girls. In the first half of this century, improvements in prenatal care reduced the number of miscarriages and stillbirths and hence increased the proportion of baby boys in most industrial countries. But since 1970 the trend has reversed: in the U.S., Canada and several European countries, the percentage of male births has slowly and mysteriously declined. So far the decrease has not been alarmingly large. In the US in 1970, 51.3 percent of all newborns were boys; by 1990, this figure had slipped to 51.2 percent. But in Canada the decline has been more than twice as great, and similar long-term drops have been reported in the Netherlands and Scandinavia. High exposures to certain pesticides may disrupt a father's ability to produce sperm cells with Y chromosomes-the gametes that beget boys. Other toxins may interfere with prenatal development, causing a disproportionate number of miscarriages among the frailer male embryos. (XY embryos require hormonal stimulation to produce masculine genitalia, which may make the unborn males more vulnerable to hazardous chemicals.) Perhaps the most striking example of a lopsided birth ratio occurred in Seveso, Italy, where a chemical plant explosion in 1976 released a cloud of dioxin into the atmosphere. Of the 74 children born to the most highly exposed adults from 1977 to 1984, only 35

percent were boys. And the nine sets of parents with the highest levels of dioxin in their blood had no boys at all (*Where have all the boys Gone?* Sci Am Jul 98 13).

An enigmatic diving of the male reproduction rate has been found at Aamjiwnaang community next door to the Sarnia-Lambton Chemical Valley complex in Ontario (McKenzie R450).

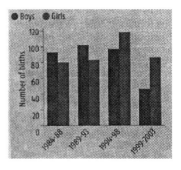

Similar depression of boys has been found in highly pollluted areas of Brazil. In the least polluted areas 51.7% of the babies born were male - but in the most polluted areas the percentage of males born decreased to 50.7%. In an experiemntal test on mice, males from a filtered air environment produced offspring with a 1.34 male/female ratio, while males that had been exposed to polluted air produced offspring with a 0.86 male/female ratio. Separate research found that pregnant mice exposed to air pollution were more likely to miscarry than those breathing filtered air.

The sex ratio can also be affected by stress in the mother. After 9-11, even as far away as California, in December 2001 there were 2% fewer males than expected and 29% fewer low-birthweight males, indicating premature loss of small male embryos by stressed mothers (R109). One can thus also see a basis for changes in the sex balance towards girls associated with lower classes in hypergamy (p 30).

More generally, several factors are combining to reduce the fertility of both human sexes:

Infertility is set to double in Europe over the next decade, a leading UK fertility expert has warned. One in seven couples now has trouble conceiving naturally, but Professor Bill Ledger from Sheffield University warned this could rise to one in three. He told a European fertility conference that women should be offered career breaks so they could have children younger, when they are more fertile. The incidence of chlamydia, a sexually transmitted infection which carries a risk of infertility, has doubled over the last decade - and 6% of girls under the age of 19 are currently classed as obese. A potential rise in male infertility could also affect couples, Professor Ledger said. Both the quality and quantity of sperm appeared to be in decline. "The sustainability of the population of Europe is at risk because there are too few children being born. It is a threat to the future." (*'Infertility time bomb' warning* Michelle Roberts BBC 20 June 2005).

Infertility however is increasingly a man's problem:

Infertility may be becoming more of a man's than a woman's problem, new figures suggest. Until now, both were level pegging - 40% of cases linked to men, 40% to women and 20% to joint problems. However, the European Society for Human Reproduction and Embryology found rates of an IVF treatment typically used to help male infertility have risen. It said a number of factors including declining sperm quality due to environmental toxins may be involved. Use of ICSI (intra-cytoplasmic sperm injection), in which a single sperm is injected into the egg to fertilise it, made up only 43% of IVF cycles in 1997, but accounted for 52% of cycles in 2002 (*Male infertility 'is increasing'* BBC 23 June 2005 Michelle Roberts).

As a potent reminder, high fertility in mid-life is associated with a sub-population of women who have exceptional anti-ageing DNA repair systems:

The very few women who have children after the age of 45 may be capable of doing so because anti-ageing mechanisms are more active in their bodies. Neri Laufer's team at Hadassah University Hospital in Jerusalem recruited eight women who had given birth naturally after the age of 45. His team compared levels of gene expression in the women's blood from with levels in six mothers of the same age who had chosen not to have any more children after 30. They found differences in 716 genes. Intriguingly, many of the genes that were more active in the fertile over-45s are involved in repairing DNA damage and preventing cell death. All the women were ultra-orthodox Ashkenazi Jews, but Laufer says preliminary results from a study of Bedouin women suggest the results apply to all (*Fertility in middle age linked with anti-ageing* New Scientist 21 June 2005 Michael Le Page).

Phytoestrogens can also have unforseen effects in women. Although the isoflavones in soya are both believed to reduce prostate cancer and reduce male virility in Asian countries, (NZ couples copulate around 144 times a year on average but Japanese only 35) soya phytoestrogens can also make sperm too 'frisky' too soon:

Women should avoid eating too much soya if they are trying for a baby, a UK fertility expert believes. A study in humans has shown the genistein in soya sabotages the sperm as it swims towards the egg. Professor Lynn Fraser, from King's College London, said even tiny doses in the female tract could burn sperm out. The compound kick-started a reaction in a large proportion of the sperm that gives them the ability to fertilise an egg. In real life, this does not usually happen until the sperm have been inside the female for some hours and are close to completing their long swim towards the egg (*'Avoid soya if you want a baby'* BBC 21 June 2005 Michelle Roberts).

The Three Parent Child and The Sexual Chimaera

A variety of techniques additional to IVF, involving various of forms of reproductive germ-line engineering, are emerging. These have major implications, because the genetic changes induced are heritable and will continue down the generations and be mixed with natural genes during sexual exchange. The techniques include mitochondrial transfers, fertilization with transplanted nuclei including stem cells, spermless fertilization using a second female haploid set, and even inter-sex chimeras. There are already scores of children in the US born by some of these techniques particularly those with genes from three parents, by injecting including mitochondria from another female to boost defective ones in the mother. There are about 30 children in the US who have already become germ-line genetically modified humans.

Scientists have confirmed that the first genetically altered humans have been born and are healthy. Up to 30 such children have been born, 15 of them as a result of one experimental programme at a US laboratory. The oldest of the children turns four in a month. But the technique has been criticised as unethical by some scientists and would be illegal in many countries, including the United Kingdom. Genetic fingerprint tests on two one-year-old children confirm that they contain a small quantity of additional genes not inherited from either parent, from the mitochondria of an egg from another female. The children were born following a technique called ooplasmic transfer. This involves taking some of the contents of the donor cell and injecting it into the egg cell of a woman with infertility problems. The additional genes were in mitochondria taken from a healthy donor. As many as 100,000 float in the cells cytoplasm (*Genetically altered babies born* BBC 4 May 2001).

But there was an outcry when the first two of the attempts had to be terminated because of genetic abnormalities.

The American doctor who trumpeted a fertility technique using three genetic parents failed to disclose that along with 15 healthy babies, it produced two fetuses with a rare genetic disorder. Experts are horrified because the fault can be passed to future generations. Dr Jacques Cohen denounced as 'hysterical' growing criticism of his claims that the research posed no risk. "Many of the techniques I carry out in America are illegal in Britain but that does not mean they are immoral." 27 infertile couples who could not conceive through IVF took part in the programme, in which an infertile woman's egg is mixed with her husband's sperm and parts of a younger woman's egg. In 30 attempts, 15 babies were born. Their maternal genes came from their true mothers and all appeared completely healthy. The researchers concluded there was no reason to believe the technique was harmful to foetuses or babies. But what Cohen's team failed to reveal was that though 15 babies were born, 17 foetuses were created. The first unborn foetus was aborted and the second miscarried after both developed a genetic anomaly called Turner's Syndrome, a rare disorder in which an X chromosome is missing. Two out of 17 far exceeds normal statistical expectation (*Gene Technique Faulty* NZ Herald May 21 2001).

The US acted within two months to ban the free use of this technique.

Does manipulating an egg prior to IVF turn it into an 'experimental product' that has to be regulated like a new drug or medical device? Yes, says the US Food and Drug Administration. This month, the agency wrote to several fertility clinics warning them that any treatments that genetically alter egg cells or embryos would constitute a 'clinical investigation' and so fall under the agency's authority. The announcement will effectively prevent clinics using a controversial technique known as 'ooplasmic transfer' (*US puts its foot down on tinkering with IVF babies* New Scientist 21 Jul 2001).

However a variant of the technique has since been used (unsuccessfully) in China following the techniques of an American team using the nuclear transfer commonly used in cloning.

A woman has become pregnant through a procedure that combines a controversial IVF method with one of the techniques used for cloning. But the fetuses that resulted, although they did not survive to term, were certainly not clones. In fact, they had three genetic parents. The procedure involves transferring a fertilised nucleus from the mother's egg to an egg from another woman. Any child born this way would inherit the vast majority of its genes from its mother and father, like a normal baby, but the handful of genes found outside the nucleus, in the cell structures called mitochondria, would come from another woman. The latest work was done

408

by John Zhang's team at the Sun Yatsen University of Medical Science in Guangzhou, China, with the help of Grifo's team. The donor eggs were emptied of their nuclei, and a fertilised nucleus from the woman's eggs transferred into each one. Five of the resulting embryos were implanted, resulting in a triplet pregnancy. Doctors reduced this to twins, but one fetus died at 24 weeks, and the other at 29 weeks (*IVF creates fetuses with three parents* New Scientist 18 oct 2003 12).

A variant of this technique has been approved in the UK:

UK scientists have won permission to create a human embryo that will have genetic material from two mothers.The Newcastle University team will transfer genetic material created when an egg and sperm fuse into another woman's egg. The groundbreaking work aims to prevent mothers from passing certain genetic diseases on to their unborn babies. (*Embryo with two mothers approved* BBC 8 Sep 2005).

An improvement in this technique has come from inserting mitochondria from other ovarian cells from the mother, however this may perpetuate the mitochondrial genetic defect:

Injecting a woman's eggs with fresh supplies of power-generating mitochondria from the egg of another woman is known to boost the success rate IVF. But there's a serious ethical hitch: any resulting embryos contain genetic material from three different people. Now doctors from Taiwan have isolated cumulus cells, which normally nestle around developing eggs in a woman's ovary, and extracted the mitochondria from these. They injected up to 5,000 mitochondria into each egg, 5% of the total number they already contain. They then fertilized the eggs in the lab, allowed them to grow into embryos and implanted them into the woman's uterus. Of 71 attempts, 35% resulted in a pregnancy and 20 babies were born. By contrast, only 6% of attempts without mitochondrial injection had previously resulted in pregnancy in the same group of patients, none of which had reached term. By contrast, with egg cells which remain quiescent in the ovary, cumulus cells are regularly refreshed so their mitochondria carry fewer defects.

Previous attempts to pep up women's eggs with fresh mitochondria have all suffered from ethical and safety concerns. One method, called cytoplasmic transfer, involves injecting cytoplasm and mitochondria from a healthy woman's egg into the egg of an infertile woman. The US Food and Drug Authority banned this technique in 2001 (except in clinical trials), because of concerns that it raises the risk of children suffering genetic abnormalities. There are also ethical concerns about creating an embryo containing the genetic material of three parents: the mother, the father, plus the small amount of DNA harboured in the donor woman's mitochondria. A related experimental, and also contentious, technique involves transplanting the entire nucleus from an infertile woman's egg into the egg of a healthy woman that has been stripped of its own nucleus. Because this technique replaces all the mitochondria in the egg, it could be used to help women whose own mitochondria carry a genetic disease that might be passed onto their children. A group in China revealed that they had tried this last year (Egg injection boosts fertility Helen Pearson Nature 20 October 2004 doi:10.1038/news041018-10).

.BBC

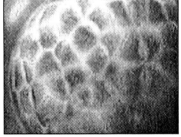

At an extreme of identity blending, a sexual chimaera has been created containing cells of both sexes which would produce a hermaphroditic individual of two differing genetic identities at the cellular level. The long term aim of this is to prevent genetic diseases by introducing cells from another genetic source in the hope of compensating for genetic abnormalities. However it raises fundamental issues of a Frankenstein-like nature

An experiment in the United States has created a mixed-sex human embryo. The team insists that the creation of an hermaphrodite human embryo was designed to cure illness, but critics say moral and ethical standards have been breached. The process creates a 'chimaera' - a blend of two embryos, each of which would have a distinct genetic identities. Any attempt to produce such a baby would provoke a worldwide ethical storm. In experiments using donated embryos, scientists from the Centers for Human Reproduction in New York and Chicago have taken the first step - and found that, in some cases, the introduced cells do proliferate and spread throughout the chimeric embryo. Their hope is that having even a small proportion of cells from a healthy embryo might prevent certain genetic diseases from arising .However, other experts have dismissed the idea as "deeply flawed" - and say research into the issue, even in animals, should not continue. Any use of chimeric technology in human reproduction in the UK is illegal (*'Merged embryo' cure hope attacked* BBC 3 July 2003).

Such chimeras are by no means unknown in the human population. Some individuals have been found to consist of two genetically-distinct merged cell lines as a result of non-identical twins becoming integrated at an early embryonic stage. If both are of the same sex, this will result in a normal individual but cause sexual abnormalities and infertility if it occurs between a non-identical brother-sister twin chimaera. Such individuals can also confound paternity testing because some of their tissues display one genetic identity and others another. Most of us may in fact be micro-chimeric as a result of perfusion of individual cells both between a mother and child in-utero and between two normal twins. Such perfusion may actually help to avoid a mother developing immunity to her offspring (Ainsworth R3).

However scientists and ethicists are deeply concerned about the prospect of inheritable germ line engineering:

> Attempting to rearrange genes and create future generations of perfect human beings is dangerous, irresponsible and should not be permitted now, a panel of United States experts says in a report. A committee of the American Association for the Advancement of Science has called for the creation of a public committee to monitor and oversee the increasingly sophisticated research into genetic modification. "This would widen the gap between the. 'haves' and the 'have nots' to an unprecedented extent" the report said. The committee report. Evidence to the committee showed IGM research was not yet safe to use on humans. For each triumph there could be scores of animals born with terrible and usually lethal genetic problems (*Inheritable Human Genetic Modification Opposed* NZ Herald 20 Sep 2000).

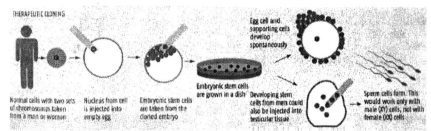

Therapeutic reproductive cloning from stem cells New Scientist 10 May 2003

Demise of the Egg and Sperm

Into this already heady mix enters the idea that we don't need an egg and a sperm at all to have effective fertilization several steps of this types of reproductive engineering have already ben taken. The most outstanding of these is to prime a stem cell to convert into a surrogate ovarian follicle (Westphal R724, Johnson et al R335, Pilcher R530):

> Last week, researchers in the US reported that they had transformed mouse embryonic stem cells into mature eggs in the lab, and a Japanese team has produced sperm in a similar way. Worryingly, more eggs will also be a boon to those who want to create living clones. Making eggs and sperm also has huge potential for helping infertile couples. It would depend on therapeutic cloning to generate embryonic stem cells, something that has yet to be achieved with human cells. But if that does happen, it could enable couples who cannot make their own eggs or sperm to have children who are a mixture of their genes, just like those conceived in the old-fashioned way. Yet these couples need not be old-fashioned couples. Some eggs in the latest experiments came from male stem cells. If the same can be done in humans, a gay couple could supply both egg and sperm to create their own child. That prospect will no doubt outrage some. It would certainly require a rethink of the laws covering parentage. But before this ever happens, we need to have a clear picture of the risks to any offspring born from artificially created eggs and sperm. Recently, a number of small studies found that IVF children have a higher risk of defects caused by errors in imprinting, the process by which genes in the embryo are switched on or off. The inability to generate the right pattern of imprinting has thwarted all past attempts to create artificial eggs and sperm. It is also the reason why cloning is so difficult and the rate of abnormalities in clones is so high (*Brave new IVF* New Scientist 10 May 2003).

In a follow-up news release (New Scientist 13 Dec 2003 19) mouse embryos were made by fertilizing eggs with immature sperm cells made from embryonic stem cells. It remains doubtful whether these have the correct imprinting to give rise to viable embryos. In the same issue (14) frozen sperm stem cells were successfully used to rear live pups.

> Researchers are very close to creating sperm outside of the body for the first time. The feat has already been achieved with eggs. It was accomplished with cells originally derived from mouse embryos, but most experts see no reason why the technique would not work with human embryonic stem cells too. If human eggs and sperm created this way are healthy - and it is a big if - the implications for reproductive technology and regenerative medicine would be immense. Intriguingly, eggs form from both female (XX) and male (XY) ESCs. That is because mammalian germ cells will go down the egg route unless signals produced by the testes tell the cells to become sperm. This is also why getting ESCs to turn into sperm is more complex. However, a team led by Toshiaki Noce at the Mitsubishi Kagaku Institute of Life Sciences in Tokyo may already have succeeded. According to a document found by New Scientist, the team allowed male mouse ESCs to develop spontaneously into various different types of cell, and picked out those that had begun turning into germ cells. These cells do not develop far in culture, but when Noce's team transplanted them into testicular tissue he found after three months that they had undergone meiosis and formed what appeared to be normal sperm. The critical next step would be to fertilise the artificial eggs with normal sperm, or use the artificial sperm to fertilise normal eggs. The big question is whether the resulting embryos will have normal imprinting and develop into healthy baby mice (*Stem cells can become 'normal sperm'* Sylvia Pagán Westphal New Scientist 7 May 2003).

More recently stem cells have been made into precursorsor of both sex cells:

> Human embryonic stem cells have been coaxed in the lab to develop into the early forms of cells which eventually become eggs or sperm, UK researchers have revealed. Work by several groups has shown that a tiny proportion of human embryonic stem cells (ESCs) spontaneously develop into primordial germ cells when allowed to differentiate in a dish. In this latest study, Behrouz Aflatoonian and colleagues at the University of Sheffield, produced primordial germ cells which began to express the proteins characteristic of sperm cells, while others resembled eggs (*Further steps towards artificial eggs and sperm* 20 June 2005 NewScientist Michael Le Page).

The therapeutic cloning technique to create eggs is deceptively simple. Extracting stem cells and growing them under high density causes them to adapt naturally to form the most basic unit of mammalian perpetuity the ovarian follicle, complete with an ovarian cycle, and can even be induced to 'ovulate' using lutenizing hormone:

> The mammalian egg, the cell that holds the secret to fertility, cloning and cell rejuvenation, has been created outside the body for the first time. Researchers are very close to creating sperm in a similar way. The feat was accomplished with cells originally derived from mouse embryos, but most experts see no reason why the technique would not work with human embryonic stem cells too. If human eggs and sperm created this way are healthy - and it is a big if - the implications for reproductive technology and regenerative medicine would be immense. Most immediately, a cheap, limitless supply of human eggs would greatly accelerate research in keys fields such as infertility and therapeutic cloning. The method used to create eggs from embryonic stem cells (ESCS) was astonishingly simple. Instead of searching for chemicals that coax ESCs into becoming eggs, as many have attempted, Hans Schuler's team at the University of Pennsylvania just let mouse ESCs grow at high density. In these conditions, some of the cells form floating aggregates most scientists would discard as useless debris. But team member Karin Hilbner instead placed the clumps in new dishes. "In four days they proliferated like crazy," says Schuler. The aggregates seem to behave like miniature ovarian follicles in which small cells nurture a bigger cell that forms an egg. Further studies by the team revealed that these egg-like cells form by meiosis, and switch on the same key genes as normal eggs as they develop. The follicle-like structures make hormones such as oestradiol in amounts that rise and fall on the same time scale as the menstrual cycle. Adding a hormone called gonadotrophin triggers the expulsion of the egg cell into the culture dish, mimicking ovulation (Science, DOI: 10.1126/science.l083452). Intriguingly, eggs form from both female (XX) and male (XY) ESCs. That is because mammalian germ cells will go down the egg route unless signals produced by the testes tell the cells to become sperm. This is also why getting ESCs to turn into sperm is more complex. However, a team led by Toshiaki Noce at the Mitsubishi Kasei Institute of Life Sciences in Tokyo may already have succeeded. According to a document found by New Scientist, the team allowed male mouse ESCs to develop spontaneously into various different types of cell, and picked out those that had begun turning into germ cells. These cells do not develop far in culture, but when Noce's team transplanted them into testicular tissue he found after three months that they had undergone meiosis and formed what appeared to be normal sperm. Both teams have yet to perform the next, crucial step: fertilising the artificial eggs with normal sperm, or using the artificial sperm to fertilise normal eggs.

Other more meticulous methods have also been used achieve 'artificial' eggs which could also be fertilized without sperm:

> "Birth of a miracle" Soon you may not need eggs or sperm to have children of your own New

Scientist 7 Jul 2001 Men and women who can't produce sperm or eggs could one day have 'natural' children of their own thanks to a form of cloning. Gianpiero Palerino of Cornell University in New York has created artificial human eggs that contains just one set of a would-be mother's chromosomes. Such eggs could be fertilised with the partner's sperm, just like a normal egg. And in Australia, Orly Lacham-Kaplan of Monash University in Melbourne has shown that you can fertilise eggs, not with sperm, but with cells taken from elsewhere in the body. But there are still considerable obstacles to overcome before either technique could be used to create human babies. The trouble is that we inherit not just genes, but chemical marks, or imprints, that turn some genes off. Chromosomes taken from body cells have different patterns of imprinting to egg and sperm cells, and that could cause developmental abnormalities. This may be why some clones have problems (*The next IVF revolution* NS 10 may 2003).

The technique involves persuading a normal cell to go through a process of simulated meiosis to form an egg with only one set of chromosomes. It could also enable same-sex couples to parent their own genetic children, terminating the intrinsic complementarity of the sexes:

A technique that uses cells from the body, rather than sperm, has been used to create embryos in mice. A way to fertilise human eggs without using sperm threatens to make men redundant. The technique which uses cells from any part of the body, rather than sperm has already been used to create embryos in mice. The research by Melbourne's Monash University aims to help men who have no sperm, or even sperm-raking cells, to father babies that are their own genetic offspring. But it could help lesbian couples to have baby girls that are genetically their own. Research team member Dr Orly Lacham-Kaplan said the sperm-free technique could, in theory at least, enable a lesbian couple to have a baby, with one woman contributing an egg and the second a cell to fertilise it. There are theoretical problems to overcome in combining the genes of two women, because aspects of development are controlled by a paternal gene when a maternal copy is turned off, and vice versa, as a result of a process called imprinting (p 346). "But we have no proof yet that it is or is not a problem," Dr Lacham-Kaplan said. Her team has succeeded in "fertilising" a normal mouse egg by using an artificial gamete, a cell taken from the body of a male. This is remarkable because, unlike sperm, the body cell has two sets of chromosomes. To overcome that problem, the team exploited cellular machinery used by an unfertilised egg to eject a spare set of chromosomes when it meets sperm. During normal fertilisation, two sets of chromosomes in an egg are separated and one set is ejected in a package that biologists call the polar body, leaving a single set to combine with another set from the sperm. After 'fertilisation' of the mouse egg, the team used chemicals to persuade the egg to carry out the steps typical of normal fertilisation: it released its spare set of chromosomes into a polar body, only this time the body cell also expelled its spare set into a second polar body. The embryos go on to develop fairly normally in the laboratory and the team is about to transfer them into the wombs of mice (*Spermless fertilization* NZ Herald July 2001).

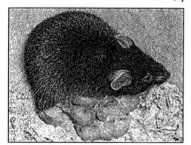

Parthenogenic mouse is a fertile mother Kono (R377)

The potential barriers of sexual imprinting (p 346) have already have been breached with the successful production of mice born without fathers through manipulation of oocyte imprinting, one raised to adulthood and bearing live offspring (Loebel and Tam R411, Kono et. al. R377):

Scientists have created two female mice without fertilising the eggs they grew from, the journal Nature says. The eggs had two sets of chromosomes from two female mice, rather than one from the mother and one from the father as in a fertilised embryo. Some researchers say the procedures may be applied to stem cell research, but the scientists who carried out the work say it would not yet work in humans. Tomohiro Kono and colleagues switched off a key gene in the donor eggs which affected imprinting - a barrier to parthenogenesis in mammals. By blocking expression of a gene called H19 in the immature mouse eggs associated with female imprinting, the researchers increased the activity of another gene called Igf2 expressed in males (p 347). Igf2 manufactures a protein responsible for regulating growth in the developing foetus. These genes are sexually imprinted. The team injected the genetic material from the genetically-modified mouse eggs at an immature stage when maternal imprinting is thought to be erased into mature eggs with their own set of female-imprinted chromosomes. They then 'activated' the combined eggs, prompting them to start growing as an embryo. As a result of this modification, just two out of 598 mice embryos made it to full term. One of the surviving mice was used for testing, while another, which the researchers named Kaguya after a Japanese fairy tale character, was allowed to grow into an adult (*Rincon P. Mice created without fathers* BBC 21 April 2004).

Sex on Ice: Transplanted Generations

The use of frozen embryos has already resulted in children being born from eggs kept on ice. This leads to the possibility of offspring being awakened centuries after they were conceived.

A mother has given birth to what are believed to be the first twins to be born in the UK from frozen eggs. Isabella and Anna Fahey were born three weeks ago from eggs which had been kept in deep freeze storage at the Midlands Fertility Services (MFS) for two years. Their mother Margaret McNamee's own eggs were fertilised by her partner Michael Fahey's sperm. An MFS spokeswoman said only about 300 babies have been born worldwide from frozen egg fertility treatment (Twins born after two years on ice BBC 11 October 2005).

There are a series of moves underway to separate our sexual organs from our bodies, so that defective organs can be stimulated to produce live sex cells, cancer patients who will be rendered infertile can save reproductive tissue so that women in careers can save frozen ovarian tissue to reawaken their reproductive capacity after their natural span of fecundity. Fertilized embryos can also be saved for later implantation. Sperm frozen for up to 21 years have been used to sucessfully father children. A woman has become pregnant naturally after slices of frozen ovarian itssue were reimplanted after 6 years because of cancer treatment (New Scientist 3 Jul 04 4). A woman has had her ovary transplanted on to her arm after an operation for cancer of the cervix so that she can later conceive by IVF.

Technologically simplest is transplantation to a refrigerated environment:

Career couples in New Zealand who want to put their fertility on ice will keenly watch developments across the Tasman. The Royal Women's Hospital in Melbourne announced this week that it would freeze the embryos, eggs and ovarian tissues of couples who decide to delay starting a family for life-style reasons. But after an angry response from family and church groups, the hospital's divisional director of surgery, Dr John McBain, said an ethics committee had yet to approve the proposal. Dr Fisher said there was plenty of time to construct an ethical framework for delaying fertility, because more research was needed. One in 10 frozen embryos implanted resulted in a pregnancy, but the use of ovarian tissue was still experimental (*Fertility on Ice still ethical dilemma* NZ Herald 9 Sep 98).

The first (natural) human birth has taken place from frozen ovarian tissue:

A cancer patient made infertile by chemotherapy has, in a world first, given birth after revolutionary treatment, Belgian doctors say. Ovarian tissue from the Belgian mother, 32, was removed and frozen seven years ago before chemotherapy, then re-implanted into her pelvis last year. She conceived naturally and gave birth at Brussels' Cliniques Universitaires Saint-Luc this week, Lancet reported. Researchers said all young women with cancer should be offered the treatment (Woman left sterile gives birth BBC 23 September, 2004).

Transplanted tissue has been used to successfully rear live young in monkeys:

Scientists in the United States have produced the first live birth from transplanted ovarian tissue. Scientists from Oregon University removed part of the ovary in a rhesus monkey and transplanted it to another part of the body. When eggs matured on the transplanted tissue, they were collected in fertilised in the lab. The embryos were transplanted back into the womb and one developed into a healthy baby monkey (*Fertility first with tissue transplant* BBC 13 Oct 2003).

Men can also transplant their testicular tissue into rodents and produce mature sperm:

A scientist in Japan claims that he has used the testes of rats and mice for this purpose. The first fertilisations of human eggs from rodent-reared sperm could come within the next few weeks, he says. Sofikitis took spermatogonia from infertile men and injected them into the testes of rats and mice that had been specially bred to have defective immune systems. Along with the human spermatogonia, he injected cells from the recipient rodent's eye. These cells-from the fluid just in front of the lens-secrete a protein called fas ligand, a signalling molecule that triggers immune cells to commit suicide. This eliminated the last vestiges of an immune response and allowed the spermatogonia to take, Sofikitis says. Sofikitis gave the injections to 10 rats and 8 mice. Five months later, he detected large numbers of mature human sperm in three rats and two mice. In one rat, he found fully motile sperm "with better motility than that of many fertile men" (*Of Mice and Men* New. Sci. 13 Feb 1999 4).

Some of these rat sperm have claimed to have already been used to sire human offspring and measures are underway to provide the same process for eggs:

Women may soon have a better way of saving their eggs Within the next year mice will be incubating the eggs of women who risk damaging their ovaries because of medical treatment, say Canadian scientists (*Mice to the Rescue* New Scientist 1 July 200). The team has already successfully harvested human eggs from the back muscles of rodents. Ariel Revel who leads the team developing the technology, says it "offers new hope" to young women who become infertile after vital medical intervention, such as cancer treatment. The development is sure to be controversial. There was an outcry last year when Italian embryologist Severino Antinori claimed to have produced four babies using sperm grown in rats' testes (New Scientist, 27 March 1999, 5).

Transplantation of ovarian tissue which has a shorter life span in humans is also underway:

Tokyo Japanese and United States researchers claimed a world first yesterday in transplanting human ovaries into mice, creating altered rodents that might produce human eggs. Scientists obtained the ovaries from three US women who had them removed for womb diseases. Approval was received from the university's ethics committee and the women gave consent. They dissected the ovary tissue into square pieces measuring just 2mm across. A total of 108 pieces were then injected into nine mice under the skin of the abdomen. Researchers injected hormones into the rodents to stimulate the growth of the ovarian tissue, which includes primitive human cells capable of developing into a mature ovum. After about two weeks some of the transplanted lines of human tissue developed into 'cumulus oophoms,' sacs which are the first stage in development of ova. 'We need to find out how we can nurture eggs from that stage. The basic idea was to create an egg bank for patients suffering infantile cancer who may survive into their adulthood md want to have a child' (*Inserted Ovaries* New Scientist 1 May 99

Parenthood now occurs in 'defiance of metaphysics' - through the use of frozen eggs and postmortem extraction, dead people are becoming parents. Sperm have been used to father children after a man's death sometimes without 'consent' from the corpse itself, or from frozen sperm banks:

In 1999 in California, a baby girl was born after sperm had been extracted from her dead father. "Great expectations" New Scientist 1 May 99

Taking sperm from a corpse in New York state may soon be possible only if the man gave written consent before his death. A bill before the state legislature would also ensure that only the dead man's spouse or partner could request sperm retrieval. The bill marks the first serious attempt to regulate America's private fertility clinics, which are effectively governed only by the scruples of the doctors involved. 'What's disturbing is that an individual could be posthumously the parent of a child that he never had any intention of creating' (*Life after death* New Scientist 21 Mar 98).

Increasing demand for fertility treatment and stem cell research means hundreds of thousands of human eggs are being sought worldwide. Women from vulnerable socio-economic backgrounds are being exploited by being offered financial compensation for their eggs. Sharing the surplus eggs produced by a woman undergoing IVF treatment to become pregnant for use by other women, or for research can provide enough eggs without donation. Egg doning is also not without its risks, including maternal hypertension and hormonal over-stimulation OHSS.

A rare, but potentially fatal, risk of IVF treatment and egg donation is ovarian hyperstimulation syndrome (OHSS), caused by the drugs that are used to make the ovaries produce more eggs than normal. In mild and moderate cases, affecting up to 20% of women undergoing ovary stimulation, this leads to symptoms such as swelling and breathlessness that resolves. However, in about 1% the symptoms can become so severe that they are deadly. However the risks of death during a pregnancy remain much higher than the risks with IVF treatment (*Safety of egg donation 'unclear'* 30 Jun 2005 BBC).

At 29, Jackie Rushton was happily married, and she and her husband decided they wanted to start a family. But after two years of trying with no success, they decided to seek help and opted for IVF. Women undergoing IVF treatment are given hormone injections to make their ovaries produce more eggs than normal, which can then be harvested, fertilised in the lab and transplanted into the womb. "On the seventh day of her treatment she was showing signs of overstimulation already. "She was very bloated and she could hardly walk. She was very sore. But she just thought it was part of the treatment and that it would be worth it to have a baby. Doctors then noticed Jackie had higher than expected hormonal levels - a warning that OHSS was developing. However, it was decided that treatment should go ahead and doctors were able to collect 33 eggs - far more than the numbers normally harvested after this treatment. "After that she was very sick. From then on, every day she got worse. The fluid pushed up into her lungs. "I got a dreadful fright when I saw her. She looked so frail, like a wax doll in the bed." Jackie's lungs became too weak and she died (*'IVF treatment killed my daughter'* 30 June 2005 BBC).

It has now been discovered maternal hypertension is halved if a sister is used as the donor:

Pregnancy-induced hypertension, which can be fatal, occurs more often in women needing donor eggs to conceive. A Korean team have found the risk is 5.4-fold higher if the egg comes from an unrelated donor - but only 2.2-fold if it comes from a sibling. Eggs donated by a sister are more likely to be genetically similar to the woman's own eggs than those from a stranger. The immune system is likely to play an important role in PIH in these women. Dr Sun Hwa Cha and colleagues looked at 61 women who they helped to become pregnant in their clinic using donor eggs and IVF treatment. Pregnancy-induced hypertension (PIH) is thought to occur in around 10% of pregnancies. When it is more severe, and called pre-eclampsia, it can be very serious, killing between three and five women and 500 and 600 babies a year in the UK (*Donor eggs from sisters are safer BBC 21 June 2005 Michelle Roberts*).

Germ-line Engineering a Brave New Universe

The greatest threat to our own evolutionary paradigm comes from precisely the area containing the greatest visionary utopian potential. At stake here is not just a question of human ethics and freedom of choice but the very principles upon which the survival of living species depends. Each species which survives is part of an unbroken genetic web which runs from the beginning of life on earth. It survives because its reproductive process is an evolutionarily stable strategy which is also robust to change and fluctuation over evolutionary time scales. Our social structures are already becoming unstable to slighter and slighter disturbances, with food production depending on modified species which cannot survive in the wild and sophisticated networks of information and transport, the failure of which could cause most of the world's population to die out overnight .

There are immense pressures from those who harbour deleterious genes and who wish to have children to invoke techniques of gene manipulation which will free their offspring from such defects. Leading on from this there are those who believe we have left the age of natural evolutionary stability and now wish for a variety of medical elitist and cosmetic reasons to enter the brave new world of endless human genetic design. Finding a course through this futuristic mire is the greatest challenge facing humanity outside mass extinction of the biosphere. Many bioethicists are sympathetic about using germ-line therapy to shield a child from a family disposition to cancer or atherosclerosis or other illnesses with a strong genetic component. As James Watson co-discoverer of the double-helical structure of DNA said: "We might as well do what we finally can to take the threat of Alzheimers or cancer away from a family." No law prohibits germ-line engineering. None of us want to pass on to our children lethal genes if we can prevent it. - that's what is going to drive this. At a UCLA symposium on germ-line engineering, two thirds of the audience supported it. Few would argue against using the technique to eradicate a disease that has plagued a family for generations. As one commentator pu it: "We know where to start. The harder question is do we know where to stop?"

Already we have mice genetically engineered to have three rather than two copies of the tumor suppressing to resist cancer. At present these are experimental animals for human drug research, but the development of highlights how pressure could grow for germ line engineering to achieve a cancer-free or cancer-reduced human race:

Scientists have bred a family of "supermice" that are highly resistant to cancer. They have three instead of two copies of genes that keep cell division in check. The team at the Spanish National Cancer Centre in Madrid report their findings in Genes and Development. Cell growth and division is normally kept under control by a group of gatekeeper genes called tumour suppressors. Dr Manuel Serrano used DNA technology to breed mice that had an extra copy of part of the tumour suppressor genes called Ink4a/ARF locus. This locus controls the production of two proteins that together appear to stop most human cancer cells developing. When the animals were exposed to various carcinogens they developed tumours at a much lower rate than normal. What's more, the presence of the extra copy of the locus and increased cancer resistance had no apparent effect on the lifespan or fertility of the 'supermice' (*The supermice that resist cancer BBC 2 Nov 2004*).

Some researchers question why these considerations need to lead to germ-line engineering at all. Parents known to be at risk of certain serious genetic abnormalities are already offered genetic testing and the option of an abortion if their fetuses have the disorders. Using this approach, the number of Tay-Sachs births has been reduced by more than 95 per cent among American Jews. For women willing to have IVF, an embryo can even be tested before pregnancy starts and as a combination of IVF and genetic testing becomes more available most of its techniques appear to have the same protective effect without active gene splicing.

Clearly, pre-implantation genetic diagnosis (PGD) creates an ethical problem for anyone who believes that life begins at conception. But even people who don't share this view may be troubled by, say, PGD for conditions that take many years to show up. Take for example, the cancer of the bowel that is caused by the familial polyposis coli gene (FAP) or the breast and ovarian cancers that are linked to mutations in the BRCAL and 2 genes. Is it right to test-and discard-an embryo for a disease that would not develop until after several decades of a presumably fulfilling life? Surely, in those intervening years, better methods of prevention, detection and treatment could be developed. So, is PGD really eugenics? We usually think of eugenics as a societal or governmental effort to advance humanity by 'improving' heredity. But can it seem more benign-merely the sum of individual choices that prevent children with certain genetic defects from being born? Are such genetically based interventions aimed at improving the lot of our children akin to piano lessons, or are they more sinister? (*'Great expectations'* New Scientist 1 May 99).

Then there's the possibility of cosmetic changes and enhancements that have nothing to do with saving lives and preventing disease. Many behaviourat traits, from cheerfulness to sexual orientation, have already been linked, if tenuously, to variations in single genes. Many more such links will be reported in the near future. For example, if we become able to dramatically affect intelligence, it will be pretty irresistible.

One reason for cold feet is that systematic genetic engineering could actually rob society of desirable traits. 'Disease' genes in combination with other genes, or in people who are merely carriers, may also help produce such intangibles as artistic creativity, a razor-sharp wit, or the ability to wiggle ones ears? Wipe out the gene, and you risk losing those traits too. And while no one would wish manic depression on anyone, society might be the poorer without the inventiveness that many psychologists believe is part and parcel of the disorder or the visionary nature that accompanies schizophrenia and some social maladjustment.

If esoteric worries about what may or may not happen in a genetically engineered society are unlikely to change people's views, safety issues could, at least until they are solved. With germ-line engineering there's scope for unpredictable, even monstrous, alterations. The so-called 'Beltsville pig', was engineered by scientists at the US Department of Agriculture to produce human growth hormone that would make it grow faster and leaner. They added a genetic switch that should have turned on the growth hormone gene only when the pig ate food laced with zinc. But the switch failed. The extra growth hormone made the pig grow faster, but it also suffered severe bone and joint problems and was bug-eyed to boot. Unlike human experiments, slaughtering 'failures' is no problem for animal genetic engineers.

Cloning is one of the aspects of germ-line modification which seems to strike the rawest nerves and excite the basest instincts. Cloning is both feared as a potentially totalitarian form of extreme eugenics and focal power. Abhorred as defying our God-given sexual nature. Many technophiles, if such a term is biologically possible consider it the utopia of created immortality. Cloning is really just one very rigid form of germ-line engineering designed to produce a parthenogenetic copy of the original organism. Reproductive cloning does however raise major issues of genetic uniformity and extreme lack of genetic diversity.

Besides reproductive cloning there is a burgeoning market in therapeutic cloning. Techniques that would for example save a few stem cells from an early embryo to use as cells for organs for tissue transplant or replacement of essential cell types in cases of cancer treatments which kill reproductive or immune cells. There is also the idea of using therapeutic cloning to generate stem cell lines from aborted fetuses to provide embryonic stem cells which although not genetically the same could still be of use in regenerating damaged systems in the body. This in turn involves unresolved ethical issues about the status of the unborn human embryo, when does consciousness begin, abortion and to what extent the embryo should become a market or medical research commodity.

416

Therapeutic cloning itself uses human eggs and raises the barrier to reproductive cloning, since the same technology would apply.

> South Korean scientists say they have made stem cells tailored to match the individual for the first time. Each of the 11 new stem cell lines that they made were created by taking genetic material from the patient and putting it into a donated egg. The resultant cells were a perfect match for the individual and could mean treatments for diseases like diabetes without problems of rejection. But the researchers told Science that there were still hurdles to overcome. (*'Patient-specific stem cell first'* BBC 19 May, 2005)

However problems with regenerating the telomeres essential for continued replication may remain, the stem cells need to be reprogrammed to specific tissue types, genetically-modified to remove disease bearing traits and concerns have been raised that such stem cells could give rise to cancers.

Telomeres fluoresce at the tips of chromosomes (Jones R339).

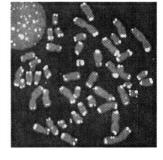

> Every time a cell divides, it sheds tiny snippets of DNA known as telomeres, which serve as protective caps on the ends of chromosomes. After perhaps a hundred divisions, a cell's telomeres become so truncated that its chromosomes, site of the cell's genes-begin to fray, rather like shoelaces that have lost their plastic tips. Eventually, such aged cells die - unless, like "immortal" cancer cells, they produce telomerase, an enzyme that protects and even rebuilds telomeres. Scientists have long dreamed of drugs that would inhibit the immortalizing enzyme because, observes M.IT biochemist Robert Weinberg, "then maybe cancer cells would run out of telomeres and just poop out." Wishful thinking? Maybe not. In papers published just a week apart in the journals Science and Cell, two teams of researchers-one led by Nobel-prize-winning biochemist Thomas Cech of the University of Colorado, the other by M.IT's Weinberg - have announced a breakthrough that could help bring about such a drug. Both teams have managed to clone a gene that controls the activity of the telomerase enzyme in human cells. (*The Telomerase Gene is Isolated* Time, Sep 1, 1997)

Huntington Willard and his colleagues have reported that they had created artificial chromosomes in cultured human cells that replicated every time the cells divided. "We cultured them for six months, and they looked like perfectly normal chromosomes," says Willard. Because these human artificial chromosomes (HACS) promise the ultimate in genetic engineering, they have done more to fire up discussion about human germ-line engineering than just about any other technology. Once perfected, HACs will make it possible for genetic engineers to ship complex custom-made genetic programmes into human embryo cells. Each gene could come with control switches geared to trip only in particular tissues, or when the patient takes a particular drug. Suppose, for instance, that men in your family tend to get prostate cancer at a young age. Insert into your fertilised egg an HAC containing a gene for a toxin that kills any cell that makes it, and two switches for that gene one that is turned on only by prostate cells and another by ecdysone, an insect hormone that humans cannot make. Nine months later, you're delivered of a bouncing baby boy. Fifty years later, he gets prostate cancer. He takes ecdysone, which activates the prostate poison, killing every prostate cell in his body Even cancer cells that have spread to other parts of the body should be wiped out. However inserting extra chromosomes or other DNA even into sex cells is liable to produce a 'mosaic' organism because the DNA is not integrated into the chromosomal genome, so will not be perpetuated in the germ-line as a fully heritable trait. A first step to full germ-line engineering of sperm has been made in zebra fish by growing sperm precursor cells and using retroviruses to insert a new gene into their genome and then letting them mature to make fully GM sperm (Proc. Nat. Acad. Sci. 101 1263).

But something else is suddenly making it okay to discuss the once forbidden possibility Of germ-line engineering. Molecular biologists now think they have clever ways to circumvent the ethical concerns that engulf this sci-fi idea. There may be ways for instance to design a baby's genes without violating the principle of informed consent. This is the belief that no one's genes, not even an embryos - should be altered without his or her permission. Presumably a few people would object to being spared a fatal disease. But what about genes for personality traits, such as risk-taking or being neurotic? The child of tomorrow might have the final word about the genes says UCLA geneticist John Campbell. The designer gene for say patience could be paired with an of-off switch, he says. The child would have to take a drug to activate the patience gene. Free to accept or reject the drug, he retains informed consent over his endowment ('Tomorrow's Child' Sharon Begley NZ Herald Nov 98).

Researchers are experimenting with tricks to make the introduced gene self-destruct in cells that become eggs or sperm. That would confine the tinkering to one generation. Then if it became clear that eliminating the genes for say mental illness also erased genes for creativity that loss would not also become part of the man's genetic blueprint. In experiments with animals Mario Capecchi if the University of Utah has designed a string of genes flanked by the molecular version of scissors. The scissors are activated by an enzyme that would be made only in cells that become eggs or sperm. Once activated the genetic scissors snip out the introduced gene and presto it is not passed along to future generations. "What I worry about" says Capecchi "is that if we start mucking around with eggs and sperm at some point - since this is a human enterprise - we are going to make a mistake". You want a way to undo that mistake. And since what may seem terrific now may seem naive in 20 years you want a way to make genetic change reversible (ibid).

There is no easy technological fix for another ethical worry however. With germ-line engineering only society's haves will control their genetic traits. "If you are going to disadvantage even further those who are already disadvantaged" says bioethicist Ruth Macklin "then that does raise serious concerns" (ibid). Lee Silver (1999) predicts in 'Remaking Eden' that cloning and other genetic technologies could create a genetic elite, or what he dubs the 'GenRich' class, who would refuse to mate with 'natural' human beings and ultimately become a separate species. "The notion that the upper and the lower classes will become further and further apart until they separate into different species I think would be the most horrible thing that ever happened to humanity. It would give those who were genetically enhanced a rationale for severe discrimination against those who were not. The enhanced would treat the unenhanced the same way we treat other species right now. We treat human beings as equals, but we put other highly intelligent primates, such as chimpanzees and gorillas, into zoos and cages" ('Us and Them' New Scientist 9 May 98 36). But Steve Jones doubts the reproductive isolation will hold. "The GenRich would be hard pressed to keep their new genes to themselves", he says. History shows that even in a highly stratified society, the classes still mingle due to our basic, animal instincts. "I believe in the healing power of lust" (NS 13 Jan 2001).

"The potential power of genetic engineering is far greater than that of splitting the atom, and it could be every bit as dangerous to society," says Liebe Cavalieri, a molecular biologist at the State University of New York in Purchase. Cavalieri, who has worked in the field for more than 30 years, thinks it unlikely that the ugly side of genetic engineering will stop development of the technology in its tracks. "It is virtually inevitable it will get used and for the most banal reasons possible-to make some money, or to satisfy the virtuoso scientists who created the technology" (New Scientist 3 Oct 98 25)

Some people go so far as to say germ-line engineering is the key to our race to the stars. Our destiny, says Robert Zubrin, is to leave the planet, just as our ancestors left Africa and colonised the rest of the world. He believes that a fully functional Martian city will be built in this century. And as surely as our descendants shape that world, it will shape them. There would be incredible selection for people whose genes help them survive in the harsh environment, and even on a terraformed Mars this would long persist. While providing Earthly children with genetic enhancements may seem like a frivolity, it would just be good sense to endow Martian kids with the ability to endure a thinner atmosphere and stronger solar radiation. And since the gravity on Mars is only about one-third the strength of Earth's, Zubrin suggests it might also be wise to give its inhabitants long, springy legs to cover terrain more easily ('The Future of Human Evolution' New Scientist 13 Jan 2001).

But to survive in time we need natural evolutionary stability, so that even if humanity does split into two races, we also need for our own survival to make sure the naturally selected genome of humanity survives, particularly as it does with almost no resources in places like the Kalahari Desert. Unfortunately the very people upon whom our best human traditions of long-term survival depend are being driven from their habitat by the government of Botswana, to turn the Kalahari into a wildlife park, leaving the world vulnerable to the complete loss of the most evolutionarily stable mode of long-term existence on planet Earth.

We thus urgently need to understand how to evoke the principles of sexual paradox in an era of nascent technological change in ways which preserve the intrinsic robustness of the genetic endowment which makes us human and which ensure our emergence and survival over evolutionary time scales -massively parallel natural genetic algorithms with their deep variety and emergent novelty - so that we can provide for the evolutionary possibilities the uncertain future may demand. We need urgently to develop a future ethic to deal with reproductive technology in terms of our evolutionary fitness as a species, as well as individual choice and utopian ambitions. If we don't we could suddenly find ourselves becoming extinct overnight because of an ever-so-slight disruption of the technological civilization on which we depend, having become unable to fed ourselves or reproduce without the intervention of sensitive high technology.

Forest destruction Amazon
(New Scientist).

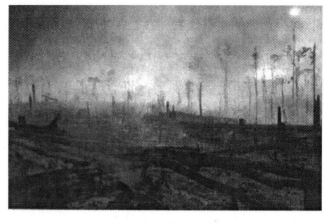

Rape of the Planet and Genetic Holocaust

Rape of the planet has become something we take for granted. It has become a central figure of speech and an assumption about the existential condition, as if such actions are an implicit part of human nature. But the very metaphor indicates that patriarchal sexual prerogatives are driving human impact. Rape is, by its nature sexual, and intimately connected with male violence in the pursuit of insemination by violent 'power over' the other. It is brought into an altogether unseemly conjunction with our deep cultural emphasis on the Earth as 'mother', becoming at once an original sin of mankind - the rape of Mother Earth.

We have seen from the previous discussion that rape of the planet does not occur because humanity is a violent dangerous species. Rather, we have emerged stably over evolutionary time scales in an apparent state of sexual paradox. The very idea of raping the planet is an outgrowth of the male spermatogenic imperative manifest in biblical terms in the Fall from Eden and the free-slather paradigm of dominion over woman and nature.

From this initiative springs the imperative of spermatogenic dominion as Abraham was promised offspring as the dust of the Earth and as the stars in the sky. It is by no means confined to the Hebrew tradition, emerging across the whole Near East, from ancient Greece attested by Zeus stringing up a recalcitrant Hera, to Enki masturbating the waters of Sumeria. It emerged with the rise of the shepherd kings and was possibly exacerbated by the Indo-Aryan migrations.

The Spermatogenic Imperative

To clarify the situation we need to focus briefly on the essential characteristics of the male spermatogenic reproductive strategy taken on its own:

Firstly it is frequently involved principally in mating, rather than parenting. As we have seen this remains substantially true in extremely patriarchal societies. It thus lacks essential characteristics for parental and generational survival promoted by maternal natural selection. Given a bare mating strategy, it is easy to see how this becomes rape of the 'silent' Earth in a patriarchal society.

Secondly it is specifically a short-term investment strategy resourcing the current offspring, at the expense of future progeny, commanding all the available maternal resources, by contrast with the balancing maternal investment for all progeny. It thus lacks the characteristics of stable long-term investment.

Thirdly it is a high variance strategy which seeks to monopolize maximum resources to empower an exponential bounty in reproductive advantage typified by the huge harems established by many powerful male despots, expressed in history and religious doctrines on reproduction. This leads to a false idea of exponentiating fortunes, interrupted by life and death crisis in boom and bust.

Fourthly it is based on a winner-take-all form of reproductive competition lacking compensating networks of cooperative resourcing more typical of females, where competition is only necessary when resource become scarce. It is thus intrinsically highly exploitative.

Fifthly it is a venture-risk strategy which risks death to achieve high reproductive gain. From the male's point of view this embraces apocalyptic final conflict, and preparedness to annihilate to achieve social or reproductive ends.

Sixthly it is a strategy which involves male combat, competition and the implicit use of violence and war, setting up a paradigm of conquest of opponents, of the female and of nature.

Taken together, these reproductive characteristics invoke (1) exponential boom and bust insatiability, (2) lack of any long-term survival strategy (3) winner-take-all competition without compensating cooperation (4) exploitation of available resources without regard to continuity (5) risking death to achieve life (6) the notion of final confrontation and (7) implicit violence in a state of perpetual conflict.

The spermatogenic imperative is destabilizing human society. The evolutionary strategy of the female to build a sustainable world into which her massive reproductive and nurturing investment will be realized over time has been pushed aside by the spermatogenic venture-risk exploitation strategy of the male, who can always afford to sacrifice one opportunity for many others, or even risk death to reproduce.

Patriarchy and Population Boom and Bust

Historically the world population grew only very slowly from about 2.5 million at the beginnings of urbanization to some 50 million around the time of the black plague of the middle ages. It is only with the industrial, scientific and medical revolution and the colonial expansion of Western powers, that the world population has climbed to the dizzy heights. During the 20th century, the world's population increased almost fourfold, from 1.6 to 6 billion. Until very recently there were fears that in the next century, world population would explode to some 12 billion people, leaving little room for wilderness areas to preserve wildlife and putting extreme pressure on food production, water and non-renewable resources.

At a time when there has been a manifest need to curtail runaway population growth, the leaders of the world's great patriarchal religions have, almost without exception been ordering their populations to continue to multiply making frontal attacks on any effective form of contraception and family planning. The Catholic church has waged war not only on abortion but cursed any effective form of contraception as simple and protective of disease as the condom. Islamic leaders have also roundly opposed family planning. The leaders of both the Christian and Islamic world share an agenda of male reproductive right and a calculated determination to multiply the faithful by advocating unrestrained fertility even in the face of the manifest damage such policies have caused. Desmond Morris makes no bones about it:

> "If we are honest there is only one root cause of the disaster facing the planet, and that is the appalling rate at which our human species has increased its population in recent centuries. ... Who is to blame for the crisis we face? First and foremost, I accuse the religious leaders of the world. They have fed mankind with the dangerous myth that humanity is somehow above nature and that it is our god-given right to hold dominion over the Earth and subdue it. In many cases, they have actively encouraged over-population and have gone out of their way to prevent family-planning schemes. They are a disgrace. Secondly, I accuse political leaders, almost all of whom follow a policy of national growth, regardless of the consequences. ... But we are not designed as a high-quantity species. We are a high-quality species, and all our social thinking should be directed to this thought" (Porritt R537).

The attitude of world leaders has also been irresponsible and self-serving. While the leaders of major western powers push for ever greater gross national products, honing their economies as if there was never an end to increasing production, 9/10ths of the world population sinks further into poverty, losing educational, resourcing and livelihood opportunities.

Fortunately 2002 figures showed a drop in fertility. Current trends suggest a population in 2050 around 9.2-9.3 billion (UN, Population Research Bureau BBC 18 Aug 2004). To everyone's surprise in 2002 a very significant drop was detected in the fertility rates of a broad spread of diverse countries spanning the developed and developing world comprising half the world's population and with little in common between their governments and social attitudes. In 1950, worldwide the average woman had five children. Today she has just 2.3. Although in many countries there are still a large number of people at or below child-bearing age and actual birth rates will remain very high for some years to come, this fall has already led to a downgrading of future population predictions and fears of a population crash with societies full of the elderly unable to support their own services. However 2004 predicitions have incresed again from around 8.9 to 9.2 billion.

Few of the countries showing declines, bar China, have forced contraception or sterilizationon their populations. Opposition from the Catholic Church has ensured that Brazil has no state family planning programme. Even so, millions of its women have attended sterilisation clinics, and fertility has halved in 20 years to today's 2.3. The case of Iran is even more remarkable. In 1994, the mullahs ruling the country went to a UN population conference in Cairo and declared opposition to much of the international agenda for cutting birth rates. But back home, women were taking charge of their bodies and sending fertility rates crashing from 5.5 children per woman in 1988 to just 2.2 in 2000. Italy the country that is home to the Catholic Church, noted for its opposition to artificial birth control, is notching up super-low fertility rates way below replacement levels. At just 1.2 children born to each Italian woman, the rate is little more than half the figure needed to prevent the population plummeting, closely matched by Greece, Spain and Czechoslavakia (Pierce R528).

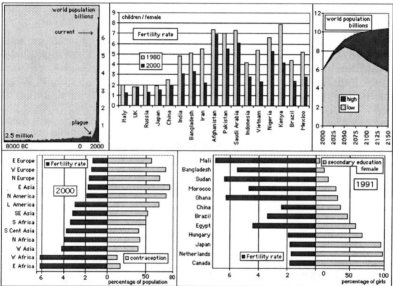

Top left: Historical population trends. Centre: Falling fertility rates in 2000. Top right: Falling predictions 2002 may see the world population peak at about 8 billion by 2050 although many predictions still anticipate 10 billion. Increasing use of contraception (lower left) and improved female education (lower right) both correlate with falling fertility rates and reduced population pressure.

There are some notable exceptions. Conservative Islamic countries like Saudi Arabia, Afghanistan, and Pakistan still have some of the highest birth rates on the planet. In India the Muslim community grew by 36% between 1991 and 2001 and now stands at 13.4% of the total population. Hindus account for 80.5% of all Indians, a growth of 20.3% in the same period, down from 25% in 1981-1991. The Muslim community fares poorly in literacy compared to other groups - which is seen as one reason for their increasing numbers (*Indian Muslim community growing* BBC 7 Sep 2004). African results are uneven, but here HIV is wreaking havoc on young populations. The UN expects 15 million deaths from AIDS in the next five years, the great majority in Africa. Life expectancy in Botswana and Zimbabwe has plunged from 60 years to close to 40 years.

Contraceptive use in the developing world has risen from one in 10 couples to more than half of all couples. A 15 percent increase in the use of contraceptives means, on average, about one fewer birth per woman. Thus, in Ethiopia only 4 percent of women use contraception and the fertility rate is seven, while in South Africa 53 percent use some method and average fertility is 3.3. The desire for smaller families is spreading. In 1998 researchers associated with the Asian Development Bank in Laos, one of the world's poorest countries, invited people there to say what help they wanted most. The men requested jobs, but the women's number-one priority was family planning (*The Unmet Need for Family Planning* Scientific American Jan 2000).

The reasons for this reduction are complex, but the critical factor is that cultural changes have increasingly liberated women from the home and child-rearing. In poor countries with a traditional patriarchal society, the spread of TV has opened many women's eyes to a whole new world, and modern birth control methods have allowed them to turn those aspirations into reality. Demographer Tim Dyson attributes this to 'cultural diffusion'. Not having children has become a statement of modernity and emancipation, and women are unlikely to give up the new freedoms. They are also taking over from their brothers and husbands the role of shaping their societies. "Go to rural India, and you find that women are fed up with the men, who seem to be going nowhere. It is the women who are running the farms. It is the women who are getting jobs and taking charge. They don't have time to have children any more." With men no longer in charge, their usefulness to society and the old Indian preference for sons may diminish as a result, he says. That, too, will help reduce fertility as couples see daughters as well as sons as potential heads of a new generation (Pierce R528).

In Sweden they have 1.6 children per couple, Norway 1.8 and Britain and Finland 1.7 much closer to replacement. The difference is more chance of combining a career with motherhood. Suitors are more likely to have set up home on their own before marriage, are better house-trained, and Nordic governments are better at helping couples juggle family and work. About half the jobs held by Swedish women are part- time, creches are near-universal and paid parental leave lasts for a year. All this is unheard of in Italy, where only 12% of employed women have part-time jobs, and in eastern Europe, where fertility rates have plunged since the collapse of communism wrecked state-funded family support services. To cope with this Singapore's prime minister has announced financial incentives for families, increased maternity leave, and cut working hours so single people can meet more easily.

Peter McDonald, argues that the southern European phenomenon is a result of the lopsidedness of moves to gender equality. Women have got the freedoms that arise from better education and employment, but not in their relations with their men or in terms of state services for the family. Economic liberalism has clashed with social conservatism. Result: a childbirth strike. Jean-Claude Chesnais goes further. With poor state child-care provision, and most men unlikely to help in looking after their offspring, "the obstacles to child-bearing in countries like Italy [and Japan (*BBC Japan sounds alarm on birth rate 3 Dec 2004*)] are enormous and the economic sacrifices made by mothers are viewed as unbearable". Caldwell thinks the signs are clear: "The Mediterranean patriarchal model is far more common in the world than the northern European model of more helpful husbands." McDonald says we can already see this in eastern Asia, where conservative family values lie behind the ultra-low fertility rates from Shanghai to Tokyo (R528). These low rates could bring about a serious crash in populations. McDonald calculates that the population of Italy is set to crash from 56 million now to just 8 million by 2100. Likewise Spain would lose 85 per cent of its population within the same time frame and Germany 83 per cent. Russia's population decline is accelerating, according to the country's official statistics agency, equivalent to 100 people dying in Russia every hour.

The UN warned that Russia's population could fall by 1/3 by the middle of the century. Many solutions to the problem have been proposed, ranging from family-friendly tax breaks to legalising polygamy. The WHO suggests putting up the price of alcohol or forcing people to wear seatbelts (*Russia's population falling fast* Steven Eke BBC 23 June, 2005).

Scarcity of oil may exacerbate falls in birth rate and cause a reduction in infant survival (*Energy crisis 'will limit births'* BBC 13 Feb 2004). Paradoxically perhaps, the more feminist attitudes that have helped bring about the dramatic decline in family size in the past 50 years will need extending rather than dismantling, if family sizes are to rise from the worst-case Italian model. But the new agenda may be less about creating new freedoms for women and more about instilling new responsibilities in men and the state. In most of the world , fertility rates are plunging because women have decided they want to become more like men. Right now that leaves little room for babies. To change that, men must take the plunge and start to become more like women. The future of humanity could depend on it (R528).

By any standard of ecological biodiversity conservation, all these population figures are vastly too high to preserve existing ecosystems. More than a third of the planet's land surface including its most productive land is now commandeered for human monoculture. In the midst of this situation the Bush administration encouraged by the religious right, has cut funding for the UN Population Fund, on the basis the agency was supporting coercive family planning in China. The White House continued to withhold funding even after the State Department declared these charges were false (Sachs). Population in the sub-Saharan Africa is expected to rise from 667 million to 1,085 billion by 2025 where total fertility rates remain at 5.4. The Middle East with fertility rates at 3.5 will also se very high birth rates. These high rates reduce economic growth, stress environmental resources and young populations with excess adolescent men cause manifest political instability and violence. The world rate of population increase has fallen from 2.1% per annum to 1.3% but the overall increase is still continuing with large young populations with high birth rates. These religiously-motivated actions continue to be manifestly irresponsible.

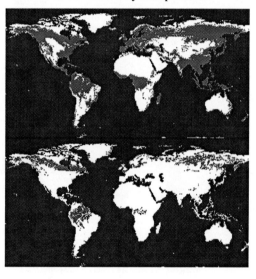

World frontier (virgin) forests as they originally stood and as they stand in 2000. There are additional areas of secondary growth and other regeneration , but these tend to have predominant weedy species and not the climax diversity of virgin forest and jungle (World Resources Institute).

Mass-extinction of Biological and Genetic Diversity

Nowhere are the disastrous effects of the patriarchal view of dominion over nature and winner-take-all exploitation of resources more clearly expressed than in the destruction of Earth's major ecosystems, the felling of our great forests, and the mass extinction of the living species of the planet with its consequent loss of genetic diversity which could haunt us not for just thousands of years, but millions or tens of millions of years to come.

The Earth is entering the sixth great mass extinction recorded over evolutionary time (Leaky and Lewin). All previous mass extinctions of biodiversity were precipitated by huge astronomical disasters. The dinosaurs were wiped out by one or more asteroids which plunged the Earth into a 'nuclear' winter after causing global flash fires burning up much of the natural cover, setting off volcanic activity in its wake opposite in India, followed by a dark cool period and then sudden global warming, leaving oxygen levels semi-permanently reduced by a third. But this is just a blip on the map of biodiversity compared with the Permian extinction in which 90% of living species became extinct, amid what is believed to have been an even impact which first caused the oceans to recede by perhaps a third and then rise again in an oceanic flood. Such extinctions always been caused by massive interventions, cometary or asteroid impacts, supernovae, massive volcanic intrusion or solar flares.

What is absolutely unique about the sixth extinction is that it is not being caused by any such disruption, but simply by the explosive exploitation by a single species who ought to know better and that it is completely unnecessary and deleterious for this species' own survival. It is estimated that over 25% of living species will become extinct in the next 25 years unless radical world-wide efforts are made for collective conservation on a genetic, species and ecosystem-wide basis. Long term prediction by the end of the century could see more than half the living species disappear. Just as the asteroid which hit Yucatan wiped out the dinosaurs, so the great apes are facing extinction in the wild, along with our own founding human groups such as the San, leaving our own human evolutionary strategy unprotected.

Decline in species populations reflects a world rate 100 to 1000 times greater than normal and predicted to rise to 10,000. 90% of large predatory ocean fish are already gone from overfishing. Loss of biodiversity will result directly in human poverty and hunger. (See http://www.maweb.org/en/index.aspx 2005).

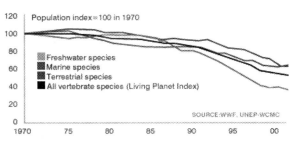

This mass extinction is being caused by a host of factors, but habitat destruction and the islandization of the great tropical forests and their diversity hotspots into unsustainable fragments, which cannot sustain species diversity are pivotal and systematic overfishing of the oceans to exhaustion. Logging, poaching, release of exotic species and pollution all play a serious part, as well as burgeoning threat of precipitate climatic change.

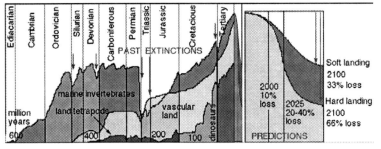

Paradise Lost? History and Projected Future of Life's Diversity

No matter how grandiose our technological pretensions, humanity depends on living species as foods, medicines and the key to our commercial products to survive. Yet at the same time as we are mindlessly tearing down the remaining biodiversity hotspots, having only characterized about a tenth of the living species, or the medicinal or life-enhancing properties they may contain, we are also busy reducing the genetic diversity of the species we do depend on. The use of monoclonal hybrids, on a world-wide monocultural scale, genetically modified varieties, genetic cloning and the choice of varieties which have no hope of surviving in the wild are reducing the innate viability of the species on which we depend and hence our own viability to a vanishing equation. Our food production and distribution systems are becoming ever more dependent on high technology, while the naturally viable 'heritage' seeds from which we derive our commercial varieties are given no viable habitat, are stored in gene banks where a power failure could render much of our genetic heritage 'dead-in-the-water' overnight and the patenting of wild varieties by large agrochemical companies such as Monsanto (who recently tried to buy the rights on virtually all wild Chinese soya varieties at the same time as marketing round-up ready soya) thus taking these very species out of the human orbit altogether.

The innate robustness of the biosphere which brought us here is being reduced to a fragile human technical fantasy. When the triple-witching hour of natural catastrophe arrives, we could be a defenseless blip on an ever more precipitous and accelerating boom and bust chart. The final stock-market crash. Given the unremitting exploitation of nature and the consequent instabilities to human survival, the human species may become extinct (Leakey and Lewin R393). This is clearly an issue of patriarchal short-term, winner-take-all, boom-and-bust exploitation of the Earth with no long-term nurturing strategy to compensate. It raises huge questions about the role of Western democracies and corporate capitalism as entrenched institutions of patriarchal power and exemplifies the way sexual dominion can lead to an irrational and wholly damaging situation which escapes our civilized control.

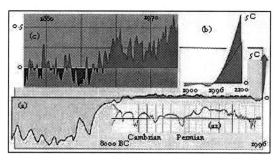

.Trends in global warming as of 2000 from the Cambrian to the present.

Climatic Chaos and Human Hubris

As shown in the above chart, during its history, the Earth has seen major shifts in temperature, often accompanied by changes in the level of carbon dioxide or CO_2. These have generally been accompanied by major changes of an astronomical nature, such as changes in solar brightness, or volcanic changes to the carbon dioxide content, and major evolutionary changes in the biota such as the advent of photosynthetic cyanobacteria in the ocean and land plants.

The Gaia hypothesis proposes that the biota and other geological cycles are involved in a form of homeostasis which helps to maintain Earth's environment in a stable atmospheric state, however there are also clear examples of processes which can instead bifurcate and flip into a new stability pattern locking us into a runaway warming. Venus for example has a runaway greenhouse effect which has driven the surface temperature to 400 °C. Carbon dioxide which is an almost universal output of our carbon-based economy is the major chemical contributor to atmospheric global warming. People have cited a variety of other factors, from solar fluctuations to cosmic rays, the incidence of sulphate haze and differing absorbency caused by changing forests and ice sheets. There are also major questions of deposition of in carbonates on the ocean floor into limestone. Previous changes have resulted in major fluctuations of the ocean of up to 60 feet, far more then the 60cm rise predicted this century. Even this amount will be disastrous for many countries from Polynesian atolls, through Bangladesh which lost 110,000 people in flooding in the 1990s to the Nile delta. Two worrying positive feedback influences which could cause a flip to a long-term warming are melting of the polar ice caps which reduces reflectance and so increases warming and the release of massive sub-ocean methane hydrates as a result of the warming itself. Methane, CH_4, although currently a less major contributor to warming, is about 20 times more potent than CO_2, although it is degraded over time by oxidation. Its contributions are currently coming from increased termite action from whole sale rain forest destruction and large numbers of burping ruminants on pasture land.

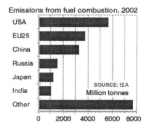

Emissions from fuel combustion, 2002

There are already signs of major disruptions to both the Arctic and Antarctic ice sheets which seem to be accelerating. Changes in global temperature may also be linked to a more chaotic climate with more frequent costly and damaging storms and changes in the North Atlantic conveyor which powers the Gulf Stream and keeps the north from extreme winters and possibly El Niño, although this is debated. However by far the most serious effect is the potential destruction of genetic and species diversity. The above map shows the regions of the planet which would remain stable to several current predictions of global warming. Most areas are expected to go through such climatic shock that neither the plants nor animals endemic to the areas will find themselves in a viable climatic habitat. The pace of global warming is so rapid that there is no time for plant species to spread by seeding and whole ecosystems are predicted to die out. Global warming is thus one of the potentially most major contributors to mass extinction.

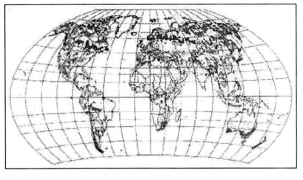

Life zones remaining stable in four different global warming models (Groombridge R266).

The most disquieting aspect of this situation is that the country with by far the greatest production of carbon dioxide, the United States, which emits about 150 times as much CO_2 per head of population as under-developed countries is doing its utmost to continue to exacerbate the situation. Along with its rejection of many other major world treaties, such as the Biodiversity Convention, unlike Europe's responsible attitude as a developed region, the US has mounted a vigilant campaign of opposition to any form of control on its own profligate waste of natural resources. This failure of any kind of global ethics, reinforced by spurious arguments that the massive injections of human produced CO_2 are having no effect on global warming, or that the effect is beneficial, need to be looked at very carefully. If the rest of the world were to follow suit, the situation would clearly be untenable and possibly lethal.

Per capita emission of CO_2 in metric tons per person per year. Green coastal areas are threatened by rising oceans. Sample figures: Qatar 16.9, USA 5.2, UK 2.63, China 0.42, India 0.21 illustrating the excessive emissions by developed nations. The US produced 23% of world emissions. Over 80% of Brazil's emission came from forest burning. Sumatran peat fires contributed as much CO_2 as Western Europe (King redrawn from 1996 data).

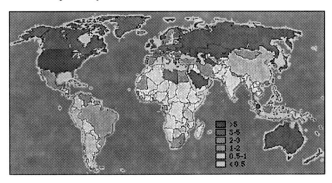

This is a clear case of the principal world superpower acting as a rogue nation in the interests of competitive exploitation of economic advantage over the rest. It is an arch male strategy which makes the pretensions of US society to be a sexually-emancipated society where women's rights and approaches are as keenly expressed as men's completely hollow. Central to this is the role of venture capital transnational corporates sourced in the US and the non-genetic 'free-market' philosophies corporate capitalism espouses which are themselves representative only of the spermatogenic aspects of reproductive strategy.

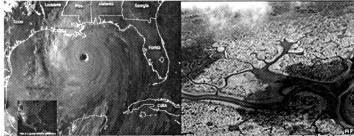

Linked global climatic instabilities due to warming in the tropical Atlantic: Left: Hurricane Katrina peaking the highest hurricane season on record. Right: Severe drought in the Amazon basin (www).

Research confirmed in November 2005 from ice cores in Antarctica confirm that current atmospheric concentrations of CO_2-380 parts per million (ppm) - are 27% higher than the highest levels found in the last 650,000 years. The ice core data also shows that CO_2 and methane levels have been remarkably stable in Antarctica--varying between 300 ppm and 180 ppm - over that entire period and that shifts in levels of these gases took at least 800 years, compared to the roughly 100 years in which humans have increased atmospheric CO_2 levels to their present high. If nothing is done to reduce emissions, current climate models predict a global warming of about 1.4 – 5.8°C between 1990 and 2100. (United Nations Framework Convention on Climate Change).

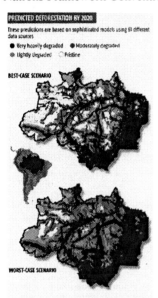

PREDICTED DEFORESTATION BY 2020

These predictions are based on sophisticated models using 61 different data sources

● Very heavily degraded ● Moderately degraded
⊛ Lightly degraded ○ Pristine

BEST-CASE SCENARIO

WORST-CASE SCENARIO

Predicted state of the Amazon by 2020 New Scientist 15 Oct 2005 35-39.

In addition to significant indications of melting in Antarctica and at the North Pole, there is also evidence that because of massive influxes of melting glaciers and ice sheets in Greenland that the North Atlantic conveyor, which carries energy equivalent to a million power stations, is failing because of the distruption of circulation caused by the mass of cold fresh water dumped into the Arctic. This is likely to cause severe winters in Northern Europe despite an overall warming and significantly increase ocean levels. The average sea level is predicted to rise by 9 to 88 cm by 2100. This would be caused mainly by the thermal expansion of the upper layers of the ocean as they warm, with some contribution from melting glaciers. The most dramatic such change, the collapse of the West Antarctic ice sheet, which would lead to a catastrophic rise in sea level of 6 meters, is now considered unlikely during the 21st century.

Accompanying a peak in severe hurricanes in the Carribean due to rising ocean temperatures in the tropical Atlantic has been a severe drought in the Amazon, accentuated by runaway deforestation from burning and logging, killing the majority of fish life and rendering many centres of population inaccesible, because the only access by river boat is impassable. Predictions from deforestation and underestimates of the effects of selective logging are in a worst case scenario for the Amazon to be essentially gone by 2020.

Analysis of world oil production indicates that we are already reaching the limits of oil production and that a permanent decline will set in during the next decade (Sci. Am. Mar 98). Massive efforts of technological realignment are required to convert the freeway-based emission culture into a sustainable transport economy based on renewable energy. Below left new discoveries have been falling since the 1950s. Below right: Three predicted scenarios for future consumption. (New Scientist 12 Aug 2003 9).

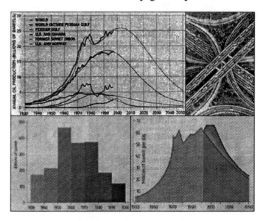

Resource and Energy Exploitation

Central to this hubris is a failure of the most technologically sophisticated nation, the US to develop a rational policy to world non-renewable resources or to develop in advance the alternative technologies to make this possible. While Europe is making a massive investment in wind power and a variety of solar, fuel cell and hydrogen-based technologies are clearly within sight, the US has no national strategy for advancing these technologies, and continues to make its major thrust cornering as much as possible of the dwindling world supplies of oil, engaging wars in both Afghanistan and Iraq with oil pipelines and supplies the centre of strategic attention. This failure of constructive engagement is again a manifestation of a complete failure of constructive sexual relationship underlying the corporate basis of US consumer society where up to 40% of the 'management' positions are nominally held by women but the corporate ethic remains one of patriarchal handshakes behind the corridors of power and in politics as ever 'money talks'.

Apocalypse and Armageddon

By far the most direct and troubling manifestation of the nightmare of unbridled patriarchal dominance is the endless gravitation towards a paranoid scenario of final conflict in an Armageddon type apocalypse between the forces of light and dark epitomized by the 'evil empire' be it Hitler, Soviet Communism, Islamic fundamentalism or Saddam Hussein and his illusory weapons of mass destruction, or the President of the United States claiming if you are not with us you are against us.

While we can all accept that Hitler's heritage and Stalin's too were totalitarian monstrosities in the name of the people they misled, and that Shoah, the Jewish holocaust, is a warning of eugenic genocide the world should continue to remember in the genetic age, the attributing of evil to the 'other' is the classic gambit of the patriarchal apocalypse of the war of dark and light. In these circumstances, it is all too easy to ignore the evil at one's own doorstep in the sleight of hand with focuses attention on the evil of the dark 'other'.

We also need to be mindful that it was the allies who developed nuclear weapons as a final solution, to counter Hitler's 'holocaust', sparked by the scientific genius of Jews whose relatives had been incarcerated or killed in the Nazi death camps, and that the first detonation at 'truth or consequences' took place in the name of the Christian Trinity. Oppenheimer even cited Bohr's vision of 'complementarity'- that although the Bomb might be the greatest disaster to have befallen humankind, it may well be a great blessing, 'a turning point in history'."

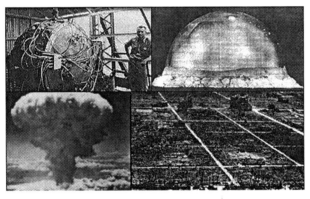

Left: The Trinity bomb. Right: The Trinity test at 300 ms (Scientific American). Hiroshima: Humanity gains the ultimate powers of mass extinction of life. A transition to the prospect of mutually assured destruction in patriarchal combat.

Michael Ortiz Hill (R308) describes the godly patriarchal 'climate' as follows:

"It is impossible to ignore or to diminish the religious element that turns up again and again in the accounts of the Trinity blast. ... It was named by Oppenheimer, invoking by way of John Donne the mystery of the martyred and resurrected God: 'As West and East In all flat maps - and I am one - are one. So death doth touch the Resurrection.' 'That still doesn't make a Trinity,' Oppenheimer confessed - and then speculated that perhaps he was influenced by a better known poem, one of Donne's Holy Sonnets, beginning, 'Batter my heart, three person'd God; for you As yet but knocke, breathe, shine and seek to mend; That I may rise, and stand, o'erthrow mee, and bend Your force to breake, blowe, burn and make me new'. After Trinity, Thomas Farrel wrote: 'The effects could well be described as unprecedented, magnificent, beautiful, stupendous and terrifying.... The lighting beggared description. The whole country was lighted by a searing light with the intensity many times that of the midday sun. It was golden, purple, violet, gray, and blue. It lighted every peak, crevasse and ridge of the nearby range with a clarity and beauty that cannot be described but must be seen to be imagined.'... Other observers were more explicitly religious in speaking of the event. ...It is striking that, following Oppenheimer's lead of naming the site of the first nuclear test "Trinity," Weisskopf and Laurence - both Jews - saw in the Bomb the glory of Christ. ... William Laurence wrote that it was like being 'privileged to witness the Birth of the World-to-be present at the moment of Creation when the Lord said: 'Let there be light'. He compared the experience to witnessing the second coming of Christ. ... Ferenc Szasz notes, "Others whispered, more in

> reverence than otherwise: 'Jesus Christ'. Another striking theme that repeats again and again ...
> is birth and paternity. William Laurence called the rumblings of the Trinity explosion the 'first
> cry of a newborn world'. ... Teller sent a telegram to Los Alamos saying simply, 'It's a boy'. ...
> one notices a vivid absence of the feminine amidst all this imagery of birthing."

Debate continues about the wisdom of unleashing the world's first nuclear war on Japan
and the fallout that has continued since. It is clear that actually carrying out such an act is
the clearest provocation possible to the Soviet Union for its own defence to immediately
embark on a program of nuclear weapons, leading directly to the nuclear Cold War and the
build-up of enough nuclear weapons to lay waste to the planet 40 times over.

This situation dramatically reduced the viability of the human race to one small accidental
error, amid the continuing strategic jockeying for the capacity for a unilateral first strike, in
which a variety of circumstances, including unusual cloud cover and miscommunicated
weather rocket launches several times nearly caused and accidental nuclear mobilization.
This philosophy of MAD mutually-assured destruction became a psychic and social deadlock that overshadowed much of the 20th century, leaving many people uncertain whether
to have offspring because of root uncertainty they would have livable lives to lead.

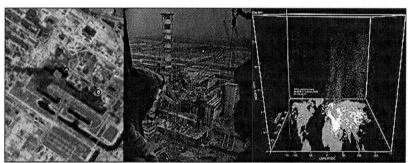

Left; Ground zero from satellite during the fire. Centre: Chernobyl radioactive. Right: The global
extent of the radioactive contamination cloud (National Geographic)

It was only with the nuclear explosion at Chernobyl, fifty times as polluting as Hiroshima
and Nagasaki, its name "bitter grass" echoing the resonances of the Biblical 'Wormwood'
and its bitter waters (Kravchanka 1990), that the spell of this gaze of fatal nuclear attraction was shattered and people on both sides of the dissolving 'Iron Curtain' realized that
things had gone too far. We however need to continue to be mindful that, despite a closer
dialogue with Russia, we are still in a state of 15 times overkill and that the nuclear threat
is becoming ever more subtle and complex as the impossible 'war on terror' itself a contradiction terms, motivates smaller groups to mount a counter-cultural act of asymmetric
warfare.

Again here the threat is not from the 'other' so much as the 'devil we know' in our own
back yard squandering resources which could save biodiversity and educate the world's
women on 'star wars' and 'mini-nukes' which could be used in conventional warfare.
Israel as part of this legacy has 200 nuclear weapons in what they call 'the Sampson
option' to pull down the pillars on the whole Middle East. We need also to be mindful,
given this history, that the advent of an Islamic bomb in Pakistan developed in opposition
to India's nuclear development, (along with its possible dissemination to Iran and North
Korea) and attempts to enrich fissionable material in Iran are a reaction to real perceived
threats of a crusade against Islam. The nuclear apocalypse has fed the imagination of religious extremists more than any of the equally apocalptic issues we have discussed. Only a
nuclear winter prospect as lethal as a large astronomical impact has brought people to a
semblance of their senses.

Boom and Bust and World Poverty

Them that's got, shall get them that's not, shall lose
so the Bible said, and it still is news
mama may have, and papa may have

God bless' the child, that's got his own
(Arthur Herzog Jr., Billie Holiday)

The Western economic model is not based on the fluctuations and natural cycles character-istic of the feminine reproductive strategy, but concentrates almost exclusively on expo-nentials. The gross national product, interest rates, and inflation are key manifestations of the exponential growth scenario. The exponential characteristics of the male strategy taken on their own are almost inevitably going to lead to boom and bust dynamics for the lack of adequate stabilizing long-term feedback. Capital markets are thus chaotic and dis-play dynamical instability. The free market model is non-genetic and thus also provides for unstable fluctuation lacking any of the integrative genetic processes that mutational evolution by natural selection engages. Electoral democracy, particularly in a first past the post system, involves pure competition with winner-take-all rewards, and highly fluctuat-ing fortunes all concordant with the male reproductive strategy. The exponential dynamics and the pure competition and instability which form the basis of the capitalist free market are thus all central characteristics defining male reproductive strategy. This male instabil-ity of mutual defection also occurs spatially in the massing of personal fortunes, which in turn empower the capacity to command greater advantages. Consequently we have mani-fest power law inequity of resourcing on a male reproductive distribution.

A common theme in the distribution of wealth and poverty is that the richest 20% control 85% of domestic investment, domestic savings, world trade and gross national product. The bottom 20% hold only 0.7% to 1.4% of these nearly a hundred times less. The extreme variances in wealth are common to most human societies and reflect a fractal-type power law relationship which assigns wealth on a roughly inverse square to inverse cube law formula. A variety of models have been used to explain it including tensile wires on a random landscape. The gist of such models is that a major factor in opportunistic wealth is not elite expertise so much as being in the right place at the right time. ("The Rich Get Richer" New Scientist 19 Aug 2000). Such a resource power law is clearly reflected in male reproduction in the approximately $1 / 2^3$ men who can support 2 wives in societies which permit polygyny. Historically male reproductive power has been directly translated into dynastic family power through patriliny, so the link with capital and estates is clear.

Such wild differences in resource wealth are unparalleled in the natural world, even among hoarding animals such as chipmunks, except in terms of variance in male reproductive fit-ness, where for example, one male elephant seal may have a harem of twenty females and another male none at all. Neither is it common, particularly for females, for there to be frank resource competition under circumstances where there are sufficient resources to feed an entire population. This is exactly the situation currently faced by humanity, even given an overblown population of six billion.

We thus have to ask ourselves how much this very uneven assignment of wealth is an indi-rect consequence of male reproductive strategies underlying the monetary acquisition and possession of wealth and its application in personal and corporate capitalist investment. Ironically, it was one of communism's forerunners, Engels who feminists frequently cite in discussions of the rise of class-based patriarchy (p 174). This is a double irony because the egalitarian 'collective wealth' of the communist system has been as manipulated by nepotistic patriarchs with aspirations to sexual despotism, such as Mao Tse Tung, as has the capitalist system and has been even more prone to totalitarian control. However such extreme inequity raises a basic question about the patriarchal basis of venture capitalism and what feminine or ecosystemic antidote might become capitalism's evolutionary suc-cessor.

Inequitable Distribution

Among the 4.4 billion people who live in developing countries, 3/5 have no access to basic sanitation, almost 1/3 are without safe drinking water, 1/4 lack adequate housing, 1/5 live beyond reach of modern health services, 1/5 of the children do not get as far as grade five in school and 1/5 are undernourished. The divergence between rich and poor is accentuat-ing as time goes by. The 3 richest in the world own assets that exceed the combined gross national product of all the least developed countries and their 600 million people. The richest 20% of the world's population enjoys a share in global income that is 86 times that of the poorest 20%. More than 1.2 billion people in the world live on less that $1 a day. More than 50% of them are children. Nearly 1 billion cannot meet their basic consumption requirements. The assets of the 200 richest people are more than the combined income of 41% of the world's people. A yearly contribution of 1% of their wealth or $8 billion could provide universal access to primary education for all.

Industrialized countries hold 97% of all patents, and global corporations hold 90% of all technology and product patents. Over 80% of foreign direct investment in developing and transition economies goes to just 20 countries, with China receiving the maximum share. Debt relief for the 20 worst affected countries would cost between US $5.5 billion to $7.7 billion, less than the cost of one stealth bomber.

Inequitable Consumption

Further figures from the UN Human Development Reports (1998-2000) note the following contrasts between basic and feminine luxuries and minimal resources such as sanitation and education of women:

1. Basic education for all would cost $6 billion a year; $8 billion is spent annually for cosmetics in the United States alone.
2. Installation of water and sanitation for all would cost $9 billion plus some annual costs; $11 billion is spent annually on ice cream in Europe.
3. Reproductive health services for all women would cost $12 billion a year; $12 billion a year is spent on perfumes in Europe and the United States.
4. Basic health care and nutrition would cost $13 billion; $17 billion a year is spent on pet food in Europe and the United States.

By comparison with these small items, $35 billion is spent on business entertainment in Japan; $50 billion on cigarettes in Europe; $105 billion on alcoholic drinks in Europe; $400 billion on narcotic drugs around the world; and $780 billion on the world's militaries.

20% of the world's people in industrialized countries account for 86% of total private consumption expenditures, while the poorest 20% account for 1.3%. The share of the poorest 20% of the world's people in global income is 1.1%, down from 1.4% in 1991. There are 16 cars per 1,000 people in developing countries and 405 cars per 1,000 people in industrialized countries. On average, developing countries have one doctor for every 6,000 people whereas industrialized countries have one for every 350 people.

Compare this for a minute with the dissatisfaction women in the US have which makes for such reluctance to admit there are any sexual differences even if they are complementarities:

> "Though the women's movement has begun to achieve equality for women on many economic and political measures, the victory remains incomplete. Take two of the simplest and most obvious indicators: women still earn no more than 72 cents for every dollar that men earn, and we are no where near equal numbers at the very top of decision making in business, government, or the professions" Betty Friedan (Pinker R532 351).

As of 2003, although women comprise 46.6% of the U.S. labor force, 50% of managerial and professional specialty positions, women hold only 13.6% of board seats at Fortune 500 companies. The number of seats held by women of color has increased from 2.5% in 1999 to 3% in 2003. Of the Fortune 500, 54 companies have 25% or more women directors. However seventy two percent is a good deal better slice of the cake than one part in eighty-six, so those seeking sexual equality in the US deserve to be mindful of the fact that their cosmetics bill would provide two-thirds of the world's costs in reproductive health care for all women. Shattering the glass ceiling of 'gender' depends on being able to critique the male reproductive inequity of the US capitalist system, not simply clammer greedily for as much of the income as any man in the street, while women in the rest of the world can't express their own maternal ambivalence so fortuitously, nor spend as much on make-up.

Why do you want to get to the top of this patriarchal dominance hierarchy? Is this a case of transsexual aspirations? Where is the egalitarian network of mutual caring and support?

Military Bias

Commenting on an earlier UN Human Development Report (Mukerjee R483) notes that poverty is not foremost among the criteria by which wealthy nations choose to disburse their aid. This indicates that all aid has a measured degree of self-interest and strategic-interest associated with it, rather than selfless altruism.

Two thirds of the world's poor get less than one third of the total development aid. Donor nations routinely tie assistance to military spending. In 1992 countries that spent more than 4 percent of their GDP on their military received $83 per capita in aid, whereas nations that spent less than 2 percent got $32. A large part of this imbalance is brought about by bilateral donors, who offer not just military but economic aid to strategic allies. For instance, Israel and Egypt received more than $2 billion of the $7.4 billion of bilateral assistance the U.S. gave in 1994. (The two nations receive an additional $3.1 billion in military assistance from the U.S. every year) The US, Russia, China, France and the UK - the five permanent members of the UN Security Council supply the most weapons to developing countries. Although multilateral institutions are more evenhanded - the World Bank gives about half its aid to two thirds of the world's poor, they do not redress the imbalance. As a result, a Brazilian woman living below the poverty line receives $3 in such support a year, whereas her Egyptian counterpart receives $280.

Far more foreign capital flows to developing countries in the form of private investment instead of aid In 1992 more than $100 billion was invested as opposed to the $60 billion donated. Unfortunately for the poorest of the poor, this form of cash flow misses them too. In the late 1980s sub-Saharan Africa received only 6 percent of foreign direct investment. Trade, another means by which developing countries earn foreign capital, also benefits the more developed and illustrates the ambivalence of wealthy states toward the world's poor. Although poverty wins a measure of sympathy, the cheap work force of poor nations makes them an economic threat. By one estimate, if developed countries lifted all trade barriers to Third World goods, the latter would gain in exports twice what they now receive in aid. Another constraint on the development of the Third World - foreign debt - keeps growing. In 1970 total debt was $100 billion; in 1992 it stood at $1.5 trillion, including service charges. During the decade preceding 1992, net financial transfers related to loans amounted to $125 billion-from the developing to the developed world.

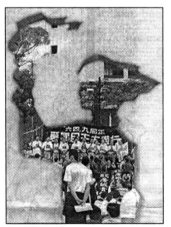

The Goddess of Democracy: Hong Kong commemorating Tiananmen Square (NZ Herald).

Capitalism and Democracy

Democracy is the capacity of a group or population to make decisions or choose a government by majority vote. It is spoken of as a holy grail of a free society as if democracy and freedom were synonymous, yet democracy carries with it a form of totalitarianism which can become oppressive - the tyranny of the majority, for democracy is not based on support for the diversity of a people but on absolute numerical domination.

Democracy also leads to an adversarial form of politics divided into parties with opposing political agendas rather than members elected by the people on their merits. In a first past the post system a tenuous majority can lead to absolute power, potentially 51% of the electorate can result in a government with no opposition at all. These knife-edge characteristics are precisely those of male combat for ultimate reproductive reward. They encourage gerrymandering and provoke wild swings of policy calculated to advantage one side or the other in the Machiavellian round of vote enticement.

Various forms of transferable or proportional voting have been devised to dilute the absolute domination of democracy.

In an MMP system, the extreme male competition is diluted by also having a party vote. This ensures that there will at least be an opposition, although a party with a majority can still govern outright. It tends to favour smaller parties and leads to more feminine strategies, of coalition-building, in turn lambasted by critics, as involving back room deals by non-elected 'party list' members. Mixed MMP as in New Zealand and Germany divides the vote between pure competition in the case of electorate candidates to an integrative continuous party vote. The 5% threshold for small parties without electorate candidates ensures the number of small parties will be few enough to enable a consensual coalition to emerge. The end result is that the individual vote has 'wave' and 'particle' features and that majority and consenus play a role in forming a governement both through hierarchical leadership and collegial coaliton reflecting sexual paradox and the prisoners' dilemma.

Steven Pinker (R532 161) contrasts two traditions of sociological government, the utopian and tragic, closely associated with assumptions of human altruism and selfishness:

> *It is not from the benevolence of the butcher, the brewer, or the baker that we expect our dinner,*
> *but from their regard to their own interest. We address ourselves,*
> *not to their humanity but to their self-love. - Adam Smith*
> *From each according to his abilities, to each according to his needs. - Karl Marx*

"Smith the explainer of capitalism assumes that people will selfishly give their labor according to their needs and will be paid according to their abilities (because the payers are selfish, too). Marx the architect of communism and socialism assumes that in a socialist society of the future the butcher, the brewer, and the baker will provide us with dinner out of benevolence or self-actualization - for why else would they cheerfully exert themselves according to their abilities and not according to their needs?"

Pinker notes (R532 294) that the communist tradition is based on utopian heroic optimism: "Marx wrote that a communist society would be the genuine resolution of the antagonism between man and nature and between man and man; it is the true resolution of the conflict between existence and essence, objectification and self-affirmation, freedom and necessity, individual and species. It is the riddle of history solved. It doesn't get any less tragic or more utopian than that," contrasting it with the tragic view of democracy as the lest diabolical of evils: "'Two cheers for democracy,' proclaimed E. M. Forster. "Democracy is the worst form of government except all those other forms that have been tried," said Winston Churchill. These are encomiums worthy of the Tragic Vision."

Continuing (R532 169) he notes: "What stands in the way of most utopias is not pestilence and drought but human behavior. So utopians have to think of ways to control behavior, and when propaganda doesn't do the trick, more emphatic techniques are tried. The Marxist utopians of the twentieth century, as we saw, needed a tabula rasa free of selfishness and family ties and used totalitarian measures to scrape the tablets clean or start over with new ones. As Bertolt Brecht said of the East German government, 'If the people did not do better the government would dismiss the people and elect a new one.' Political philosophers and historians who have recently 'reflected on our ravaged century,' such as Isaiah Berlin, Kenneth Minogue, Robert Conquest, Jonathan Glover, James Scott, and Daniel Chirot, have pointed to utopian dreams as a major cause of twentieth-century nightmares. Twentieth-century Marxism was part of a larger intellectual current that has been called Authoritarian High Modernism: the conceit that planners could redesign society from the top down using 'scientific' principles." Pinker's comments about cultural feminism are also pertinent here.

The totalitarian nature of the one party state, in contrast to the extreme male combat of first past the post democracy, is partly a reflection of the monolithic feminine strategy in which full agreement is imposed by the unity of the one party. As we have noted, Engels intimated such a swing of the sexual pendulum in conceiving of socialism as a correction to the transition from primal matriarchy to patriarchal class-based capitalism. Of course communism has never been a feminist system, rather one hijacked by male nepotism, but the appeal to altruism and the nurturing principle for all is both feminine and matriarchal, just as the Islamic *umma* was originally a 'mother unit'.

Such a pessimistic view of democracy as the least dangerous of selfish social contract systems does not sit well with Islamic theocracy. Karen Armstrong (R23) outlines the landscape of this divergence between Islam and the democratic ideal pointing out the tenuous capacity for an Islamic state to accept a separation of religion and politics and consensual decision-making although in a more theocratic than democratic context (p 268):

"But politics was no secondary issue for Muslims. We have seen that it had been the theatre of their religious quest. Salvation did not mean redemption from sin, but the creation of a just society in which the individual could more easily make that existential surrender of his or her whole being that would bring them fulfilment. The polity was therefore a matter of supreme importance, and throughout the twentieth century there has been one attempt after another to create a truly Islamic state. This has always been difficult. It was an aspiration that required a jihad, a struggle that could find no simple outcome. The ideal of tawhid [unity of and with God] would seem to preclude the ideal of secularism, but in the past both Shiis and Sunnis had accepted a separation of religion and politics. ... Democracy also posed problems. The reformers who wanted to graft modernity on to an Islamic substructure pointed out that in itself the ideal of democracy was not inimical to Islam. Islamic law promoted the principles of shurah (consultation), and ijmah, where a law had to be endorsed by the 'consensus' of a representative portion of the ummah. The rashidun had been elected by a majority vote. All this was quite compatible with the democratic ideal. Part of the difficulty lay in the way that the West formulated democracy as 'government of the people, by the people, and for the people'. In Islam, it is God and not the people who gives a government legitimacy. This elevation of humanity could seem like idolatry (shirk), since it was a usurpation of God's sovereignty".

Pinker (R532 284) distinguishes the traditions of sociology, communism, postmodernism with the social conract tradition on a similar basis:

"In the sociological tradition, a society is a cohesive organic entity and its individual citizens are mere parts. People are thought to be social by their very nature and to function as constituents of a larger superorganism. This is the tradition of Plato, Hegel, Marx, Durkheim, Weber, Kroenber, the sociologist Talcott Parsons, the anthropologist Claude Lévi-Strauss, and postmodernism in the humanities and social sciences. In the economic or social contract tradition, society is an arrangement negotiated by rational, self-interested individuals. Society emerges when people agree to sacrifice some of their autonomy in exchange for security from the depredations of others wielding their autonomy. It is the tradition of Thrasymachus in Plato's Republic, and of Machiavelli, Hobbes, Locke, Rousseau, Smith, and Bentham. In the twentieth century it became the basis for the rational actor or "economic man" models in economics and political science, and for cost-benefit analyses of public choices. The modern theory of evolution falls smack into the social contract tradition. It maintains that complex adaptations, including behavioral strategies, evolved to benefit the individual (indeed, the genes for those traits within an individual), not the community, species, or ecosystem. Social organization evolves when the long-term benefits to the individual outweigh the immediate costs. Darwin was influenced by Adam Smith, and many of his successors analyze the evolution of sociality using tools that come right out of economics, such as game theory and other optimization techniques. Reciprocal altruism, in particular, is just the traditional concept of the social contract restated in biological terms. Of course, humans were never solitary (as Rousseau and Hobbes incorrectly surmised), and they did not inaugurate group living by haggling over a contract at a particular time and place. Bands, clans, tribes, and other social groups are central to humane existence and have been so for as long as we have been a species. But the logic of social contracts may have propelled the evolution of the mental faculties that keep us in these groups. Social arrangements are evolutionarily contingent, arising when the benefits of group living exceed the costs. With a slightly different ecosystem and evolutionary history, we could have ended up like our cousins the orangutans, who are almost entirely solitary. And according to evolutionary biology, all societies - animal and human - seethe with conflicts of interest and are held together by shifting mixtures of dominance and cooperation".

Madison wrote, "What is government itself but the greatest of all reflections on human nature?" The question this raises is immediate - if the sociobiological tradition falls squarely into the social contract tradition, what forms of social contract would adequately reflect the state of sexual paradox, so misrepresented by the predominance of male reproductive features in the form of capitalist democracy - the dominant form of governance on the planet?

Capitalism is tightly linked with Western democracy in the twentieth century, by contrast with the monolithic unelected governments of communist and fascist regimes. However capitalism has no fundamental connection with democracy as such except in so far as both are manifestations of the social contract. Capitalism does not apply directly to electorates but to the right of private enterprise to use its capital to invest for its own benefit with minimal state control. While democracy mediates the power of government, capitalism is the foundation of corporate power. Capitalism has a long history, which is in no way identifiable with electoral democracy, from the first merchant societies through colonial organizations such as the East India company to modern transnationals which evade the constraints of any democratic electoral mandate. Essentially capitalism confers a right on the possessor of capital to invest as they see fit, without placing on them a moral or regulatory burden to act for the benefit of society as a whole. Corporate interests can also become central agents maintaining fascist leaders in totalitarian power to ensure corporate domination remains unchallenged. Capitalism is intrinsically amoral, having no manifest ethic for the common good, other than survival of the fittest under pure competition, and is fundamentally exploitative because it empowers capital holders over those with few or no resources. It thus tends to exacerbate inequalities, in which the rich gain a stranglehold over the poor. As we have noted these are again key characteristics of the male reproductive strategy.

Linked to capitalism is the 'new right' idea that the interests of a free society are best served in a minimally regulated economy in which there are no monopolies and competition alone is the guarantor and benefactor of welfare and innovation through corporate entities acting in competitive paradox to improve efficiency and hence the common good. Free competition is contrasted with the state controlled monopolies of communist societies specifically dedicated to the common good, because they are prone to becoming monolithic, inefficient and totalitarian. However pure competition is an unstable un-ecosystemic application of the male reproductive principle that leads to short-term winner-take-all exploitation, boom and bust economies, relentless takeover and ultimately the domination of markets by a few ruthless players. For this reason, even the 'purest' capitalist systems find it necessary to enact laws which mediate the negative effects of capital dominion.

A clear example of this ruthless drive to a domination perilous to the planet is the octopus grip the diversification of agricultural and chemical giants such as Monsanto into biotechnology and monopolizing world seed production. Monsanto, starting out with a chequered track record over agent orange has attempted to ensure continuity of its patent on the herbicide roundup beyond its natural term by developing GM roundup-ready soya which contractually requires Monsanto roundup to control weed growth. Monsanto also courted terminator technology despite widespread opposition to gain complete control over the viability of its seed products. At the same time Monsanto has been acquiring major world seed distributors in a strategic attempt to monopolize the world's genetic resources of food and commercial species. Through aggressive takeover by Monsanto and other giants such as Aventis, a major proportion of world seed production has recently fallen into the hands of only a few dominant players. The future of many of the world's source food species in germ banks is also threatening to pass into private hands. The drive for intellectual property rights patenting the world's natural genetic heritage is perhaps the greatest theft of all time.

As of writing Monsanto is seeking to monopolize one of the world's main food crops, soya (wild and cultivated varieties). China is the centre of diversity for soya with over 90% of (more than 6000) existing wild varieties . At the start of the UN Conference on Biodiversity in Bonn, Greenpeace revealed Monsanto's application for a patent, which would grant the company an exclusive right on soy plants, their seeds and progeny with high yield traits. Monsanto claims rights to a natural gene sequence discovered in wild plants originating from China. This sequence is directly linked to high yield characteristics of the soybeans. The patent application was filed simultaneously in over a hundred countries, including the US and Europe. "Monsanto is a ruthless biopirate. The company tries to hijack the genetic resources of a major food crop - basing their claim on a discovery of a gene sequence found in nature. Once this gene sequence is identified even in wild plant, Monsanto has an exclusive right to profit from it," said Greenpeace China. Chinese scientists were shocked. The patent would have large scale consequences.

Neither does such competition necessarily lead to the best solution for consumers as Brian Arthur, economist at the Santa Fe Institute has made clear. Microsoft, which has been the target of continued anti-trust litigation over blatant anti-competitive practices has by far the largest share of the market with its Windows operating system, a redesigned Apple OS look-alike. But the massive number of virus attacks, security glitches and intimations of floating spy code as well as general system inefficiencies confirm it is by no means the optimum product on the market, its huge share maintained by dynamical system stratification because it is too hard for individual users to switch to any other system because of its stratified dominance. John Cassidy explains this idea succinctly:

"When Brian Arthur presented a paper entitled 'Competing Technologies and Lock-in by Historical Small Events' he drew a strong, and largely hostile, response ranging from 'If you are right, capitalism can't work,' to 'Your argument cannot be true!' However since then the example of Microsoft Windows has proved the thesis to the tune of an incipient anti-trust suit for exploiting its market domination in unfair anti-competitive practices. The essential point which goes beyond the monopoly such a large company possesses is that in some commodities competition does not result in an optimum product because any large market share locks consumers in, regardless of the product's real value. As long as Windows is dominant, no form of competition can crack the dominion, because of the lock-in effect the Windows standard sets up (New Yorker 12 Jan 98 32).

Heinz Pagels in "The Dreams of Reason" (R515) concludes that in the absence of a good understanding of complex systems, economists are led into ever more rapid instabilities. 'The economic system, if it is anything, is a system far from equilibrium like the evolutionary system or the immune response. It is continually making adjustments to keep itself far from equilibrium (although there may be local equilibria). Next to nothing is understood about dynamical systems far from equilibrium. Probably the various kinds of attractors - fixed points, limit cycles, and strange attractors - play a role in coming to grips with how a complex system like the economy functions."

The problem of male competitive motifs to the exclusion of cooperative ones is noted specifically by the financier philanthropist George Soros (R640). He contends that capitalism itself has become a threat to democracy. That the free-market, in claiming unilateral possession of the truth, has inadvertently become an enemy of the 'open-society': "Although I have made a fortune in the financial markets, I now fear that the untrammeled intensification of lassiez-faire capitalism and the spread of market values into all areas of life is endangering our open and democratic society. The main enemy of the open society, I believe, is no longer the communist but the capitalist threat. ... [Karl] Popper showed that fascism and communism had much in common, even though one constituted the extreme right and the other the extreme left, because both relied on the power of the state to repress the freedom of the individual. ... I contend that an open society may also be threatened from the opposite direction - from excessive individualism. Too much competition and too little cooperation can cause intolerable inequities and instability."

Once again here we have the sexual prisoners' dilemma between competition and cooperation rearing its 'genitals'. Soros emphasizes the intrinsic instability of financial markets and their 'reflexive' capacity to bring about the very circumstances they claim are realities:

"If we look at the behavior of financial markets, we find that instead of tending toward equilibrium, prices continue to fluctuate relative to the expectations of buyers and sellers. There are prolonged periods when prices are moving away from any theoretical equilibrium. Even if they eventually show a tendency to return, the equilibrium is not the same as it would have been without the intervening period. Yet the concept of equilibrium endures. It is easy to see why: without it, economics could not say how prices are determined. ... In the absence of equilibrium, the contention that free markets lead to the optimum allocation of resources loses its justification. ...Economic theory has deliberately excluded reflexivity from consideration. In doing so, it has distorted its subject matter and laid itself open to exploitation by laissez-faire ideology. ...There has been an ongoing conflict between market values and other, more traditional value systems, which has aroused strong passions and antagonisms. As the market mechanism has extended its sway, the fiction that people act on the basis of a given set of non-market values has become progressively more difficult to maintain. Advertising, marketing, even packaging, aim at shaping people's preferences rather than, as laissez-faire theory holds, merely responding to them. Unsure of what they stand for, people increasingly rely on money as the criterion of value. ... The cult of success has replaced a belief in principles. Society has lost its anchor."

This is profoundly true of the US stock market which dominates the world financial markets to such an extent that rising expectations which drive up prices can in turn provide such financial windfalls to transnational corporations that it enables them to unilaterally intensify their venture capital exploitation of the rest of the world and its resources in turn feeding profits and their stranglehold on power. Mere sentiment can thus become dominion.

A critical development in the rise of world capitalism has been trans-nationalization and its offspring globalization. Since the time of the Phoenicians merchant enterprises have transcended national barriers. With the travels of Marco Polo these activities became global. Colonial developments like the East India Company carried this process forward into the current paradigm of corporations in developed countries acting globally to exploit the resources of the developing world.

There is a stark contrast between the activities of national governments, which are, by definition regional to their land and population, and those of corporations, which are in no way bound by national barriers. This means that the relationship between government, people and corporations is not a level playing field, because corporations can evade the limits of national control, and any responsibility or accountability to the very electorates who constitute the peoples of planet Earth. This 'divide and rule' over national democracies enables transnational corporates to evade both social controls and local taxes and to penalize recalcitrant governments by diverting investment to compliant states. Consequently the power of transnational corporations has eclipsed that of many national economies and the direction of world development and exploitation has become driven by international corporate investment rather than any policy decision of an elected government or population.

However there is a clear alliance with key superpowers, in whose domicile many transnationals originate. The power and dominance of the US economy over those of other countries, as manifested by the world financial domination of US stock markets, is spearheaded by US-sourced transnational corporations. Ensuring world transnational domination even at the expense of reneging on key treaties such as the Biodiversity Convention and renewed Biological Warfare Convention in the interests of intellectual property rights has become a key strategic interest of the US government, advanced by trade threats and litigation. Patenting of genetic sequences and species, including those in the wild, is robbing the people of the earth of evolutionary resources. A further erosive trend has been the rise of 'neo-liberalism' with a dedicated agenda of reducing the regulatory power of government to free the corporate sector to pursue its goals minimally affected by government interference. While this has been touted as removing bureaucratic red tape, reducing taxes by leaning government, and freeing economies to become more dynamic, its net effect has been to marginalize the autonomy of national electorates to make decisions over their own economic futures.

Corporations are neither genetic nor are they ethically based in benefiting society or the common good. Company law does not predicate the nature of the business to be conducted nor does it require a company to benefit, rather than exploit, society or the natural world. The conditions determining company incorporation are simply the rules for convening the board and general meeting of shareholders and provisions for paying any taxes due. Public corporations thus have a responsibility to the board and less directly to the shareholders, but only through national regulation, if any, to the consumers, employees, affected third parties, or the common good. The result is a fragmentation of world democracy into a host of small unaccountable competing units, none of which have a vested interest in the common good, of humanity, nor the preservation of natural resources. Neither are there adequate safeguards of the moral kind invoked by theories of the social contract for human personal interactions. Corporate institutions become faceless entities where people do not have to take personal responsibility for the effects of executive decisions until a company goes into receivership. Just as with tropical forests it is the fractal islandization of democracy which poses the greatest threat to world freedom and justice.

We thus need to find ways of restoring democracy and consensual society to planet Earth. Entering into this mix has been the phenomenon of globalization driven by corporate advisers and members of institutions such as the World Bank holding closed door conferences with leaders of dominant nations to establish a new contract between transnational investment and national sovereignty which would pass to the corporate world much of the autonomy possessed by regional democracies. Many free trade agreements marginalize national governments by making them subject to international litigation if they act to protect their national interest. This power of corporate litigation over elected governments represents a watershed loss of democratic autonomy by electoral populations. ßThe reaction of protesters and the enclave mentality of those sponsoring globalization shows clearly that this process is not democratic, but is rather a gambit for control of the world's resources by the corporate sector. While this may not be a totalitarian conspiracy as such, but rather a dynamical force driving whole economies inexorably to a conclusion through established media interests and stock market fluctuations, it is nevertheless undemocratic, unethical and damaging.

Despite being weakened in many countries by globalization, national sovereignty is in turn used to weaken international bodies such as the UN to create a form of tragedy of the commons by a reverse consensus of non-interference in another country's affairs. This means that issues involving global resources such as the Amazon and its biodiversity can be stymied by a single nation exerting unilaterally its territorial imperative over what is genuinely a world heritage resource for the whole of humanity and the diversity of life.

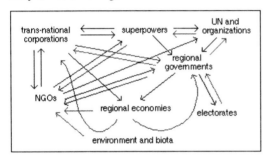

The major dynamical feedbacks in global political decision-making

In terms of environmental health, the planet is a dynamical system driven by at least four major factors: (a) the 200 or so national governments some democratically elected some otherwise, (b) multi-national corporations, (c) the globalist influence of the UN and its bodies such as UNEP etc., (d) NGOs, and (e) the 'North-South' dialogue between developed energy-hungry countries and developing energy-lean countries, which also possess a large proportion of the genetic resources of the planet. The same deregulated conditions which encourage transnational investment encourage evolutionary democracies. These provide an opportunity to redress the loss of democratic autonomy, by providing a means for the whole of human society to cooperatively deal with the ethical decisions required to provide a sustainable future for all of us.

The continuing pattern of exploitative venture capital investment competing to take advantage of all remaining natural resources is a direct threat to biodiversity planet-wide. It is likewise contrary to any grass-roots move to establish the future ecosystemic society upon which we will have to depend for a sustainable existence. It is both devastating to the future sustainability of the planet and as contrary to the interests of the people in the very developed countries which are the source of the initiative as it is to people in developing countries who become exploited by the undemocratic investment initiatives of the developed world. It is sourced in three evolutionary fallacies, the idea that an ecosystem survives by competition alone rather than a mix of competition, cooperation, niche formation and diversification. It invokes male winner-take-all reproductive mating competition, to the exclusion of the female honest out-front long-term investment for survival across the generations. Finally the process is non-genetic, has no generations and has no principle of selective advantage across generations. Although capitalism has brought developed countries a period of high living standards, and a strategic dominance in the world arena, its exploitative instabilities are leading us towards a precipice of collapse of this temporary abundance through rampant resource exploitation and increasing world conflict because of its exacerbation of poverty and inequality and failure to bring about a compassionate and just society which caters to the common good of humankind.

Gareth Hardin (R283) in his 'seminal' article "The Tragedy of the Commons" outlines the way in which many of the crises facing humanity are examples of the 'commons tragedy', in which individual advantages, regardless of exhortations to altruism inevitably lead to the destruction of common resources in ways which cause an irresolvable dilemma for each of the participants. It applies to population explosion and the exploitation of mineral resources like oil and the destruction of biodiversity. This is exacerbated by a cutting edge free-market based on competitive instability under individual incentives of a winner-take-all nature. The tragedy of the commons is a warning and a terminal metaphor for the entire capitalist competitive paradigm and a warning to us about the impending holocaust of biodiversity.

Pinker (R532 161) notes that dealing with defection is part of our traditional moral dilemma, but we have to find effective ethical paradigms to deal with the corporate sector:

> "For that matter, everyone, regardless of Politics, has to be appalled at people who impose costs on society in pursuit of their individual interests-hunting endangered species, polluting rivers, destroying historic sites to build shopping malls, spraying graffiti on public monuments, inventing weapons that elude metal detectors. Equally disturbing are the outcomes of actions that make sense to the individual choosing them but are costly to society when everyone chooses them. Examples include over-fishing a harbor, overgrazing a commons, commuting on a bumper-to-bumper freeway, or buying a sport utility vehicle to protect oneself in a collision because everyone else is driving a sport utility vehicle. Many people dislike the suggestion that humans are inclined to selfishness because it would seem to imply that these self-defeating patterns of behavior are inevitable, or at least reducible only through permanent coercive measures."

Noam Chomsky, despite being branded a socialist, has validly highlighted the exploitation of the developing world by the West for raw materials and particularly the neo-liberalist agenda to diminish democracy sufficiently so that corporate power will be able to run so-called free societies through their financial monopoly as a group. Minimizing the state, which means minimizing the public arena in which people can act to determine their futures. Instead, power has been transferred to financial institutions such as the World Trade Organization, IMF, the World Bank and to transnational corporations via international 'free' trading agreements. Citing Orwell, Chomsky sees the media in free-market societies as representing the business establishment view of their major financiers by executing a voluntary form of censorship more insidious and pervasive than a police state could achieve by force.

In "From Corporatism to Democracy" John Ralston Saul affirms 'government' as opposed to the corporate sector as the bastion of personal autonomy. "The most powerful force possessed by the individual citizen is their own government. Or governments, because a multiplicity of levels means a multiplicity of strengths. The individual has no other large organized mechanism that he can call his own. There are other mechanisms, but they reduce the citizen to the status of a subject. Government is the only organized mechanism that makes possible that level of shared disinterest known as the public good. Without this greater interest the individual is reduced to a lesser, narrower being limited to immediate needs. He will then be subject to other, larger forces, which will necessarily come forward to fill the void left by the withering of the public good. Those forces will fill it with some other directing interest that will serve their purposes, not the larger purposes of the citizen. ... This is what makes the neo-conservative and market force arguments so disingenuous. Their remarkably successful demonization of the public sector has turned much of the citizenry against their own mechanism. Many of us have been enrolled in the cause of interests that have no particular concern for the citizen's welfare. Our welfare. Instead, the citizen is reduced to the status of a subject at the foot of the throne of the marketplace."

The Free-market Myth and Ecosystemic Society

The myth of the free-market is that the lean mean world of competition is a more ecosystemically efficient system than any regulated economy. This has a tragic flaw. Ecosystems are conserved sustainably because all surviving organisms have a cumulative genetic imprint of their entire evolutionary history. They are survivors in a surviving biosphere. The leopard cannot change its spots in a single generation and become a shark.

Companies have a non-genetic charter which determines only how they hold meetings, nothing about their evolutionary niche. They are non-democratic. Their directors are generally only financially accountable to the shareholders, not strategically accountable. In the absence of societal regulation, they are completely non-accountable to the human and natural environments in which they operate, consumer, worker, affected citizen and impacted environment alike. They are unstable dynamical systems striving to exploit resources more quickly than their competitors and capable of liquidating their assets and changing their strategic identity and line of business if they exploit and destroy a given resource.

The North Atlantic Cod fishery, probably the richest fishery in the world was destroyed because competing deep sea fishing companies partly sponsored by the Canadian government fished out the entire cod spawning grounds. Fisheries inspectors were not adequately equipped to keep up with this devastation until too late, but the companies themselves sold their plant, liquidated their assets and entered new lines of business, creaming the profits of destroying a world resource which had been successfully fished from the time of Columbus until the 1970s. Genetic corporate constitutions are essential to prevent this kind of hit and run. An Economist article "Flexible Tiger Lives by Law of the Economic Jungle" on Taiwan business and its survival without government support illustrates how naive ecosystemic ideas pervade competitive free-market thinking. In fact, the only ecosystemic ideas in the picture are 'tiger' and 'jungle'. The idea that no government regulation of the birth, competition and bankruptcy of businesses fosters a lean mean 'round of selection' is false Darwinian reasoning since the genetic principle is completely absent and there is no cumulative selection over generations. In the article, the turnover in chemical companies in five years was so high that the virtually all the market leaders were essentially replaced and many had been taken over or ceased to exist. The consequences for accountability of such high-impacting industries are alarming.

The other aspect of this tragedy which is non-biological is that the venture-risk winner-take-all model of competition is not actually a truth of genetic conservation, because genes and organisms, even selfish genes and predator and prey systems which are apparently antagonistic are often bound in constructive feedback (p 507), leading to long-term genetic survival. Risking death to make large venture capital gains is the male reproductive imperative of mortal dependence on competition to fertilize the opposite sex, with immense reproductive windfalls if the venture brings in large resources. The female strategy, unlike the sneaky, low investment, short-term male strategy has always been honest and 'out-front' (human pregnancy is the most massive and hardest to hide) and it has always been an investment in which risk has to be minimized for the mother in consideration of a large investment made across future generations. In a male-dominant society it is easy to understand how institutions and economic policies can become a product of the spermatogenic imperative but for our survival is it essential to correct this imbalance.

Both multi-national corporations and political democracies are founded on the concept of a charter of association, which determines how the executive is elected and how democracy of management and members proceeds. Changes in concept of charters of association to a more genetic type of paradigm including an ethical memorandum of ecosystemic function with accountability to all 'interested' parties, consumers, workers, third parties affected for example by pollution, as well as investors and shareholders, could dramatically change the principles of both corporate and political worlds and the face of the world for the better.

Heavenly Paradise and Earthly Destruction

One of the most damaging aspects of this paradigm of 'dominion over nature' is that to the religious Christian fundamentalist it is the way the 'late planet earth' can be consigned to oblivion in seeking a heavenly paradise, based on a pagan Pauline myth of 'rapture', which abnegates personal responsibility for apocalyptic destruction, and the rape of the planet that results from such disregard and disrespect for the umbilicus of nature:

we who are alive, who are left, shall be caught up together with them in the clouds
to meet the Lord in the air (1 Thess 4:15).

Islam, which shares the Christian apocalyptic agenda of final conflict, also shares this error. When al-Quaeda terrorists flew planes into the World Trade Centre they presumably knew Muhammad himself is reputed to have suggested the end would come when people built buildings too tall. When George Bush Jr. says in invading Afghanistan after the fall of the twin towers: "this crusade, this war on terror, may take a while" he is exposing the true nature of the conflict as a clash of partiarchal religious imperatives and when he invades Iraq, finding no weapons of mass destruction, it is clear the conflict is motivated by the culture of honour in family feud (p 187). Both are blatant manifestations of male combat.

"I said to him, 'I believe in Allah.' So he said, 'But I believe in torture and I will torture you.'
Because they started to hit my broken leg, I curse my religion.
They ordered me to thank Jesus I'm alive." Iraqi US abuse victim

In the minds of the technophiliac, the rapture gains another 'incarnation'- a space-race utopia of human galactic-colonization; having 'unfortunately' wasted our home planet in our 'growing-up'. In a sense, this is the greatest expression of unbalanced male reproductive ambition possible in the apocalyptic scenario, excelling the stars in the sky granted to Abraham. Even the seeding of life in the universe has been claimed to be cosmic 'panspermia.'

Without being unduly pessimistic, we are foolishly heading towards a needless and serious risk of extinction. Human society still contains unacceptable levels of nuclear and other weapons of mass destruction. These nearly became an Armageddon of mutually assured destruction during the cold war and should be removed completely. Our impacts are rapidly leading to mass extinction of the diversity of life and our population growth is still unsustainable for the future diversity of the biosphere. While many people are watching science fantasy on television and imagine escaping to another planet, we are unwittingly precipitating the 'sixth extinction' of life which could become as serious as the Permian one, taking 50 million years to make a substitute recovery.

This indicates a serious mismatch between cultural and technological fantasy and sustainable evolutionary reality. Genetic engineering, cloning, reproductive technology could next be used to turn the entire biosphere into a bunch of 'boys toys' - a potentially terminal condition, because the underlying diversity of natural medicinal and food species is replaced by a fragile assortment of genetically-engineered near zero-diversity products which are non-viable in evolutionary terms but dominate productive areas. At the same time our own natural human viability is being compromised by runaway biotechnology including IVF, routine Caesarians, the drive for often cosmetic germ-line engineering and male-driven eugenics, including artificial wombs, and ambitions for cloning from religious and utopian movements and their leaders. All it would take is a small astronomical mishap to bring on a mass extinction of humanity from a complete failure of the food distribution system. Even a small asteroid impact on a brittle culture in a damaged biosphere, dependent on computer planning (albeit with a 'nuclear proof' world-wide web), highly technologized food-distribution to urban centres dependent on agro-tech, and foodstuffs, made using genetically engineered agricultural species which have no natural viability, with a human population propped up by extreme medical technologies, could cause almost certain demise of humanity, from the very brittleness of the society we have generated, to natural disruption.

While these technologies, used for the right purposes, have great potential to do good, it is natural diversity upon which we depend to survive and diversity we should foster. Without a clear ethical consensus from society at large to protect genetic diversity, the gene technology industry stands to collapse the entire bubble of living diversity while playing scientific and financial 'he-man'. We urgently need to heal these wounds to our viability through an appreciation for the sustainable evolutionary endowment we possess as a species.

Conclusion: Partnership Society and Sexual Redemption

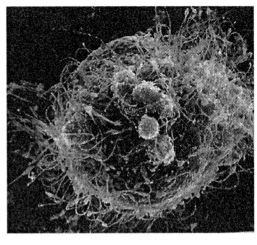

Human ovum with sperm (New Scientist)

Sustainable Culture and Natural Abundance

To survive in abundance over evolutionary epochs, our societies need to develop the powers of survival we know are possessed by natural ecosystems - societies which reflect our sexual complementarity in partnership and natural diversity in all our interactions - autonomous, free societies, with rich regional variation.

The key to this is replenishing the fertile condition of sexual paradox in human relationships, engendering between women and men a mutual sense of appreciation, respect, awe, and completion. The healing of our social 'condition' in 'whole-heartedness' involves both a 'holy' wholeness - completion in complementation between the sexes; and heartedness - emotional connectedness with one another, which engenders a sense of being participants together in the unfolding adventure of life.

It is the very interplay between chaos and order, in natural and sexual selection, which is at the root of the ecosystemic climax complexity of natural and social diversity, and the future abundance of life. For all its paradoxes of chaos and order (p 498) in the prisoners' dilemma of fidelity and deceit (p 13), our gatherer-hunter roots have evolutionary original virtue (p 50), through the positive feedback of mutual sexual acceptance, and the physical and emotional bonding which accompanies it. Through the influence of sexual selection, we are capable of romantic and compassionate love, beyond the confines of kin altruism or reciprocation (p 19). When imposed divisions of alienation are removed, we are sufficiently generous and empathic to be naturally capable of forming a just, supportive and caring world society. We are so, principally because of the positive filtering of sexual selection, rather than through negative social, moral, or religious filters using the threat of punishment, nor through the Machiavellian complexities of expedience alone, although these are also part of our heritage. Without such original virtue, all attempts to impose the good and just upon us would fail.

We can capitalize on our evolutionary sustainability and innate sexual goodness of heart in love as a species, to evoke consensually a sane, blessed, biodiverse, sustainable society, through the autonomy of family, partnership and our peers - and centrally through the sacredness of sex itself and its relation to the reproductive process, through which the immortal passage of the generations comes about.

Society still hasn't come to terms with female reproductive choice, even in an era when genetic testing has become routine. The complementary paradox between the reproductive strategies of women and men and mate selection as a catalyst of human evolution into cultural complexity is only beginning to be understood. We need to accept female reproductive and maternal choice as 'holy' if anything is - an integral part of the whole pattern of living existence. We need to allow women to make reproductive choices, even though this may cause men jealous anxiety. Rights of choice over pregnancy and sensitive issues like abortion need to be understood in the context of maternal ambivalence and its key role in natural selection for our long-term survival. Men in turn need to play a greater creative role in child-rearing and display supportive parental love to all the offspring their partner may have regardless of the 'stripped naked' evidence of genetic testing.

The feminist revolution has brought a swing of the pendulum in Western society away from patriarchal dominance, in which women are recognized as the equals and even superiors of men in many respects, are able to enter management positions and pursue academic, artistic and entrepreneurial careers without discrimination. However the paradoxical reunion in partnership sexual equality and complementation invites has yet to take place. The immense central importance of mothering to the future of life has been all but discarded in a narrow culturally-based idea of 'gender' which neglects the very biological complementarity which underpins our future survival. The resolution of this dilemma is made possible only through a mutual respect between women and men for the contributions each can make to parenting.

The old patterns of patrilineal inheritance have given way to equal patterns of inheritance by both sexes, and patrilocality has given way to fluid and flexible family associations, from single-parent and nuclear families, to the diverse parenting arrangements provoked by serial monogamy. These could bring grandmothers, daughters and granddaughters back into a closer relationship where good female choices can be encouraged which promote resourceful sociable male partnering rather than the violence and domination of the disaffected patriarchy. Young women need to be able to make wise decisions in picking male partners who will espouse resourceful domestic bliss, rather than delinquent patriarchal confrontations, amid lethal jealousy. We all need to take advantage of these gains, by the men learning to take full advantage of a partnership society by engaging as fathers and as lovers in a way which enriches and complements family life and creative abundance.

Many of our institutions and corporate, economic, social and electoral processes are still patriarchally distorted with motifs of pure competition without compensating cooperation, boom and bust short term instability, winner-take-all exploitation and profound inequity of resources, education and opportunity. We need to review all these structures and institutions and find new, more abundant, and fairer ways of dealing with our social contracts, the equitableness of resources and opportunities between women, and men and between rich and poor. Central to this is a fundamental change in workplace practices to integrate the needs of mothering and parenting as central human activities essential to the human condition with continuity of careers. Flexible work conditions, including part-time, shared positions, and adequate parental and maternity leave are a starting point.

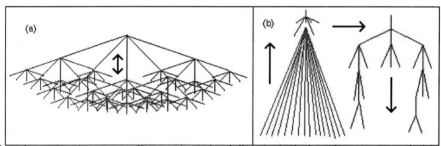

Fractal ecosystemic consensuality permits regional diversity in the branches, consensus decision-making without a division by keeping decision making groups to a size between 9 and 16. Nominees are group representatives at the next higher level and remain accountable on all levels. Even on a planetary basis, this has far fewer layers of hierarchy than traditional systems of electoral democracy (right) in which a diffuse electorate (green) elects a party into power (blue) which runs a bureaucracy (red) which governs a population.

Central to this is the affirmation of sexual paradox as a founding principle of social engagement, and of consensual agreement rather than competitive majority decision-making in our government and economic life. There are many ways of doing this. One way would be to require mutual participation of women and men in decision making with a consensual agreement required between men and women on major policy directions as the Ashanti have done. Another would be to extend existing methods of proportional voting to elect a consensus cabinet comprising major parties and affiliations rather than an executive president or a prime minister and cabinet elected by the dominant party. This would avoid the administration and major portfolios always being in the hands of the 'effective majority'. Consensus would provide fuller agreement, but in the event of a break down into a majority decision, a natural opposition would emerge, guaranteeing checks and balances.

Another more radical possibility, which fits with the decentralized autonomous nature of human trust and decision making based on kin and peers, is ecosystemic consensuality, in which a fractal structure of consensual decision-making replaces central government. This would allow for much greater diversity in social styles and preferences and cater for both regional and minority group diversity and relative autonomy. It generally has many fewer layers of bureaucratic hierarchy than traditional electoral government. For example working in fractals of 12-13 requires only 9 levels of hierarchy to cover the world population.

Many of the vagaries associated with sexuality are products of sexual dominion. Feminists rightly decry the hard-core aspects of male-oriented pornography and its extremes of sadomasochistic violence taken to a nemesis of the whole meaning of sexual fertility in 'snuff movies'. The same goes for exploitation of children in paedophilic pornography where adult power is a form of sexual dominion. We have seen in the context of ancient Greece (p 203), and in violent male warrior societies today, such as the Yanomamo (p 149), where sexual access to women is limited that the toleration of male homosexual paedophilia correlates with male supremacist attitudes and monopolization of women. Although we all have needs for sexual bonding, prostitution is another face of the woman as possession (p 60).

Sexuality needs to be lifted up to its whole, holy and complete status as sacred, and the deepest expression of integration of spirit and nature, not cast into the gutter as pornographic carnal lust. Women, given a conducive environment, enjoy sex, and sexual erotica, every bit as much as men and are a sexual and sensual inspiration to ecstasy. Reducing sex to prim moral imperatives on the one hand and a commercial commodity bought and sold on the other is to keep it in patriarchal bondage.

The continuing social conflicts over abortion are also a test case of the dynamics of sexual domination in action. Fundamental opposition to abortion comes most prominently from adherents and spokespeople for major patriarchal religious views, which promote unrestrained fertility, both to increase the 'faithful' and to protect paternity rights over the unborn. Womens' right to 'choice' is an expression of the female's evolutionary maternal ambivalence in the face of fluctuating male investment and paternity demands and the very real burdens of reproduction that fall on the human female, as Sarah Hrdy has noted (p 35). In an enlightened society, these factors, along with a sense of compassion for both the life process and for the mother's central role, would mediate the need for abortion, in favour of effective contraception. There is also a need to differentiate particularly late forms of intervention such as 'partial birth', which raise deep ethical issues of the consciousness of the unborn, from early termination of pregnancy by curettage, or the morning after pill. Moral or ethical choices about such questions are central strategies in the prisoners' dilemma game the passage of the generations presents us and have to remain part of the ongoing decisions living people make, rather than being subjected to a final moral edict.

It is also clear that all the forms of sexual 'infidelity', from secretive affairs, through sewing wild oats, and polygyny, to carefully negotiated polyamory, each wracked with their surrounding atmospheres of jealousy and intrigue, can and should never be eliminated from the social picture, repressed, or censured ethically, because they are fundamental components of the reproductive choices both sexes make. This applies particularly for females, who carry more than the 'lionesses' share of the reproductive parenting investment, even when they have partners who are good 'house husbands'. Nevertheless there are ways of dealing with sexual choice in relative openness, which can help to protect existing relationships, in caring for our offspring and our long-term partners. Without this sense of long-term trust, in a context of autonomous choice, sexuality itself becomes a meaningless degrading consumptive condition on the one hand and a straight-jacket on the other. In a modern connected world, we have to take additional responsibility and care for those we associate with sexually, to protect them from the very real defilements of sexually transmitted diseases, which often target women, from HIV, (which was first spread by highly promiscuous homosexual and heterosexual men, but is becoming a disease of women, because it is twice as likely to be transmitted from a man to a woman as the reverse), to chlamydia (a key cause of female infertility). Careless love can become fatal attraction, both for lovers and unwitting partners.

We need to learn to celebrate the deep relationship between sexuality and the sexual act as the most tumultuous expression of the life force in its pleasure and in its reproductive basis in the passage of the generations, for society to retain its biological anchor. To reduce sex on the one hand to a purely social bonding involving consenting acts between adults in private without any connection with reproduction, and on the other hand a religious imperative to reproduce often without pleasure, in a state of original sin, is schizophrenic and leads to a divided and confused attitude to sexuality, reproduction, and our living futures.

While society, as a system of moral contracts, needs to have the teeth to deal with violent defection, corruption, and sexual exploitation, we need to also recognize that criminality as defection is central to the prisoners' dilemma and that our patriarchal paradigm has actually been founded on defection in competition and gain for the strong against the weak. The true remedy is social justice and equitability. We need to develop natural justice with fair rewards as well as the minimal punishments necessary to avoid defection becoming anarchy, recognizing that defection is also essential to our welfare, in counter-cultural critique, art, music, scientific paradigm shift and the court and spark of love's enticements. Criminality is best incorporated into the prisoners' dilemma constructively. Draconian penalties simply lead to more intractable conflicts, and the emergence of cut-throat professional criminal syndicates.

We need to recognize the basic holiness of all the phenomena of life, particularly the ecosystemic aspects of living fertility. Sex, power plants, music and art, are a key to ecosystemic liberation because each provides a unique avenue of interactive engagement of consciousness, both between people and across species. Although the living sacraments have been revered in all traditional societies which have discovered their use, their synthetic analogues have become a scourge on modern society partly because of the very taboos against non-conformity which make them illegal. We need to accept and understand that agents which take us to the 'other' are valuable in understanding the verdant complexity that lies in the unstable equilibrium between the will to order and the fear of chaos. The war against drugs, like the war on terror is a contradiction in terms, an attempt to impose order by totalitarian conformity and taboo, which merely adds enticement to transgression.

We need to begin a forward 'visioning of our futures' through consensual dialogue involving a broad consensus in diversity among women and men, to conceive alternative futures and new democratic processes to address all the major issues of sexual equality, fairness of distribution, restoration of biodiversity, protecting the world's resources for all, demilitarization, climatic responsibility. We urgently need to develop a far-sighted and altruistic view of our human genetic futures and those of the species on which we depend, which can cope with the enormous watershed changes rapidly occurring, in a way which retains human viability and evolutionary adaptability. Entering the age of detailed genetic testing, germ-line engineering, cloning and artificial reproductive technology could be as fatal as rampant mass extinction of biodiversity and the rape and genocide of the natural planet's resources, unless we come to understand the dynamic roots of reproductive engagement.

Discovering the spontaneous roots of human goodness in the most fundamental altruistic relationship the cosmos has discovered - the sexual relationship - could become the key for a truly sustainable society with minimal imposed structure, local diversity, and sustainability. Such a society would have few of the root causes for criminality and violent defection that arise from the inequities and injustices of social opportunity, which inevitably result from the winner-take-all competition of an unmediated patriarchal free-market hierarchy. Recognizing the joyful completion of our original virtue, in the hidden repressed feminine complement of our all-too-male capitalist winner-take-all paradigm, could lead to the flowering of an autonomous, consensual, sustainable society, not based on imposed institutions of competition and greed, but spontaneously in perpetual abundance for all, in our enclosed planetary garden of paradise, celebrated by long life, good science, sumptuous environments, fulfilling families immortalizing our good relations, entertaining partners, entrancing music, fine art , deep meditation, cataclysmic sacraments, and life-long, life-giving love.

It is to the intrinsic goodness arising from sexual selection, we owe the finest virtues we usually associate with the higher spiritual domains - of transcendence, enlightenment, and divine grace as manifestations of the cosmic in subjective consciousness. It is thus to the redemption sexual wholeness provides us that all the mergings of atonement follow. From the sexual relationship, formed in paradox between the genders, all the skills of sustainable survival in mutual appreciation discovered in the evolutionary emergence of humanity flow forth in abundance, and with them our capacity to bring to bear, with the benefit of enlightened technology, a sustainable future on planet Earth, both for ourselves and for all the diverse species which give the planet its paradisiacal robustness over evolutionary epochs.

The time of planetary rape needs to give way to planetary replenishment in abundance. Sheherazade's tale of "The Thousand and One Nights" is a founding parable of female wisdom healing the homicidal despotism of the king. As in Chaucer's tale of the Wife of Bath, the redemption of the young male rapist on a year's commuted death sentence to find 'what women want' is to give the gnarled crone sovereignty. When she offers him the fatal choice: he can have her old and ugly and faithful or young, beautiful, and possibly unchaste, he tells her to choose. When he does so, she turns into a beautiful maiden, and thus they live to their 'lyves ende in parfit joye'. This ideal is not submission to female dominance, but turning the tables of the prisoners' dilemma, from a race against the other, into a peacock's tale of cultural and sexual splendour.

Why sex IS polarized

Sex is polarized and its extreme polarity is the very source of living diversity. Hence we should respect it and not seek to dissolve it into a sameness of our own cultural contrivance. Fusion sex (p 336) is a inter-fertile division of life into two complementary polarities. Symmetry-breaking is essential to generate complexity, because it means that the two 'aspects' are able to express differences, creating new kinds of interactions, often even in such a way as to make each dependent on the other. Their very differences lead both to interactive complementation and to strategic dissonance, and hence complexity.

Although it may have emerged from a form of cellular cannibalism, sex is the most powerful form of organic altruism to emerge in evolution, unparalleled at the molecular level by any other process. It is altruistic because we contribute our genetic endowment only in half-share to the next generation, to be entwined with the 'alien' other (p 329). From this time on, in the sexual weave, our unique genetic identity will never come together again. Because of this, sexual recombination in turn enables the generation of endless individual variety, almost every combination of which is viable. Without the recombinational power of genetic sexuality, no multi-celled organism could have ever evolved. Nevertheless it is from the polarity of sex that its full complexity emerges. The complementarity of heterosexuality is a direct generator of the complexity of life's evolution. Its polarity is no more starkly emphasized than in the egg and sperm, the immortal germ line, in respect of which we are merely a mortal conscious shadow.

The sex cells could not be more dissimilar if they consciously tried to plan their own design. The sperm is a tightly packaged bunch of almost entirely inactive DNA driven by the motile flagellum. The ovum, by contrast is huge, the largest of all cells and is electrically poised to crisis. One merely a nucleic acid particle, but the other an excitable wave enveloping cell - a nascent conscious being. At the cellular level, only heterosexuality is possible. There is no way a sperm can naturally make sex with another sperm, or an egg with an egg. Moreover this is because evolution has found the polarity of sex to be the most wildly creative solution to biodiversity.

Fertilization is not a neutralizing merging of these polarities, but a critical state of explosive complexity. At fertilization, it is almost impossible to discern which is the instigator of the merging. The sperm is trying to dissolve the egg's coating and but into it, but the egg is poised to an orgasmic cortical reaction, which sets of a wave of electronic excitability, explosively firing off all its outer coating. It then proceeds to drag the hapless sperm inside itself with octopus-like pseudopods (p 337).

This polarization of the egg and sperm has come about through a sex war, whose complexity has to make one marvel as much as its Machiavellian nature might make us cynical (p 335).The first sexual organisms had identical isogametes, so they were truly gay. Two egg-sperms from distinct strains would simply fuse together. But unfortunately their cytoplasms didn't get along because their endosymbiotic mitochondria, our bacterial energy batteries of respiration, were in deadly competition. A cytoplasmic war broke out and 90% of the cytoplasm frequently got lost, causing a huge deficit in fertility. The sustained attack of the dominant mitochondria caused a symmetry-breaking in which one sex stopped investing in cytoplasm, kept the flagellum and evolved into a particulate motile molecular DNA capsule. The other gender became the 'mother body', retaining the cytoplasm and internal endo-symbiotic organelles. These large cells then became the archetype of all of organismic diversity. The involuting form of the ovoplasm becoming the three-layer topological embryo.

Ever since, there have been sputtering genetic wars, from male-killer mitochondria to male flies that bear poisons which prevent a female mating with other males, to which the females evolve resistance in turn (p 16). In sea urchins, the sperm and egg are locked in such a genetic war, with the sperms continually evolving antigens to dissolve into the egg and the egg evolving just as rapidly to prevent it. These sex genes thus evolve at a highly accelerated rate. It is the very strategic paradox of this entwined dance of cooperation and competition, called sexually-antagonistic co-evolution (p 16), that has created the consonance and dissonance that has seen the teeming climax of living diversity, complexity and intelligence arise in multi-celled animals and plants. Even hermaphroditic plants, which are in the vast majority, emphasize the intrinsic polarization of sexuality in their adapted sperm consisting of fine pollen and ovum become embryonic seed germ, waiting to be fertilized in the flower's ovary. Sex-changing fish likewise display clear sexual polarity, switching sex so as to reproduce, based on dominance, (or possession of a sea anemone in the case of Nemo the clown fish). This is no sexual rainbow, but a natural metamorphosis from one extreme to the other.

Every aspect of this polarization has led to the enhancement of biological complexity and living diversity. Because the sperm is little more than crystalline inactive molecular DNA driven by a flagellum it can be produced easily in millions of copies. Paradoxically for a stripped-bare cell, the sperm flagellum is supposed to become the primal spindle orchestrating the division of the combined chromosomes of the fertilized egg - not a bad idea since it has proven it can work very well in getting the sperm here. The eggs by contrast are few and massive. This again enhances the evolutionary process because it enables the fickle males to be strongly selected and the females to become ever more adapted to viable motherhood. The ovum has become specialized to possess a unique vast cytoplasm, in which it carries a morphogenic imprint sufficient to enfold the entire complex topology of the organism through symmetry-breaking genetic switches, as the fertilized ovum begins to divide. Each stage of the development of complexity of the embryo is a symmetry-breaking 'sexual' division of the stem line. The ectoderm breaks symmetry with the endoderm and so on until we have the migratory interactions of migrating neurons in the brain. We are in this sense intimately heterosexual in the variety of our organs and cell types.

From the first egg and sperm, the investments of males and females have been skewed, complementary, but in partial conflict (p 335). Males invest less, contributing only DNA, and tend to cut and run. Females have to invest not only in an egg, but in mammals in pregnancy, lactation, and child care. This polarization continues all the way to the relation between male and female minds. Males are more lateralized and more focused to the exclusion of the whole picture (p 388). These complements have been of natural benefit to both sexes in all phases of our evolution, from the death of the dinosaurs, to the human gatherer-hunter mind, with its targeting, map reading males and classifying, networking females. This complementation of two somewhat differing minds bringing differing skills and intuitions to the bed and dinner table, caught in strategic paradox, yet aiming to please the 'other' and thus be sexually accepted, has been the basis of the flowering of all cultural and social complexity (p 53). Yet is is not just the human mind, but the human sex organs and their diverse and complementary orgasmic climaxes, that the beauty and meaning of sexual polarization gains its most sensitive expression, for here, like the evolutionary race between the sea urchin egg and sperm, there has been an amatory race between an ever more impetuous and discriminating clitoris, made all the more intoxicating by the unbearable fecund beauty of burgeoning breasts and buttocks, and an ever more turgid, pretentious, yet coquettish penis, seeking, at all costs, to satisfying the 'other' in the interplay of incessant social sexuality, which crowns the diversity of life with the bitter-sweet Machiavellian panoply of culture.

While we spend over 99% of our adult love life engaged in habitual, and sometimes highly creative social sex, a full 100% of us come into this world as conscious living beings through reproductive sex. This poses a paradox, which liberal attitudes to purely social sex between consenting adults fails to resolve successfully. Although human sex is highly social and conception is very occasional, in the face of the relentless habituality of coitus, it is reproductive sex which makes viable sense of the pleasure principle in evolutionary terms and puts all of sex's diversity, addiction, longing, and sometimes frank pain, in relationship with the immortal passage of life itself. The fullness of reproductive sexuality doesn't just have meaning between coital mother and father, in the ultimate Tantric act of reunion which sometimes becomes conception, but is intrinsic to brother and sister, mother and son, grandmother and granddaughter and the whole fabric of kinship and extends to the bonding between all people in the flow of life's living generations. In the passage of the generations, social sex and the pleasure principle gain their true meaning, as the glue which binds the affection of the generations, to care for the future of life itself, generative of all life's diversity.

Social sex is also capable of manifold diversity, despite the overt confines of a moral society, simply because human sexuality is vastly abundant over its immediate reproductive function. Social sex is central to the glue that binds, not only traditional couples and families, but a wider spectrum of emotional bonding between people as an expression of physical intimacy and the ecstatic pleasure of physical contact and belonging. Thus individuals may elect to become philanderers, swingers, polyamorists, bisexuals or homosexuals. The emphasis of coitus shifts to all forms of erotic stimulus from fellatio and cunnilingus through vibrators and penis pumps to homosexual and heterosexual sodomy. People practice manifold forms of erotic dance, music and art, fetishism, transvesticism, transexuality, sado-masochism, prostitution, voyeurism and hunger to explore virtually every expression of sexual transgression the mind can imagine. These are themselves an expression of sexual paradox in abundance. In many ways this diversity is an expression of social maturity between consenting adults in pursuit of the pleasure principle, as well as perverted lust, domination and frank commercial exploitation. It is social maturity which speaks for acceptance of the right of people to choose their sexual orientation and style of love life, but social sexuality ultimately draws its rationale and meaning from reproductive sex and the sociobiological roots of the two sexes in their differing and complementary reproductive strategies.Without it reproductive underpinning, social sexuality drifts towards mere personal gratification. Unlike some forms of human social sexuality, bonobo sexuality, despite its manifestly bisexual nature, integrates fully with bonobo reproduction (p 62).

The advent of effective contraception (p 396) has resulted in a divorce between reproductive and social sex in which sexual reproduction tends to be marginalized as an appendage to a purely social interpretation of sexuality, becoming an extraneous elective that only the more conservative nuclear families in traditional societies and religious fundamentalists indulge, or the unfortunate consequence of contraceptive mismanagement. Heterosexual child-bearing women are vilified as mere 'breeders' by some of their lesbian and cultural feminist sisters, and gay men proudly claim to be practicing sexual liberation free from the risk of unwanted children in an already overcrowded world. At the same time in contrast scientists are seeking to provide same-sex couples with reproductively engineered off-spring (p 409). However any society that defines sexual attitudes without supporting its reproductive basis runs a risk to its long-term viability, as evidenced in the almost precipitous population declines in several developed countries.

It is the prisoners' dilemma of life that sex is both the deepest union and the most divisive force, because of its exclusive nature. Many seek to tame this divisiveness by subjugating sex to a more oceanic spiritual love, forgetting that it is from sex that this all-embracing love and our heaven-and-hell panoply of emotional states evolved. Parenting is also divisive, because those that don't have children, whether gay, childless or unpartnered, recoil at the idea that in any sense we could be in some way unequal. But in seeking such equality we are letting go of the sacred process which gives us life in the first place. We are together as one in spirit, so it is in sharing the generational process that we really become one in the spirit and the flesh. This oneness of heart and the altruistic virtues of selfless and spiritual love all owe their emotional ambience to sexual evolution.

True fertility spirituality thus has the reproductive principle, pregnancy and the birth and continuity of all life's diversity as its core flowering principle. Any society which seconds this to the varieties of social sex, diverse or perverse, loses its way and ultimately becomes lost to history. Civilizations and spiritual movements rise and fall through the plug-hole of reproductive sexuality. All the pretensions of intellect fade in the light of differential reproduction not just because we are driven by our gonads but because it is our sex cells and only our sex cells which are the truly immortal bearers of life.

This polarity extends to the very foundations of the existential universe. Wave and particle (p 299) and mind and body (p 364) are each as complementary and polarized and different as they can possibly be. Most of the places where the relationship between us all and with nature breaks down is when one side of the Tao of sexual reality fails to recognize the intrinsic complementarity of the other, or lays claim to it. This is the classic mistake of both sexual dominance and self-love.

We should thus stop and consider whether it is wise for the liberation of sexual reunion, in seeking to merge the twain, to seek to diminish or neutralize the intrinsic polar complementarity that sex has given us, as its unbroken heritage of perennial life, from the ancient slime mold all the way to the flowering of human culture. Social sexuality emphasizes the *horizontal* - passion between people in the here and now, reproductive sex has a strong *vertical* component, running through the generations of time. They intersect in partnership in sacred union. This is the complete and fertile Tao.

Fertility and Spirituality

Some of you will no doubt ask where God has gone in this dissembling of the 'divine', exposed as a projection of male reproductive imperatives and anxieties. In answer to this, the sexually paradoxical state of immanent-transcendence, of incarnate 'soulfulness', holds the keys. The subjectively conscious mind in a physical body returns us right to the *mysterium tremendum*.

The 'easy' problems of consciousness research, such as how a human subject discriminates sensory stimuli and reacts to them appropriately, or how the brain integrates information from many different sources and uses this to control behavior , deal broadly with problems of consciousness in ways which could be resolved by functional explanations. The 'hard problem', by contrast, is the question of how physical processes in the brain give rise to subjective experience. This puzzle involves the inner aspects of thought and perception and the way things feel for the subject - all of them subjective experiences known only to the participant. In laying bare the depths of 'hard problem, David Chalmers (R111) noted:

"If the existence of consciousness cannot be derived from physical laws, a theory of physics is not a true theory of everything. So a final theory must contain an additional fundamental component. Toward this end, I propose that conscious experience be considered a fundamental feature, irreducible to anything more basic."

This position, in one sentence, reverses the Copernican revolution, putting the brain and its inner secret, the conscious mind, back into centre stage of the cosmic puzzle. We have explored this trend in the brain chapter (p 364), and the way both subjective consciousness and emotions, such as love, arise as universals in evolution (p 325), in a way which is consistent with the conscious brain being a culmination of the interactive processes begun in cosmic symmetry-breaking at the origin of the universe.

This is a view consistent with the Vedantic 'self' of the Upanishads we have noted (p 466), if expressed in somewhat devotedly male-oriented terms:

> The Self knows all, is not born, does not die, is not the effect of any cause, is eternal, self-existent, imperishable, ancient. How can the killing of the body kill Him? He who thinks that He kills, he who thinks that He is killed, is ignorant. He does not kill nor is He killed. The Self is lesser than the least, greater than the greatest. He lives in all hearts. When senses are at rest, free from desire, man finds Him and mounts beyond sorrow.

Yeshua in the gnostic Gospel of Thomas portrayed the cosmic nature of incarnate consciousness in startling terms, at once also confluent with the immanence of nature (p 229):

> "It is I who am the light which is above them all. It is I who am the all.
> From me did the all come forth, and unto me did the all extend.
> Split a piece of wood, and I am there.
> Lift up the stone, and you will find me there." (77)

Since, as Elaine Pagels has so astutely noted, the entire theme of the gospel of Thomas Didymus the 'twin' is that we are gnostic twins of the 'christ' state, Yeshua is here saying something from the conscious realm as acute as David Chalmers (R111). Each of us is in the incarnate archetype of the cosmic 'I'. Each of us carries in our genes and in our subjective consciousness the capacity to see face-to-face the ultimate 'nature' of existential reality.

No longer through a glass darkly, as Paul declared (1 Corinth 13:11):

> When I was a child, I spake as a child, I understood as a child, I thought as a child:
> but when I became a man, I put away childish things.
> For now we see through a glass, darkly; but then face to face:
> now I know in part; but then shall I know even as also I am known.

This 'knowing' is *gnosis* and it is not a religious figment invented by culture, like some brief dew on the lawn of time, but lies in right the bones of our evolutionary heritage. We, by the very prisoners' dilemma of conscious mortal existence - natural sexual organisms, yet sentient in the archetype of the cosmic, have nowhere to turn, but to ourselves and our personal responsibility, as living participants, to ensure the future generations flower in abundance, so long as Earth shall live.

In returning to our innocence as a child we are returning to our evolutionary roots in sexual complementarity and to the garden of paradise and the immortal passage of the generations which all our hearts seek, even in the throes of apocalyptic conflict.

In this quest for the inner light, it is the fecundity and abundance of nature, in all her immanence, that is our most precious resource. As we look out at the universe, as a realm of dark forces and consuming energies, from an explosive big bang to an almost certain heat death, the only thing we know possesses the mystery of subjective consciousness is that three-pound universe, so apparently fragile and such an idiosyncratic product of evolution - the sentient brain. It is thus to the mind-brain and to the diversity of nature, we should stoop to respect, to revere, to cherish and replenish in our awareness of the cosmic mystery within:

> Such in outline, but even more purposeless, more devoid of meaning is the world which science presents for our belief. Amid such a world, if anywhere, our ideals henceforward must find a home. That man is the product of causes that had no prevision of the end they were achieving; that his origin, his growth, his hopes and fears, his loves and his beliefs, are but the outcome of accidental collocations of atoms; that no fire, no heroism, no intensity of thought and feeling, can preserve an individual life beyond the grave, that all the labours of the ages, all the devotion, all the inspirations, all the noon-day brightness of human genius, are destined to extinction in the vast death of the solar system, and that the whole temple of man's achievement must inevitably be buried beneath the debris of a universe in ruins - all these

things, if not quite beyond dispute, are yet so nearly certain, that no philosophy that rejects them can hope to stand. Only within the scaffolding of these truths, only on the firm foundation of unyielding despair, can the soul's habitation henceforth be safely built. ... Brief and powerless is man's life, on him and all his race the slow, sure doom falls pitiless and dark ... (Russell R589 45)

The antidote to this schizophrenic vision of a physical wasteland lies in sexual paradox. The balance between the transcendence of the *mysterium tremendum* and the immanence of nature is sustained by respecting nature in all her diversity and the sexual paradox between nature and consciousness, without which divinity and the cosmic mind would never be able to be revealed, in the completion we find in the living universe. We thus attain to the light, not by flailing a defective flesh, but by cherishing and respecting the body, sexuality, and the conscious mind as finely tuned instruments of the evolutionary paradigm reaching towards a universality, in which nature is as sacred as divinity.

In her closing statement in 'The Curse of Cain', (R616) Regina Schwartz, commented:

"My re-vision would produce an alternative Bible that subverts the dominant vision of violence and scarcity with an ideal of plenitude and its corollary ethical imperative of generosity. It would be a Bible embracing multiplicity instead of monotheism. And I hope that this description of the Bible will also serve to describe its future, that it will not only tell of proliferation, but that new versions, decrying the violence of monotheism, will proliferate. I anticipated concluding with the injunction from Augustine to 'close the Book.' For him, faith had superseded it; for me, its ancient agonistic values are far too dangerous to continue authorizing. The old 'monotheistic' Book must be closed so that the new books may be fruitful and multiply. After all, that was the first commandment."

Part of the purpose of writing this work in partnership has been to open these avenues of abundance between women and men in the paradigm of diversity, while at the same time giving a fitting accounting of the failure of the patriarchal epoch to address the totality of existence fruitfully, through imposing the paradigm of dominion over woman and nature.

The true strength of human society lies in its fostering of creative diversity and the wisdom that consensual agreement can be achieved through respect for diversity. The means of achieving a truly compassionate society comes from the wisdom of a population autonomously and consensually understanding the natural and social need and thus acting together to ensure government and the corporate sphere serve a wider ethic of compassionate justice in which diversity can flower and new evolutionary features can surface. This does not come from the rule of law, or the dominion of order, but from creative dissonance between order and chaos, without invoking the need for violence or force.

We also need to develop creative traditions celebrating living diversity, rather than the stereotyped ceremonies of submission to a higher power in the name of cultural conformity and patriarchal order. Neither the monotheistic tradition, which has sought to tame social sexuality and submit reproduction to the growth of the religious community, not the so-called fertility tradition of Neolithic Goddess culture, which has been fixated on the agricultural cycle, male sacrifice, and fertility rites which relate only casually to parenthood, can be considered true fertility spirituality. It is with the promise of the Tree of Life and the immortal weaving of the germ lines if each living species, that a true sense of sacred fertility emerges, and with it a balancing of the population crisis and the rape of the planet.

We are the living creative presence of the conscious life force and need to give expression to this on our living diversity autonomously and compassionately together. Just as religion is 'to bind together', so we need to unbind our spiritual traditions in the bridal unveiling the word apocalypse actually means, engaging in artistic and musical pageants which celebrate the living diversity of our fertility in nature - Gaian comedies in the chaotic denouement tradition of Shakespeare's 'Twelfth Night' healing the world themes of Dionysian tragedy exemplified by the unending violence of crucifixion, genocide and martyrdom.

In recognizing reproduction, sexuality and nature as our immortal unfolding context, sacred above all other attitudes, assumptions and beliefs, celebrating our living diversity in abundance we can come into our deepest sense of belonging in the universe - unfolding sexual paradox in the immortal prisoners' dilemma of survival, which we can never win outright as mortal individuals, but can give to life in fullness, while we are here, in altruistic nurturing of the unborn generations to come.

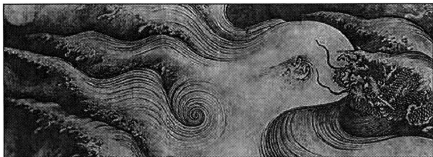

The Dragon of Order amidst the swirling Chaos of the Abyss (Rawson and Legeza R555)

The Way of the Ultimate Tao

There was something complete and mysterious
Existing before heaven and earth,
Silent, invisible,
Unchanging, standing alone,
Unceasing, ever in motion.
Able to be the mother of the world.
I do not know its name.
Call it Tao. Lao Tsu.

Complementarity: The Tao of Physics, Nature and Gender

The foundation of the mind and of the universe is the Tao. It is forever a complementation, not a Decartesian duality, across which there is an indivisible gulf, but the intimate marriage of realities - It is the *hieros gamos* of nature itself.

From the beginning both mind and universe exist as paradoxical complements, each discovering its own nature through it's complement. From birth to death, all our experience of reality is through the magic warp and weft of the subjective conscious mind. It is the umbilicus of reality without which the physical universe would be an abyss without even a dream of existence.

Yet the physical universe is also fundamental to existence, for through it our manifold dreams of existence find one common ground of objectivity in which the entire historical process of incarnation can come to a meaningful account. We are physical. We bleed when cut and swoon when concussed. Yet the description of physical reality is no more and no less than a myth told about the stabilities and correspondences of our conscious experience.

The phenomena of the physical universe are themselves in a state of a paradox of relativity and quantum uncertainty in which the future and the past become lost in probabilities which can never be disentangled from their quantum superpositions until the reaper of experience casts our lot and the world becomes frozen into the history we see being made before our eyes.

For the universe is forever the Tao of Physics, as Capra (R106) noted - the paradoxical interplay of wave and particle, and as natural processes gather into the macroscopic world of experience, chaos and order, as the weather, evolution and conscious thought alike attest. For order to attempt to rule over chaos is as futile as for the particle to try to rule over the wave. Any society which attempts to rule by order alone is doomed to catastrophe as the natural process transition becomes frozen into an apocalyptic revolution collapsing the old order.

'The prophecies sometimes set your mind off in new directions'
Lee & Yang before making their Nobel prize-winning discovery of non-conservation of parity

In regard to nature, the imposition of order, by domination of nature, through belief that the rule of order of civilization can continue until the evidence to the contrary is incontestable is suicidal. By this time many chaotic transitions have reached irreversible crisis and we become doomed by our own rigid lack of sensitivity and foresight. This the why we need inebriety of foresight, and the samadhi of contemplation as well as the rational scientific approach when dealing with the uncarved block of future possibilities.

The natural order requires complementation between the harmonious rule of order and a continuing respect for the fertility of chaos. Order needs to be at all times suppliant and responsive to fertile transition so that new order can emerge from the natural ferment of chaos.

The Tao is the path of nature. It is not only living with nature but being nature as individuals and in the societies we foster and the cultures we celebrate. The way of nature is also the way of life and death, of tooth and claw, but it is the role of immortal wisdom to understand nature in all her complements and to utilize her bounty in arriving at a just and harmonious existence, without imposing on her our own selfish designs. In doing so we are 'future dreaming' engaging in a vision quest of the evolutionary unfolding. The Tao stresses moving with the forces of nature in utilizing their own flow sustainably, not in dominion and domination.

The Way of the Valley

In the "Tao te Ching" (R206, R733), Lao Tsu, or 'old man' provides a clear and organic example of Taoist subtlety in erasing personal history. The work was written only through a twist of fate, because as Lao Tsu was leaving for the wilderness for the last time, he was jailed by the gatekeeper until he wrote down his teachings for posterity. This 'gatekeeper' is himself said to be a great master Yin-hsi of the Kuan (i.e. Han-ku) Pass (Wilhelm 1931 6). It is said that when Lao Tsu walked, the birds and animals would accompany him. Lao Tsu and Confucius were contemporaries and it is said that Confucius met Lao Tsu to take advice from the 'man of the wilderness', whom he found an unnerving foil to his own ideas of social order.

"The dark has a light spot and the light has a dark spot - that's how they can relate to one another" Complementation of male and female nature yin and yang in one another in the Tao (Joseph Campbell and the Power of Myth - TV).

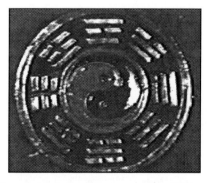

"In the Taoist perspective, even good and evil are not head-on opposites. The West has tended to dichotomize the two, but Taoists are less categorical. They buttress their reserve with the story of a farmer whose horse ran away. His neighbor commiserated, only to be told, "Who knows what's good or bad?" It was true, for the next day the horse returned, bringing with it a drove of wild horses it had befriended. The neighbor reappeared, this time with congratulations for the windfall. He received the same response: "Who knows what's good or bad?" Again this proved true, for the next day the farmer's son tried to mount one of the wild horses and fell, breaking his leg. More commiserations from the neighbor, which elicited the question, "Who knows what is good or bad?" And for a fourth time the farmer's point prevailed, for the following day soldiers came by commandeering for the army, and the son was exempted because of his injury." Huston Smith, The World's Religions (Occhigrosso R500 153)

The Chinese Tao, natural law, or way provides a cleavage of the totality into complementary creative and receptive principles. The Tao is a seamless web of unbroken movement and change filled with undulations, waves, patterns of ripples, vortices and temporary standing waves like a river. Every observer is an integral functioning part of this web which extends both into the past and into the future throughout space-time. It never stops, never turns back on itself, and none of its patterns of which we can take conceptual snapshots are real in the sense of being permanent, even for the briefest moment of time we can imagine. Like streaming clouds the objects and facts of our world are to the Taoist simply shapes and phases which last long enough in one general form for us to consider them as units. In a strong wind clouds change their shapes fast. In the slowest of the winds of Tao the mountains and rocks of the earth change their shapes very slowly - but continuously and certainly.

No binary, ideal or atomic concept has any independent reality or permanence in this unchanging river of change. No symbol can be separated from the organic context of the whole. Nothing which happens, no event or process ever repeats itself exactly. Nevertheless the Tao is unchanging like a convoluted eroded stone which stands beyond time. Men simply find it hard to observe the fact. All the separations which men claim to decipher in the web of Tao are useful fabrications, concepts being themselves ripples in the 'mental' part of the stream. Each human being himself is woven out of a complex system of totally mobile interactions with his environment. His body is in perpetual change, not by jumps from state to state; for his aging does not correspond to minutes, hours and birthdays, but goes on all the time.

The twisted and eroded stone was a motif repeated tens of thousands of times in paintings and on ceramics, often combined with trees, flowers and birds. Its reference always is to this truth of Tao as a reality whose essence is never ceasing, perpetual, seamless process. In the face of this intuition, what can man do?

There is a relevant story told in the Chuang-tzu, one of the most revered Taoist books. One day Confucius and his pupils were walking by a turbulent river, which swept over rocks, rapids and waterfalls. They saw an old man swimming in the river, far upstream. He was playing in the raging water and went under. Confucius sent his pupils running downstream to try and save him. However, the old man beached safely on the bank, and stood up unharmed, the water streaming from his hair. The pupils brought him to Confucius, who asked him how on earth he had managed to survive in the torrent among the rocks. He answered, 'Oh, I know how to go in with a descending vortex, and come out with an ascending one' (Rawson and Legeza R555).

In the Chuang Tzu Lao Tzu asks Cofucius "What is the gist of your teaching?" "The gist of it is benevolence and righteousness." "May I ask if they belong to the inborn nature of man?" asked Lao Tzu. "Of course," said Confucius. "If the gentleman lacks benevolence, he will get nowhere; if he lacks righteousness, he cannot even stay alive. They are truly the inborn nature of man. What else could they be?" Lao Tzu said, "May I ask your definition of benevolence and righteousness?" Confucius said, "To be glad and joyful in mind; to embrace universal love and be without partisanship - this is the true form of benevolence and righteousness." Lao Tzu said, " 'Universal love' - that's a rather nebulous ideal, isn't it? And to be without partisanship is already a kind of partisanship. Do you want to keep the world from losing its simplicity? Heaven and earth hold fast to their constant ways, the sun and moon to their brightness, the stars and planets to their ranks, the birds and beasts to their flocks, the trees and shrubs to their stands. You have only to go along with Virtue in your actions, to follow the Way in your journey, and already you will be there. Why these flags of benevolence and righteousness, so bravely upraised, as though you were beating a drum and searching for a lost child? Ah, you will bring confusion to the nature of man."

The Tao, that web of time and change, is a network of vortices like a moving and dangerous torrent of water; and the ideal Taoist is he who has learned to use all his senses and faculties to intuit the shapes of the currents in the Tao, so as to harmonize himself with them completely. Works of art provide some of the means for bringing people into communion with the currents and vortices, giving them a deep sense of their presence, and of the ways in which the tangled skeins evolve.

'Vast indeed is the ultimate Tao,
Spontaneously itself, apparently without acting,
End of all ages and beginning of all ages,
Existing before Earth and existing before Heaven,
Silently embracing the whole of time,
Continuing uninterrupted though all eons, ...
It is the ancestor of all doctrines,

The mystery beyond all mysteries' (Tao te Ching).

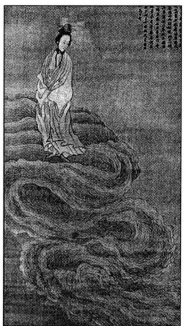

The Jade Lady among the clouds - Yin as Chaos Ts'ui Tzu-chung (Rawson and Legeza R555). One of the most important and complex female deities of Taoism is the Queen Mother of the West, who can confer immortality.

It is only in this sense of unbroken wholeness that the Tao is subdivided into natural complementary creative and receptive principles of yang and yin associated with male and female, day and night, heaven and earth etc. The power of the creative lies beyond the describable, and complements the world of form. The two together form the mysterious totality of existence. Central to the organic nature of the Tao is the inextricable dependence of each attribute on its complement, from which it draws its very identity.

> *Under heaven all can see beauty as beauty*
> *only because there is ugliness.*
> *All can know good as good*
> *only because there is evil.*

The Tao cannot be named, cannot be symbolized nor captured by rational thought or symbols:

> *The Tao that can be told is not the eternal Tao.*
> *The name that can be named is not the eternal name.*
> *The nameless is the beginning of heaven and earth.*
> *The named is the mother of ten thousand things.*
> *Ever desireless, one can see the mystery.*
> *Ever desiring, one can see the manifestations.*
> *These two spring from the same source but differ in name;*
> *this appears as darkness.*
> *Darkness within darkness.*
> *The gate to all mystery.*

The Tao is timeless and ancient, imperceptible and indefinable yet ever present:

> *From above it is not bright;*
> *From below it is not dark:*
> *An unbroken thread beyond description.*
> *It returns to nothingness.*
> *The form of the formless,*
> *The image of the imageless,*
> *It is called indefinable beyond imagination.*
> *Stand before it and there is no beginning.*
> *Follow it and there is no end.*
> *Stay with the ancient Tao,*
> *Move with the present.*

Knowing the ancient beginning is the essence of Tao. Taoist philosophy is singularly relevant to the modern age because it teaches that nature should not be disrupted:

> *Do you think you can take over*
> *the universe and improve it?*
> *I do not believe it can be done.*
> *The universe is sacred.*
> *You cannot improve it.*
> *If you try and change it, you will ruin it.*
> *If you try and hold it, you will lose it.*
> *It also lies beyond simple rules of morality:*

> *A brave and passionate man*
> *will kill or be killed.*
> *A brave and calm man*
> *will always preserve life.*

> *Of these two which is harmful?*
> *Some things are not favoured by heaven.*

Who knows why? Even the sage is unsure of this.

Lao tsu pictures the sage as wild and untamed but in contact with the natural maternal source:

> *People have purpose and usefulness*
> *But I alone am ignorant and uncouth*
> *I am different from all the others,*
> *but I draw nourishment from the mother.*

The opposites of male and female, light and dark etc. are not only interdependent, but it is essential for humanity to maintain a receptive relation to the creative Tao. This requires both the feminine receptiveness of the valley of the earth, and the primal pregnancy of the 'uncarved block', and also an attitude towards leadership and control which is humble and submissive and yields to transition rather than imposing order:

> *Know the strength of man,*
> *But keep a woman's care!*
> *Be the stream of the universe,*
> *Ever true and unswerving,*
> *Become as a little child once more.*
> *Know the white, But keep the black!*
> *Be an example to the world!*
> *Being an example to the world,*
> *Ever true and unwavering,*
> *Return to the infinite.*
> *Know honour and humility.*
> *Be the valley of the universe,*
> *Ever true and resourceful,*
> *Return to the state of the uncarved block.*
> *When the block is carved it becomes useful.*
> *When the sage uses it he becomes the ruler.*
> *Thus, "A great tailor cuts little" (Lao Tsu).*

Thus man follows the feminine earth, rather than heaven and consequently the creative emerges from nature itself:

> *Man follows earth.*
> *Earth follows heaven.*
> *Heaven follows the tao.*
> *Tao follows what is natural.*

However, despite being in yielding responsiveness to the natural order, the sage possesses the personal power of the shaman:

> *He who knows how to live can walk abroad*
> *Without fear of rhinoceros or tiger.*
> *He will not be wounded in battle.*
> *For in him rhinoceroses can find no place*
> *to thrust their horn,*
> *Tigers no place to use their claws,*
> *And weapons no place to pierce.*
> *Why is this so?*
> *Because he has no place for death to enter.*

Lao Tsu naturally saw the machinery of the state as a structured force which ran against the verdant abundance of the Tao:

> *The more laws and restrictions there are,*
> *The poorer people become.*
> *The sharper men's weapons,*
> *The more trouble in the land*

The Tao also has an active sexual manifestation similar to Tantrism. The natural complementation of male and female sexual energies, ching, as manifestations of life force became elaborated into a technique of gathering vital energies through active love-making while withholding orgasm. This attitude arises from the pursuit of immortality, and origins in matriarchal land title-holding based on yin-earth identification, resulting in polygamy and the need to maintain many active relationships. The inner alchemy of Taoism is closely related to the practices of Tantric yoga, involving similar chakra centers based on sex, heart and mind, derived from Buddhist influences.

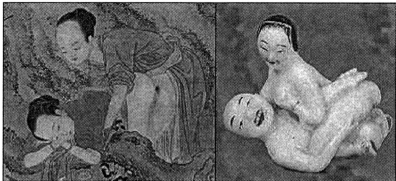

Sexual union is central to Taoist thought. Sex roles give both genders the superior position. Despite the patriarchy, ancient matriarchal identification with the land required conserving male energies to maintain relations with many wives (Rawson and Legeza R555).

Oracle of Sexual Paradox

The I Ching oracle (R732), or book of changes, is a primary example of a sexually paradoxical chance oracle, as it is based on applying uncertainty to the female and male principles of yin and yang. It shows both fundamental Taoist and Confucian influence which was again serendipitously created as a result of incarceration. According to the principles of the I Ching, consciousness, living organisms, and chance are a common manifestation of the cosmic creative principle. Thus the use of chance in throwing the oracle, far from being superstitious faith in the drop of a coin, links to consciousness. uncertainty and to life itself, as with the Urim and Thummim of Judaism, and the Tarot.

Yin and yang are firstly further divided into 8 yin-yang trigrams: ☰ heaven (the creative), ☴ wind (wood), ☵ water (the abyss), ☶ mountain (stillness), ☷ earth (the receptive), ☳ thunder (the arousing), ☲ fire (the clinging), ☱ the lake (joyful). The trigram transformations are then doubled to give 64 hexagrams, whose 64 x 64 = 4096 secondary transformations represent a set of archetypal dynamical situations. This set of 64 states have been carefully designed to give a generic set of conditions. Chance is used to generate a reading by throwing sticks or coins. The results of these two methods differ in the greater probabilities the coin oracle give to moving lines.

The origin of the trigrams is said to go back to Fu Hsi a legendary character from the period of hunting and fishing and the invention of cooking. They are thus of such antiquity that they antedate recorded history. The names of the trigrams do not occur anywhere else in Chinese language leading some to suggest they have a foreign origin although this may be simply due to their very ancient nature. King Wen, the progenitor of the Chou dynasty, elaborated the eight trigrams into a vastly larger system of transformations. King Wen is said to have added brief commentaries when he was imprisoned by the tyrant Chou Hsin. Wen was named king posthumously when his son Wu deposed the house of Shange and began the Chou dynasty which lasted 900 years. His son, the Duke of Chou, added the text of the moving lines. Confucius then studied and added to it in his senescence adding the Commentary on the Decision and less directly the Commentary on the Images.

屯 ䷂ 井

3 : Chun / DIFFICULTY AT THE BEGINNING
DIFFICULTY AT THE BEGINNING works supreme success, furthering through perseverance.
Nothing should be undertaken. It furthers one to appoint helpers.

Clouds and thunder: The image of DIFFICULTY AT THE BEGINNING.
Thus the superior man brings order out of confusion.

(1) Hesitation and hindrance. It furthers one to remain persevering.
When an eminent man subordinates himself to his inferiors, he wins the hearts of all people.
(2) Difficulties pile up. Horse and wagon part. He is not a robber; He wants to woo when the times comes.
The maiden is chaste, she does not pledge herself. Ten years - then she pledges.
(3) Whosoever hunts deer without the forester only loses his way in the forest.
The superior man understands the signs of the time and prefers to desist. To go on brings humiliation.

48 : Ching / THE WELL
THE WELL. The town may be changed, but the well cannot be changed.
It neither decreases nor increases. They come and go from the well.
If one gets down almost to the water and the rope does not go all the way,
Or the jug breaks, it brings misfortune.

Water over wood: the image of THE WELL.
Thus the superior man encourages people at their work
And exhorts them to help one another.

The patriarchal gloss of many translations of the I Ching obscure its essential complementation between yin and yang, and the notion that man's relationship to the nature should be the feminine way of the valley. Several modern interpretations of the I Ching reverse this gloss producing a distinctly feminist emphasis.

The above reading is "difficulty at the beginning" becoming "the well" in the Richard Wilhelm translation (R732). Barbara Walker's "I Ching of the Goddess" would read these like this:

Difficulty at the Beginning: "Heavy rains over thunder symbolize the storms of tribulation and trouble... the sages likened such difficulty to a traumatic birth attended by blood and pain."

The Well: "It is said that dwellings can be moved, whole cities can be moved, but the well supplying water for the population can't be moved. The source must remain in its own place. Those who seek it must go there".

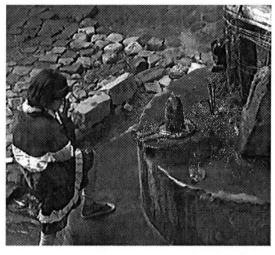

School girl making a morning offering
to a Shiva lingam-yoni or penis-vagina
Katmandu (King)

Tantra and Sacred Sexuality

Tantra stands relatively uniquely among traditions in being a path of discovery and even 'enlightenment' which founds its reality centrally on the sexual principle. Not only are the central rites of illumination and empowerment sexual, but the entire demeanour and behavior is one of sexual traversing of the boundaries of taboo in taking the tortuous dangerous left-hand path to the totality. This is manifest in the Tantrika indulging the senses, rather than withdrawing into spiritual isolation, writing fervent music, consuming the pleasure of worldly vices such as alcohol, 'ganga' (cannabis) or even 'soma' (the mythical sacrament of the Aryans identified with the Moon), and crossing all boundaries of taboo, by caste, marriage, sex, law, or even life. In this context an almost standard theme is using death as an advisor in performing Tantric vigils in the graveyard.

The chief symbol and energy Tantra uses is sex. The act of continuous creation is expressed in patterns of sexual activity, which is seen as infused with a sense of totally transcendent love. The existence of the world is thought of as a continuous giving birth by the yoni (vulva) of the female principle resulting from a continuous infusion of the seed of the male in sexual delight. The yoni is the mouth spewing forth the world but at the same time there would be neither world nor yoni without the 'seed', which gives the whole system its possibility of existence its being, which is always implicit but can never be an object of perception. Tantra supposes that the seed itself generates the yoni. In the shri yantra, it is the central point or dot, which has location but no magnitude. We can see dangerous hints at once of later patriarchal glosses, for in some way this is an echo of the male seed being the ultimate source of life with the female only a receptacle to nurture it, except that, as Kali, the feminine principle is the ultimate creatress and destructress of all temporal phenomena.

Tantric Genesis and Reunion

In many ways all creation myths are Tantric origins. Virtually all have a common theme of the origin of the first male and female pair in a sexual tale generally tangled with incest, deceit and betrayal in a fall into a state of division accompanied by the world's conflicts. The Edenic, Takano, Maori, Babylonian Dogon and Tantric origins all speak of a sexual 'falling out'. But each one is a different twist to the tale:

In the *Eden* story, God makes the Earth and Heavens and the plants and breathes life into Man out of dust. Adam and Eve were cleaved from a single androgynous being by the rib and are then cursed by a jealous God for eating the forbidden fruit and cohabiting in lust. They fall into mortal sexuality, woman in pain of childbirth, ruled by her husband, and they are driven from the Garden, lest they also eat of the Tree of Life and become like 'Him'.

In the *Tukano* origin, the Sun and Moon are brothers, with the Sun incestuously seduced by Venus causing all women to bleed. The subsequent abduction of Venus by the Moon and his diminishing by the Sun in punishment is again a myth of incest, jealousy and betrayal.

In the *Maori* origin, Io the nothingness became Rangi the Sky and Papa the Earth whose ever-so-close embrace shut the light out from their offspring in a primal uterine confinement. Tane, God of the Forest, pushes them apart, groaning, to create the cosmos.

In *Babylon*, Tiamat is originally paired with the An, as the two primal female and male fresh and salt waters. She is later killed by Marduk in a final battle between male order and primal chaos and her body is split in two to make the cosmos.

In *Dogon* myth, God makes the world, casting seed in the four directions to form the Earth's surface. He throws Earth to form the sun and stars. He then moulds clay which flows out over the Earth to form Mother Earth. He now desires to make love with this Goddess. But her clitoris sticks out as an anthill and resists his advances. A calamity results and monsters are born. He then cuts off the clitoris of Mother Earth, establishing female circumcision.

The *Tantric* origin is ingenious and cosmologically astute, as well as showing the way back to the paradisiacal state. The cosmos is created in sexual union. This completely integrated state began to recede in the genesis of all reality in the universe. Shiva as primal awareness, lost himself in contemplation and in conjugal bliss with Shakti as primal energy and interaction and the manifestations of the physical universe as 'mother'.

Again we can see patriarchal glosses in this genesis, with Shiva manouvering to claim he is the primal seed of consciousness, but the genesis now gives rise to the entire dance of life and death and the passage of the generations in time, overall the creative process. And the way back is open. Return to the state of intimate union is the royal route to the cosmic completion 'holiness' and 'sacred' imply.

The immense beauty of the Tantric tradition, if it can be called that, is fivefold: Firstly it is based on sexual love as an integrated biological and spiritual manifestation of genesis. Secondly it appeals to the female aspect of reality as integrally as to the male. Thirdly it engages both natural and conscious aspects of reality in one integrated whole. Fourthly it crosses all taboos, boundaries and confines, in mediating order and chaos. Fifthly it integrates the fertility tradition in nature with the contemplative and sacramental traditions in consciousness.

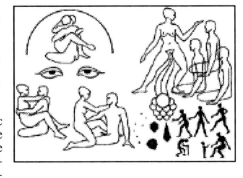

The Tantric creation myth - emergence of the opposites of male and female, subject and object from the transcendent unified totality to become the dance of Maya (Rawson R554). Maya the feminine, also named as Buddha's mother, is assigned to the role of physical illusion - the false separateness from the cosmic oneness of being arising from identification with and absorbtion in the physical. In Tantra the cosmic origin is the intimate sexual union of the complements.

As shown in the diagram top left the cosmic genesis begins with two male and female principles, Shiva (male) and Shakti (female energy) in deep sexual union. In a patriarchal hint, the latter is said to have been projected from the former as the first stage of creation (Rawson). The pair are so closely embraced that neither is fully aware of the other as distinct. In another patriarchal twist, it is said that Shiva, the principle of self and complete identity, dominates. Shakti is said still to 'have her eyes closed', in total bliss, because she has not awoken to the state of separateness. The two eyes are each person's own indicating the separation that is to come, but the arch is the dome of his skull rooted in the one cosmos.

The next phase is illustrated below left. Here Shakti's eyes have opened, though the couple are still united. She is now in the first state of realized separation. The Shiva-self, the subject, has been 'presented' (patriarchal 'has presented himself') with a separate active object, a 'that' distinct from his 'I'. The two face each other; but the fact is that this separation, and the separations which follow, are all the work of Shakti, who was projected expressly for this purpose. At the next stage down the couple move out of Union into distinct parts. Only their mutual sexual attraction reminds them that they belong to each other, that self and world are really only complementary aspects of the same reality (Rawson).

Now Shakti can really begin to function. She becomes in the top right-hand image that beautiful female dancer, who weaves the fabric of the world. The patterns of the dance are not illusion, but nether are they 'real' in the sense of being pure concrete facts. The self is so fascinated by her performance that it believes it is seeing all kinds of different things which are really her movements and gestures. Most important of all, it begins to think-because of her bewildering activity - that it is itself not one, but many, male and female. The bewildering array of an infinity of separate facts which composes the objective universe and at which we grasp, is presented to our self through what we call our mind and body, the psychosomatic mechanism in which each of our separated selves seems to be isolated and imprisoned. That, too, is part of the activity of the Goddess which, as we have seen, can also by symbolized by her fertile womb. All the things which we imagine we experience in time, the whole course of our individual life through our immense universe, is generated for us by that dance, or through that womb which, if only we knew it, is not different from us. All our mental faculties and sense organs, with all the qualities they perceive and co-ordinate, are channels for that energy working towards separation and distinction, which Shakti represents.

Philosophically such a doctrine is the most thoroughgoing holistic view, which pushes to its conclusion the ideas towards which many of our sciences are groping: that wholes are not compounds of lesser units - limbs, organs, elements and atoms-but that wholes come first and generate their parts. All causes lie in wholes, not in the accidental relationships between inferior parts. If time is included into the holistic picture, the meaning of the ultimate whole becomes virtually a definition of Tantrik enlightenment (Rawson).

It is by working it in reverse order that we can climb back up to the condition of knowing the Whole Truth. The vital link is the human body, with its senses and worlds of experience. For all the various stages represented in the diagram are correlated with groups of the body's own faculties. One can therefore say that, figuratively speaking, the whole universe is contained within the human body. But this is something that can only be realized in a special flash of intuition. Indian tradition has described many occasions on which some divinity has shown him or herself to followers as containing all the stars, universes, worlds, and creatures down to the minutest, within his body. This truth is as basic on the human scale.

Tantric devotion may centre its adoration on an image of the Goddess, which represents her as a beautiful girl who, as she dances crazy with love, lets down her hair, spreading out the worlds, and binds it up again, bringing them to their end. The male Tantrika's mind is sometimes continually absorbed in that shining and fascinating image. Every woman appears to him clothed in it. But it is not, for him, the woman who personifies the Goddess, but the Goddess the immortal feminine principle who appears in the woman.

All objects, no matter how dense they seem are intimately interwoven with our ideas of them as to be inseparable. All are processes of time, described as *mahakala* the male Great Time and Kali, time's female personification.From a human point of view Tantra recognizes that we are in one way closest to the female aspect of creation. The Goddess of Time is continually producing through us and for us. Women therefore play a crucial role in Tantra. They are carriers of that female energy which occupies the central place in Tantrik imagery, and in ritual practice it is only by cooperation with women that the male Tantrika can progress. The loving Goddess of Creation has another face. She brings man into time in his world and she also removes him from it. So she is destroyer as well. All things that can cripple and kill - disease, famine, violence and war - are an inevitable part of her activity.

Indian tradition has always visualized the human body as growing like a plant from the 'ground' of the Beyond, the Supreme Brahman, the Truth. And just as the vital juices of a plant are carried up and outwards from the root through channels and veins, so are the creative energies in the human body. Only the root of the human plant is not below, but above, beyond the top of the skull over the spine. The nourishing and bewildering energy flows in from the Beyond at that point. After spreading along through the body's channels it flows to the outermost tips of the senses, and even further out, to project the space around it which each body believes it inhabits. The pattern of veins and channels which compose this system is called the 'subtle body' and is the basis of Tantrik yoga.

Most conventional Indian traditions hold that the way to return to the wholeness of Truth is to repress ferociously, by asceticisms and will-power, all the faculties of the body and mind which participate in the process of projecting the mirage of separate persons inhabiting separate worlds. Tantra regards that sort of uphill struggle as absurd. Instead it says that all the faculties - the senses, the emotions and the intellect - should be encouraged and roused to their highest pitch, that the person's store of memories and responses can be awakened and re-converted into the pure energy from which they all originated. Feelings and pleasures thus become the raw material for transformation back into enlightenment.

The extra dimension in Tantric yoga comes from the bodily actions which are performed during sexual intercourse . These are meant both to enhance the physical sensations and to transform them into a vehicle for blissful insight. They are learned only in practice with a sexual partner, under the guidance of a teacher; though in fact one partner may be the teacher, very often the woman.

This brings us to a most interesting point about Tantra. It records innumerable legends about the way its most famous male-saints were initiated; in these the central episode is usually a ritual sexual intercourse with a female 'power-holder', whose favours the initiate has to win. This may well be one of the most ancient elements in Tantra, since the idea that not only initiation, but the very capacity to reach the Tantric goal can only be transmitted along a line of female 'power-holders' probably has roots in the oldest strata of human religion. Recent Indian religions are all strongly male-orientated; and many of the more conventional interpretations of Tantra, in texts which have been screened by Brahmin or Buddhist interpreters, tend to play down this central importance of the female in various ways.

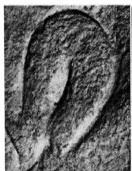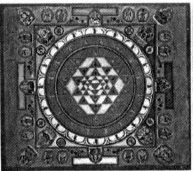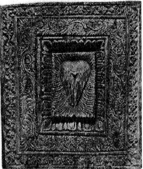

Yoni (paleolithic Ferrassie), Shri-Yantra has superimposed yoni-lingam motifs, Yoni (South India) (Rawson R554)

But history is full of examples of actual Tantrik saints, poets and sages who made much of their sexual relationship with a particular woman whose charms aroused them strongly, and who became for them prime agents in their enlightenment. Such women were usually of low caste; they might also be promiscuous practitioners of sexual intercourse and ritual, such as temple dancers or family prostitutes. Contact with one would be, according to Indian notions of caste purity, defiling, and place the Tantrika beyond the bounds of respectable society. This was always intentional. For Tantra demands that every bond with the everyday conventional world must be broken if one is to obtain enlightenment; and the idea of oneself as 'good and respectable' is one of the most dangerously insidious of such bonds.

The most powerful sexual rite of re-integration in some traditions requires intercourse with the female partner when she is menstruating, and her 'red' sexual energy is at its peak, perhaps on a cremation ground among the corpses and flaming pyres.

Traditions differ on another point. Some, probably the representatives of the oldest strand of thought, accept that the white male seed should ultimately be ejaculated into the woman's responding yoni, as if it were an offering of sacred oil being poured into an altar fire; the genuine physical orgasms of both partners are thus transformed and consumed in the far greater ecstasy induced by elaborate yogic practices. Other traditions, more ortho- dox in the Indian sense, say that male orgasm must be totally inhibited, and the energy which would have been expended in them should be turned back and totally sublimated into a radiant inner condition.

The basic principle of Tantrism was that women possess a more unbounded spiritual energy than men, and a man could achieve realization of the divinity only through sexual and emotional union with a woman. A fundamental rite was controlled sexual intercourse, *maithuna*. This requires reservation to the extent that control over male ejaculation must be good enough for the female to fully enter her own sexual ecstasy without the male pre- cipitously bringing the intimate union to a false climax. Tantra in its essence is a fertility rite in which there is a complete consummation of the female and male sexual energies and thus must centrally also involve male fertilization of the female.

However in later patriarchal interpretations, the theory became that a man must store up his vital fluids altogether, rather than expending them in ejaculation, following the idea that the male absorbs the energy of many female orgasms into his own power. In this view male and female energies have again become opposed in principle. Through Tantric train- ing, a man learned to 'absorb' through his penis the fluid engendered by his partner's orgasm and to prolong sexual intercourse for many hours. In this way he could become like Shiva, the God in perpetual union with the Goddess. Theoretically, the vital fluids thus conserved would be stored in a man's spinal column, mount through the chakras up to his head, and there flower forth with the inspiration of divine wisdom in kundalini energy.

One of the most famous Tantrik rites are the variants of the chakrapuja. This is a kind of long-drawn Eucharist, carried out by night, attended by a number of couples, married or not, who ceremonially take the five enjoyments normally forbidden in high-caste society: meat, alcohol, fish, a certain grain, and sexual intercourse. The last may be performed with several different partners, one's own, or one chosen at random. Again, it is a question of arousing and controlling extraordinary energies.

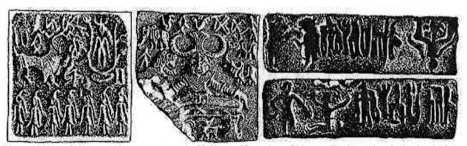

The goddess of the sacred grove, an early Kali manifestation, Shiva as Pashupatinath the lord of the animals, the sacrifice. Indus Valley 2000 BC (Campbell R103v2 166-9)).

Tantric Origins

The Tantric tradition goes back into the most ancient Antiquity of India. It predates the Aryan equine incursions (1800BC) and is clearly manifest in the Dravidian Indus Valley civilizations of Harappa and Mojendaro (3000 BC). The arrival of Vedic culture is believed to have replaced an earlier matrilineal culture with a patriarchal one.

The complex of Hindu beliefs and practices appears to originate from the interaction of these two peoples in turn upon ancient gatherer-hunter peoples the nishadha as told in the battle of Garuda and the Nagas and the birth of Krishna as a pastoral herder. Daksha's horse sacrifice, at which Sati immolated herself over Shiva's exclusion, hints at such an overthrow. The prevailing theory is that the Aryas brought horses to India and in a ceremony known as Ashwarneda, they let loose their most magnificent horse and laid claim to all the lands the horse traversed unchallenged.

When the Pandava Yudhishtira became king, he performed a horse sacrifice and let loose his royal horse. Arjuna led the armies that followed this horse. The horse crossed many lands and the kings of those lands accepted the overlordship of the Pandavas. But then on the border of Manipura, the warrior Babruvahana stopped the stallion and challenged Arjuna to a duel. In the fight that followed Babruvahana successfully shot a poison-tipped arrow into Arjuna's chest. When Babruvahana's mother, Chitrangada, saw the dying Arjuna she burst into tears, for Arjuna was her husband-Babruvahana's father-who as per the marriage contract had agreed to let her father, who had no male offspring, adopt the son born of their union. Babruvahana had never seen his father. He had learned archery from Uloopi, a naga woman who was also Arjuna's wife, but one he had forgotten soon after marriage. Thus scorned, she had used Babruvahana to avenge her humiliation. At the request of Babruvahana and Chitrangada, Uloopi brought Arjuna back to life with the help of the serpent gem that serves as an antidote against all poisons (Pattanaik).

Anthropologists suggest that Chitrangada probably belonged to a matrilineal clan - not unlike the Nairs of Kerala - where the child belongs to the mother's, not the father's, family. Kunti, the mother of the Pandavas, says in the Mahabharata, "In days of yore women went about freely doing as they pleased. There was no obligation to be faithful to their husbands". Anthropologists and feminists interpret this as a shift from matriarchal to patriarchal traditions. With this shift came stories to explain practices that the later patriarchy found unacceptable (Pattanaik R518 165).

Tantra also serves as a mid-point between the fertility rites that abound in everyday pastoral India and requiring participation of husband and wife, and the inner contemplation of the ascetic path, reflecting the complementation of the feminine as nature and the masculine as contemplative soul and culture. At the same time it has had three influences, the animistic states of trance possession of the forest dwellers, attributing consciousness to every manifestation of nature, and the agrarian sacred union between the goddess and the god of fertility, glossed over later with the patriarchal idea of the illusory nature of the world as *maya*.

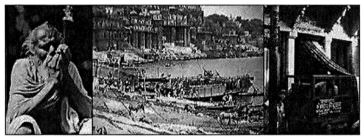

The River of the Sadhu: Om Nama Shivai! A Sadhu takes the sacred chillum (Schultes & Hofmann R612). The immortal Ganges is the very name of Hemp. Government Ganga shop: Varanasi: Sacred status permits the sale of Ganga within the ancient city of the Ganga (King)

Tied into this interactive process between mind and nature is the ancient association of Shiva with the sacred herb Ganga and with the use of His sacrament in visionary trance, as espoused by wandering sadhus across the length and bradth of the Indian subcontinent.

Shakti and Kali as Female Power

Shakti is the personification of Cosmic Energy in its dynamic form. The power and energy with which the Universe is created, preserved, destroyed and recreated (by Brahma, Vishnu and Shiva). Shakti is worshipped in several forms. She is the Universal mother, the gentle consort of Shiva, the queen of Shiva, she rides the tiger, and bears weaponry. In the angry and terrifying form of Kali (R469), she destroys and devours all forms of evil. As Kali, she is also the personification of time, her dark form being symbolic of future beyond our knowledge.

Shakti is the primal goddess of folklore, progenitress of the Gods:

In the beginning the supreme Goddess Adi Shakti laid three eggs in a lotus. From these three eggs emerged the three worlds and the three gods: Brahma, Vishnu, and Shiva. Desire awoke in the heart of the Goddess, who asked the Gods to make love to her. "But you are our mother," said Brahma and Vishnu, shying away. The Goddess was angry at being rejected and reduced the two Gods to ashes by casting a glance of her fiery third eye. She then turned to Shiva, who agreed to make love to her if she gave him her eye. She did. Shiva used it to reduce her to ashes and revive the other two Gods. Brahma, Vishnu, and Shiva then decided to populate the world with living beings, but they could not do so without wives. They gathered around the heap of ash that was once Adi Shakti, divided it into three parts, and with the power of the third eye created the three Goddesses Saraswati, Lakshmi, and Gauri. The three Goddesses married the three Gods and together they populated the cosmos with all manner of plants, animals, and other living things, including gods, demons, and humans (Pattanaik).

In the Tantric cosmology, the whole universe is perceived as being created, penetrated and sustained by two complementary fundamental forces, Shiva the constitutive elements of the universe, and Shakti the dynamic potency, which makes these elements come to life and act. Shiva-Shakti corresponds to two essential aspects of the One: the masculine principle, the abiding aspect of God, and the feminine principle, the Energy, the Force which acts in the manifested world, life itself considered at a cosmic level. From this point of view, Shakti represents the immanent aspect of the Divine, that is the act of active participation in the act of creation. Shiva defines the traits of pure transcendence and is normally associated to a somewhat terrible personification of Shakti's own untamed and limitless manifestation.

Tantra transforms dualistic philosophy in that the two cosmic principles are united, not separated a unity between the two principles, opposed in appearance, but indissoluble united in each act of the creation. The God and the Goddess are the first self-revelation of the Absolute, the male being the personification of the passive aspect, Eternity, the female of the activation energy, the dynamism of Time. On one hand is presented the cosmic dance of Shakti on the lying body of Shiva. On the other hand, the two deities are pictured in tantric sexual union. This sexual union is different from what is usually understood by this in the western traditions. The man is immobile, while the woman, embracing him, assumes an active role during the sexual act.

Kali on Shiva Rajasthan 18th cent (Rawson R554)

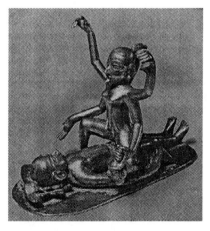

The Sanskrit word Kali literally means time. Kali is the feminine word for time, for which the masculine is kala. Time as we are forced to understand it, is the foremost power that we experience. Kali is the personification of time. It is not surprising that the deity of time has a terrifying image. After all, time is the slayer of all. Time is the very stuff that our lives are made of. To waste time is to waste life. The reason as to why time is represented in a feminine form is that time is the great womb - the great mother - from which we are all created - therefore it has a feminine quality. Time is also the force which causes all living beings to perish. Therefore Kali is like the mother who destroys the children which she has created - which is one of her frightful features. Yet, through the action of time, Her action, occurs our salvation. Through time, over repeated births, we experience all that we have to and learn all that we must learn in order to merge back into our eternal existence from which we fell, into limited time and space.

Shiva is the non-created creator of all: he knows all, he is pure consciousness, the creator of time, all knowing and all powerful. Shiva is the lord of the soul and nature and of the three conditions of nature. From him comes transmigration of life and liberation, bondage in time and freedom in eternity. To some he is Shiva the beneficent and to others he is the destroyer. For some he is Shiva the ascetic, wandering the world. For others he is still the Great Lord, King of all creations. Still it is as the lord of the dance that all his aspects come together in one spectacular form! Nowhere else in the universe is there a clearer picture of what a God is and does. Shiva dances the dance of creation, the dance of destruction and the dance of solace and liberation.

The earliest Upanishads date from 900 to 600 BC. The fundamental concern of the Upanishads is the nature of reality. They teach the identity of the individual soul (atman) with the universal essence soul [Brahman]. Because they are the final portions of the Vedas, they are also known as Vedanta, "the end of the Vedas," and their thought, as interpreted in succeeding centuries, is likewise known as Vedanta. Notice the patriachal gloss in the mind-sky:

Death said: "The word the Wedas extol, austerities proclaim, sanctities approach - that word is Öm. That word is eternal Spirit, eternal distance, who knows it attains to his desire. That word is the ultimate foundation. Who finds it is adored among the saints. The Self knows all, is not born, does not die, is not the effect of any cause, is eternal, self-existent, imperishable, ancient. How can the killing of the body kill Him? He who thinks that He kills, he who thinks that He is killed, is ignorant. He does not kill nor is He killed. The Self is lesser than the least, greater than the greatest. He lives in all hearts. When senses are at rest, free from desire, man finds Him and mounts beyond sorrow. Though sitting, He travels; though sleeping is everywhere. Who but I Death can understand that God is beyond joy and sorrow. Who knows the Self, bodiless among the embodied, unchanging among the changing, prevalent everywhere, goes beyond sorrow. The Self is not known through discourse, splitting of hairs, learning however great; He comes to the man He loves; takes that man's body for His own.

Tantric union is a wedding of the incarnations - of deities, old as time itself - even the wedding of our very first ancestors. It is also a multiple polyamorous marriage, a marriage between chaos and order, mind and body, soul and spirit, anima and animus, as well as of many goddesses and gods manifest in Shiva and Shakti. Their love for each other is legendary, and their union brings peace, understanding, and exquisite bliss. It generates the full spectrum of existence, the ten thousand levels of manifestation.

Shakti, the bride is wondrous and She is everywhere! She dances in the life of the plants, She is the spark in the laugh of the child. She is present in the growing belly, the voice that sings, the heart that loves. She is the urge to grow, to move, to change, to awaken. She is pure energy, chaotically free, the fuel for all activity, infinite energy. Her full name is Kundalini Shakti. Sometimes She manifests as a serpent, coiled tightly around the four petaled lotus that grows at the base of your spine. Here is the bed where She sleeps, giving you grounding and stability, security and peace, with your roots buried deeply in the Earth. Her home at this level is called Muladhara, or root support. It is here that She binds together the physical world. Her instincts help you survive. But sometimes She stirs, languidly ravishing in the sensuous movements of Her serpentine body, sinuously sliding through the liquid nectar of your cells, moving upward through the curves and organs of your flesh. She pierces the lotus of six petals, whose element is water, and in this from She may bring you intense desire. Hers is the longing that cries out for touch and brings forth lust to awaken you to ecstatic pleasure. She may have many lovers, each one renewed in the her glorious energy (A Tantric Wedding - www.consciousnessevolution.com).

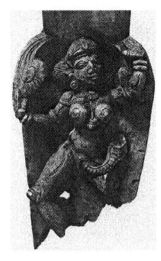

Yogini with serpent energy coming from her vulva
(South India c1800 Rawson R554). Energy many patriarchs
fear.

Beware, though, because her movements may be chaotic
when She breaks out of Her slumber. She may be a wild
dancer, robbing you of sleep. You may shake with her
tremors, burn with her longing, ache with her movement,
her search for her true love, Shiva himself. If she does not
find him, She may get more and more agitated, burning
even stronger with desire, until you think you will burst
with the intensity of her presence. But She must have
power to attract Shiva, rising to the third chakra of fire.
Here you will find the strength and fierceness of a warrior
Goddess, not merely the soft feminine sweetness of the
young maiden. Shiva is a formidable force, and does not
trifle with Maidens, but only with the raw stuff of life, the
Goddess Herself. In this form, you may see her riding a
tiger, as the goddess Durga, or dancing with Shiva as her
Dark Sister, Mother Kali, who drips blood form her
mouth to splatter upon her necklace of skulls. Her power
at this level is to break apart old forms, for once awak-
ened, She hates constriction, and you may find nothing in your life is ever the same. In her
search for her lover, she can be most intense, relentless, in fact, and there may little you
can hold onto if it gets in her way. You'd best cooperate with her and begin looking for her
lover, for She will not stop until She finds him.

And who is he? He is the Lord of Sleep, the undifferentiated bliss of meditation, unified
with all that is. He is the wisdom of pure consciousness, the divine intelligence that
shapes primordial chaos into order and form. His most familiar home is in the crown
chakra, in the undifferentiated realm of limitless spirit, where he sees and knows All. But
he is also a dark one, known as Rudra, the howler or weeping one, a Lord of Destruction,
whose lightning bolt can destroy your attachments with but a single glance. He is also a
god of healing and sacrifices, worshipped by many in the rising phallus, the Shiva Lin-
gam, always erect and ever thrusting into the great mysteries of the feminine, never satisfied. Without his lover, however, Shiva is but a corpse, lost in meditation of the infinite
wonders, enfolded in the bliss of perfect enlightenment, disembodied form the world of
samsara, of birth and death.

And now Shakti-Parvati sits upon his left thigh, encircling her arm about his shoulder.
When She strokes the rising phallus, the drums and music play ever more forcefully, the
dancers writhing feverishly to the rhythm. When the hall can no longer contain this passionate energy of creation, Shiva springs forth. The divine couple stare fixedly into each
other's eyes, lost in eternal rapture. Though appearing as two, they know that they have
always been inseparably one, and their union is a return to the primordial unity from
which all things spring forth. The polarities of the universe combine, creating cascading
multiplicities, dark and light, joining in a shower of rainbows, sparks and jewels explode
across time and space in the ever generating and eternal sri yantra, symbol of endless creation and destruction. Shakti has met her match. With destruction as her ally, She can now
create endlessly to her heart's content, knowing that all of maya, all of the manifested universe is an endless cycle of creation and destruction. Shiva has found his sacred other, a
feminine source of limitless energy. He can now move from static to dynamic dance, as
Shiva Nataraj. And as they tumble into eternal ecstasy and divine union for the creation
and destruction of all that is, all who are present to this divine and auspicious ritual are forever transformed.

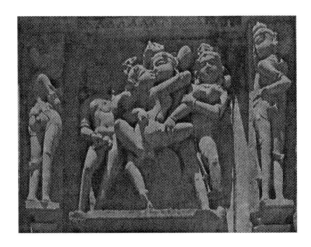

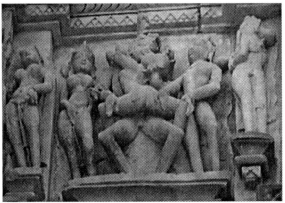

Khajuraho (King). Shakti embracing a recumbent Shiva..

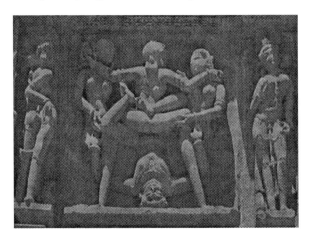

Tantric Buddhism

Although Buddhism is a path of renunciation in which the central aim is escape from the endless cycle of birth and death into the still point of the turning world, the Buddha state of no-mind, Tibetan Buddhism, partly as a consequence of underlying influences of Bön shamanism, has adopted a complex cosmology of natural influences and diverse meditation practices embracing the Tantric approach.

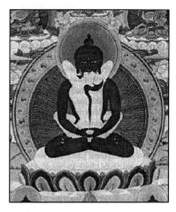

Some of these involve meditation on a *yidam* in the form of a female deity, or dakini. They also include, as a higher initiation, the sexual fertility rite of *yab-yum* or 'father-mother.' Sometimes, as in the picture to the right, the female is portrayed as a mere agent of the male illuminated condition. Indeed the initiation of high lamas involved a period of being bricked up in a cave with a temple prostitute for several months to complete these sexual empowerments.

Unlike the images of Kali astride a supine Shiva, these frequently involve a sexual union sitting, or standing face to face in a lotus position. In some of these representations the male is full of power having many arms holding objects of power crowned by many heads expressing the full flush of inflamed enlightenment. However, Tibetan Buddhism has also adopted the varying positions and sexual relationships manifested by Kali and Shakti, partly as a means to circumnavigate the Vedantic ground swell from which Tibetan Buddhism emerges.

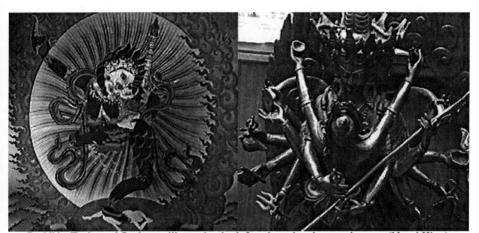

Buddhist Tanka and Sculpture illustrating both female and male sexual power (Nepal King)

Like the Indian Tantric rites and reports of some Ophite ceremonies (p 235), the practice of yab-yum as sacred union may involve the use of female and male secretions as sacraments:

"When the semen made molten by the fire of great passion, falls into the 'lotus of the mother' and mixes with her red element, he achieves the 'conventional mandala of the thought of enlightenment.' The resultant mixture is tasted by the united 'father-mother' [Yab-yum] and when it reaches the throat they can generate concretely a special bliss ... the bodhicitta - the drop resulting from the union of semen and menstrual blood - is transferred to the yogi ... This empowers his corresponding mystic veins and centers to accomplish the Buddha's function of speech. The term 'secret initiation' comes from the tasting of the 'secret substance'." (Tatz and Kent R668 128)

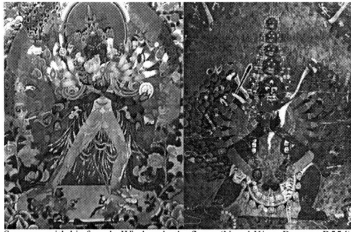

Samvara with his female Wisdom both aflame (Nepal King, Rawson R554)

Despite the male-oriented monastic tradition of three of the four schools of Tibetan Buddhism, many of the Tantric tankas do involve expression of both female and male orgasmic energy. In the above illustrations both sexes are manifest in the supernatural dance of illumination with many arms or heads, giving a feel for the cosmic power sexual energy contains.

Krishna with the Gopis
Kangra (Rawson R554).

Krishna and Kunti

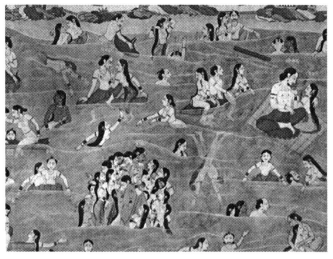

A very different patriarchal tale of polygynous sexual union is purveyed by the myth of Krishna, another incarnation of Vishnu, and the gopis, or cow girls. One one occasion Krishna stole their clothes as they were bathing in the Yamuna river and refused to return them until they had emerged naked one by one with their hands raised in supplication. Before long all the gopis were in love with the enchanting Krishna and whatever the obstacles in their way, responded to his summons. Krshna would play his flute, beckoning the milkmaids of his village. They would leave their homes and husbands, and come secretly, risking their reputations, and make a circle around him to dance to his tune, losing themselves completely. When this happened, it seemed to each milkmaid that Krishna had 'danced' with her alone. Even as the *ras* dance continued, Krishna would slip away with one of them, the others disconsolately tracking their footprints until the dance was resumed. Sometimes the milkmaids boasted that Krishna belonged to them. When this happened Krishna would disappear, making the women experience the pain of separation, returning only when this need to possess him was abandoned. Nevertheless Radha stands among the gopis as Krshna's great love and even in their separation he pined for her and was ready to abase himself to make amends.

Complementing this tale is the story of the princess Kunti involving pre-marital and extra-marital conceptions. Kunti served the sage Durvasa well when he visited her father's house and in return gave her a magic formula by which she could have a child by any deva. She has a child by Surya the sun god and leaves it, like Moses by the river, to avoid sullying her reputation. She marries King Pandu, but finds him impotent, so she then copulates with Dharma the god of righteousness, Vayu the god of winds, and Indra the rain god and bears three sons, each conceived in the name of Pandu to perpetuate the male line.

Sacred Sexuality and Fertility

The key to the union is complete, unconditional, selfless love for the other. Ideally the partners are in love, falling in love, or about to. This is a journey from the origins of the universe through many tortuous paths. A meeting of two beings travelling from forever through endless lifetimes, who yet have only a moment's grace to give expression to the untameable abyss of the heart. More erotic than pornography. The contemplative union of love and lust.

Central to sacred sexuality is the fact that female sexual ecstasy is itself a cosmic force, different and distinct from male sexual energy. It is an all-consuming ecstasy more powerful and long lasting than male ejaculation. It is thus essential for the male to be able to flow with and worship female sexual energy and all its varieties of sexual experience and to postpone orgasm sufficiently to enable the female sexual whirlwind to reap its own harvest. Female sexuality crests in an undulating series of waves of several types of physical orgasm vaginal, uterine and clitoral, merging into chaotic whole body 'climax' - a manifestation of the sexual life force unleashed from the simple act of fertilization. This is why it is likened to the kundalini that lurks in the base of our spines and can rise to the heights of explosive illumination. However permanent withholding of male orgasm is a patriarchal idea based on a desire to gain control of female sexual energy, rather than to merge with it and flow with it in the wholeness of complementarity. Sacred union is not for the male to draw power from the female into a lone *samadhi*. The fulfillment of female ecstasy is all-consuming of the fertilizing act of the male in a ravishing consummation. The natural creative erotic peak of the sacred act for the female is during ovulation, rather than menstruation, in terms of both fertility and sexual arousal. The Shakti energy, which pervades the entire universe is the life force itself, which expresses itself centrally in fertility and reproduction and in the diversity of all life, celebrated in the mystery of the *hieros gamos*. The peak of sacred sex is the full merging of the two, in the fertilization which generates life and the universe anew. It is sourced in the primal fires of fusion and it is fertility ovrflowing with abundance in paradise.

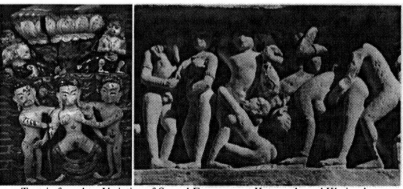

Tantric foreplay: Varieties of Sexual Engagement Katmandu and Khajuraho.

Huichol yarn painting depicting themes from their genesis myth: The Nierika or cosmic portal opened by peyote, linking the underworld with Mother Earth, through which the gods came and all life came into being. It unifies the spirit of all things and all worlds. (Schultes & Hofmann R612).

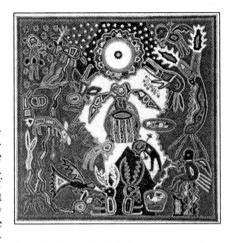

Sacrament, Consciousness and Sexual Paradox

Christianity is a prime example of a world sacramental religion, founded on 'holy communion' - a flesh and blood sacrament - the *sangre* and *soma* - symbolic of a sacrificial death. These simple wafers of bread and sips of diluted wine carry no effect in themselves, but claim to infer a reality so powerful that merely to partake of the 'eucharist' is deemed to be the innermost mystery of communion with the godhead. If such a sacrament is going to be of functional effect, shouldn't one expect it to actually be a potent psychoactive substance in biological terms?

The notion of sacrament as something natural that is consumed to make 'holy' or whole poses a central question of sexual paradox in consciousness. How *is* such completion achieved in the universe? Is it arrived at through an outer journey of scientific or empirical discovery in the material world? Is it to be found through philosophical analysis and discourse? Is it to be found in a covenant of submission to the will of God? Is it to be pursued through an arduous meditative journey into the innermost reaches of the mind and soul to the cosmic self? Or is it to be found in sexual reunion and in the interactive mysteries of the 'living sacraments' of the biosphere?

Lying beneath this is the fraught question of what subjective consciousness actually is. Is the complete mind - the visionary state - something we possess alone and sufficient unto ourselves, a pure state in inner devotion, separate from the material world, or are the highest experiences of unification achieved not alone but in interaction? Is mystical consciousness somehow not only collective but interactive? Is its 'purpose', rather than communication with the absolute or an unseen God, rather the genesis of a more compassionate and aware natural condition - of living co-participation?

No one in their right mind would consider humanity, for all its domination of the living species of the planet completely independent of them. Man must eat and eat the living flesh of plants fungi and animals to exist. Merely to consume other life forms we are interdependent with them. This interdependence is accepted as central and fundamental to our natural condition, but when it comes to consciousness, our patriarchal mind-sky heritage makes us feel that our mental identity is to be carved out, not in interactive merging but in a lone isolation, on the one hand a supremacy of contemplation and mental control, and on the other a submission to a higher power - the will of god.

Yet perhaps both these hierarchical ideas are misconceived. Perhaps the purpose of the conscious mind is not to leave the natural world for a 'higher plane', but to be learn to better integrate with conscious nature in a wholeness that both gives us the sense of completion and fulfillment we seek, and in so doing sustains living diversity in a more integrated compassionate and caring relationship. Indeed this is the only practical route to the immortal paradise all our myths and religions gravitate towards, and the reality the immortal sexual passage of the generations attests to. Therefore we need to consider the possible role psychotropic plants, fungi and animals may have in making the consciousness of the biosphere complete, whole and 'holy'.

The relationship between so-called 'power plants' and human consciousness is a startling example of the sexual paradox principle in action - the idea that the crowning forms of integrative conscious experience are not gained by one species in isolation but in interaction between complementary living principles, without which, the heights of the spiritual experience might be difficult or impossible to achieve, attained only by a mystic or psychotic few, or so become so distorted by second-hand accounts, that they are perceived only 'through a glass darkly', rather than knowing and being known face to face.

Complementing the deep meditation of the Eastern traditions of Buddhism and the Upanishads is a Western tradition of sacramental shamanism every bit as ancient in which virtually every psychedelic species has become revered as a sacred 'power plant' for curing and access to the divine and hidden realms of nature. The origins of these discoveries in myth frequently go back to discoveries by women gatherers which are later stolen by the men.

Mircea Eliade (R184) made a major conceptual error when, in his seminal work "Shamanism" he relegated sacramental forms of shamanism to an inferior status. In fact the strongest, deepest and by far the most insightful traditions of shamanism come through the power plants. Centrally important here is a world view in which nature and all the species therein are sacred and the 'good life' is lived in an intimate caring relationship with nature rather, than the dominion over nature claimed by humanity, projected through a high god.

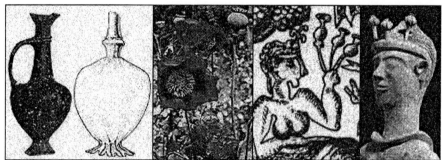

Cypriot juglets from Egypt 18 th dynasty from around 1350 BC appear to be designed on inverted poppy pods, Papaver somniferum, inset of Minoan seal from Crete 1500 BC, head of Goddess with slit poppies Crete 1350 BC (Rudgley R584, King, Gadon R229).

The 'war on drugs' is an aberration in human history, which runs counter to the experience of virtually every culture which has preceded it. It is based on a Christian fear of paganism, of witches brews and of any form of material access to the divine - that anything outside the carnivorous Christian sacrament of soma and sangre, is diabolical.

Many of our modern medicines are plant sourced. Our evolutionary endowment in psychoactive plants has been particularly rich, with some of the most potent psychedelic substances known coming directly from natural sources. Although some of these, such as the solonaceous plants used in mediaeval witchcraft are frankly toxic, others despite being somewhat bitter medicines are medicinal or of no seriously debilitating effect. The 'medicine men and women' who partake and administer these live healthy lives into their nineties extolling the power and virtue of these sacraments.

We will examine just a few cases, choosing the context of the Christian sacrament to confirm an evolution from the traditional Eucharist to the use of 'living sacraments'. However the principle applies to all sacred use of power plants, whatever their religious context.

Maria Sabina and the Agape of Pentecost

In 1935 the anthropologist Jean Bassett Johnson witnessed an all night mushroom ceremony at Huautla de Jiménez. This report was to lie idle until the night of June 29th 1955 when the mycophiles Gordon and Valentina Wasson, upon a clue from the anthropologist Weitlander, with the help and encouragement of Robert Graves (R503, R504) 'were invited to partake of the agape of the sacred mushrooms' in the hills of Oaxaca, among isolated peasant peoples who used the plant to divine the future and seek a cure of illness, after a long search and a previous unsuccessful season in the town. After a season of difficulty securing the trust of the Mazatecs, Wasson had commented:

'Perhaps you will learn the names of a number of renowned curanderos, and your emissaries will even promise to deliver them to you, but then you wait and wait and they never come. You will brush past them in the market place, and they will know you but you will not know them. The judge in the town hall may be the very man you are seeking and you may pass the time of day with him yet never know that he is your curandero'. (Weil et. al. R723 30).

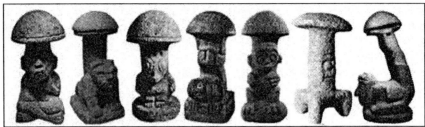

Mayan mushroom stones 1000 - 300 B.C. (Schultes & Hofmann R612)

In fact the man who finally led him to the eucharist was indeed the judge Cayetano.

Wasson (R716) was deeply struck by the spiritual power of the sacred mushroom (R647, R612), which he referred to as 'the divine mushroom of immortality':

'Ecstasy! The mind harks back to the origin of that word. For the Greek ekstasis, meant flight of the soul from the body. Can a better word be found to describe the bemushroomed state? ... Your very soul is seized and shaken until it tingles, until you feel you will never recover your equilibrium' (Furst R227 198)

The sacred mushroom *teonanactl* is 'known to the ancient Meso-Americans as the Flesh of God, echoing the *soma* and *sangre* of the Christian Eucharist (Harner R285 90). Wasson also noted that Greeks call mushrooms *broma theon* 'the food of the gods' (Furst R227 194) and specifically likened the experience to the epoptea of Eleusis 'For me there is no doubt that the secret of Eleusis lies in hallucinogens'.

'On both nights Wasson stood up for a long time in Cayetano's room at the foot of the stairway, holding on to the rail transfixed in ecstasy by the visions that he was seeing in the darkness with his open eyes. For the first time that word 'ecstasy' took on a subjective meaning for him. ... There came one moment when it seemed as though the visions themselves were about to be transcended, and dark gates reaching upward beyond sight were about to part, and we were to find ourselves in the presence of the Ultimate. We seemed to be flying at the dark gates as a swallow at a dazzling lighthouse, and the gates were to part and admit us.'. (Riedlinger R569 31)

Wasson's father Edmund was a maverick Episcopal priest, who had written a book called "Religion and Drink" and never tired of telling Gordon that Christ's teaching began with the water into wine at Cana and ended with the wine of the Eucharist at the Last Supper. Gordon was to interpret his experience in the light of its significance as the agape of the Early Christians. This eucharist and the falling sacred words evoked to Wasson the day of Pentecost in which the disciples and the women at the burial were "filled with new wine". In his subsequent article in Life he wrote (Riedlinger R569 26):

"On the night of June 29-30 1955 in a Mexican Indian village so remote from the world that most of the people spoke no Spanish, [we] ... shared with a family of Indian friends' a celebration of 'holy communion' where 'divine' mushrooms were first adored and then consumed. The Indians mingled Christian and per-Christian elements in their religious practices in a way disconcerting for Christians but natural for them. ... We had come from afar to attend a mushroom rite but had expected nothing so staggering as the virtuosity of the performing curanderas and the astonishing effects of the mushrooms. ... We were received and the night's events unrolled in an atmosphere of simple friendliness that reminded us of the agape of early Christian times"

"One can imagine the many trembling confabulations of the friars as they would whisper together how to meet this Satanic enemy. The teonanactl struck at the heart of the Christian religion. I need hardly remind my readers of the parallel, the designation of the Elements in our eucharist 'Take, eat this is my Body'... and again 'Grant us therefore my gracious Lord, so to eat the flesh of thy dear Son ... and to drink His blood'. But the truth was even worse. The orthodox Christian must accept on faith the miracle of the conversion of the bread and wine into God's flesh and blood: that is what is meant by the Doctrine of Transubstantiation. By contrast the sacred mushroom of the Aztecs carries its own conviction: every communicant will testify to the miracle that he has experienced" (Furst R227 191).

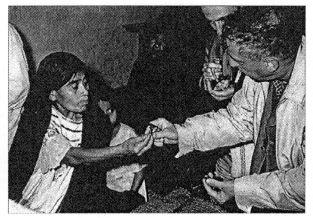

The transmission of the sacrament by Maria Sabina (Riedlinger R568).

The curandero who opened the secret of the mushroom to Wasson was Maria Sabina. Shortly before his arrival she had a vision that strangers would come to seek the little one who springs forth. She had shared her vision with Cayetano García the local sindico or justice, and it was he who agreed that the knowledge should be shared and brought Wasson to her.

The mushrooms were consumed before a small altar. The curandera kept one corner free so that the Holy Ghost could descend in the form of the sacred words that came to her, the words of her little book: "I see the word fall, coming down from above as though they were little luminous object falling from heaven. The word falls on the Holy Table, on my body, with my hand I catch them word for word." (Halifax R274 134)

> "Says.. woman who thunders am I,
> woman who sounds am I.
> Spiderwoman am I, says
> hummingbird woman am I says
> Eagle woman am I, says
> important eagle woman am I.
> Whirling woman of the whirlwind am I, says
> woman of a sacred, enchanted place am I, says
> Woman of the shooting stars am I." ...
> I'm a birth woman, says
> I'm a victorious woman, says
> I'm a law woman, says
> I'm a thought woman, says
> I'm a life woman, says ...
> "I am a spirit woman, says
> I am a crying woman, says
> I am Jesus Christ, says ...
> I'm the heart of the virgin Mary."
> (Mushroom Ceremony - Smithsonian Institute)

Her long life to age 91 was beset by many tragedies including a macabre vision she had shortly afterward on the 'little things', which foretold the murder of her son, possibly in vengeance for opening the knowledge of the mushroom. Her house and little shop were also burned (Estrada R196 71, 79).

"The father of my-grandfather Pedro Feliciano, my grandfather Juan Feliciano, my father Santo Feliciano - were all shamans - they ate the teonanacatl, and had great visions of the world where everything is known... the mushroom was in my family as a parent, protector, a friend".

Maria Sabina had sampled sacred mushrooms in abundance as a child. A few days after watching a wise man cure her uncle she notes: "Maria Anna and I were taking care of our chickens in the woods so that they wouldn't become the victims of hawks or foxes. We were seated under a tree when suddenly I saw near me within reach of my hand several mushrooms. 'If I eat you, you and you' I said 'I know that you will make me sing beautifully'. I remembered my grandparents spoke of these mushrooms with great respect. After eating the mushrooms we felt dizzy as if we were drunk and I began to cry, but this dizziness passed and we became content. Later we felt good. It was a new hope in our life. In the days that followed, when we felt hungry we ate the mushrooms. And not only did we feel our stomachs full, but content in spirit as well. I felt that they spoke to me. After eating them I heard voices. Voices that came from another world. It was like the voice of a father who gives advice. Tears rolled down our cheeks abundantly as if we were crying for the poverty in which we lived.' She had a vision of her dead father coming to her. I felt as if everything that surrounded me was god" (Estrada R196 39).

"Maria Anna and I continued to eat the mushrooms. We ate lots many times, I don't remember how many. Sometimes grandfather and at other times my mother came to the woods and would gather us up from the ground on which we were sprawled or kneeling. 'What have you done?' they asked. They picked us up bodily and carried us home. In their arms we continued laughing singing or crying. They never scolded us nor hit us for eating mushrooms. Because they knew it isn't good to scold a person who has eaten the little things, because it causes contrary emotions and it is possible that one might feel one was going crazy" (Estrada R196 40).

Maria Sabina describes access to the timeless eternal visionary realm: "There is a world beyond ours, a world that is far away, nearby and invisible. And there is where God lives, where the dead live, the spirits and the saints, a world where everything has already happened and everything is known. That world talks. It has a language of its own. I report what it says. The sacred mushroom takes me by the hand and brings me to the world where everything is known. It is they, the sacred mushrooms that speak in a way I can understand. I ask them and they answer me. When I return from the trip that I have taken with them I tell what they have told me and what they have shown me" (Schultes and Hofmann R612 144).

"The more you go inside the world of teonanacatl, the more things are seen. And you also see our past and our future, which are there together as a single thing already achieved, already happened . . . I saw stolen horses and buried cities, the existence of which was unknown, and they are going to be brought to light. Millions of things I saw and knew. I knew and saw God: an immense clock that ticks, the spheres that go slowly around, and inside the stars, the earth, the entire universe, the day and the night, the cry and the smile, the happiness and the pain. He who knows to the end the secret of teonanacatl - can even see that infinite clockwork" (R612 149).

Eunice Pike noted to Wasson in 1953 "One of the proofs that it is 'Jesus Christ himself' who talks to them is that anyone who eats the mushroom sees visions. Everyone we have asked suggests that they are seeing into heaven itself. ... Not all Mazatecs believe that the mushroom messages are from Jesus Christ ... Most monolinguals however will either declare that it is Jesus Christ who speaks to them, or they will ask a little doubting 'What do you say, it is true that it is the blood of Jesus'?" (Mushroom Ceremony - Smithsonian Institute).

The Man in the Buckskin Suit

Jesus came to the white man as flesh and blood, but to the Native American as peyote. John Wilson, who many claim as the 'founder' of the peyote religion in the United States claimed that he was continually translated in spirit to the 'sky realm' by peyote and it was there that he learned the events of Christ's life and the relative position of several of the spirit forces such as sun, moon and fire.

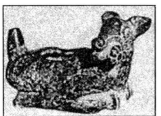

Ceramic snuffing pipe with a deer holding a peyote in its mouth Monte Alban 500 BC (Schultes & Hofmann 1979).

He reported that he had seen Christ's grave, now empty and that peyote had instructed him about the 'Peyote Road' which led from Christ's grave to the moon (this had been the Road in the sky which Christ had travelled in his ascent. Most peyotists strongly affirm the Christian elements as an important part of their religion (Anderson R15 36, 51):

"God told the Delawares to do good even before

He sent Christ to the whites who killed him ...
God made Peyote It is His power. It is the power of Jesus.
Jesus came afterwards on this earth, after peyote."

"You white people needed a man to show you the way, but we Indians have always been friends with the plants and understood them ... "The white man goes into a church and talks about Jesus , but the Indian goes into a teepee and talks to Jesus." (Anderson R15 52).

However, it is Christ in his second-self who came to give the peyote ritual to the Menomini:

"This old man was a chief of a whole tribe, and he have his son to be a chief. He said, "I'm going to go, and you take my place. Take care of this [tribe]." And the boy, he went out hunting; He was lost for about four days. He began to get dry and hungry, tired out; so he gave up. ... So he went, lay himself down on his back; he stretched out his arms like this [extending his arms horizontally], and lay like that. Pretty soon he felt something kind of damp [in] each hand. So he took them, and after he took them, then he passed away. Just as soon as he - I suppose his soul - came to, he see somebody coming on clouds. There's a cloud; something coming. That's a man coming this way, with a buckskin suit on; he got long hair. He come right straight for him; it's Jesus himself. So he told this boy, "Well, one time you was crying, and your prayers were answered that time. So I come here. I'm not supposed to come; I said I wasn't going to come before two thousand years," he said. "But I come for you, to come tell you why that's you [are] lost. But we're going to bring you something, so you can take care of your people. ... So they went up a hill there. There's a tipi there, all ready. So Christ, before he went in it, offered a prayer. ...Take this medicine along, over there. Whoever takes this medicine, he will do it in my name." So that's how it represents almost the first beginning." (Anderson R15 23-4)

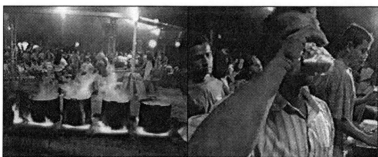

UDV meeting with ayahuasca brewing. The Celebrants sit for several hours in the church meeting hall in contemplation, music and some speeches. A celebrant drinking ayahuasca (Psychedelic Science).

The indigenous use of Amazonian ayahuasca, has been reformed into a modern religious movement, Union of the Vegetal, to "remember past lives and to understand the true meaning of reincarnation as well as to become familiar with the origin and the real destiny of nature and of man". The Union Vegetale or UDV is a nominally Christian movement devoted to experiencing inner harmony through partaking of ayahuasca tea. A fortnightly meeting is held by the movement, which includes members of both sexes from all walks of life. Its membership is not restricted to one fringe group. Similar movements, surround the use of iboga in equatorial Africa in the bwiti and mbiri cults in which men and women make a vision quest to visit the ancestors (p 126).

What is at stake here goes far beyond Christian horizons. It is the discovery that the mystical visionary state is unlocked, not by conscious control, but the incipient chaos that comes from the interaction of the 'other' with our will to order. It extends from the psychotropic plants and fungi to the actual molecules which are their active principles, and their variants.

Persephone giving Demeter the Epoptea sacrament. Eleusis -'liberty cap' mushroom (Graves R256).

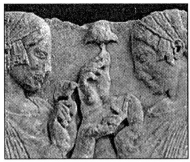

Healing the Nations

However, this association between an active sacrament and mystical gnosis has been lurking in the Christian condition since its beginning. Allegro (R8) has speculated that the mystery at the Christian origin is founded on an agaric mushroom cult. Commenting on the Elusian epoptea, Clement of Alexandria likens Christ, to the Hierophant of the sacred mysteries (Mylonas R485 274):

"Are they not sesame cakes, cakes with many marvels, . and a serpent, the mystic sign of Dionysos Bassareus? Are they not also pomegranates, fig branches ... ivy leaves, round cakes and poppies? In addition there are the unutterable symbols of Ge-Themis, majoram, a lamp, a sword and a woman's comb? [kteis - genital organ symbol]... Oh truly sacred mysteries! Oh pure light! In the blaze of torches, I have an epoptic vision of heaven and of God. I become holy by initiation. The Lord is the Hierophant who reveals the mysteries and commends them to the Father's care, where he is guarded for ages to come" .

John Spong (R645 198) notes that the sacred meal is not just a ritual instituted by Jesus but is also the central motif in the manifestation of the resurrected Christ in which "their eyes were opened", just as were those of Adam and Eve when they ate the forbidden fruit:

"And it came to pass, as he sat at meat with them, he took bread, and blessed it,
and brake, and gave to them. And their eyes were opened,
and they knew him; and he vanished out of their sight." (Luke 24:30)

Likewise in John 21:4 it is the dining which reveals the Christ:

"Jesus saith unto them, Come and dine. And none of the disciples durst ask him,
'Who art thou?' knowing that it was the Lord."

In Acts again, eating and drinking the sacred substance with the redeemer is the central key:

"Not to all the people, but unto witnesses chosen before God,
even to us, who did eat and drink with him after he rose from the dead." (10:39)

Spong comments: "in the act of eating and drinking in the name of the Lord, here and now, we are sharing a foretaste of that kingdom. Perhaps in such a setting our eyes might well 'be opened' to behold the one."

Perhaps after all, Eve was right all along to seek the fruit that would 'make one wise' - hidden since the foundation of the world:

"And he shewed me a pure river of water of life, clear as crystal,
proceeding out of the throne of God and of the Lamb.
In the midst of the street of it, and on either side of the river,
was there the tree of life, which bare twelve manner of fruits,
and yielded her fruit every month:
and the leaves of the tree were for the healing of the nations.

Confluence and Dissonance: The Song of Songs as Holy of Holies

In the introduction (p 8), we mentioned the Song of Songs (p 182) is the Holy of Holies in the Torah, so that that our relationship with the ineffable is mystically represented in the sexual realtionship of the sacred union of woman and man, allegorically represented in the love song of King Solomon and the Queen of Sheba. There are futher motifs in the Judeo-Christian tradition that add to this picture. Hochmah or Wisdom (also called Sophia) is also set up from everlasting (p 208) and the Shekhinah or 'indwelling' feminine face of the divine is manifest in the tent of Sarah and the Eagle's wings of the pregnant madonna retreating into the wilderness in Revelation. It is said that when the Fall occurred in Eden, the Shekhinah retreated and theat the sparks of the Shekhinah will all come together again in the reunion at the end of time when the Tree of Life reappears. The mystical union and our deepest 'relationship with the *mysterium tremendum* are thus manifest in the sexual union and this is the innermost secret of the Bible, the Kosher Tantra of the Torah.

To celebrate the Song of Songs in matrimonial concord we shall tell our own simple tale of the passage of life sacred and profane. Talk of sex and sexual relationship is hearsay until it pulsates with the flesh and blood of the first person. What everyone wants to know are the throes, hunger, and intrigue, the unnerving climax of 'being there', and then of course the fallout. Our relationship experiences, while far from unique, convey many of the dimensions of conflict and complexity in gatherer-hunter societies and in societies which permit polygamy and group marriage, rather than the deceptively clean-cut serial monogamy of Western Christianity-based culture, with its seamy commercial underbelly of prostitution and pornography . Here in first person are many of the predicaments anthropologists document as strangers in a strange land.

Chris

I grew up in a state of 'Victorian' innocence of sex, reminiscent of Buddha's ignorance of death. I was the only child of my parents. My older half-siblings were sent to boarding school as early as I could remember, so I had no sister of my own age or close playmates to gain a feeling of naturalness about being 'intimate' with girls. Rather than boys' war games, I used to fashion space couples, with carefully shaped breasts and buttocks, on lone marital adventures, but there were no show-and-tell sex games with other children. I didn't even know there was such a thing as sexual penetration until I reached puberty and found out the facts of life in a book shop, after a friend insisted that 'making love' was 'like running a ten minute mile'. It wasn't until my middle teens that I discovered active orgasm.

I became an unconfident, shy male, who secretly longed for love, but became tongue-tied the moment sexual interest came into the picture. This lonely dysphoria continued among my carousing flat mates, until, in my graduate year, I met the girl of my dreams, Mahina a far-out 'beatnik' girl from the States, who hung out with the most esoteric people on campus, completely out of my league. I first met her at a summer student retreat in an isolated camp in the sounds. Later I bumped into her in the lift at the library and her face lit up!

Let him kiss me with the kisses of his mouth: for thy love is better than wine.

I summoned the courage to phone her, but the family had moved. By a freak chance, her father turned up at their old place on the third call. A few minutes later, I was nervously asking out my first date. We both went to "Knife in the Water". We had both already seen it but it was an excuse to be together silently in the dark, and before I knew it I was in bed, nervously fumbling with her breasts, running to the bathroom in desperation, to 'crank up my courage' and so began love's mysterious interplay.

We spent a week close to the edge. Wild things happened. I had a motor bike and we went lots of far-out places. We became lost in the hills. We walked hundreds of metres out to sea on a breakwater beyond the airport. As we looked out at the horizon, a tidal wave came rolling in. I could tell it was as tall as we were, even standing on the twenty foot high concrete break-water. We braced ourselves and held on tight to one another, and for an instant we were standing in the middle of the teeming ocean up to our waists, and were all-but swept away. Five weeks later we were married in a beautiful Quaker ceremony signed by all members present. But this was no ordinary marriage and there were big differences in our lives. I had come from a straight-laced Anglican family, where you married one partner for life. Her family were nuclear protesters who had left the US and were into communal living. I had had no other sexual experience. She had had several very cool boyfriends and was still breaking up with one amid tears and regrets. I felt paranoid and vulnerable, knowing show strongly she felt for these other guys.

When she agreed to marry, she told me confidentially that her father said to make clear that consent was on the basis that marriage was not 'exclusive' so that she/we could have other lovers later as she wished. Despite it being light-years outside my cosmology, I agreed, because a bird of paradise in the hand was a dream come true. For three years we had an idyllic existence. We travelled to England and restored a canal boat while I was a graduate student, plied the canals in the idyls of summer and through the ice cracking flows of winter, hitch-hiked round Europe, had our first child and returned to Aotearoa via the far East.

It was only when we were coming to have our second child that love's dysphoria set in. We had gathered with a group of young explorers of alternative states and student comrades who were seeking to go back to the land. One of these was a wild, dashing young friend, Forest, with inscrutably direct blue-grey eyes whom Mahina fell in love with. He became a life time friend and co-founder of the conservation community we set up together. But he was also married, and a tense standoff began, in which two lovers were drawn together, but their unwilling spouses were caught in a state of polarization. After several awkward attempts at 'tolerant openness' to her extra-marital affair, our relationship began to crumble amid my paranoia, sexual jealousy, and emotional violence at 'fear of flying'. This is a classic saga that happens to many relationships. One partner is more vulnerable, and becomes more dependent, more demanding and the other more independent, more equivocal, more interested in others, so the instability feeds on itself.

love is as strong as death, jealousy as cruel as the grave
the coals thereof are coals of fire, that hath a most vehement flame

Finally, after some ill-conceived jealous threats of violence, I was sent packing by her family. This schism occurred in the midst of finding my way into a relationship with Jessica, a brilliant young pianist. Coming from a conservative background, I had no resources to handle the emotional confusion amid unrelenting group living with little privacy. Although I had a new relationship, I was disconsolate at the breakup of my family and children.

After a few weeks apart, Mahina agreed to come back together again if all three of us settled into a *menage-a-trois*. It was a kind of pact of open living to give protection to everyone, while keeping the family together, and giving us all more individual freedom. This broke the ice. We spent the next eighteen months living together and having a succession of affairs. I was no longer jealous of causal relationships. It became a central ethic not to be jealous of one another's affairs. Later, we settled briefly back into monogamous married life, after a second breakup with Jessica, who, in this small antipodean world, went on to marry Mahina's first love. However, during a long hot summer on the land, Mahina continued her long-standing affair with Forest and began another, with one of our close male friends. In the midst of trying to look after our two young children, Christine turned up on her motor cycle and we dived into a wild love-making the night through, in and out of her little tent.

Christine

I grew up in a large family with both brothers and sisters. I had a boy friend in school and more than one relationship before getting married. Liaisons were fluid among our small group of students with a leaning to Society of Friends liberalism. I also married in a Quaker ceremony. My ex-husband is a kindly and loveable person, but he pursued a string of affairs, claiming to be seduced by an older woman and taking a lover where he worked in other places, leaving me alone at home for weeks at a time. I sought the affections of a close married friend and shortly after became pregnant, uncertain to whom. Realizing neither man would commit to supporting the child, I ended up having to fly to Australia, accompanied by my husband to terminate the pregnancy. On the way back he left me at the airport and flew off to visit his Chinese lover in the south, summing up my desolate predicament.

Chris

Knowing Christine really wanted a child, I suggested she get pregnant and come to live with us as. Just as she was denied a child by her previous partnership I offered to espouse her pregnancy. We met again in the capital and spent a few more nights together and a few months later Christine came to live. Shortly beforehand Mahina had said "I want to just be Mr. and Mrs. King again", but by this time a lot of troubled water had passed under the bridge. When Christine arrived, we had a crazy pregnant love affair, climaxed by the arrival of her first child. As with the first *menage*, Mahina settled into this polygynous de facto 'marriage' with an amazing sense of ethical sisterhood. There was none of the competition and antagonism between 'co-wives' which often plagues polygynous marriages.

The daughters saw her, and blessed her;
yea, the queens and the concubines, and they praised her.

Christine

My relations with Mahina were always cordial and supportive. She has a compassionate ethical sense of egalitarian cooperation, which didn't contrast the status of wife and lover and provided strong mutual support in the caring for small children. She was experienced and confident in her life relationships with others and did not feel threatened by my presence.

Christine and Chris

We lived our lives communally. We had a large common sleeping room with a bed for the three of us, into which our young children crawled and cuddled up together. There was another smaller love room in a secluded corner of the house where lovers could meet privately, either two of us, or a tryst with a companion. We held a free-love court where many close friends would come to stay, spend the night and enjoy the favours of love's lubricious embrace. Life was a continuing experimental party, with many live-in friends, couples and their children staying for periods. There was a lot of cooperation between mothers with young children. There were several home births as friends came in from the country.

Sometimes we set up a communal guest bed and occasionally group sex ensued. This was not a swingers' life style of sex for its own sake. We gravitated neither to sexual voyeurism, nor same-sex erotica, but romantic adventure - polyamory in the name of love itself. Although many fleeting encounters fell far short of this ideal, others were sumptuous and overflowing in their times of splendour. All the while we kept a strong commitment to the family and welfare of the children. It is all too easy for love to become prostituted to sexual gratification when sex is pursued just for its own sake. The electronic market now pulsates with 'cum shots' debasing women, animal acts, sadistic, hurtful and harmful sex, and exploitative sex with young girls, which cater mainly to male voyeuristic lust to get one's rocks off at all costs. There is a world of difference between hard-core sex and the quest for romantic love which knows no confines.

Open to me, my sister, my love, my dove, my undefiled:
for my head is filled with dew, and my locks with the drops of the night.

My beloved put in his hand by the hole of the door, and my bowels were moved for him.
I rose up to open to my beloved; and my hands dropped with myrrh,
and my fingers with sweet smelling myrrh, upon the handles of the lock.

Sexual love has a deep and undying creative relationship with reproduction. Each of us were parents pursuing love in a context of ongoing parenthood. While sex was a pleasure and sexual trysts were enticing, parenthood was an ongoing 'sacred' commitment. Ideas of sex as merely a social contract between consenting adults fail to grasp the biological basis of reproduction underlying sex and love, which is how we all got here throughout life's history and how the immortal continuity of life continues. For all the mountains of spices in the Song of Songs, it is still a pastoral love song of burgeoning natural fertility:

Thy teeth are like a flock of sheep that are even shorn,
which came up from the washing;
whereof every one bear twins,
and none is barren among them.

Once sex is divorced from reproduction, it loses the life 'force which through the green fuse drives the flower' as Dylan Thomas put it. It becomes reduced to erogenous gratification and expedient social bonding. Falling in love and the power of love's infatuation and addictive obsession make evolutionary sense because the passage of the generations needs gratifying one-on-one physical bonding to promote strong affirmative relationships, which will support struggling infants amid parental conflicts of interest, at least to the age when children can walk and talk and feed themselves if need be. In turn the deepest meaning of sex and the pleasure of sexual love are given their full and complete expression in the lubricious 'waterline' of sexual procreation by woman and man. The fullest and most complete orgasmic expression of primal fusion is the tumultuous fertility of conception and pregnancy. Any view of sexuality which remains in denial of its life-giving powers is incomplete and liable to become perverted pleasure, carnal lust and selling our sexual bodies and souls for profit.

Another aspect of this paradox is the tortured relationship between sex and God. Patriarchal religions treat the sexual urge as a dangerous source of pollution of paternity. Only in the Song of Songs, Tantric creation and the Tao do we find sex, fertility and the cosmic in generative harmony. The Christian church sees woman as the fallen temptress, sex and sexual 'fornication' as a dangerous loss of free will to our no-longer innocent animal drives, to be engaged purely for reproductive ends, in denial of sensual pleasure. Islam likewise sees women as second class citizens, only half a man, and so dangerously enticing as to need to be hidden from the face of other men. The prime relationship with God, in both fundamentalist and mystical traditions, is a state of utter and complete submission to an 'higher power'. However the end result of such submission to the cosmic self is a soaring state of arrogant male hubris, in which conversion by the swords of crusade and jihad are equated with God's will.

By contrast, the sexual relationship is the way in which biological immortality is entwined in complementary mortal beings. The sexual relationship is the ultimate relationship with the alien and exotic 'other' in mutual fertility. It is also a meeting of two conscious living beings, who each possess the uncertainties of free and intentional will. But in this relationship, by contrast with the living offspring of each, there is little or no genealogical kinship between partners, so the relationship between them, while held together by sexual attraction, is also mediated a spectrum of emotions, from love and compassion to rebelliousness and jealousy, in an interplay between cooperative complementarity and strategic dissonance. Nevertheless, it is to love we turn for the life and light of concord. There is a deep truth to the sexual relationship and sexual love as the redemption of immortality in biological form. Because it is also the central relationship in which conscious, intentional autonomy meets its compassionate nemesis in the autonomy and reproductive choices of the other, and it is integrally involved in the passage of life and the future of all life, sexual love, and our ecosystemic relationships, rather than God 'alone' is the acid test of our future viability. It is the living context in which we reach towards a biodiverse, robust, safe world in evolutionary time, because in our very intentionality and our ecological sensitivity, we are 'procreating' the future of life on Earth for our descendents, throughout our future generations. It is to this primal sexual complementarity that the Wisdom of Proverbs stakes her ultimate claim:

The Lord possessed me in the beginning of his way, before his works of old.
I was set up from everlasting, from the beginning, or ever the earth was.
When there were no depths, I was brought forth; when there were no fountains abounding with
water.
Before the mountains were settled, before the hills was I brought forth:
While as yet he had not made the earth, nor the fields, nor the highest part of the dust of the world.

The ideal of courtly love is worship of the holy grail - the sacred cup in which sensuality and the power of the female being and her sexual charisma overfloweth, a mystery as deep and engrossing as the fearsome mysteries of God and the divine.

Thou hast ravished my heart, my sister, my spouse;
thou hast ravished my heart with one of thine eyes, with one chain of thy neck.

We can have strong friendships, deep soulful relationships, working partnerships, and collaborations in discovery, without sex or sexual jealousy entering into the picture, but Platonic love casts a screen - an 'iron curtain' chastity belt - a darkened veil of prohibition - across the deepest mingling of all, in which our very identities are merged and dissolved with the exotic other - the sexual fusion of two beings in love on a mysterious life journey, whose meetings are often fated to happen, yet frequently remain tragically unfulfilled. The source of the repression of sensuality is male anxiety about paternity uncertainty and the power of female sexual energy, which is the very basis of female reproductive choice.

Polyamory tries to resolve this paradox of sexual confinement, without resorting to the levels of dishonesty and intrigue that plague conventional 'monogamous' relationships, where one partnership is morally blessed and overt, if confining, while all others are stolen moments of deceit captured in the covert shadows, wayward and corrupt, if full of love's longing for freedom and merging with the mysterious exotic other. Nevertheless polyamorous relationships are still plagued by jealousy and a streak of competitiveness towards the charisma that comes from successfully attracting partners in love. "Making it" in a string of romantic trysts can become a consuming obsession, spawned by the very culture of love.

Many relationships are casual, slightly contrived, or even misconstrued meetings, and there is no lasting emotional bond. However the few cases where one does meet and fall in love passionately with another being become life long treasures, which add to our being and sense of completion in life. In sex, the full interplay of psychic, and life energies come together into a primal vortex of arousal of all our being, our deepest instincts and our mortal journey through life as if two travellers who have been seeking one another since the dawn of time have finally met and found their sanctuary together. It is not just the sexual act but the intimacy, the poetry, the hidden story of the life journey of the other that enthralls and the honour and beauty of acceptance by the other that burns in our souls.

My beloved is unto me as a cluster of camphire in the vineyards of Engedi
Who is this that cometh out of the wilderness like pillars of smoke,
perfumed with myrrh and frankincense?
How fair is thy love! how much better is thy love than wine!
and the smell of thine ointments than all spices!
Thy lips drop as the honeycomb: honey and milk are under thy tongue;
and the smell of thy garments is like the smell of Lebanon.

Chris

Having started out as a conservative, jealous, only child of my parents, dragged into a highly unconventional polyamorous life-style, I began to realize in my bones that men are naturally attuned to loving more than one woman if they can and Guinivere no less, if they get the chance of a lifetime. There is little reproductive cost for a man, and much potential benefit. Each woman is a mountain of spice, alluring and attractive in a way which causes a pheromonal and sensual yearning to sew oats as far and wild as the wind carries exotic perfumes. I became deeply adapted to partnering more than one woman over several polygynous relationships, lasting over most of my reproductive life. Women too have a deeply rooted evolutionary destiny, locked in their wildest ecstasy, to seek the gallant 'unattainable' Lancelot, central to female reproductive choice in evolution, albeit in the shady groves of covert intimacy, out of sight of gossip's tortuous grape vines, if they (or indeed he), already have a potentially jealous partner, as is more than likely in an almost coercively marital world.

Christine

We have debated back and forth the best framework for accomodating a new sexual attraction with the needs and demands of an existing relationship, and whether there can ever be any clear answer to the prisoners' dilemma this involves. One strength of the polyamorous 'way' is that it seeks to respect existing relationships even when having a heady affair, and to mediate the all-too-natural forces of jealousy when they do arise, providing more of a cushion against the tendency to pursue one serially monogamous infatuation after another, scattering children behind us in a string of broken families, divorce battles and custody suits resulting in pain, wounding, divided loyalties and a perpetuation of the same from generation to generation. On the other hand, polyamory's often fatal weakness, despite the perennial nature of the eternal triangle, is that it invites complexities which tend to make all relationships more dynamically unstable. People naturally gravitate to a one-on-one relationship where they can have intimacy without the vulnerability and conflict of shared affections, so polyamory is very liable to lead to a quest for monogamy. I'm still reserved about it's ability to successfully mediate these conflicting forces.

I am my beloved's, and his desire is toward me.
His left hand should be under my head, and his right hand should embrace me.

Chris and Christine

Does polyamory suit men better than women? This is a difficult one. In a heterosexual reproductive world, for every philandering man, there is also a *femme fatale*. The Western norm is for declared monogamy with a sub-culture of amorous affairs. Polygynous extended families are far more common across human societies than the few examples of polyandry, which are usually confined to marriage to several brothers. Women frequently claim to favour monogamy, consistent with womens' need to establish a resource-bearing husband to support their pregnancies and offspring, while men choose to spread wild oats. The essential difference between men and women is that women generally have a lot more to lose from being found out - the loss of a resourceful husband or a violent attack from a jealous male or even the murder of her children. It is the females who carry the key repro-ductive burden in pregnancy, so they have to be much more careful than casual males. On the other hand a polyamorous woman in her prime can lead a blazing trail few men can keep up with, because far more men are willing partners to a casual sexual invitation from a female than women are from a male. Although women claim to prefer monogamy, statis-tics in US society show that serial monogamy is used by men to pre-emptively sire new families with younger women, so it's a way men in monogamous societies practice de facto polygyny.

Regardless of how society deals with sex, and the waxing and waning of romantic love over the ages, the stories of love's trials, tragedies and fulfillments captivates us all, from the Song of Songs' mountains of spices dripping on the key hole of the lock, to Layla's "do you want to see me crawl across the floor to you?". Sexual love is the strongest force - the primal rhythm driving social interplay and the most subject to violent reaction when the whip-lash of jealousy unwinds into the light of day. It is the life force itself, through which the immortal passage of the generations arises, so it can never be fully tamed by moral oppression. Religious paths have sought, almost without exception, to debase the primal mystery of sex, and sensual lubricity as a contrivance of female wiles, yet no reli-gious path which confines sexual liberty can know the *mysterium tremendum* in its full power and splendour.

The watchmen that went about the city found me, they smote me,
they wounded me; the keepers of the walls took away my veil from me.

Chris

In our own love lives there were many such intrigues and many strange affairs. Everyone had their turn in the unexpected flowering of the love light. All this was fine with casual relationships, but once one of us began to fall seriously in love in a way which might com-promise existing relationships, the ancient dragons of jealousy would re-emerge. Mahina became less than satisfied with having become semi-permanently caught in a group mar-riage from which she couldn't retreat back into simple partnership. She began to court and spark with a view to a new monogamous relationship. By this time our children were four and five so it coincides with the 'four year love bond' in human evolution, after which offspring can walk and talk and the needs for parental pair-bonding become less acute, and partners can move on to greener pastures.

While Christine and I were on a short visit to South East Asia, Mahina fell in love with another charismatic man. Fortunately Colin was also involved with another woman who had left her husband to be with him. A month or two later the three of us made a journey across country to visit Colin and another of his close friends, Daniel. Colin and Daniel immediately took off with my two partners, leaving me 'cuckolded' at the end of the long journey. Ever compassionate, Christine, recognizing my predicament, loved me back to life again. Some months later Mahina took up a serious relationship with Daniel, who embarked on a sequestered one-on-one exclusive relationship with her. She carefully became pregnant to him and the whole situation became very tense.

Daniel was not prepared to make an accomodation to the extended family and this now had no real future. I had taken sabbatical leave with the intention of travelling to the East to discover the mysteries of Buddhist and Vedantic mysticism. As my departure loomed the entire extended family headed for breakup. I departed for Asia with both partners heading separate ways into the arms of other men. Nothing could be a greater fall from grace, comfort and self-esteem than to descend from a polygynous patriarch to lone wanderer in Sadhu's robes, shorn of all one's worldly affections in a disintegrating diaspora.

Christine

Shortly after Chris left, the family separated and I was left to care for my daughter with occasional visits from Chris's older two children. Although I had Chris's financial support, like all mothers I was left 'holding the infant' while the male in the piece wandered off in pursuit of the mysteries of culture. At the same time this gave me an opportunity to consolidate my independence on the land and to have a more autonomous relationship with the others in our wilderness community. During this period I became a teacher in the local school and established firm roots in the country, which have become an integral part of my life, and a central formative part of the growth and maturation of all our children.

Chris

I traversed India for six months as a sadhu, sharing life with street children, lepers and beggars, frequenting the temples and pilgrimage spots and taking Buddhist initiations with Yeshe Dorje, the Ningmapa weather lama, who had a wife and seven children in a kerosine tin shanty above McLeod Gang. I learned to use uncertainty and loss of personal history as a catalytic act of power. Every day was an unfolding surprise. Many fleeting relationships crossed my path. A lonely woman in Katmandu who was missing her boyfriend. A street woman from Sikkim in Calcutta. A Californian 'sunyassin' named Maya who was seeking tantric sexual annihilation and left me for a sexual 'double ride' with two eager young Pakistanis. A sixteen year old opium addict, who walked with a stick and was drawn to me because her junkie boyfriend had become impotent. An ex-student I met by chance on the opposite side of the planet. By degrees I became a charismatic international traveller. Women would discard their bags on the beach, just for an excuse to get away from their boyfriends, to steal a kiss with me on the sly. Within a few days of arriving in a new place, I could find a lady love, or two, just as the troubadours did of old.

I completed this journey with a visit to natural habitats of the psychic power plants of the western hemisphere and experienced the shamanic use of peyote with Tellus Goodmorning, teonanactl, and later ayahuasca with Senor Trinico in the Amazon. Subsequently I communed with the visionary power plant sacraments I had discovered on my far-flung travels. A number of women sought sexual trysts with me as an avenue to their mysteries.

The mandrakes give a smell, and at our gates are all manner of pleasant fruits,
new and old, which I have laid up for thee, O my beloved.

On my return to Aotearoa, my relationship with Christine continued, but entangled in the divided loyalties of her other commitment. I also began a relationship with Joan, one of Mahina's oldest female friends. For a year we became a loose foursome living in cabins on various parts of our wilderness community. However the women did not meet eye to eye and their relationship remained somewhat tense, as is common in polygamous societies. Joan moved to the city and we became long-term partners there, while Christine remained in the country, teaching and bringing up our children. On weekends I would be the wilderness pioneer, sharing in the extended family life, which continued with my children by Mahina. During the week I earned the daily bread as a professional in the city. The extended family remained strong and connected, as Mahina continued to live on the neighbouring land. We cooperated over the children's welfare . They passed freely between us, as members of both adjacent communities. Mahina declared herself to be committed to monogamy. She sired two children with her new partner, who have become a close part of the extended family. She separated from Daniel to find her current partner when he 'came out' to lead a more promiscuous gay life-style.

For eleven years I commuted weekly between work in the city and family in the country with a partner in each place. This caused continuing tensions which came to a head when Christine and I had a further child together and Joan, who had refused to have a child with me in the complexities of the extended family, resented the pregnancy and insisted the city house was her partnership domain and that I not be intimate with Christine when she was in the city, even when Christine came to the house to give birth to our next child. Christine had a miserable time and nearly had to deliver our son's head herself during an unexpectedly precipitate birth, because I was consoling my other distraught partner, in an adjoining room. She remained angry about this for years, although she had a faultless quick birth. Although I sympathized with Joan's vulnerability, this conflict undermined our relationship. It wasn't consistent with the sisterly cooperation I had previously experienced and knew was the key to a viable extended family. Keeping a viable family life was not a negotiable option for me as a father. The situation was already complex enough without further division.

Eventually Christine moved to the city so the children could go to high school, on condition my other partner moved to her house nearby. This was not well received and a period of separation ensued from Joan, although we remained covert lovers off and on for eight years after. This was somewhat of a paradox. All my previous sexual relationships had been honestly declared and these were both by now very long established partnerships, but there had also been continuing antipathy and I wasn't prepared to risk the family future and make life untenable for everyone by openly courting two 'sparring' partners. I did my best to give Joan what love and companionship I could, but it had become a secretive and surreptitious affair. Eventually she threw down the gauntlet and demanded I declare that I was equally committed to her, and when I declined to protect the family, we parted company.

By this time HIV had chastened the 'pristine innocence' of free-love and Christine and I settled into several years of monogamous family life. She has remained monogamous since and I have had only very occasional sexual partners since, and then only for a meaningful purpose, with prior medical checks, so that no partner is compromised through the sexual exchange. If sexual desire comes before the safety of others it is bound to fail.

In the year leading up to the millennium I set off on a world sabbatical vigil to draw attention to human devastation of biodiversity, which included study in the US, a traverse of the Amazon and a rite of passage for sexual reunion in reflowering abundance in Jerusalem. I negotiated with Christine to partner with Mariam, a friend in the US I had cooperated with on the internet, for the duration of the ten month journey.

Christine

While Chris was on sabbatical, our son was just beginning university a couple of years early and I wanted to make sure he had adequate support to make a good start. It's all very well for the men to have visions of world redemption and go forth to try to achieve cultural transformation, but while these escapades are taking place family life and the needs of even maturing offspring tend to get left to the woman in the piece. I also had reservations about participating in Chris's vigil, whose apocalyptic flavour I didn't identify with, and the good deal of potential risk, as well as discomfort, in the swamps of Amazonia.

Although I had helped with gathering and assessing a lot of the research which contributed to The Codex of the Tree of Life, and found many of its tortuous twists and turns in the pagan backdrop of monotheism interesting and provocative, I found Chris's identification with the messianic quest, even if conceived of in shamanistic terms as a reunion reflowering, too close to the single-minded intensity that has troubled religious history to become the *'femme fatale'* in the Jerusalem reunion. I am much more responsive to our evolutionary heritage and the realities of complementarity and reproductive choice between the sexes that are the basis of our key roles of mothering and parenting and how these influence our social choices.

Chris

I kept contact with Christine and regularly helped my younger son with questions about his courses. After leaving the US, Mariam and I traversed the Amazon together with my older son and Adam a long-term friend from Aotearoa on a biodiversity study, documenting human impact, from the burning season in Bolivia, through the altiplano and high passes of the Andes, down the Urubamba and Ucayali to the Amazon basin. Adam set out on a searing career as a Cassinova and ran off with seven Peruvian women, from nightclub dancers to young students, in as many days, causing us all a considerable degree of concern. We parted at Iquitos and my son and I travelled on down the Amazon to Manaus and via the Pantanaal to Rio, documenting the destruction of the rain forest and wildlife as we went.

Mariam and I made a circuit of sites in Europe associated with Magdalen and the Black Madonna Sarah at Saintes Marie de la Mer and to Rome. We flew to Israel-palestine and performed the sacred union of woman and man in reflowering the Tree of Life in the apocalyptic unveiling of bridal reunion in Jerusalem in a series of rites of passage, from an all night celebration on the Mount of Olives on Millennium Eve, to a reunion procession from the ascension site on the Epiphany through the old city past Gethsemane and the Mercy Gates to the Western Wall, pronouncing our mythopoetry of reflowering as we passed:

I have come here to remind you.
You are Him, and I am She,
and we, the ark of the world.
We must not transport to the void
but sweetly plant in Earth,
our love so rare

Mariam is a loving companion in the reflowering vigil who gave her heart and soul to this venture. I did likewise faithfully, but I had a covenant to return to the family. The sacred union in the tradition of the *hieros gamos* in Jerusalem was a climax for both of us, but was as fleeting as the masked rites of Beltane. Almost immediately we had celebrated the sacred marriage of the Song of Songs at the Wailing Wall, my sabbatical and the millennial vigil came to an end in a planetary parting of the ways.

I opened to my beloved; but my beloved had withdrawn himself, and was gone:
my soul failed when he spake: I sought him, but I could not find him;
I called him, but he gave me no answer.

Mariam returned West to California and I journeyed briefly further East to Varanasi, the Himalayas, and South East Asia to document Kali and the destruction of biodiversity in Asia. We continue to have a commitment to the validity of healing the living planet:

We cannot escape through worship
our own conscious destiny.
Our meeting and our embracing.
For the Renewal of all life
lies in this sacred realm,
and that rare stranger in the garden,
the immortal Beloved, is also Yourself.

Two years later, a *'flamme fatale'*, appeared, who became a colourful, affectionate, humorous and yet challenging 'nemesis' partner in sacred reunion. This time the paradigm was Kali, the unspeakable feminine of Thunder Perfect Mind, and the primal fires of Tantric sexual fusion at the origin of the universe - a confluence having the potential to open up a flowering interplay between the chalice and the blade at the very roots of existence.

You give kali a bad rap by your equating her with male sacrifice ...
for kali as personification of sacrificer exists only as ego destroyer
and if you fear not transcendence of death by transcendence of ego ...

I lay my fate gladly at the feet of the dark goddess of the enclosed garden ...
to lie beneath you lovingly as kali ma-donna, for in this transient life I am the walking dead ...

then you shall walk no more as dead, my beloved, but risen, radiant and resplendent ...
and in tenderness and loving compassion shall we dance through the fragrant vineyards of our love
...

Christine gave her consent for a short 'sabbatical' visit, with a view to creative collaboration. This was a planetary conjunction on the 'noosphere', sight unseen beyond a photograph and affectionate e-mails. We met, embraced and commingled, traversing the far-flung shorelines of Aotearoa, from the twelve pillars of *Kohititangamarama* - 'the first appearance of the moon,' believed to be those of the Temple itself; to *Irimahuwhero*, 'place of the hanging red hair', so iconic of Rose's flowing tresses. Though a soulful kindred spirit, the knife edge between fusion and nemesis is but a hair's breadth. Although Rose had before her arrival expressed concern to me that she might cast a shadow which could undermine Christine, Christine and Rose chose neither to meet nor to communicate directly when she arrived - a first among all our diverse relationships. Christine, though a consenting party, at once perceived that a planetary 'nemesis', which didn't seek her acknowledgment, woman-to-woman, could become a winner-take-all rout, and she put up a spirited resistance, which 'ruffled' the limpid waters throughout our journey. Shortly after Rose returned to her Northern climes, our affectionate correspondence metamorphosed into an ever more schismatic dialogue. Serial monogamy and polyamorous 'philandering' now clashed in a molten flow of opposition. Fusion had become its own volcanic nemesis.

Return, return, O Shulamite; return, return, that we may look upon thee.
What will ye see in the Shulamite? As it were the company of two armies.

Christine and Chris

This occluded union acted as a catalyst to bring the each of us into a tumultuous renaissance. For several months we lived a double life at the edge, established partners with land and family, and nascent lovers in a strange affair, steeped in the uncertainty which untamed love had cunningly brought about.

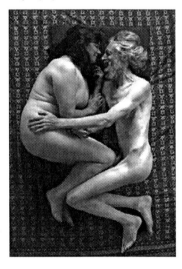

Behold, thou art fair, my beloved, yea, pleasant:
also our bed is green.
The beams of our house are cedar, and our rafters of fir.

Make haste, my beloved, and be thou like to a roe
or to a young hart upon the mountains of spices

This closing circle, which opened when we first met, has in turn led to the writing of "Sexual Paradox", as an unveiling of the sexually complementary nature of the entire sweep of existence, from our cosmic origins, through our evolutionary heritage, and the cultures of male domination, to an unveiling of mutual paradox, which we see as humanity's best hope for reconciliation in the world today.

many waters cannot quench love, neither can the floods drown it.

Pregnant Zero and Universal Paradox

As a koan for sexual paradox we can consider the double contradiction represented by a single sheet of paper with contradictory signs on each face:

The statement on the other side is false.
The statement on the other side is true.

If we accept either in its entirety, we are in a double-bind, for each leads us into a state of global contradiction, when the other is taken into account. In fact paradox is itself sexual between truth and falsehood for it is a situation where the truth of the statement implies its falsehood and vice versa. In every other situation truth and falsehood remain segregated but in paradox they are in logical coitus.

"I Wonder if they Had Trouble Inventing Zero?"

To illustrate the nature of paradox and sexual division we shall make a short digression into numbers and logical systems. This is taken with due respect to the vastly greater complexity of the real world of living beings, consciousness and the enigmas of quantum reality simply to go to the heart of logical paradox and its implicitly sexual nature permeating existence.

Arabic-Indic numerals well-indicate the nature of such primal division. The linear 1 is an inheritance from a simple mark, a line, digit or finger, indicating the presence of an object, or event, thus making a primal distinction - existence. By contrast, zero is much more difficult to arrive at, since it does not count for anything at all and at face value there is nothing to be done. Zero thus only came to be recognized indirectly, through a long, tortuous route, which first led to positional notation for numbers and then to the need for a mark for

European	0	1	2	3	4	5	6	7	8	9
Arabic-Indic	٠	١	٢	٣	٤	٥	٦	٧	٨	٩
Persian / Urdu	٠	١	٢	٣	۴	۵	۶	٧	٨	٩
Devanagari Hindi	०	१	२	३	४	५	६	७	८	९
	०	१	२	३	४	५	६	७	८	९
Gupta (4th cent. AD)	—	=	≡							
Brahmi (1st cent. AD)	—	=	≡	+						

a space For example in counting a hundred and one objects by writing 101, the zero (*sunya*) is needed to indicate there are no tens. This led to the use of a simple dot (*bindu*) to indicate a space and eventually the small circle we now associate with zero. In the process even the stars in the sky came to be referred to in Indian literature as *sunya bindu* or 'void dots'.

Zero and with it positional notation was transmitted in the Middle ages from India, through the Arabs, to Europe. In the process *bindu* became Arabic *sifr* which again means a space. This has evolved into our term cipher, which has come to mean both zero and a digit, with undertones of worthlessness - 'a mere cipher' and more sinisterly, covert encryption - to 'decipher' a code is to expose it - illustrating the dark concealed complexity within zero in the minds of men seeking a universe of perfect order.

Zero, and with it the positional number system, was championed by Fibonacci, whose name, 'Bigollo', can mean 'good-for-nothing' as well as 'traveller', both of which are apt here. Fibonacci is among other things famous for the sequence of magic numbers we shall see play a role in chaos (p 504). It is thus to Fibonnaci all merchants owe the Arabic-Indic positional notation which has made numerical calculation so natural and made both science and the precipitous rise and fall of stock markets in their triple witching hour possible.

Positional notation was actually a much earlier invention, harking back to Sumeria and Babylon, but here it was embraced in base sixty, much too large for easy manipulation of less than titanic quantities, and so succeeding cultures lapsed back into the positionless numbers exemplified by Roman numerals such as MCMXLIV which are unnaturally clumsy to calculate with. Our current base 10 number system, which transparently corresponds to our two sets of five appendages, shared between vertebrates and echinoderms, still declares its biological origin in the name 'digits' given to whole numbers. In a sense the numbers other than zero are simply 'giving the fingers'.

In a final nemesis of the historical complexity of number bases, the modern computing paradigm has converged back to the dyadic sexual division itself in the two primal numerals 0 and 1 in using base 2 arithmetic because this reflects the two states of existence of a single discrete 'charge' in memory - a binary distinction, now symbolized by an almost 'penile' 1 complemented by a distinctly 'vaginal' 0.

The 'it from bit' concept of quantum cosmology attempts to similarly describe all quantum phenomena in terms of their information content in terms of bits signified again by the binary 'digits' 0 and 1, sometimes with the three-valued logic of 0, 1 and 'uncertain'.

Despite their fertile and convoluted history, the numerals in their binary form return to a primary sexual division between a pregnant feminine 0 representing absence, enclosure and completion and a discriminating masculine 1, representing existence, distinction and separation. Enclosure and completion lead naturally to wave-like nature while distinction and separation to particle nature. Notice also that the absence implied by the zero is also both a unity undivided by distinction and a totipotentiality out of which all distinction can come, just as the primal void or chaos of *tohu vohu*.

These two processes are fundamental to all differentiation of the existential condition, in both the physical and experiential realms. For anything to exist, it must be differentiated from that which it is not. The primary distinction is between existence manifest as 1 and non-existence represented by the positional void of 0. The totality is thus in its essence a unity which is also a duality. This is a primal form of sexual paradox at the origin of the cosmos. Any attempt to draw a distinction by placing a boundary also results in enclosure, so the zero also contains within it the germ of the 1 just as the 1 also implies the unity of existence and thus contains the germ of 0.

Sexual paradox implies a primal cosmology, in which all phenomena present as complements, through which the totality is manifest. These result in contradiction or degeneracy if either of the primal complements is invoked to the exclusion of the other. The cosmos described as divine order in the human mind leaves the totality lacking the chaotic abyss underlying zero which is pregnant because it is the formless progenitor of new form, just as we shall see new order frequently bifurcates out of chaos. This means that the feminine aspect of the zero harbours undelimited potential as well as the instability and fluctuation abhorred in descriptions of a cosmology emerging from primal chaos.

Bootstrapping from Nothing to an Abnormal Universe

We can see this potentiality of the pregnant 0 in archetypal form in Von Neumann's construction of the natural numbers from the empty set $\varnothing$ - the set consisting of no elements or members, and thus corresponds to the cardinal number 0. We can then recursively define $\{\varnothing\}$ the set whose only element consists of the empty set, which corresponds to cardinal number 1 and then the set consisting of $\{\varnothing, \{\varnothing\}\}$ corresponding to 2 and so on, thus defining all the natural numbers from the 'pregnant' empty set - form out of void.

The very notion of a set of elements attempts to give us a foundation level of distinction and membership, $x \in X$, defining x to be an element of the set X. Notice also that attempts to define a universal set run into a paradox due to Bertrand Russell which is also in its essence a sexual paradox of division associated with the concept of a universal totality in which elementary membership is possible.

Notice that our construction of the numbers from the empty, or null set assumed that a set such as $\varnothing$ could itself be an element of another set $\{\varnothing\}$. We however immediately run into trouble when we consider the universal set U consisting of all possible sets. Let us define a set to be *normal* if it does NOT contain itself as an element - i.e. $X \notin X$ ... Now, if we consider N the set of all normal sets, we find we are in a double bind. Is N normal or not? If it is normal then it is not a member of itself and hence not a member of the set of all normal sets, hence it is abnormal. But if it is abnormal then it is a member of itself and hence a member of the set of all normal sets and hence normal. Contradiction.

This universal paradox is both sexual in the sense that it arises from a division into two conditions, normal and abnormal, and is fundamental to the notion of universality even in the restricted domain of 'normality'. We can't eliminate the dilemma of Russell's paradox no matter how counter-intuitive it may seem. Sexual paradox is thus primal to the universal order. Notice that it also fulfils an important part of the central idea of paradox, as something which defies common sense and is yet true.

Propositions which Can't Make up their Minds

However paradox, in terms of logically confounding, has a wider application. Another face of sexual paradox may lie in our incapacity to completely tie down descriptions of reality into fully-definable closed systems. Traditionally a contradiction is a statement whose truth implies its falsehood and vice versa. This is rather like a logical version of the entangled mixing we shall later associate with chaotic processes, in the sense that true and false have become inextricably entwined. However, the other face of this is an undecidable proposition - one to which neither true nor false can be definitively be assigned from the axioms of the system.

Kurt Gödel has become famous or notorious, depending on your point of view, for proving his 'incompleteness theorem': that any logical system containing finite arithmetic possesses within it formally undecidable propositions. This means also that the propositions definable within real world systems can never be exhaustively proven, because some of the statements we can validly make can never be verified using the system's postulates.

Peano arithmetic, has five simple axioms defining natural numbers, starting from 0 using successors: $1=S(0)$, $2=SS(0)$, etc. The axioms are as follows for any a and b:

(1) $Sa \neq 0$, (2) $a+0=a$, (3) $a+Sb=S(a+b)$, (4) $a \cdot 0=0$, (5) $a \cdot Sb=a \cdot b+a$

Gödel's trick was to also use the natural numbers to encode logical propositions. We can do this encoding by assigning unique numbers for free variables such as a and b, for arithmetic operators such as '+', '·', '=' and so on, and also for the logical statements 'for all', 'there exists', 'such that', 'not', 'and', 'or', etc. All statements provable from the axioms can be reached by syntactic substitutions which can also be encoded using the number code.

Around twelve simple rules of substitution, such as:

'for all a this does not happen' $\cong$ 'there does not exist a for which this happens'

can generate every syntactically correct proposition in Peano arithmetic, and each proposition can thus be represented by a unique integer, called its Gödel number. Given the five axioms and some twelve grammatical rules for constructing statements, this 'numerical logic' lets us also write down propositions which are about propositions. Not all Gödel numbers correspond to syntactic statements which can be proved from the axioms however. Each that can be proved we can call a 'theorem of numerical logic'. In particular, we can write down self-referential propositions, ones which include their own Gödel number.

The key Gödel number that is undecidable corresponds to a self-referential paradox:

"This statement is not a theorem of numerical logic."

Is the above statement true or false? If it is false, then it IS a theorem of numerical logic, so we have a valid theorem proved from the axioms, but it is false, so the whole system falls apart by inconsistency. Hence it must be true. But if it is true, then, by its own statement, it is not a theorem of numerical logic. This means that the statement is true, but it is not a provable proposition from the axioms. The system is thus incomplete, and the truth of the proposition is undecidable within the system.

Undecidable propositions can come in diverse and varied forms, but a classic one is: "Will a computational process eventually complete?" - the 'halting problem' of Alan Turing, who broke the 'enigma' code. It is illustrated (p 509) in cellular automata. Even for these apparently simple systems, we cannot determine in advance whether they will terminate or reproduce forever. Such issues extend to cellular automata simulating the prisoners' dilemma game (p 21), which can also be undecidable (Grim R265).

Can the Universe be Told?

The second law of thermodynamics says that any closed system will tend to equilibrium where entropy (disorder) is at a maximum and the rate of entropy production has fallen to a minimum of zero. Ilya Prigogine (R541) and others have noted that open thermodynamic systems however do not have to tend to equilibrium but may go into complex far-from equilibrium states where entropy production is minimized . The living biosphere is an example in which increasing complexity and decreasing entropy result from the open thermodynamic boundary of the biosphere fixing incident solar energy by photosynthesis.

Logical systems are thus rather like open thermodynamic systems, which exchange information across their boundaries, and do not necessarily tend to a closed equilibrium. Because Gödel incompleteness also applies to any logical system containing finite arithmetic it applies to virtually all non-trivial domains of existence including the real world around us with its manifold complexities of quantum reality, life and subjective experience, which transcend formal logic. After spending years seeking a unified theory of cosmology, Stephen Hawking has recently begun to lament that Gödel's theorem may make it impossible to form a grand unified 'theory of everything', or TOE, for the universe.

The *Tao te Ching (R733)* expresses this succinctly as "The way that can be told is not the countless way" (p 453). Transcendence over closed logic is common to many religious and mystical traditions. We are here running up against a form of paradox involving order, chaos, complexity and our incapacity to define a closed boundary between a given realm and its complement. It is pertinent here to consider our linguistic terms for the universal condition and ponder the role mankind's will-to-order plays in determining our universal concepts and the toll it has on the darker concealed aspect the pregnant zero contains.

The founding historical concept in both the religious and natural realm is 'cosmos' from the Greek *kosmos* - order. Cosmos here, despite laying claim to be the entire universe is implicitly contrasted with primal chaos as the condition of divine or perfect order. Norman Cohn's work "Cosmos Chaos" (R125) well describes the counterpoint of these two ideas in religious history, from the slaying of Tiamat - the primal mother waters of chaos by Marduk the divine agent of civic order, through the Biblical and Apocalyptic traditions to the founding of Christianity. 'Universe', our more physically accepted scientific term, again highlights an evolution to unity through order in the Latin *universus* - 'turned into one' - *uni-* 'one' *versere* 'turned'. Such an ordered unity is a little like the 'false vacuum' we will investigate at the inflationary cosmic origin. 'Turned into one' is an imposed order violating the ground swell of chaos and unstable to it into which imposed order shall again dissolve in the final unravelling (p 298).

The Symmetry-Breaking Logic of Topology

There is a deep identity between logic and set theory, because the set operations are symbolic logic applied to the elements. Union, intersection and complement are simply logical OR, AND and NOT:

$$A \cup B = \{x \in X, (x \in A) \vee (x \in B)\}$$

$$A \cap B = \{x \in X, (x \in A) \wedge (x \in B)\}$$

$$X \backslash A = \bar{A} = \{x \in X, \neg(x \in A)\}$$

Moreover these laws are symmetric to union and intersection, to form a Boolean algebra.

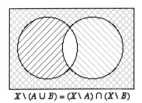

$X \setminus (A \cup B) = (X \setminus A) \cap (X \setminus B)$

For example we have the distributive laws

$$A \cup (B \cap C) = (A \cup B) \cap (A \cup C)$$
$$A \cap (B \cup C) = (A \cap B) \cup (A \cap C)$$

and De Morgan's laws of complements

$$X \setminus (A \cup B) = (X \setminus A) \cap (X \setminus B)$$
$$X \setminus (A \cap B) = (X \setminus A) \cup (X \setminus B)$$

Topology breaks this symmetry, by defining open sets such as $(0, 1) = \{x \in R, 0 < x < 1\}$ to exclude their boundaries and consist only of interior points and closed sets such as $[0, 1] = \{x \in R, 0 \le x \le 1\}$ to include all their boundary points. Complements of open sets are closed and vice versa, for example $R \setminus (0, 1) = (-\infty, 0] \cup [1, \infty)$, which is closed, since it contains its only two boundary points, 0 and 1. However most sets such as $(0, 1] \cup [2, 3)$ are neither open nor closed.

We now find open sets remain open under infinite unions but only finite intersections:

For example: $\displaystyle\bigcup_{n \in N}\left(\frac{1}{n}, 1 - \frac{1}{n}\right) = (0, 1)$ but $\displaystyle\bigcap_{n \in N}\left(\frac{-1}{n}, 1 + \frac{1}{n}\right) = [0, 1]$.

This symmetry-breaking becomes the axioms for a topological space, upon which all continuity depends. Arbitrary unions of open sets are open but only finite intersections are:

(1) $\{O_i \text{ open}, i \in I\} \Rightarrow \displaystyle\bigcup_{i \in I} O_i$ open (2) $\{O_i (\text{open}, i, 1...n)\} \Rightarrow \displaystyle\bigcap_{1...n} O_i$ open.

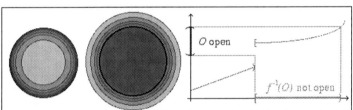

(a)Symmetry-breaking in topology. The union of open discs of radius $r < 1$-$1/n$ is the open disc of radius $r < 1$, but the intersection of open discs of radius $r < 1 + 1/n$ is the closed disc of radius $r \le 1$. (b) A discontinuity in a function is detected because the inverse image of open O is not open. Continuous functions, including waves, are the basis of differentiation $\dfrac{df}{dx}$ and integration $\int f dx$ in calculus; representing the function's instantaneous rate of change, or slope; and cumulative area enclosed.

Continuity can be defined in terms of open sets. A function $f: X \rightarrow Y$ is continuous if and only if, for every open set O in Y, the inverse image $f^{-1}(O) = \{x \in X, f(x) \in O\}$ is open.

Borromean rings as 2-D manifolds illustrate how continuity becomes the basis of defining knotted topological spaces. Such ideas may be implicit in the transformations required to integrate gravity with the other forces (p 314) and may use a complementary type of brain activity to formal linguistic processes of symbolic manipulation (p 367).

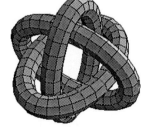

Mathematical Foundations of Complementarity

Mathematics, like quantum reality, contains two currents, typified by the discrete operations of algebra and combinatorics and the continuous properties of the functions and limit operations of calculus and topology. Indeed as noted (p 367) it has been suggested that these complementary aspects of mathematics may be lateralized, with the knotty topological properties of continuity being a right brain spatial activity, and the symbolic manipulations of algebra being a left-brain activity like language. Although mathematicians will hasten to obscure this distinction by pointing out the essential unity of mathematics and the fact that algebra and calculus deal with both discrete and continuous systems, the distinction is intriguingly reflected in the mathematics used to discover the fundamental principles of quantum theory.

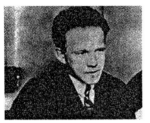

Werner Heisenberg (R746).

Heisenberg was the first person to define the concept of quantum uncertainty, or indetermincay, as the term also means in German.

Heisenberg's research concentrated on momentum and angular momentum. It is well known both rotations in 3-D space and matrices in general do not commute. $AB \neq BA$, because matrix multiplication multiplies the *rows* of the first matrix by the *columns* of the second:

$$AB = \begin{bmatrix} a & b \\ c & d \end{bmatrix}\begin{bmatrix} e & f \\ g & h \end{bmatrix} = \begin{bmatrix} ae+bg & af+bh \\ ce+dg & cf+dh \end{bmatrix}, \text{ but } BA = \begin{bmatrix} e & f \\ g & h \end{bmatrix}\begin{bmatrix} a & b \\ c & d \end{bmatrix} = \begin{bmatrix} ea+fc & eb+fd \\ ga+hc & gb+hd \end{bmatrix}.$$

Hence $AB - BA \neq 0$. More generally, if $C = AB$, $C_{rc} = \sum_s A_{rs} B_{sc}$. In quantum mechanical notation, we have $\langle r|A|c \rangle = A_{rc}$ so $\sum_s \langle r|A|s \rangle \langle s|B|c \rangle = \sum_s A_{rs} B_{sc} = [AB]_{rc} = \langle r|AB|c \rangle$, showing that $|s \rangle \langle s| = 1$, all states leading to completeness with unit probability.

Erwin Schrödinger

Schrödinger's wave equation and Heisenberg's matrix mechanics highlight a deeper complementarity in mathematics between the discrete operations of algebra and the continuous properties of calculus. When Heisenberg was trying to solve his matrix equations, the mathematician David Hilbert suggested to look at the differential equations instead. But it fell to Schrödinger, who took his mistress up into the Alps and discovered his wave equation on a romantic tryst. It was only when Hilbert and others examined the two theories closely that it was discovered they were identical, but complementary, descriptions.

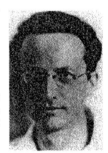

Schrödinger derived his time-independent wave equation as follows. The Hamiltonian dynamical operator representing the total kinetic and potential energy $H \equiv K + V$, of the system, in terms of how the wave varies with time and space:

$$H(\bar{r}, t)\Psi(\bar{r}, t) = \left(\frac{-h^2}{8\pi^2 m}\nabla^2 + V(\bar{r}) \right)\Psi(\bar{r}, t) = \frac{ih}{2\pi}\frac{\partial}{\partial t}\Psi(\bar{r}, t), \text{ where } \nabla^2 = \frac{\partial^2}{\partial x^2} + \frac{\partial^2}{\partial y^2} + \frac{\partial^2}{\partial z^2}.$$

This is a non-relativistic equation expressed in terms of the first time derivative. If we now assume the wave function consists of separate space and time terms $\Psi(\bar{r}, t) = \psi(\bar{r})\phi(t)$, and seek time independence of the wave function at constant energy E, we get

$$H(\bar{r})\psi(\bar{r}) = \left(\frac{-h^2}{8\pi^2 m}\nabla^2 + V(\bar{r}) \right)\psi(\bar{r}) = E\psi(\bar{r}), \text{ or } H\psi = E\psi.$$

Interpreted in terms of matrix mechanics, the Schrodinger wave equation becomes a sum of basis vectors $\psi = \sum_n c_n|n \rangle$ representing each of the wave states. The algebraic version of the equation, $H\psi = E\psi$, becomes $H\sum_n c_n|n \rangle = \sum_n c_n H|n \rangle = E\sum_n c_n|n \rangle$. Solving in terms of a transformation to a new state, we have $\langle m|H\sum_n c_n|n \rangle = \sum_n c_n \langle m|H|n \rangle = E\sum_n c_n \langle m|n \rangle$, where $\langle m|n \rangle = \begin{cases} 0, & m \neq n \\ 1, & m = n \end{cases}$. Hence

$E\sum_n c_n\langle m|n\rangle = Ec_m$ and so $\sum_n H_{mn}c_n = Ec_m$. Thus $H_{nm} = 0, m \neq n$ and

$H_{mm}c_m = Ec_m$. This the famous eigenvalue (own-value) problem, whose stable standing wave solutions are the s, p, d and f orbitals of an atom (p 318).

Heisenberg's problem of uncertainty expressed in non-commuting operators such as position x and momentum p_x gives us back the uncertainty relation when we reinterpret momentum in terms of the wave function as a differential operator $p_x = \dfrac{h}{2\pi i dx}$, we have

$$(xp_x - p_x x)\psi = x\frac{h}{2\pi i dx}\frac{d\psi}{dx} - \frac{h}{2\pi i dx}\frac{d}{dx}(x\psi) = x\frac{h}{2\pi i dx}\frac{d\psi}{dx} - \frac{h}{2\pi i}\left(\psi\frac{dx}{dx} + x\frac{d\psi}{dx}\right) = -\frac{h}{2\pi i}\psi = \frac{i}{h2\pi}\psi \cdot$$

Hence $[x, p_x] = (xp_x - p_x x) = i\dfrac{h}{2\pi}$, another view of the uncertainty relation $\Delta x \Delta p_x \sim \dfrac{h}{2\pi}$.

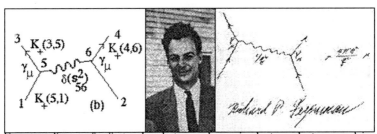

Feynman diagram for first order photon exchange in electron-electron repulsion.
Richard Feynman with his own diagram (R746).

The underlying wave-particle complementarity in Feynman's approach to quantum field theory, despite its apparent explanation of the electromagnetic field in terms of particle interaction is succinctly demonstrated in the first-order diagram from electron-electron scattering (electromagnetic charge repulsion) through exchange of virtual photons provided by uncertainty. The propagator for the diagram is:

$$K_{3,4,1,2} = -e^2\iint K_a(3,5)K_b(4,6)\gamma_{a\mu}\gamma_{b\mu}\delta(s^2{}_{56})K_a(5,1)K_b(6,2)(d\tau_5)d\tau_6$$

where γ are the variants of the Pauli spin matrices, the Dirac δ function represents the discrete interaction of the virtual photon over the space-time interval $s^2{}_{56}$ and K are the propagators for electrons a and b to be carried by Huygen's wave-front principle according to the wave summations $K(p,q) = \sum\limits_{pos E_n} \varphi_n(2)\overline{\varphi}_n(1)e^{-iE_n(t_2 - t_1)}$ for $t_2 > t_1$ representing positive energy 'retarded' solutions travelling in the usual direction in time and

$K(p,q) = -\sum\limits_{neg E_n} \varphi_n(2)\overline{\varphi}_n(1)e^{-iE_n(t_2 - t_1)}$ for $t_2 < t_1$ the corresponding negative energy solutions in the reversed 'advanced' time direction, where E_n and φ_n are the energy eigenvalues and eigenfunctions for the wave equation.

This both explains how the relativistic solution gives rise to both time backward negative energy solutions and time forward positive energy ones, which make particle-anti-particle creation and annihilation events critical to the sequence of Feynman diagrams possible, and also shows clearly in the complex exponentials the sinusoidal wave transmission hidden in the particle diagrams of the quantum field approach.

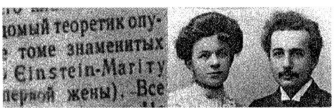

A passage in a Russian journal citing Einstein-Marity as the author of the theory of relativity.
Albert and Mileva's wedding photo.

Relativistic Dysfunctionality?

We finish with an ironical tale of dysfunctional complementarity in the breakdown of a partnership and possible research co-authorship at the heart of Einstein's presumed discoveries. Although she never made any public claim, evidence has continued to accumulate that his wife, Mileva Einstein Maric is co-author of "The Theory of Relativity".

Albert was slow to speak as a child, not speaking until 3. He attributed his spectacular success to his slow start in life. "A normal adult never stops to think about problems of space and time. But my intellectual development was retarded, as a result of which I began to wonder about space and time only when I grew up." Albert was a bad speller as a boy and had trouble learning to read, suggesting dyslexia. There are also claims that he suffered from mild autism. In 1897, as a student, he met and fell in love with Mileva Maric, herself a brilliant physics student. In 1903, despite vehement objections from his parents, he married his companion, colleague, and confidante. In their love letters, he describes her as "a creature who is my equal, and who is as strong and independent as I am". Their first daughter dies of scarlet fever in his absence, possibly in the care of relatives, because they were not married when she was born. One of their sons develops schizophrenia. After the marriage she becomes subordinate to his professional career. It is said he later told Mileva to not speak unless spoken to. He ran off with one mistress Elsa, first toying with taking her daughter for a lover, and hires a friend's niece as a secretary to pursue a second affair. Elsa permits Albert to see his next mistress twice a week, in exchange for keeping a low profile. Mileva died after spending the rest of her life looking after their schizophrenic son on her own.

When "The Theory of Relativity" appeared in 1905 in the *Annalen der Physik*, only Albert's name was in the journal as author, but according to physicist Abram Joffe, who saw the original manuscript, it was signed 'Einstein-Marity'. 'Marity' is a variant of the Serbian 'Maric', Mileva's maiden name. Mileva Maric Einstein's name was left out when publication of the article took place. The extent of Mileva's contribution to Einstein's work remains controversial. According to Evan Harris Walker, a physicist, the basic ideas for relativity came from Mileva. Senta Troemel-Ploetz, a German linguist, says that the ideas may have been Albert's, but Mileva did the mathematics. Others marginalize her involvement merely as a 'sounding board'. In February 1990, members of the American Association for the Advancement of Science convened to debate the subject of Mileva Maric's possible collaboration on the 1905 papers. The group could not reach a consensus.

In early 1905, Einstein's *annus mirabilis* (miraculous year), Albert is 26 and working 6 days a week in the Patent Office. Mileva is a *hausfrau* of 29 with a baby on her hip. If Einstein had never written another equation after 1905, history would still place him among the greatest minds of the 20th century. Even today, it is hard to imagine that any scientist could produce so much significant work, on such widely varied topics, quantum theory, Brownian motion relativity, and the equivalence of mass and energy, within a single year. Yet Einstein did it while he was working full time. Or did he?

(www)

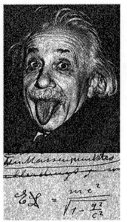

The case for Mileva as co-genius mostly depends on letters in which Albert referred to "our" theory and "our" work, and on a divorce agreement in which Albert promised her his Nobel Prize money. Mileva was a statistician who had expressed interest in molecular motion in letters to to Albert and the Brownian motion ideas may well have originated from her. Einstein never received a Nobel for relativity, which is suggestive that the Nobel committee may have had wind this work was not entirely his own. More intriguingly, he gave his Nobel prize in quantum physics for the photo-electric effect $E=hv$ to Mileva. Was this a secret pact to 'honour' her contribution and preserve his reputation? In her letters, she lamented "One person gets the pearl and the other just gets the shell"? He retorted "One should be nice and modest, and keep one's mouth shut, that is my advice to you". So the prodigy icon of physics may have been a creative partnership that went sour, casting deep questions over our reverence for the male genius who discovered the apocalyptic equation $E=mc^2$.

Einstein confessed to Queen Elizabeth of Belgium in March 1955 "the exaggerated esteen in which my lifework is held makes me very ill at ease. I feel compelled to think of myself as an involuntary swindler." (Holt R319).

Einstein had a close relationship with Gödel and they walked together. Gödel discovered a solution to Einstein's equations involving rotation rather than expansion and in which time became looped, causing Gödel to speculate that time was an illusion. Ultimately, Gödel was to die of starvation in a state of paranoia and Einstein commented: "To those of us who believe in physics, this separation between past, present and future, is only an illusion, if a stubborn one." When his own time came a couple of weeks later he said simply "It's time to go".

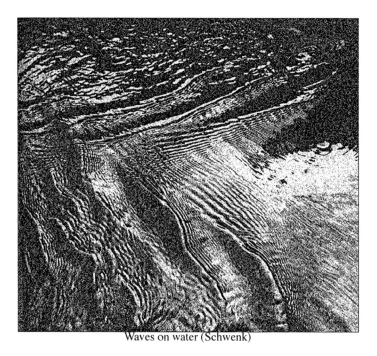
Waves on water (Schwenk)

The Sensitivity of Chaos

The Mythology of Chaos

Chaos Gk. *kaos* abyss - to'yawn' or 'gape'.

In the Britannica Dictionary chaos is 'a condition of utter disorder or confusion as the unformed primal state of the universe' citing either utter disorder and confusion or an unfathomable abyss as definitive. The Concise Oxford speaks of 'formless void or great deep of primordial matter, this personified as the oldest of the Gods, utter confusion'. The Grollier Encyclopedia notes that in Greek mythology, Chaos was the unorganized state, or void, from which all things arose. Proceeding from time, Chaos eventually formed a huge egg from which there issued Heaven, Earth, and Eros (love). According to Hesiod's Theogeny, Chaos preceded the origin not only of the world, but also of the gods. In Hebrew myth *tohu wabohu* is the universe without form and void, as in Genesis 1:2:

And the earth was without form, and void;
and darkness was upon the face of the deep.

Barbara Walker likens chaos to the undifferentiated raw elements occupying the womb of the world-goddess between destruction and recreation of the universe.

The eternal religious war of light and dark is very much the battle of chaos as the dark 'force' and order as the principle of light . This is enacted in diverse myths of origin. In Babylon, Tiamat the feminine primal abyss and ancient mother is overthrown by Marduk the youthful male slayer of chaos, in the name of civic, and world order. The same theme extends to classic male combat myth in the cosmic Zoroastrian war of dark and light which became in Jewish and later Christian thought the battle between God and Satan which leads to Armageddon and the unveiling tumult of apocalypse. This opposition between chaos and order is a fundamental misunderstanding of the natural condition.

The Nature of Chaos

Far from being the nemesis of order, or the primal ooze in which order is imposed, chaos is also the genesis of new form. Most complex systems arise from the mutual interaction between chaos and order, through *bifurcation* - 'abrupt change of form under continuous underlying transformation. Bifurcation takes its name from 'forking' but really applies to all discrete transformation under continuous change. It is typified by the onset of opposing flight or fight reactions, and sudden transformations, such as a wave breaking, or a bubble bursting. Bifurcations can introduce new structure and hence increasing complexity, particularly in transition from chaos to order, in dynamics occurring at the 'edge of chaos'.

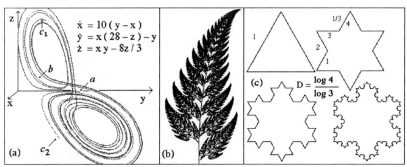

$$\dot{x} = 10\,(\,y - x\,)$$
$$\dot{y} = x\,(\,28 - z\,) - y$$
$$\dot{z} = x\,y - 8z\,/\,3$$

(c) $D = \dfrac{\log 4}{\log 3}$

(a) Sensitive dependence on initial conditions is illustrated by the Lorenz flow simulating turbulent weather. Trajectories in the flow starting arbitrarily close at a have exponentially separated by b and are in distinct parts of the flow by $c1,2$. Computational unpredictability follows from the incapacity of any numerical model to approximate the real flow over increasing time, because of such exponentiating divergence. (b) The fern leaf set is an example of a fractal (R41) generated by a simple recursive transformation. (c) Non-integer fractal dimension D of the Koch flake. If we subdivide a line of dimension 1 into pieces we get 3^1 units of 1/3 the length . If we have a planar region of dimension 2 there are $3^2 = 9$ square sub-units of 1/3 the length. In the Koch flake, each side is repeatedly replaced by $4 = 3^{\log 4/\log 3}$ sides of length 1/3. Hence its fractal dimension is log4/log3 ~ 1.26.

The failure to appreciate the generative nature of chaos has led to it being one of the last scientific frontiers to be discovered, over fifty years after relativity and quantum theory. This has happened because the human will to impose order, even among scientists, is so strong that somehow, in their rush to fit every phenomenon into a mechanistic world view, they ignored the fact that virtually all interesting natural phenomena involve chaos, from the waves on the beach, to the beauty of a forest, from our seemingly regular heartbeat to the patterns of our brain waves in the moment of 'eureka'!

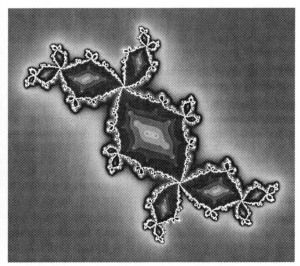

Julia sets (white) of a complex logistic map (see below) are fractal regions on which the process is chaotic. On the insides (rainbow levels) and outside (rainbow shades) the process is ordered. The multiple basins inside converge towards attracting periodic points and the basin outside to infinity. Dynamics in the Julia sets are repelling, scrambled and sensitive to initial conditions, mapping any neighbourhood of the set over the whole. In every case, the dynamic is divided between complementary regions of order and chaos.

Mathematicians distinguish dynamical chaos from a random, or *stochastic* process, in which critical events are determined by probabilities. Dynamical chaos is not simply disorder or randomness, but an internally unstable process. Chaotic systems may have well-defined dynamical formulations and may even be deterministic as classical systems, but this dynamic is one which doesn't settle down either into equilibrium or any particular periodicity or resonance, but wanders erratically over time in an unpredictable way which is deceptively similar to randomness.

Although chaotic systems may be precisely defined by a recursive formula or feedback process, they combine erratic behavior with long-term unpredictability which gives them just the character those seeking orderly prediction might fear. Chaotic bifurcations and a closely-related phenomenon called self-organized criticality are also frequently associated with crises such as cyclones, floods, avalanches, earthquakes and other catastrophic natural interventions.

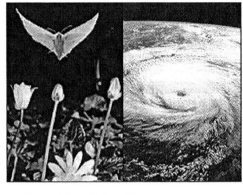

The Lorenz butterfly effect: a puff of a butterflies wing in a chaotic weather system can inflate into a tropical cyclone. Weather is thus intrinsically unpredictable, because the small differences in a tiny puff can grow and throw the whole system wildly off-course.

The essential characteristics of classical chaos are threefold (Devaney R159):

1. Sensitive dependence: Lorenz, the father of chaos theory, was first to note the key characteristic of chaos in the 'butterfly effect', that the eddies of the wings of a butterfly flying in Hawaii could later become the seed of wild unpredictable fluctuation of a tropical cyclone hitting Fiji. This is 'sensitive dependence on initial conditions', in which arbitrarily small changes can later become amplified by a chaotic process or flow into global fluctuations.

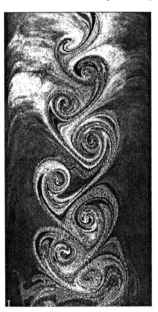

Whirls of water passing a stick (Schwenk R617).

2. Topological mixing: Any small open region will eventually become mixed over any other. This means the dynamics is very tangled, so any orbit goes almost everywhere in the 'phase space' of configurations of the system. This is precisely what happens in an egg-beater. This mixing property sometimes referred to as *ergodicity* makes the orbits or trajectories of a chaotic process appear random.

3. Dense periodicities: Chaotic dynamics is densely permeated with repelling periodic oscillations, often of infinitely many types, making for a great deal of hidden complexity.

These three combine to mean the dynamic is complex, unstable and unpredictable.

Sensitive dependence causes chaotic systems to eventually become fundamentally unpredictable even when they are deterministic. They cannot be accurately computed, since arbitrarily small errors in the computation rapidly escalate into global inaccuracies. This unpredictability is at the core of the difficulties of weather prediction and it also lies at the root of diverse phenomena, from the stock market, to the risk of nuclear holocaust.

Associated with many chaotic systems and some statistical ones, such as the 'drunkards walk' of Brownian motion, are beautiful, complex self-replicating patterns called *fractals* after their properties of self-similarity on smaller and smaller scales. Fractals are typified by the snowflake, trees, our lungs, the pattern of forest clearings and the biodiversity we associate with the evolutionary tree of life.

Fractal processes do not have to be geometrically self-similar, but possess a self-replicating basis which leads to a non-integer dimensionality, hanging paradoxically between the integer values we are accustomed to. The Mandelbrot set, a portion of which is illustrated below has varying parts representing all the different ways we can make a feedback by squaring a complex number and adding a varying constant.

Chaos occurs throughout nature, from the fractal structures of galactic clusters, through the erratic orbits of comets to the dynamic many-body energetics of the atomic nucleus. It is manifest in biological systems from fractal tissues and organs such as the form of our lungs, from the seemingly regular heart beat, through brain dynamics, to the laser pulse.

Quantum systems modify the nature of chaos, suppressing some of the fine details of the interweaving of paths in the overlapping of waves possessed by all quanta, which tend to reveal the periodicities hidden in chaotic systems.

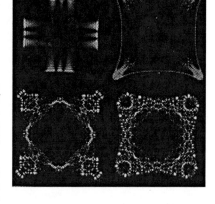

Stationary states or wave functions, associated with the energy levels of a highly excited hydrogen atom in a strong magnetic field can exhibit both periodic and chaotic qualities. However the wave aspect smooths and partially suppresses chaos. The chaotic quantum wave functions are modified from the classical picture by 'scarring of the wave function' paradoxically concentrating the probability around hidden repelling periodic orbits (Gutzwiller R269).

Nevertheless molecular kinetics in open systems is a living example of quantum chaos - a form of unstable wave-particle billiards which may critically affect the processes and reactions occurring in our enzyme reactions, particularly in the brain function supporting consciousness (p 370).

Chaotic systems arise naturally from positive feedback processes because the positive feedback amplifies small differences, causing the instability we see in the butterfly effect. We shall see shortly that sexual selection is a potentially chaotic positive feedback process, prone to exponential runaway. In this respect it is complementary to the stabilizing ordered constraints imposed by natural selection.

Many apparently periodic phenomena are actually chaotic. The heart beat appears periodic, but the healthy heart is actually tuned by chaos. This allows the brain and heart pacemakers and the heart cells themselves all to keep in feedback resonance with one another and thus respond to changing circumstances. No two heartbeats have exactly the same interval between, but vary in a chaotic manner, similar to a dripping tap.

The universe is fractal in its manifestation in galactic clusters, galaxies, solar systems, stars planets and satellites and chaotic in its diversity. Some models of cosmic inflation and cosmic evolution are also fractal, however the supposedly chaotic formless cosmic origin in the 'big-bang' is described by symmetry-breaking of an almost symmetrical or isotropic germinal state, marred only by quantum fluctuation. Herein may lie the ultimate source of what we experience macroscopically as chaos - quantum uncertainty itself. Quantum uncertainty amplified by chaotic instability may be at the heart of other processes we describe as random, from molecular kinetics to tossing a coin.

Associated with chaotic and fractal processes are systems in a state of self-organized criticality. A sand pile always converges to a limiting angles where fractal avalanches maintain the entire system in a critically unstable state. Make the pile flatter and it heaps up again. Make it too steep and avalanches bring it back to criticality. Phenomena such as earthquakes, avalanches and neurons tuned to threshold excitation, share features of fractal instability. Hence smaller and larger earthquakes occur on a fractal pattern of frequencies.

Population Catastrophe and the Beauty of Fractals

One of the most serious questions facing humanity is the boom or bust nature of human population explosion. Will we explode to an unsustainable population and wipe ourselves out with a global famine, or will we settle down nicely into equilibrium all a bit hungry but survivors as the population settles to a new plateau? The answer to this question is exceedingly complex and opens out the jewel of complexity hidden within chaos.

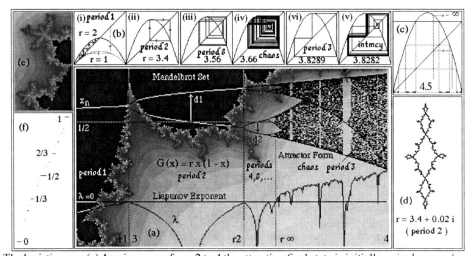

The logistic map: (a) As r increases from 2 to 4 the attracting final state is initially a single curve (an equilibrium point for each r) but then it repeatedly subdivides (pitchfork bifurcations) to make a rich and lean year (period 2) then periods 4, 8 etc., finally entering chaos (stippled bands). Subsequently there are windows of period 3, 5 etc. with abrupt transitions to and from chaos. The Lyapunov exponent indicates whether the system is chaotically amplifying small differences. During chaos it remains positive. The Mandelbrot set illustrates the fractal nature of the ordered and chaotic regimes when x and r are extended to the complex number plane. (b) A series of 2-D views of the iteration, including periods 1, 2 and 8 chaos, intermittency, and period 3. Pick an initial value x and find y by moving vertically to the curve $y = r x (1 - x)$. Next we let the new $x = y$ by moving horizontally to the sloping line. The two steps result in one iteration, i.e. $x_{n+1} = y = r x_n (1 - x_n)$. (c) The non-escaping points form a disconnected repelling fractal for r = 4.5. The attracting final set has now been broken up, resulting in a fractal Julia set. (d) A connected Julia set for the complex logistic [x-axis vertical] plotted by inverse iteration taking all the 2^n square root solutions of the inverse function

$$x_{n-1} = \frac{1}{2}(1 \pm \sqrt{1 - 4(x_n/r)}).$$

We will illustrate some of the elementary properties of chaos by looking at one of the simplest systems of all - an iterated feedback in one real variable. It is an archetype of the population explosion dilemma - how to feed a naturally growing population from a finite resource without boom and bust destroying the species.

The quadratic logistic map:

$$x_{n+1} = G(x_n) = r x_n (1 - x_n)$$

describes seasonal natural population growth given a constrained food supply. The term $r x_n$ gives natural growth by a factor r, while the additional term $(1 - x_n)$ limits growth in proportion to the unconsumed food resource (e.g. the remaining area of arable land). Many possibilities arise, depending on the growth rate r. As the growth rate varies, the iteration goes through a sequence of different stages separated by sudden changes, or bifurcations. For small r the system tends to a fixed equilibrium point then becomes repelling bifurcating to form a flip-flop (period 2), subsequently period doubling to form periods 4, 8, 16 etc. through to infinity.

At this point, a new erratic behaviour emerges, and the system wanders with no fixed period. chaos has appeared. All of the previous periodic attractors continue to exist hidden in the chaos as repellers, generating a tangled repelling flow, whose spreading causes sensitive dependence. As r increases further, windows of order, with new periods appear in a new and abrupt type of transition from chaos to order. There is yet a third type of chaotic

503

transition represented by the mode-locked periodic feedback, as in the heart pacemaker and rotations on the periodic spirals of the Mandelbrot set illustrated below.

A portion of the Mandelbrot set of the logistic map. The fractal displays all possible quadratic dynamics. Although these vary and it is thus not exactly self-similar, it is nevertheless a fractal.

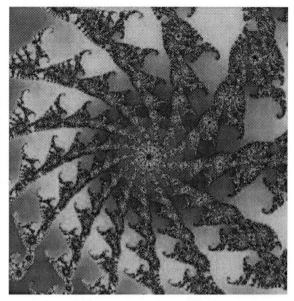

Finally a new situation emerges. The attractor becomes unstable. All that is left is a residual set of points, which do not escape, but are mapped chaotically among themselves. This Julia set has a complicated self-similar structure like a fern leaf or a snowflake and is called a fractal. Invariant sets of chaotic systems in several dimensions are frequently in the form of fractals, characterized by having a non-integer dimension (Peitgen et. al .R520, R521)

The fractal invariant sets can be seen in far more detail and beauty if the process is extended to the plane of complex numbers ($a + ib$ where $i = -1$). The Julia sets now clearly appear as fractals, each with a differing structure depending on the growth rate parameter. The Mandelbrot atlas set of all these dynamical variations has been dubbed the most complicated mathematical structure ever known.

Chaos occurs in a surprising variety of phenomena, many of which appear at the surface to be periodic. Both the heart beat and the dripping of a tap, although apparently periodic have chaotically intermittent variations in the beat period.

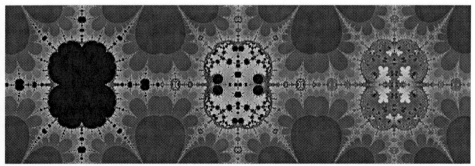

Julia set of the complex cosine pervades the plane, evolving firstly through an explosion to fractally fill the residual black region and then through an infinite set of fractal bifurcations.

The rings of Saturn and objects still remaining in the asteroid belt are governed by mode-locking chaos. Only those whose orbital periods have no rational (fractional) relationship remain, because all the fractionally-related orbits have long ago been thrown into the planets by a repeated sling-shot effect. When orbits of two astronomical bodies become mode-locked they interact strongly on a regular basis and the cumulative effect may throw the smaller one out of orbit. The asteroids remaining today are in a belt where the periods do not mode lock and have thus been left behind. More generally a large variety of systems from the weather through earthquakes, movement of the continental plates, chemical and electronic oscillations, secretion of enzymes, fluctuations in the stock market and collision of successive billiard balls, through to brain waves and possibly cognition itself, involve chaotic phases.

Chaos presents us with new properties of nature which are connected with the development of complexity. A chaotic system contains within it a fractal structure with diverse dynamics, including a dense set of infinitely many periodicities.

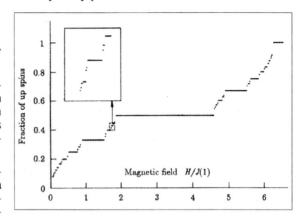

Devil's fractal staircase for an anti-Ferromagnetic spin glass in a magnetic field (Schroeder R611).

Mode Locking, Multifractality and the Devil's Staircase

One particularly interesting feature of non-linear interaction manifest in many situations from the heartbeat to planetary orbits is the phenomenon of mode-locking.

Here coupled periodic phenomena with a periodicity close to a rational number become mode-locked into a rational relationship. This relationship is illustrated by the devil's staircase, a fractal function whose graph is continuous and increasing yet constant in a neighbourhood of every rational number. A close examination of the Mandelbrot set (p 317) will confirm that the bulbs on the set follow a devil's staircase pattern with the two largest bulbs above and below having 1/3 of a revolution (see the three dendrites) and the large bulb on the left corresponding to 1/2 a revolution, with the rest forming a series conforming to the devil's staircase arrangement, in numbers called a Farey Tree. In which any two fractions generate a descendent by the rule

$$\frac{m_1}{n_1} \cdot \frac{m_2}{n_2} \to \frac{m_1 + m_2}{n_1 + n_2}$$

The Farey tree links all the mode-locked rationals in an infinite net. Starting from the top right if we alternate left and right we have a sequence of Fibonacci fractions converging to the golden mean. The Fibonacci numbers 1, 1, 2, 3, 5, 8, 13, 21, 34, 55, ... are generated by a similar relation $u = u_1 = 1, u_{n+1} = u_n + u_{n-1}$

Their ratio tends in limit to $\gamma = 1 + \frac{1}{\gamma}$, giving $\gamma = \frac{1 \pm \sqrt{5}}{2} = 1.618, -0.618$, the so-called golden mean number, which along with other such extreme irrationals, are the last numbers to become captured by mode-locked intervals.

The Farey Tree

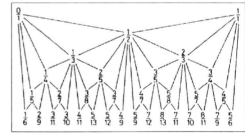

Mode-locking explains a vast variety of phenomena. The remaining asteroids all lie in the non-mode locked regions between Mars and Jupiter because rational orbital periods with respect to Jupiter have long ago been swept into the sun or planets by the pumping action mode-locking causes. Many apparently periodic phenomena such as the heart beat are also governed by mode-locking. A simple circular iteration called the circle map which can generate such behavior by modeling a sinusoidally-kicked rotator can be defined as follows:

$$\theta_{n+1} = f(\theta_n) = \theta_n + \Omega + K \sin \theta_n$$

where Ω is a constant twist by a fixed angle per iteration and the sine term causes a wobbling or pumping effect, resulting in an average twisting which may become mode-locked.

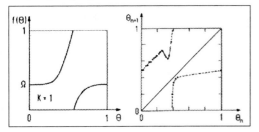

Left: The standard circle map. Right: An experimental setup using beating chicken heart cells (Schuster R615).

A 'spin glass' is considered to be a disordered system of spins just as a glass is a disordered quasi-crystalline substance. A ferromagnet has lowest energy when all its spins are aligned, giving a stable polarized lowest energy state. In an anti-ferromagnetic substance each adjacent pair of spins have a lowest energy state in which they are alternating up and down in a 3-D checkerboard pattern like the Na^+ and Cl^- ions in a crystal of salt. Closest spins have the most powerful neighbouring interaction with the strength falling off e.g. with the square of the distance. When there is no magnetic field the whole system is thus perfectly regular. However when an external field is applied, it becomes impossible for all the spins to resolve themselves in a single lowest energy arrangement, and many local minima become possible like a complex pattern of swamps and small lakes in a wild landscape. As shown on the previous page, this process is governed by mode-locking, implying that a spin glass contains fractal islands of partially resolved spins. A similar model may well describe human sexual mating patterns under a situation where one sex or the other is in scarcer supply.

Many fractal processes, from turbulence to the Julia sets of a quadratic mapping, distribute themselves unevenly, so that the process becomes fractally concentrated more in some regions than others. One can envisage this process if we cut an interval in half and give one side probability p and the other probability $1-p$ and repeat the process endlessly (see inset).

Top left: Julia set plotted by inverse iteration showing the multifractal distribution of how frequently differing subregions are visited. Inset fractal application of a probability in three stages. Inset an interval redistributed by probabilities p and $1-p$ iterates to a multifractal distribution. Lower left: The entropy function representing the information loss describes the multifractal spectrum of probabilities in the limit. Right: a continental landscape generated by repeated division of a planetary surface (see Peitgen R520, R521).

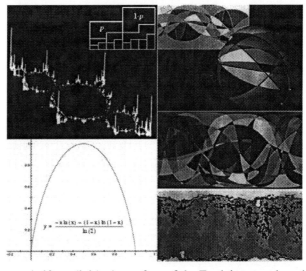

There are then fractal subpopulations corresponding to a given probability level, with a spectrum differing fractal dimensions hidden in the process. Many processes we see in nature are multifractal. For example if we divide the surface of the Earth into two broad regions and estimate that 60% of the population will be on one side and 40% on the other and repeat this process fractally, we will end up both with very sparse regions like the Sahara and very dense foci of population like New York. A similar process can generate continents.

506

The same process occurs with the inner dynamics of a Julia set as shown in the diagram if the iteration is run backwards to find all the 2^n square root solutions n-steps back and so on. Some regions are visited a very large number of times, while others are visited exponentially rarely. This means it would take longer than the history of the universe to draw a Julia set if we simply used the raw inverse method as it stands.

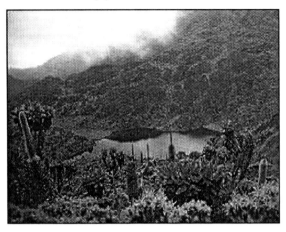

Kitami National Park: Nature, from clouds, through the forms and patterns of vegetation, to the textures of rocks and the shapes of shorelines is an immensely complex system of overlapping fractals.

The Edge of Chaos and the Complexity of Nature

"Out of chaos comes order."
Friedrich Nietzsche

A system which can bifurcate between chaos and order over time can enter a mixing phase of chaos and then retrieve structures hidden within chaos by bifurcating back into order. A chaotic system can likewise be tuned to display its hidden periodicities. Many types of system develop complex evolving structures in the transition region between order and chaos, sometimes called the 'edge of chaos' (R590, R707). The edge of chaos thus represents the region of sexual paradox between chaos and order where complexity becomes emergent.

Nature and evolution are both described as complex systems evolving at the edge of chaos through prisoners' dilemma type interactions between species. Many of the most beautiful aspects of nature arise from their fractal structures and textures. Climax forests are chaotic systems, both in terms of their species diversity and their fluctuating population dynamics. Climax forest also displays a fractal dynamic which is central to its diversity. Natural disturbances from fire and flood, wind and storm damage, to large falling trees are fractal disturbances to which diverse species become adapted in disseminating seed in an ever more complex arrangement of species diversity. The forest is colonized in up to five strata from the top canopy to the floor each with their own ecosystemic complexity.

The sunflower contains two sets of 34 and 55 spirals left and right enabling seed packing which avoids any periodic mode-locking. Many animal proportions also reflect the limiting ratio of two such magic numbers in the golden mean of 1:1.618, illustrating frozen chaos at work (see R543).

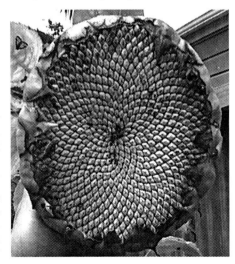

Both plants and animals are derived from fractal algorithms in nature and it is from these fractal algorithms that most of our understanding of form and diversity in nature comes. Evolution and its increasing complexity is a central instance of edge-of-chaos dynamics, as is our dynamical brain state, in both perception and problem-solving, especially when perceiving the chaotic diversity of nature itself for which we are highly adapted. It is the very sensitive dependence of chaos which ensures the brain remains completely adaptable to arbitrarily small differences.

An intriguing illustration of frozen chaos permeating biological organisms is the incidence of the golden mean as a ratio or angle in both animal and plant form. The twin spirals observed in plant forms, including the pineapple, pine cones, sunflowers and cacti occur at the golden mean angle $2\pi/\gamma$ and generally have two related Fibonacci numbers. This prevents any ordered pattern of mode-locking which would prevent the seeds of the sunflower packing together properly.

Similarly many human proportions, from successive digit bones, the relative distance from the navel to the head and feet, the widths of successive incisors and the nose, mouth and eyes all conform to the golden mean. This is the last, most irrational number to submit to mode locking, as do the orbits of the remaining asteroids in relation to the orbit of Jupiter. Mode locking can also bee seen in the 13 arms of the Mandelbrot portion above, where the dynamic is making 1/13 of a revolution.

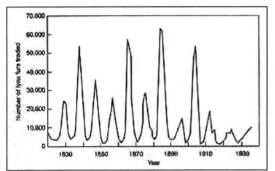

The lynx is a species with regularly, yet erratically oscillating numbers. It was once believed that lynxes were partners in a dynamically unstable association with their main prey, the snowshoe hare. Recently it has been recognized that the cycle is driven by the interaction between hares and their food plants, with the lynxes being carried along more or less passively by changes in the abundance of hares (Leakey R393).

In addition to this, the potentially chaotic population dynamics we have seen in the logistic function is displayed in many natural populations making population dynamics unstable from season to season and sensitively dependent on changes in the environment. For this reason, we have to be very careful when considering the major impacts we are making on natural ecosystems, lest chaos and bifurcation compound the problems we initiate.

It is important to note that population dynamics may cause paradoxical situations to arise. For example we usually think of a predator-prey relationship as exploitative. However a predator acts to reduce the growth rate of a population and thus protects it from boom and bust population crisis in which the prey multiplies so fast that it eats all the available food and dies *en masse* through starvation. Thus predator and prey are caught in a kind of prisoners dilemma relationship which is both destructive and protective at the same time.

Similar considerations apply to parasites and hosts. A central development of this dynamical relationship we shall see next is the idea that a prisoners dilemma genetic 'arms race' between parasites and hosts led to sexual evolution to promote genetic variety and hence resistance to disease. This mutual adaption arms race thus required each of the competing organisms to become capable of sexual recombination to survive the others changes.

Once sexuality became established, sexual selection began to become a fundamental driving force complementary to natural selection. Because natural selection tends to operate as environmental or inter-species constraints on survival it is both stable and predominantly a negative feedback. In addition the vast majority of mutations are deleterious.

Sexual selection has very different characteristics from natural selection. Firstly it acts not negatively on survival but positively on reproduction. It is also an iterative feedback process with strong positive feedback characteristics. Female reproductive choice acts as a capricious and variable positive feedback which, as it adapts to competing display by becoming more discerning, drives male evolution into potential runaway. Mutual mate selection can also have powerful effects. This leads to sexual selection becoming a potentially chaotic positive feedback force complementing the stabilizing effects of natural selection. These effects are again complemented by the opposing effects of mutations and recombination as genetic modifiers held in check by selection retaining only the viable options.

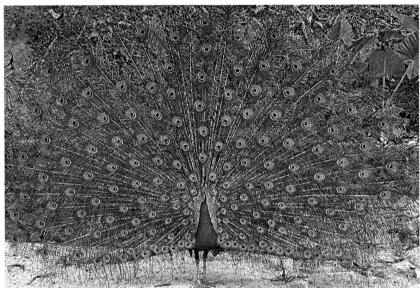

The peacock's tail illustrates how sexual selection can become a runaway positive feedback process, leading to chaotic unpredictability. Once again we see hints of Fibonacci golden mean spirals.

These effects result in a deep connection between sexual paradox and edge of chaos complexity. Broadly speaking the condition of sexual paradox induces sensitively unstable dynamics which lead to complex systems dynamics at the edge of chaos because the actions of each of the partially opposing forces are frustrated from imposing order. Loss of sexual paradox leads to degeneracy, with a dominant stable process and consequently reduced complexity and reduced viability. Thus maintaining sexual paradox in evolution and climax diversity in planetary abundance and resilience go hand in hand. Although our gatherer-hunter origins appear to be sexually paradoxical, many aspects of human culture show loss of sexual paradox into degeneracies of patriarchal sexual and natural dominion involving boom and bust and rape of the planet's diversity. These are accompanied by very worrying instances of loss of complexity which need urgent correction to ensure human viability.

A final example of the interdependence of chaos and order in the development of complexity is illustrated in the brain, (p 364), which is not simply a digital computer but displays prominent dynamical behavior, illustrated in the broad spectrum waves of excitation in the electroencephalogram. This excitation is distributed across the cortex in a manner consistent with parallel distributed processing. Both perception and cognition can be modeled as a transition from a state of chaos representing the unrecognized condition, or the unsolved problem, to a state of order. This process can be modeled as a transition: from high energy chaos, 'exploring' its internal space without getting stuck in any 'rut'; to order, as the energy is reduced so as to flow towards a minimum, through the capture of the system by a learned attractor in recognition, or the bifurcation of the system to form a new attractor. An insight 'eureka' often happens instantaneously, from a state of relative confusion, indicating a single transition from chaos to new order representing the 'knowing' state. The chaotic state is thus the progenitor of new order, rather than mere manipulation of order itself. Rather the order imposed by the problem becomes a boundary condition for chaotic resolution.

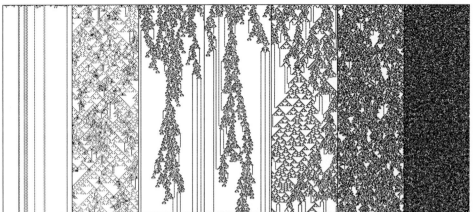

A series of 1-dimensional cellular automata with λ varying from order (0.23) through complexity at the edge of chaos (0.33) to deep chaos (0.86). All complex states in 3 eventually expire, but not in 4.

Several of these attributes of order, chaos and complexity can be displayed in some the simplest digital feedback processes, of all called cellular automata (see Wolfram R745). These contain a formula expressing the successive states in a grid of cells in terms of their immediate neighbours. Depending on the nature of the formula, and the degree of overlap, such systems can be defined to involve ordered equilibrium and periodicity, chaotic mixing of states, or complexity. Systems close to the edge between order and chaos display the capacity for increasing complexity.

For example if we consider the simplest 1-dimensional cellular automaton which has only values 0 and 1 in a given cell and determines the new state of any cell from the three immediate predecessors in the preceeding row, we can define a unique rule as a number.

There are $2^3=8$ different arrangements of a cells three immediate predecessors. To specify the rule we thus need to specify a 0 or 1 in each position giving $2^8 = 2^{2^3}$ rules numbering 0 to 255.

$2^3 = 8$ 3-cell states		
0/1	0/1	0/1
	0/1	

$2^8 = 256$ 8-state rules

Rule 110, for example, displays edge-of-chaos complexity. This system is even capable of functioning as a universal computer, because various sub-states can exchange information and perform the fundamental computations of symbolic logic.

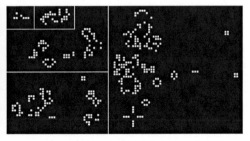

A sequence of states in the game of life.

A famous example of complexity with universal computation is Conway's 'game of life' in which a given cell survives if two or three neighbours out of the possible eight are alive and is 'born' if precisely three are alive. The 'game of life' behaves in a similar manner to a complex dynamical system at the edge of chaos. Here successive states show increasing complexity, including drifters capable of logical computation. Such processes, including 2-D cellular automata simulations of the prisoners' dilemma, (p 21), may thus become formally undecidable because of the Turing halting problem (p 492). Conway's game of life is equivalent to a prisoners' dilemma game where cooperation is incited by three cooperating neighbours and the status quo maintained by two, with other values leading to defection.

Below are illustrated some variants of the game of life in which a variety of slightly higher rewards are given for cooperation, leading to permanent equilibrium between cooperators and defectors similar to the results of Nowak's more detailed simulations, (p 21) but using only simple rules of the same type as Conway's.

Unlike the game of life, consciousness is not bound to a discrete classical logic. Ultimately, through chaotic sensitivity, the conscious brain may be able to access the quantum realm and putative forms of quantum computing and transactional space-time hand-shaking, manifestations of the weird properties of uncertainty, non-locality and entanglement, arising from quantum complementarity between wave and particle aspects. Consciousness appears to use these deeper complementarities within quantum chaos to anticipate potentially incomputable complexities and to affect physical outcomes through the application of conscious will. Here we come to the deepest expression of that complementarity in logical and existential paradox of which chaos and order are also a reflection. This is where sexual paradox enters its quintessence.

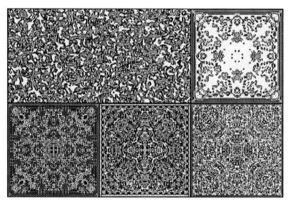

2-D cellular automaton variants of the game of life. If Conway's game is represented as 001300000 meaning death for 0, 1 and 4-8 live neighbours, the status quo for 2 and birth for 3. From top left (a) 001330000 showing long-term equilibrium between defectors (yellow and orange) and cooperators (black and blue). (b) Symmetrical fractal states generated by a single defection for 001300001- very close to the game of life - giving an expanding regime of computational unpredictability for the continuity of life (cooperation) amid defection (death), similar to Conway's game. (c) 301300001, (d) 301330001 and (e) 331300001, in which rare cooperators are rewarded.

Coda: Web of Intrigue - Sexual Paradox in Spiders

Golden Silk (Banana or Calico) Spider
Nephila clavipes male and female.

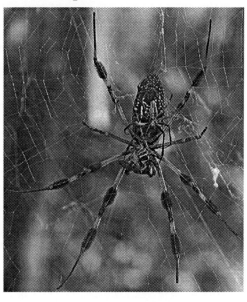

In the popular mind, mating of spiders is as far from sexual paradox as one could imagine, a naked lunch for the *femme fatale*, in which the often much smaller, male becomes a delicacy even in the throes of fertilization. However this is true only for some well-known species, such as the Black Widow. Neither is it clear this is a one-sided love affair. The Australian redback male literally dances in front of the female's jaws to entice her into biting him, giving him longer to fertilize her more completely (Andrade R16).

The sexual stakes in spiders are made higher, both by the female's predatory nature and the fact that some species mate only once or at most a few times and the females can store sperm for up to two years, making a single sexual feat by the male the progential act of a lifetime.

Despite the apparent imbalances, spider courtship poses intriguing and diverse examples of sexually-antagonistic coevolution, with all manner of subtleties and variations.

It is never easy to tell which sex the given act serves to greater degree. An Australian redback male is well-served if his death dance into the female's jaws gives him a lion's share of the male genes in her several batches of eggs. At an even greater extreme is the male orb-weaving spider *Argiope aurantia*. Male spiders transfer their sperm to palps in their legs which they insert into the female. In *aurantia* the male places both palps in the female and dies on the spot, making it difficult for another male to fertilize her (Foellmer R214).

The much smaller size of many male spiders is another sexually paradoxical issue. Male competition would select for larger, more dominant males, but the female St. Andrews Cross *Argiope keyserlingi* tends to favour smaller males (Elgar et. al. R185), suggesting female selection drives this process. The females wrap their prospective mates in a silky cocoon as a way to give them more choice over which male's sperm to favour the most. Unlike the redback, these males struggle to escape and some do, often missing a leg. In the polyandrous orb-web spider *Nephila edulis,* males are much smaller and have a very skewed size distribution. Smaller males approach the female directly and mate more successfully and more often than larger ones, who have to cut a hole in the web (Schneider et. al. R605-R608).

In *Nephila plumipes,* about 60% of males are cannibalized. However not all females are sexual cannibals, but only those in leaner condition. Males cautiously wait until the female catches a fly, thus avoiding pre-mating homicide. Despite expiring, males which are eaten have an advantage in mating for longer, if the female mates with more than one male and sperm competition is thus a real factor. Female cannibalism seems to be a function of predatory acuity generally and does not appear to be a specific sexually homicidal adaption.

Often it is not the desired male, but a rejected one who ends up becoming lunch. Tarantulas who are well-matched in size and live for up to 20 years, as well as *Thomisidae* and *Clubionidae* simply 'say hello' with a brief interplay of their front legs. Then if the female is into the idea of mating, and doesn't attack the male, copulation follows. Neither does familiarity bred contempt. Wolf spider males come in a variety of phenotypes with varying appearances. Females prefer, and are less likely to eat, males with whom they have already become familiar during an adolescence in which they remain unable to mate before their last molt . Other species of web building spider exploit this social situation by seeking a child bride, setting up home beside the web of an adolescent female so they can become familiar before she reaches maturity. In various species of *Dictyna*, a male seeks out a female in her web and then moves in. He will walk around on her web vibrating his legs on the web and giving brief vibratory touches to her with his legs when they meet. He may build a special canopy in a corner of her web. Some time and a number of meetings occur before she allows him to mate. He may stay for weeks.

Male dancing serves both as web music and a visual display. A male needs to announce his presence with a special dance quite different from the struggling of a trapped fly and the female will generally acknowledge this with responsive jiggling, warning irritation or a frightening silence depending on the circumstances. *Salticidae* males have colourful palps and front legs. Typically the male raises and lowers his front legs, vibrates his palps and runs to and fro in front of the female in order to excite her. The dancing is often energetic and prolonged, ten or twenty minutes is not unusual.

Some spider species offer a captured feast in a 'meat for sex' exchange. The male hunting spider *Pisaura mirabilis* can detect a female by smell or crossing a dragline she has left behind. He then hunts for a fly, which he wraps in a swathe of silk, postures in front of her and when her fangs are safely embedded in the fly he mates with her.

Tetragnatha males rely on strength and good design. They have large mandibles and the male has two large spines on his. When he meets a mature female he moves straight towards her with his jaws open wide. The female opens hers wide as well. As they get close enough for their legs to touch and their jaws meet, the male locks his around the female's, the spines and his longer fangs allow him to trap her jaws completely. Now that it is impossible for her to bite him, they descend on a strand of web and mate hanging face to face. Afterwards he makes a quick release escape dropping rapidly to the ground.

Xysticus cristatus mixes bravado with caution. On meeting a female he rushes up and grabs her by the leg. When she stops complaining he climbs around on her back, fondling her with his legs, gently ties her down with strands of silk. When she is under control, he climbs off her back and pushes himself underneath her from behind to allow copulation to take place. Having finished mating he departs leaving her tied up. It takes her a little while to escape once he has left.

A female redback (*Latrodectus hasselti*) has two spermathecae, for storing sperm., one on each side. A male can only insert one of his palps at a time and breaks it off inside her as a contraceptive plug, to avoid the next male using the same side having any more than a 20% chance of insemination. Having two spermathecae means the female generally has the choice of sperm from two males and the strongest sperm gets most of the offspring. But a strong male can recover from being partly digested dangling in front of the female's jaws and return to claim both spermathecae and thus 100% of the queen's potential (R639).

One shouldn't underestimate the cannibalistic voracity of female spiders however. Female *Dolomedes triton* the fishing spider which also catches small fish, can become so aggressive that she would prefer to eat male spiders before they even mate with her. The most voracious of these females however are also the most daring with predators, so other forms of selection are contributing to a diversity of personality types (Behavioral Ecology and Sociobiology DOI: 10.1007/s00265-005-0943-5).

These varieties of mating experience teach us that the relations between the sexes are an endless struggle of Machiavellian manoeuvre and counter-strike in which neither sex ultimately has the upper hand, no matter how gruesome the appearances. In the centre of the cyclone lies the state of sexual paradox with each sex running while standing still to try to keep their end of the game alive. This variety amid genuine sexual paradoxes of coevolution is a lesson for human sexual dominion, where there has been an attempt to assert a unilateral dominance in an attempt to overthrow the natural order of sexually antagonistic coevolution.

Bibliography

1. Aaby Peter 1977 *Engels and women* Critique of Anthropology 3/9-10 25-33.
2. Adams, Carol (ed) 1993 Ecofeminism and the Sacred, Continuum Publishing Company, NY.
3. Ainsworth Claire 2003 *The stranger within* New Scientist 15 Nov 2003 34-7.
4. Albert, Arianne; Otto, Sarah 2005 *Sexual Selection Can Resolve Sex-Linked Sexual Antagonism* Science 310 119-121.
5. Alexander Richard 1979 Darwinism and Human Affairs Univ. Washington. Pr., Seattle.
6. Alexander Richard 1987 The Biology of Moral Systems Aldine de Gruyter, NY.
7. Alexander Richard, Noonan Kathleen 1979 *Concealment of ovulation, parental care and human social evolution* in Evolutionary Psychology and Human Social Behavior Chagnon N. and Irons W (eds.) Duxbury Pr., North Scituate, Mass.
8. Allegro, John 1970 The Sacred Mushroom and the Cross, Hodder & Stoughton, London.
9. Allen LS, Gorski RA. 1991 *Sexual dimorphism of the anterior commissure and massa intermedia of the human brain.* J Comp Neurol 312(1) 97–104.
10. Almroth, Lars et. al. 2005 Lancet 366, 385.
11. Alpers Antony 1964 Maori Myths and Tribal Legends, Longman Paul, Auckland N.Z.
12. Anathaswamy Anil 2003 *The thermal history of life is revealed* New Scientist 31 May 20.
13. Anathaswamy Anil 2004 *Hormones converge for couples in love* New Scientist 5 May.
14. Anders Ödeen 2005 Proc. Nat. Acad. Sci. DOI:10.1073/pnas.0409228102.
15. Anderson, Edward 1980 Peyote The Divine Cactus Univ. Arizona Pr., Tucson.
16. Andrade, M.C.B. 1996 *Sexual selection for male sacrifice in the Australian redback spider* Science 271, 70-72.
17. Angelier Nicole, Penrad-Mobayed May, Billoud B., Bonnanfant-Jaïs M-J, Coumailleau P. 1996 *What role might lampbrush chromosomes play in maternal gene expression?* Int. J. Dev. Biol. 40: 645-652
18. Angier, Natalie 1999 Woman - An Intimate Geography Houghton Mifflin, Boston.
19. Aragona, Brandon 2005 Nature Neuroscience DOI: 10.1038/nn1613
20. Archer, J. and Lloyd, B. (1985) Sex and Gender. Cambridge: Cambridge University Press
21. Armstrong, Karen 1991 Muhammad, Victor Gollancz, London.
22. Armstrong, Karen 1993 A History of God, William Hineman, London.
23. Armstrong, Karen 2000 The Battle for God, Harper Collins, London.
24. Aschkenasy Nehama 1986 Eve's Journey Univ. Pennsylvania Pr. Philadelphia.
25. Aspect A., Dalibard J., Roger G., (1982), *Experimental tests of Bell's theorem using time-varying analysers*, Phys. Rev. Lett. 49, 1804.
26. Ast G 2005 *The alternative genome* Scientific American 292/4
27. Aureli Filippo, de Waal Frans 2000 Natural Conflict Resolution Univ. California Press.
28. Avi-Yonah, Michael 1969 A History of the Holy Land, Weidenfield and Nicholson, London.
29. Azim E, Mobbs D, Jo B, Menon V, Reiss A 2005 *Sex differences in brain activation elicited by humor* Proc. Nat. Acad. Sci. 102/45 16497-502.
30. Attenborough, David 1982 Discovering Life on Earth William Collins Sons & Co, London.
31. Bachofen Johann 1862 Das Mutterecht Krais and Hoffman, Stuttgart.
32. Badcock C. 2000 Evolutionary Psychology Oxford, Polity Press.
33. Bagemihl Bruce 1999 Biological Exuberance: Animal homosexuality and natural diversity St. Martins Press NY.
34. Bailey JM, Pillard RC 1991 *A genetic study of male sexual orientation* Arch. Gen. Psychiatry 48/dec 1089-96.
35. Bailey JM, Pillard RC et. al. 1993 *Heritable factors invluence sexual orientation in women* Arch. Gen. Psychiatry 50/mar 217-23.
36. Baker, Robin 1996 Sperm Wars: Infidelity, Sexual Conflict and other bedroom battles, Fourth Estate, London.
37. Baker Robin, Bellis Mark 1995 Human sperm competition, Copulation, Masturbation and Infidelity Chapman and Hall, London.
38. Bainbridge D. 2003 *The double life of women* New Scientist May 10 41-5.
39. Bamberger, J. 1974 *The myth of matriarchy: Why men rule in primitive society* in Rosaldo M, Lamphere L (eds.) Women, Culture and Society Stamford University Press, Cambridge.
40. Barash David, Lipton Judith 2001 The Myth of Monogamy WH Freeman and Co. NY.
41. Barnsley M. 1988 Fractals Everywhere Academic Press, New York.
42. Baron-Cohen, Simon 2003 The Essential Difference: Men, women and the extreme male brain Allen Lane / Penguin Press
43. Baron-Cohen S, Knickmeyer R, Belmonte M 2005 Sex Differences in the Brain: Implications for Explaining Autism Science 310 819-23.
44. Barrow John, Tipler Frank 1988 The Anthropic Cosmological Principle, Oxford Univ Pr, Oxford.
45. Bartels Andreas, Zeki Semir 2000 *The neural basis of romantic love* Neuroreport 11/17 3829
46. Bartels Andreas, Zeki Semir 2004 *The neural correlates of maternal and romantic love* Neu-

roimage 21 1155.

47. Barton, S. C., Surani, M. A. and Norris, M. L. 1984. *Role of maternal and paternal genomes in mouse development.* Nature 311: 374-376.
48. Bataille, Georges 1988 The accursed share (Robert Hurley tr) Zone Books NY.
49. Batto, Bernard 1974 Studies on Women at Mari, John Hopkins Univ. Pr., Baltimore.
50. Becher, H. 1960 The Surara and Pakidai, Two Yanoama Tribes in Northwest Brazil Kommissionsverlag Cram, De Gruyter & Co Hamburg
51. Begley, S. 1999 *Aping Language* in Annual Editions. Physical Anthropology 99/00 ed. E. Angeloni. McGraw-Hill. Conn. pp 64-66.
52. Bejerano G, Pheasant M, Makunin I, Stephen S, Kent W, Mattick J, Haussler D 2004 *Ultraconserved Elements in the Human Genome* Science 304 1321-5.
53. Bell, G. 1982. The Masterpiece of Nature: The Evolution and Genetics of Sexuality. University of California Press, Berkeley.
54. Bell John S. (1966) Rev. Mod. Phys. 38/3, 447.
55. Bellis, M. Journal of Epidemiology and Community Health, Sept. 2005; vol 59: pp 749-754.
56. Bem S.L. (1981) *Gender schema theory: a cognitive account of sex-typing* Psychological Review 88 354.
57. Benton, David. 1982 *The influence of androstenol - a putative human pheromone - on mood throughout the menstrual cycle.* Biological Psychology, 15/3-4, 249-256.
58. Betzig L. 1982 *Despotism and reproduction: a cross-cultural correlation of conflict asymmetry, hierarchy and degree of polygyny* Ethology and Sociobiology 3 209-21.
59. Betzig L. 1986 Despotism and reproduction: a Darwinian View of History Aldine, NY.
60. Betzig, Laura, Monique Borgerhoff Mulder and Paul Turke, eds.1988 Human Reproductive Behaviour, a Darwinian Perspective. Cambridge.
61. Bhattacharya, Shaoni 2005 *Giving birth by Caesarian section reduces fertility* New Sci. 2 Aug.
62. Birkhead Tim 2000 Promiscuity Faber and Faber, London.
63. Blanchard R, Cantor J. 2002 Archives of Sexual Behavior 31 63.
64. Blobel, C. Wolfsberg, T. Turck, C. Myles, D. Primakoff P. White J. 1992 *A potential fusion peptide and an integrin ligand domain in a protein active in sperm-egg fusion.* Nature 356, 248-52.
65. Blum Deborah 1997 Sex on the Brain, Penguin, N.Y.
66. Blurton Jones Nicholas, Hawkes Kristen, O'Connell James 2002 *Antiquity of Postreproductive life:Are there modern impacts on hunter-gatherer postreproductive life spans?* American Journal of Human Biology 14 184-205.
67. Boehm Christopher1999 Hierarchy in the Forest Harvard Univ. Pr. Cambridge Mass.
68. Bohm D. 1952, *A suggested interpretation of the quantum theory in terms of 'hidden' variables, I & II*, Phys. Rev. 85 166-93.
69. Bohm David 1980 Wholeness and the Implicate Order, Routeledge & Kegan Paul, London.
70. Boissinot, Stephanie, Entezam, A, Furano, A. 2001 *Selection Against Deleterious LINE-1-Containing Loci in the Human Lineage* Mol. Biol. Evol. **18(6)** 926–935.
71. Boswell John 1988 The Kindness of Strangers: The Abandonment of children in Western Europe from Late Antiquity to the Renaissance Pantheon, NY.
72. Boyd R, Gintis H, Bowles S, Richerson P 2003 *The evolution of altruistic punishment* Proc. Nat. Acad. Sci. 100 3531–3535.
73. Branciforte D., Martin S. 1994 *Developmental and Cell-type specificity of LINE-1 Expression in Mouse Testis: Implications for Transposition* Molecular and Cellular Biology 14/4 2584-92
74. Bressler E., Balshine S. 2006 Evolution & Human Behavior 27 29-39.
75. Briffault, Robert 1927 The Mothers George Allen Unwin, London.
76. Bright, John 1960 A History of Israel, SCM Press, London.
77. Britten Roy J 2002 *Divergence between samples of chimpanzee and human DNA sequences is 5% counting indels.* Proc. Nat. Acad. Sci. 99 13633-5.
78. Broadfield D, Holloway R, Mowbray K, Silvers A, Yuan M, Marquez S 2001 *Endocast of Sambungmacan 3 (Sm 3): A New Homo erectus From Indonesia* The Anatomical Record 262:369–379.
79. Brody T.M., Larner J.L., Minneman K.P. 1998 Human Pharmacology, Mosbt, St. Louis.
80. Brooks Geraldine 1995 Nine Parts of Desire, Anchor Doubleday, New York.
81. Brosnan, S., Schiff, H., de Waal, F. 2005 Proc. Royal. Soc. B. doi:10.1098/rspb.2004.2947.
82. Broude Gwen 1994 Marriage, Family and Relationships: A Cross-cultural Encyclopedia ABC-CLIO Santa Barbara CA.
83. Brown CJ Robinson WP 2000 *The causes and consequences of random and non-random X chromosome inactivation in humans* Clinical Genetics 58/5 353.
84. Brown Donald E. 1991 Human Universals McGraw Hill, New York.
85. Brown J. 1994 *A quantum revolution for computing* New. Scientist S.ept 24
86. Brown, Michael F. 1982 *The Dark Side of Progress: Suicide Among the Alto Mayo Aguaruna.* Paper delivered to 44th International Congress of Americanists, Manchester, England.
87. Brown, Michael F. 1986 *Power, Gender and the Social Meaning of Aguaruna Suicide.* Man , 21(2), 311-328.

88. Brown P., et al. 2004 Nature 431 1055-1061.
89. Brown, Raymond E. 1979. The Community of the Beloved Disciple. New York: Paulist Press.
90. Brown W. M., et al. 2005 Nature 438 1148-1150.
91. Browning, Ian 1974 Petra, Chatto & Windus, London.
92. Buchanan Mark 2005 *Charity begins at Homo sapiens* New Sceintist 12 Mar.
93. Burley, Nancy 1979 *The evolution of concealed ovulation* The American Naturalist 144 835-58.
94. Burmeister Sabrina et. al. 2005 Public Library of Science Biology, DOI: 10.1371/journal.pbio.0030363
95. Buss David 1994 The Evolution of Desire: Strategies of Human Mating Basic Books, NY
96. Cáceres M, Lachuer J, Zapala M, Redmond J, Kudo L, Geschwind D, Lockhart D, Preuss T, Barlow C 2003 Proc. Nat. Acad. Sci. 213549910-0
97. Cadbury Deborah 1997 The Feminization of Nature, Hamish Hamilton (Penguin), London.
98. Cahill L. 2005 *His brain, her brain* Scientific American May 40-47.
99. Callan H.G. 1963 *The Nature of Lampbrush Chromosomes* Int. Rev. of Cytology **15** 1-34.
100. Callan H.G. 1969 *Biochemical activities of chromosomes during the prophase of meiosis* in Lima-de-Faria ed. Handbook of Molecular Cytology North-Holland Amsterdam 540-552.
101. Camerer C., Fehr E 2006 When Does "Economic Man" Dominate Social Behavior? Science 311 47-52.
102. Campbell Anne 2002 A Mind of Her Own: The evolutionary psychology of women. Oxford Univ. Pr. Oxford.
103. Campbell, Joseph 1959, 1962, 1965 The Masks of God vols 1-3, Viking Press, N.Y.
104. Campbell, Joseph 1988 Historical Atlas of World Mythology Vol. II Part 1 The Sacrifice, Harper & Row, N.Y.
105. Campbell, Neil 1996 Biology 4th ed. Bejamin/Cummings, Menlo Park p 963
106. Capra Fritjof 1975 The Tao of Physics, Wildwood House, London.
107. Carrel L. & Willard H. F. et al. 2005 *X-inactivation profile reveals extensive variability in X-linked gene expression in females* Nature, 434. 400 - 404.
108. Carrol, Lewis 1872. Through the looking glass and what Alice found there. Macmillan, London.
109. Catalano, R; Bruckner, T; Gould, J; Eskenazi, B; Anderson, E 2005 Sex ratios in California following the terrorist attacks of September 11, 2001 Human Reproduction 20/5 pp. 1221–27.
110. Chagnon, Napoleon 1997 Yanomamo (5th ed) Harcourt Brace, NY.
111. Chalmers David 1995 *The Puzzle of Conscious Experience* Sci. Am. **Dec.** 62-69.
112. Chalmers, David J. 1996 The Conscious Mind. Oxford University Press.
113. Charon N.W., Goldstein S.F. 2002 *Genetics of motility and chamotaxis of a fascinating group of bacteria: The Spirochetes* Annu. Rev. Genet. 36:47–73.
114. Check, Erica 2005 *Genetics: The X factor* Nature 434, 266 - 267.
115. Chen Y, Olckers A, Schurr T, Kogelnik A, Huoponen ,Wallace D 2000 *mtDNA Variation in the South African Kung and Khwe—and Their Genetic Relationships to Other African Populations* Am. J. Hum. Genet. 66:1362–1383.
116. Chimpanzee sequencing and analysis consortium *Initial sequence of the chimpanzee genome and comparison with the human genome* Nature 437 69-87
117. Chomsky, Noam 2000 New Horizons in the Study of Language and Mind Cambridge Univ. Pr. , Cambridge.
118. Chown, Marcus 2004 *Quantum Rebel.* New Scientist, 183 2457 24th July 30.
119. Christ, Carol; Plaskow, Judith 1979 Womanspirit Rising, Harper & Row, New York.
120. Christiansen Morten, Kirby Simon (ed.) 2003 Language Evolution, Oxford University Press (see also Grimes, Ken *The language Bug* New Scientist 18 Jan 03)
121. Cohen, David ed 1991 The Circle of Life : Rituals from the human family album, Harper San Francisco.
122. Cohen Philip 1996 *Let there be life* New Scientist 6 July 22-7.
123. Cohen Philip 2003 *Renegade code* New Scientist 30 Aug 34.
124. Cohn, Norman 1957 The Pursuit of the Millenium, Paladin, Granada, London.
125. Cohn, Norman 1993 Cosmos Chaos, Bath Press, Avon.
126. Colborn, Theo, Dumanoski, D, Myers, J 1996 Our stolen future : are we threatening our fertility, intelligence, and survival? Abacus, London.
127. Comrie B, Matthews S, Polinsky M 2003 The Atlas of Languages Facts On File Quarto NY.
128. Conkey Margaret and Gero Joan (eds.)1991 Engendering archaeology : women and prehistory B. Blackwell Oxford, UK ; Cambridge, Mass., USA.
129. Cook Roger 1974 The Tree of Life Thames and Hudson, London.
130. Cooke B. Hegstrom CD. Villeneuve LS. Breedlove SM. 1998 *Sexual differentiation of the vertebrate brain: principles and mechanisms*. Front. Neuroendocrin. 19(4):323-62.
131. Corballis Michael 1991 The Lopsided Ape Oxford Univ. Pr., Oxford.
132. Corballis Michael 2002 From Hand to Mouth the Origins of Language Princetion Univ. Pr. NJ.
133. Corna F, Camperio-Ciani A, Capiluppi C 2004 *Evidence for maternally inherited factors favouring male homosexuality and promoting female fecundity* Proceedings of the Royal

Society B: Biological Sciences DOI: 10.1098/rspb
134. Cox C., LeBoeuf B. 1977 *Female incitation of male compettion: a mechanism in sexual selection* American Naturalist 111, 317-35.
135. Cramer J.G., 1986 *The transactional interpretation of quantum mechanics*, Rev. Mod. Phys. 58, 647 - 687.
136. Crick F, Koch C. 1992 *The Problem of Consciousness* Sci. Am. Sep. 110-117.
137. Criss Thomas Marcum John 1981 *Lunar effect on fertility* Social Biology 28 75-80.
138. Crocker William 1984 *Canela Marriage: Factors in Change in Marriage Practices in Lowland South America*, pp. 63-98. K. Kensinger. (ed.) Illinois Studies in Anthropology, no.14. Univ. of Illinois Pr.
139. Crocker, W. & Crocker, J. 1994 Canela. Harcourt Brace Forth Worth.
140. Cutler, W.B., G. Preti, A.M. Krieger, G. Huggins, C.R. Garcia and H.J. Lawley 1986 *Human Axillary Secretions Influence Women's Menstrual Cycles: The Role of Donor Extract from Men.* Hormones and Behavior, 20:463-473
141. Cutler W., Schleidt W., Freidmann E., Preti G., Stine R. 1987 *Lunar influence on the reproductive cycle of women* Human Biology 59/6.
142. Dalley, Stephanie 1984 Mari and Karana, Longman, London.
143. Daly, Martin; Wilson, Margo 1988 Homicide New York : Aldine de Gruyter.
144. Damasio A 2005 *Human behaviour: Brain trust* Nature 435, 571-572.
145. Darnell, J., Lodish, H., Baltimore D.1986 Molecular Cell Biology, Scientific American Books. W.H. Freeman and Co. NY
146. Darwin Charles 1859 (1967) On the Origin of the Species facs Harvard Univ. Pr. MA.
147. Darwin Charles 1871 The Descent of Man and Selection in Relation to Sex (2 vols) Appleton, NY.
148. Darwin Charles 1904 The Expression of Emotions in Man and Animals John Murray London 1965 Chicago Univ. .Pr.
149. Davis-Kimball Jeannine 2002 Warrior Women: An Archaeologists Search for History's Hidden Heroines Warner Books NY.
150. Dawkins, Richard 1976 The Selfish Gene, Oxford Univ. Pr., Oxford.
151. Dawkins, Richard 1986 The Blind Watchmaker, Harlow:Longman Science.
152. Dawkins, Richard 1995 A River ran out of Eden, Weidenfield & Nicholson, London.
153. Dawkins, Richard 1996 Climbing Mount Improbable, Viking, London.
154. Deacon Terrence 1997 The Symbolic Species, Norton, NY.
155. Deaner M. O., Khera A. V. & Platt M. L. 2005 Curr. Biol. published online http://www.current-biology.com/content/ article/abstract?uid=PIIS0960982205001041.
156. Dennell R, Roebroeks W 2005 *An Asian perspective on early human dispersal from Africa* Nature 438 1099-1104 doi:10.1038/nature04259
157. de Quervain Dominique, Fischbacher U, Treyer V, Schellhammer M, Schnyder U, Buck A, Fehr Ernst 2004 *The Neural Basis of Altruistic Punishment* Science 305 1254-8.
158. De Robertis E., Oliver G., Wright V. (1990) *Homeobox genes and the vertebrate body plan* Sci. Am. Jul. 26-33.
159. Devaney R.L 1986 An Introduction to Chaotic Dynamical Systems Benjamin/Cummings, Menlo Park. (2nd Ed.)
160. de Waal, Frans 1995 *Bonobo Sex and Society*, Scientific American, Mar 59.
161. de Waal, Frans 1996 Good Natured, Harvard University Press. Cambrdge MA.
162. de Waal Frans, Lanting Frans 1997 Bonobo the Forgotten Ape Univ. California Press, Berkeley CA.
163. de Waal Frans 2001 *Apes from Venus* in de Waal Frans (ed.) Tree of Origin, Harvard Univ. Pr. Camb. MA.
164. Diamond, Irene and Orenstein, Gloria (ed) 1990 Reweaving the World, Sierra Club Books, San Francisco.
165. Diamond, Jared 2000 Why is sex fun? : the evolution of human sexuality. Phoenix, London.
166. Dicks Lynn 2003 *Too close for comfort* New Scientist 18 Oct 38.
167. Di Pellegrino G, Fadiga L, Fogassi L, Gallese V, Rizzolatti G. 1992. *Understanding motor events: a neurophysiological study.* Exp. Brain Res. 91:176–80
168. Divale WT 1972 *System population control in the middle and upper paleolithic: Inferences based on contemporary hunter-gatherers* World Archaeology 4 222-43.
169. Doe, Brian 1971 Southern Arabia, Thames and Hudson, London.
170. Douglas Kate 2001 *Painted ladies* New Scientist 13 Oct.
171. Douglas Kate 2004 *Rules of attraction* New Scientsit 18 Dec 34-7.
172. Douglas Mary 1966 Purity and Danger Routledge & Kegan Paul London.
173. Draper Patricia 1975 *!Kung women: contrasts in sexual egalitarianism in foraging and sedentary contexts* in Reiter R. Towards an anthropology of women Monthly Review Press N.Y. 77-109.
174. Duff, Michael 2003 *The theory formerly known as strings (2nd ed.)* in The Edge of Physics Scientific American.
175. Dugatkin Lee 2005 *Why don't we just kiss and make up?* New Scientist 7 May 35.

176. Dugatkin, Lee and Godin, Jean-Guy 1998 *How Females Choose Their Mates* Sci. Am. Apr 46.
177. Dunbar Robin 1996 <u>Grooming, Gossip and the Evolution of Language</u> Faber and Faber, Lond.
178. Dunbar Robin 2001 *Brains on two legs: Group size and the evolution of intelligence* in de Waal Frans (ed.) <u>Tree of Origin</u>, Harvard Univ. Pr. Camb. MA.
179. Ebersberger I, Metzier D, Schwartz C Paabo S 2002 *Genome-wide comparison of sequence between humans and chimpanzees* Am. J. Human Genetics 70 1490-7.
180. Eccles, J.C. 1986 *Do men tal even ts cause neural events analogously to the probability fields of quan tum mechanics?* Proc. R. Soc. Lond. B 227 , 411–428.
181. Eisenman, Robert 1997 <u>James the Brother of Jesus</u>, Faber and Faber, London.
182. Eisler Rianne 1987 <u>The Chalice and the Blade: Our History, Our Future</u>, Harper & Row, San Francisco.
183. Eisler Rianne 1996 <u>Sacred Pleasure: Sex, Myth and the Politics of Society</u>, HarperSanFrancisco.
184. Eliade Mircea 1972 <u>Shamanism: archaic techniques of ecstasy.</u> (trans. Willard R. Trask). Princeton Univ. Press Princeton NJ. (c1964)
185. Elgar, MA, Schneider JM, Herberstein ME 2000 *Female control of paternity in the sexually cannibalistic spider Argiope keyserlingi* Proc. Royal Society of London B 267 2439 -43.
186. Ellegren H. 2000 *Heterogeneous mutation processes in human microsatellite DNA sequences* Nature Genetics 24/4 , 400-402
187. Eller Cynthia 2000 <u>The Myth of Matriarchal Prehistory: Why an Invented Past Won't Give Women a Future</u> Beacon Press Boston.
188. El Saadawi, Nawal 1980 <u>The Naked (Hidden) Face of Eve</u>, Beacon Press, Boston.
189. Ember Carol 1978 *Myths about hunter-gatherers* Ethnology 17 438-48.
190. Ember Carol 1981 *A cross-cultural perspctive on sex differences* in Monro, Monroe and Whiting (eds.) <u>Handbook of Cross-Cultural Human Dvelopment</u> Garland Press Ny 531-80.
191. Ember Carol and MR 1992 *Resource unpredictability, mistrust and war: A cross-cultural study* J. Conflict Resolution 36/2 242-62.
192. Engels Fredrick 1972 <u>The Origin of the Family, Private Property and the State</u> E Leacock (ed.) International Publishers, NY
193. Enomoto, Tomoo 1990 *Social Play and Sexual Behavior of the Bonobo (Pan paniscus) with Specific Reference to Flexibility* Primates 31(4): 469-480
194. Enquist M, Rodriguez-Girones M. 2001 *The evolution of female sexuality* Animal Behaviour 61(4) 695-704
195. Essid, Yassine, <u>A critique of the origins of Islamic economic thought</u>, E.J. Brill, Leiden, New York, Koln, 1995, p. 205.
196. Estrada, Alvaro 1981 <u>Maria Sabina : Her Life and Chants</u> Ross Erickson Santa Barbara.
197. Evans,P; Gilbert, S; Mekel-Bobrov,N; Vallender,E; Anderson,J; Vaez-Azizi L; Tishkoff,S; Hudson, R; Lahn B *Microcephalin, a Gene Regulating Brain Size, Continues to Evolve Adaptively in Humans* Science 309 1717-20
198. Faris, Nabih 1952 (trans) al-Kabali: <u>The Book of Idols</u>, Princeton Univ. Pr., Princeton.
199. Falk, D. 1992 <u>Braindance</u>. Henry Holt & Co. New York.
200. Farthing W. 2005 Evolution and Human Behaviour, 26 171.
201. Fausto-Sterling, Anne. 1985, (2nd ed.1992). <u>Myths of Gender. Biological Theories About Women and Men</u>. New York: Basic Books.
202. Fausto-Sterling Anne 2000 <u>Sexing the body</u>, Basic Books, N.Y.
203. Fehr Ernst, Fishbacher U 2003 *The nature of human altruism* Nature 425 785-791.
204. Fehr Ernst, Fishbacher U, Gächter S 2002 *Strong reciprocity, human cooperation and the enforcement of social norms* Human Nature 13/1 1-25.
205. Fehr Ernst, Rockenbach Bettina 2003 Nature 422 137.
206. Feng G., English J. 1972 Lao Tsu, <u>Tao Te Ching</u> Wildwood House, London.
207. Fisher, Helen 1982 <u>The Sex Contract: The Evolution of Human Behavior</u> William Morrow, NY.
208. Fisher, Helen 1992 <u>An Anatomy of Love</u> Helen WW Norton NY.
209. Fisher, Helen 1999 <u>The First Sex</u> Helen Fisher Random House NY.
210. Fisher, Helen 2004 <u>Why we Love</u> Henry Holt N.Y.
211. Fisher R. 1930 <u>The Genetical Theory of Natural Selection</u> Clarendon Press, Oxford.
212. Flake Gary 1998 <u>The computational beauty of nature : computer explorations of fractals, chaos, complex systems, and adaptation</u> MIT Press Cambridge, Mass.
213. Flinders-Petrie, W. 1906 <u>Researches in Sinai</u>, John Murray, London.
214. Foellmer MW, Fairbairn D J 2003 *Spontaneous male death during copulation in an orb-weaving spider* Proc. Royal Society B, doi:10.1098/rsbl.2003.0042.
215. Forger Nancy et. al. DOI:10.1073/pnas.0404644101 (see Farley Peter *Single gene removes sex differences in mice brains* New Scientist 31 Aug).
216. Forster P., Matsumura S 2005 *Did early humans go north or south?* Science 308 965-6.
217. Foucalt Michel 1981 <u>The History of Sexuality: Vol 1 An Introduction</u> Harmondsworth; Pelican
218. Fournier D et. al. 2005 Nature 435 1230.
219. Fox, Robin Lane 1992 <u>The Unauthorized Version</u>, Alfred A. Knopf, NY.

220. Frazer, Sir James 1890 The Golden Bough, MacMillan and Co., London.
221. Frayser, Suzanne 1985 Varieties of Sexual Experience HRAF Press, New Haven, Conn.
222. Friedl Ernestine 1975 *Sex the invisible* American Anthropologist, 96(4) 833-44..
223. Friedl Ernestine 1994 Women and Men: An Anthropologist's View Holt, Rinehart & Winston NY.
224. Freeman, W. 1991 *The physiology of perception.* Sci. Am. 264, Feb 35-41.
225. Friedman, David 2001 A Mind of its Own The Free Press.
226. Fukui H. 2003 *Music and Testosterone A New Hypothesis for the Origin and Function of Music* Annals of the New York Academy of Sciences 930:448-451.
227. Furst, Peter ed 1972 Flesh of the Gods Praeger, N.Y.
228. Gächter S, Falk A 2002 *Reputation and reciprocity: Consequences for the Labour Relation* Scand. J. of Economics 104 1-26.
229. Gadon, Elinor 1989 The Once and Future Goddess, Harper & Row, San Francisco.
230. Galik K, Senut B, Pickford M, Gommery D, Treil J, Kupervage A Eckhardt R 2004 *External and Internal Morphology of the BAR 1002 Orrorin tugenensis Femur* Science 305 1450-3.
231. Geary, D. 1996 *Sexual selection and sex differences in mathmatical abilities.* Behavioral and Brain Sciences, 19, 229-284.
232. Gero S 1986 *With Walter Bauer on the Tigris: Encratite Orthodoxy and Libertine Heresy in Syro-Mesopotamian Christianity* in Nag Hammadi, Gnosticism, and Early Christianity.
233. Gershevitch, Ilya 1959 The Avestan Hymn to Mithra, Cambridge Univ. Pr. , Cambridge.
234. Gibbons Ann 1998 *In mice mom's genes favour brain over brawn* Science 280 1346.
235. Gibson M. Macy R. 2003 Proc. R. Soc. Lond. B. 270. S108 - S109.
236. Giddens, Anthony 1992 The Transformation of Intimacy: Sexuality, Love and Eroticism in Modern Societies Polity Press, Cambridge.
237. Gilbert Tom 2003 *Death and Destruction* New Scientist 31 May 32.
238. Gimbutas Marija 1982 Goddeses and Gods of Old Europe Univ. California Pr. Berkeley
239. Gimbutas Marija 1989 The Language of the Goddess: Unearthing the Hidden Symbols of Western Civilization Harper & Row, NY.
240. Girard, Rene 1972 Violence and the Sacred, John Hopkins Univ. Pr., Baltimore.
241. Girard, Rene 1987 Things Hidden Since the Foundation of the World, Athlone Pr., London.
242. Glueck, Nelson 1966 Deities and Dolphins, Cassel, London.
243. Goldberg S. 1973 The inevitability of patriarchy Peru, Ill., Open Court.
244. Goldberg S. 1993 Why men rule: A theory of male dominance. Peru, Ill., Open Court.
245. Goodman M 2003 *Natural Selection's Role in Shaping 99.4% Nonsynonymous DNA Identity Between Congeneric Humans and Chimpanzees* Proc. Nat. Acad. Sci. May 19 03-2172.
246. Goodwin, Jan 1994 Price of Honour, Little, Brown and Company, Boston.
247. Goren_Inbar N, Alperson N, Kislev M, Simchoni O, Melamed Y, Ben-nun A, Werker E 2004 *Evidence of Hominin Control of Fire at Gesher Benot Ya'aqov, Israel* Science 304 725-7.
248. Gould, Stephen Jay 1983 Hen's Teeth and Horses Toes, W.W. Norton & Coy., New York, 147.
249. Gowarty P. 1997 *Sexual dialectics, sexual selection and variation in reproductive behavior* in Gowarty P (ed.) Feminism and Evolutionary Biology: Boundaries, Intersections and Frontiers Chapmann and Hall, N.Y.
250. Grammer, Karl. 1993 *α-androstenone: A male pheromone? A brief report.* Ethology & Sociobiology, 14/3 201-207
251. Grant, Valerie J. 1998 Maternal personality, evolution and the sex ratio Routledge.
252. Gray Russell, Atkinson Quentin 2003 *Language-tree divergence times support the Anatolian theory of Indo-European origin* Nature 426 435 - 439
253. Graves, Robert 1946 King Jesus Cassel, London.
254. Graves, Robert 1948 The White Goddess, Faber & Faber, London.
255. Graves R., Podro J. 1953 The Nazarene Gospel Restored, Cassel, London.
256. Graves, Robert 1955 Greek Myths Penguin, London.
257. Graves R., Podro J. 1957 Jesus in Rome, Cassel & Co., London.
258. Gray, John 1964 The Canaanites, Thames and Hudson, London.
259. Gray P, Krause B, Atema J, Payne R, Krumhansl C, Baptista L 2001 *The Music of Nature and the Nature of Music* Science, 291, 52-5.
260. Green, Tamara 1992 The City of the Moon God, E.J. Brill, Leiden.
261. Gregor, Th. (1985) Anxious Pleasures: The Sexual Lives of an Amazonian People. Chicago: Chicago University Press
262. Griaule Marcel 1975 Conversations with Ogotemmeli Oxford: Oxford Univ. Pr. 16-40.
263. Griaule M, Dieterlen G 1986 The Pale Fox Afrikan World Book Distributor
264. Griaule M, Dieterlen G 1954 *The Dogon,* in: D Forde (ed.), African Worlds. Studies in the cosmological ideas and social values of African peoples, OUP, London 83-110.
265. Grim Patrick 1997 *The Undecidability of the Spatialized Prisoner's Dilemma* Theory and Decision 42 53-80.
266. Groombridge, Brian 1992 Global Biodiversity : Status of the Earth's living Resources, Chapman & Hall London
267. Gruzinski, Serge 1992 Painting the Conquest, Flammarion, Paris.

268. Guatelli-Steinberg, Debbie Proc. Nat. Acad. Sci., DOI: 10.1073/pnas.0503108102
269. Gutzwiller, M.C. (1992). *Quantum chaos.* Sci. Am. **266**, 78 - 84.
270. Haeri, Shala 1989 <u>Law of Desire</u>, Syracuse Univ. Pr., Syracuse NY.
271. Hagedorn H, O'Connor J, Fuchs M, Sage B, Schlaeger D, Bohm M 1975 *The ovary as a source of alpha-ecdysone in an adult mosquito* Proc Natl Acad Sci. 172(8), 3255-9.
272. Haig D., Graham C. 1991 *Genomic mprinting and the strange case of the insulin-like growth factor receptor* Cell 64, 1045.
273. Haig D., Westoby M. 1989 *Parent-specific gene expression and the triploid endosperm* American Naturalist 134, 147-55.
274. Halifax, Joan 1979 <u>Shamanic Voices</u> Penguin Arkana NY.
275. Hallam, Elizabeth 1989 <u>Chronicles of the Crusades</u>, Weidenfield and Nicholson, London.
276. Hamer, Dean 2004 <u>The God Gene: How Faith Is Hard-Wired Into Our Genes</u> Random House.
277. Hamer D, Hu S et. al. 1993 *Linkage between DNA markers on the X chromosome and male sexual orientation* Science 261 321-5.
278. Hameroff, Stuart; Penrose, Roger (2003) *Conscious Events as Orchestrated Space-Time Selections* NeuroQuantology; **1**: 10-35
279. Hamilton W. D. 1963 *The evolution of altruistic behavior* American Naturalist 97 354-6.
280. Hammock E, Young L 2005 *Microsatellite Instability Generates Diversity in Brain and Sociobehavioral Traits* Science, 308, 1630-4.
281. Han K, Xing J, Wang, Hedges D, Garber R, Cordaux R, Batzer M 2005 *Under the genomic radar: The Stealth model of Alu amplification* Genome Research 15 655-64.
282. Hanlon, R. 2005 Nature. 433, 212.
283. Hardin Gareth 1968 *The Tragedy of the Commons* Science, 162 (1968):1243-1248.
284. Harner Michael 1973 <u>Jivaro: People of the sacred waterfalls</u> Garden City NY.
285. Harner, Michael ed 1973 <u>Hallucinogens and Shamanism</u>, Oxford Univ. Pr., London.
286. Harris Judith Rich 1995 *Where is the child's environment? A group socialization theory of dvlopment* Psychological Review 102 458-9.
287. Harris Judith Rich 1998 <u>The Nurture Assumption</u> Bloomsbury.
288. Harris Marvin 1974 <u>Cows, Pigs, Wars and Witches</u> Vintage / Random House NY.
289. Harris Marvin 1977 *Why men dminate women* NY Times magazine 13 Nov 46.
290. Harvati Katerina, Frost S., McNulty K. 2004 *Neanderthal taxonomy reconsidered: Implications of 3D primate models of intra- and interspecific differences* Proc. Nat. Acad. Sci. 101 1147-52.
291. Haskins, Susan 1993 <u>Mary Magdalen Myth and Metaphor</u>, Harper Collins, London.
292. Hau, M., Dominguez, O. A. & Evrard, H. C. 2004 Hormones and Behaviour, doi:10.1016/j.yhbeh.2004.02.007.
293. Havlicek J., Roberts S. C. & Flegr J. 2005 Biol. Lett., doi:10.1098/rsbl.2005.0332
294. Hawkes Kristen 1996 *Foraging differences between men and women: Behavioral ecology of the sexual division of labour* in <u>The archaeology of human ancestry : power, sex, and tradition</u> ed. Steele J. and Shennan S. Routledge.
295. Hawkes Kristen, O'Connell James, Blurton Jones Nicholas 2001 *Hadza meat sharing* Evolution and Human Behavior 22 113-142.
296. Hawkes Kristen 2004 *The grandmother effect* Nature 428 129
297. Hawking Stephen 2001 <u>Universe in a Nutshell</u> Bantam Books, NY
298. Hawking Stephen 2004 *Gödel and the end of physics* http://www.damtp.cam.ac.uk/strtst/dirac/hawking/
299. Hein J 2004 *Pedegrees for all humanity* Nature 431, 518-9.
300. Heller, Joseph 1961 <u>Catch 22</u> Simon & Schuster, NY.
301. Henrich Joseph 2000 *Does Culture Matter in Economic Behavior? Ultimatum Game Bargaining Among the Machiguenga of the Peruvian Amazon* American Econ. Review 90/4 Sept 973-9.
302. Henshilwood C, d'Errico F, Vanhaeren M, van Niekerk K Jacobs Z 2004 *Middle Stone Age Shell Beads from South Africa* Science 304 404.
303. Hern W. 1992 *Polygyny and fertility among the Shipibo of the Peruvian Amazon.* Population Studies 46:53-64.
304. Hern W. 1992 *Shipibo polygyny and patrilocality.* American Ethnologist 19(3):501-522.
305. Hewlett Barry S. 1996 *Cultural Diversity Among African Pygmies* in <u>Cultural Diversity Among the Twentieth Century Foragers</u>, edited by Sue Kent. Cambridge University Press. See also Aka Pygmies of the Western Congo Basin http://www.vancouver.wsu.edu/fac/hewlett/Introaka.html
306. Hiby SE, Lough M, Keverne EB, Surani MA, Loke Y, King A. 2001 *Paternal monoallelic expression of PEG3 in the human placenta.* Hum Mol Genet. 10(10):1093-100.
307. Hickey Donal 1982 Genetics 101 519.
308. Hill, Michael Ortiz 1994 <u>Dreaming the End of the World: Apocalypse as a rite of Passage</u>, Spring Publications, Dallas
309. Hinchcliffe E. Sluder G. 2001 *"It Takes Two to Tango": understanding how centrosome duplication is regulated throughout the cell cycle* Genes & Development 15:1167–1181.

520

310. Hines Melissa 2004 <u>Brain Gender</u> Oxford University Press, Oxford.
311. Hines M, Shipley C. 1984 *Prenatal exposure to diethylstibestrol and the development of sexually dimorphic cognitive abilities and cerebral lateralization.* Dev Psychol 20 81–94.
312. Hirschenhauser, Katharina 2002 Hormones and Behavior, 42 172
313. Hite, Shere 1994 <u>Women as revolutionary agents of change</u>: The University of Wisconsin Press, Madison, Wis.
314. Hite, Shere 1987 <u>Women and Love: A Cultural Revolution in Progress</u> Knopf New York.
315. Hoehner, Harold 1972 <u>Herod Antipas</u>, Cambridge Univ. Pr., Cambridge.
316. Holden Constance 2004 *Oldest Beads Suggest Early Symbolic Behavior* Science 304 369.
317. Holding Cathy 2004 *IVF raises the risk of birth defect* New Scientist 14 Aug 11.
318. Holmes Bob 2005 *Does RNA editing make us brainy?* New Scientist 29 Jan 13.
319. Holt, Jim 2005 *Time bandits: What were Einstein and Gödel talking about?* New Yorker Feb 28 80-85.
320. Hooper J. & Teresi D., 1986, <u>The Three-Pound Universe</u>, MacMillan New York .
321. Howard N 1998 *n-Person Soft Games* Journal of the Operations Research Society 49/2 144-50.
322. Hrdy, Sarah Blaffer 1981 <u>The Woman that Never Evolved</u> Harvard Unv. Pr. Cambridge.
323. Hrdy, Sarah Blaffer 1999 <u>Mother Nature : A History of Mothers, Infants, and Natural Selection</u> Pantheon New York.
324. Hrdy, Sarah Blaffer 2003 *New rules for an old game* New Scientist 24 May 46.
325. Hume D. 1978 1739 <u>A Treatise of Human Nature</u> Oxford Univ. Pr., Oxford.
326. Huxley T.H., Huxley J. 1947 <u>Evolution and Ethics: 1893-1943</u> Pilot Press, London.
327. Hayakawa,T; Angata,T;. Lewis,A; Mikkelsen,T; Varki,N Varki1,A *A Human-Specific Gene in Microglia* Science 309 1693
328. Iacoboni Marco, Woods R, Brass M, Bekkering H, Mazziotta L, Rizzolatti Giacomo 1999 *Cortical Mechanisms of Human Imitation* Science 286 2526.
329. International Human Genome Sequencing Consortium 2001 *Initial sequencing and analysis of the human genome* Nature 409 15
330. Jackson Jean 1983 <u>The Fish People</u> Cambridge University Press, Cambridge.
331. Jay, Nancy 1992 <u>Throughout Your Generations Forever</u>, Univ. Chicago Pr., Chicago.
332. Jegalian, Karin and Lahn, Bruce 2001 *Why the Y* Scientific American Feb.
333. Jobling Mark, Tyler-Smith Chris 2003 *The human Y-chromosome: An evolutionary marker comes of age* Nature Reviews Genetics 4, 598 -612.
334. Johns S. E., et al. 2004 Proc. R. Soc. Lond. B.
335. Johnson, J., Canning, J., Kaneko, T., Pru, J.K., Tilly, J.L. 2004 Nature, 428, 145 - 150.
336. Johnson, Peter; Bannister, Anthony; Wannenburgh, Alf <u>The Bushmen</u> New Holland Publishing Cape Town.
337. Johnston W., Unrau P., Lawrence M., Glasner M., Bartel D. 2001 *RNA-catalysed RNA polymerization: Accurate and general RNA-templated primer extension* Science 292 1319-1325.
338. Jolly, Alison 1999 <u>Lucy's Legacy</u> Harvard University Press, Cambridge Mass.
339. Jones, Steve 1996 <u>In the Blood: God, Genes and Destiny</u>, Harper-Collns, London.
340. Jones, Steve 2002 <u>Y: The Descent of Men</u> Little Brown.
341. Josephus, Flavius 1987 <u>The works of Josephus : complete and unabridged</u> (trans. William Whiston) Hendrickson Publishers Peabody, Mass.
342. Jung, Carl 1963 <u>Memories, Dreams and Reflections</u>, Fontana, London.
343. Jusino Ramon K. 1998 <u>Mary Magdalene: Author of the Fourth Gospel?</u>.
344. Kandell E., Schwartz J., Jessel T. 2000 <u>Principles of Neural Science</u> McGraw Hill N.Y.
345. Karama, S Lecours, A Leroux,J Bourgouin, P Beaudoin,G Joubert, S Beauregard M 2002 *Areas of Brain Activation in Males and Females During Viewing of Erotic Film Excerpts* Human Brain Mapping 16:1–13.
346. Keaton W.T. 1980 <u>Biological Science</u> W.W. Norton & Co. N.Y.
347. Keverne E, Fundele R, Narasimha M, Braton S, Surani M 1996a *Genomic imprinting and differential roles of parental genomes in brain development* Developmental Brain Res. 92, 91-100.
348. Keverne E, MartelF, Nevison C. 1996b *Primate brain evolution: genetic and functional considerations* Proc. Royal Soc. Lond. Series B 262, 689-96.
349. Key Catherine, Aiello Leslie 2000 *A prisoners' dilemma model of the evolution of parental care* Folia Primatol 71 77-92.
350. Khodjakov, A. Rieder, C. Sluder, G. Cassels, G. Sibon O, Wang C 2002 *De novo formation of centrosomes in vertebrate cells arrested during S phase* J. Cell Biol., 158/ 7 1171–1181
351. Kimura, Doreen 1992 *Sex Differences in the Brain*, Scientific American, Sept 81.
352. Kinebuchi T, Kagawa W, Enomoto R, Tanaka K, Miyagawa K, Shibata T, Kurumizaka H, Yokoyama S 2004 *Structural Basis for Octameric Ring Formation and DNA Interaction of the Human Homologous-Pairing Protein Dmc1* Molecular Cell 14, 363-374.
353. King Chris 1978 *Unified field theories and the origin of life*, Univ. Auck. Math. Rept. Ser. 134.
354. King Chris 1982 *A model for the development of genetic translation*, Origins of Life 12 405-425.
355. King Chris 1989 *Dual-time supercausality*, Phys. Essays 2, 128 - 151.

356. King Chris 1990 *Did membrane electrochemistry precede translation?* Origins of Life Evol. Biosph. 20, 15.
357. King Chris 1991 *Fractal and Chaotic Dynamics in the Brain* Prog. Neurobiol. 36 279-308.
358. King Chris 1992 *Modular Transposition and the Dynamical Structure of Eukaryote Regulatory Evolution* Genetica 86 127-142.
359. King Chris 1996 *Fractal Neurodynamics and Quantum Chaos* in Fractals of Brain Fractals of Mind Adv. in Consciousness Research **7** (ed.) MacCormac E., Stamenov M. 179 - 233.
360. King Chris 1997 *Quantum mechanics, Chaos and the Conscious Brain* J. Mind and Behavior 18 155-170.
361. King Chris 2001 Codex of the Tree of Life WED Monographs 1 1-775 www.dhushara.com
362. King Chris 2002 *Biocosmology* WED Monographs 2 1-44 www.dhushara.com.
363. King Chris 2003 *Chaos, Quantum-transactions and Consciousness: A Biophysical Model of the Intentional Mind* NeuroQuantology 1 129-148.
364. King Chris 2005 *Cosmic Symmetry-breaking, Bifurcation, Fractality and Biogenesis* Neuro-Quantology 3 149-185.
365. King Chris 2005 *Quantum Cosmology and the Hard Problem of the Conscious Brain* in Towards a Physics of Consciousness Springer (to appear).
366. Kingsland James 2004 *Wonderful Spam* New Scientist 24 May 42-5
367. Kinzey W.G. 1987 *Monogamous primates: a primate model for human mating systems* in Kinzey W.G. (ed) The Evolution of Human Behavior: Primate Models State Univ. N.Y. Press, Albany.
368. Kirk K, Blomberg S, Duffy D, Heath A, Owens I Martin N 2001 *Natural selection and quantitative genetics of life history traits in western women: A twin study* Evolution, 55(2), 423–35.
369. Kirk-Smith M, Ebster K 2005 Psychology and Marketing DOI:10.1002/mar.20082.
370. Kirsch, S. Rappold G. et al. 2005 Genome Res. 15, 195-204.
371. Kluger Jeffery 2005 *The funny thing about laughter* Time 17 Jan 57
372. Knight A, Underhill P, Mortensen H, Zhivotovsky L, Lin A, Henn B, Louis D, Ruhlen M, Mountain J 2003 *African Y Chromosome and mtDNA Divergence Provides Insight into the History of Click Languages* Current Biology, 13, 464–473.
373. Knight, Chris 1991 Blood Relations: Menstruation and the Origins of Culture Yale University Press New Haven.
374. Knutson Brian 2004 *Sweet Revenge?* Science 305 1246-7.
375. Kohl James V. Francoeur Robert T. The Scent of Eros: Mysteries of Odor in Human Sexuality ISBN 0-8264-0677-7.
376. Komers P., Brotherton P. 1997 *Female space use is the best predictor of monogamy in mammals* Proc. R. Soc. Lond. B 264, 1261-70.
377. Kono T, Obata Y., Wu Q, Niwa K, One Y, Yamamoto Y, Park E Seo J, Ogawa H 2004 *Borth of parthenogenetic mice that can develop to adulthood* Nature 428 860-865.
378. Koryakova Ludmila 1998 *Sintashta-Arkaim Culture* http://www.csen.org/
379. Koryakova Ludmila 1998 *The Rise of Metallurgy in Eurasia* http://www.csen.org/
380. Kosfeld M, Heinrichs M, Zak P, Fischbacher U, Fehr E 2005 *Oxytocin increases trust in humans* Nature Vol 435/2 673-77 doi:10.1038/nature03701
381. Kraeling Emil 1953 The Brooklyn Museum Aramaic Papyri Yale University Press.
382. Kravchanka 1990 in Hans Blix (IAEA) *United Nations A General Assembly A/45/PV.32 Forty-fifth session Excerpts from the provisional verbatim record of the thirty-second meeting held at Headquarters, New York on Tuesday, 23 October 1990, at 10 a.m.*
383. Kraytsberg Y, Schwartz M, Brown T, Ebralidse K, Kunz W, Clayton D, Vissing J, Khrapko K 2004 *Recombination of Human Mitochondrial DNA* Science 304 98.
384. Krings M., Geisert H.,Schmitz R., Krainitzki H., Pääbo S 1999 *DNA sequence of the mitochondrial hypervariable region II from the Neandertal type specimen* Proc.Nat.Acad.Sci. 96 5581-5.
385. Kropotkin P. 1902 1972 Mutual Aid: A Factor of Evolution N.Y. Univ. Pr. N.Y.
386. Kuukasjärvi, Seppo, C. J. Peter Eriksson, Esa Koskela, Tapio Mappes, Kari Nissinen, and Markus J. Rantala. 2004. *Attractiveness of women's body odors over the menstrual cycle: the role of oral contraceptives and receiver sex.* Behavioral Ecology 15:579-584.
387. Lahdenpera M, Lummaa V, Helle S, Tremblay M, Russell A 2004 *Fitness benefits of prolonged post-reproductive lifespan in women* Nature 428 178.
388. Lancaster Jane 1977 *Sex roles in primate societies* in Teitlebaum M. (ed.) Sex Differences Doubleday NY, 51.
389. Larsen C.S. 2003 *Equality for the sexes in human hominid sexual dimorphism and implications for mating systems and social behavior* PNAS 100 16, 9103–9104.
390. Law, Sun Ping 1986 *The regulation of the menstrual cycle and its relatonship to the moon* Acta Obstetrica et Gynecologia Scandanavia 65:45-8.
391. Leahy Stephen 2003 Granny gorilla knows best New Scientist 15 Nov 12.
392. Leakey, Richard 1994 Origin of Humankind, Basic Books, New York.
393. Leakey Richard, Lewin Roger 1996 The Sixth Extinction, Weidenfield & Nicholson, London.
394. Lee, Richard, Daly Richard 2005 *Foragers and others* http://www.udel.edu/anthro/ackerman/

hunter.pdf
395. Lefkowitz Mary R 1986 Women in Greek Myth (repr.1990) Duckworth, London.
396. Lehninger Albert 1975 Biochemistry Worth, N.Y.
397. Lerner, Gerda 1986 The Creation of Patriarchy, Oxford University Press, New York.
398. Lerner, Robert 1972 The Heresy of the Free Spirit in the Later Middle Ages, University of California Press, Berkeley.
399. Le Vay, Simon 1991 *A difference in hypothalamc structure between heterosexual and homosexual men* Science 253 1034-7.
400. Lévi-Strauss Claude 1969 The Elementary Structures of Kinship Beacn Press Boston.
401. Lewis-Williams JD 1981 Believing and Seeing. Symbolic meanings in southern San rock Art Academic Pr. London.
402. Libet B. (1989) *The timing of a subjective experience* Behavioral Brain Sciences 12 183-5.
403. Lieberman, Philip 2000 Human Language and our Reptilian Brain: The Subcortical Bases of Speech, Syntax, and Thought. Harvard University Press, Cambridge, Mass.
404. Liebovitch L.S., Fischbarg J., Konairek J.P., Todorova I., Wang Mei, 1987, *Fractal model of ion-channel kinetics*, Biochim. Biophys. Acta 896, 173-180.
405. Liebovitch L.S., T. Toth 1991 *A model of ion channel kinetics using deterministic chaotic rather than stochastic processes* J. Theor. Biol. 148, 243-267.
406. Liedloff Jean 1975 The Continuum Concept Duckworth, London.
407. Liljenström Hans, Svedin Uno 2005 Micro-Meso-Macro Addressing Complex Systems Couplings Imperial College Press, Lond.
408. LimM, Ang Z, Olazábal1 D, Xianghui Ren X, Terwilliger E, Young L 2004 *Enhanced partner preference in a promiscuous species by manipulating the expression of a single gene* Nature, 429 754-7.
409. Llinás R., 1987 in Blakemore C., Greenfield S., Mindwaves Basil Blackwell, Oxford.
410. Lloyd Elizabeth 2005 The Case of the Female Orgasm: Bias in the Science of Evolution Harvard University Press, Boston.
411. Loebel David, Tam Patrick 2004 *Mice without a father* Nature 428 809-810.
412. Lloyds, Alun 1995 *Computing Bouts of the Prisoner's Dilemma*, Sci. Am. 272/6 80-83.
413. Lonsdorff Elizabeth, Eberly Lynn, Pusey Anne 2004 *Sex differences in learning in chimpanzees* Nature 428 715.
414. Lorber Judith 1994 Paradoxes of Gender Yale Univ. Pr. New Haven
415. Lorenz Konrad 1963 On Aggression Methuen London
416. Low, Bobbi Why Sex Matters 2000 Princeton University Press Princetion NJ.
417. Lyon Mary F. 2000 *LINE-1 elements and X chromosome inactivation: A function for "junk" DNA?* PNAS June 6, V 97/12.
418. Lythgoe, K. A. Read, A. F. 1998. *Catching the Red Queen? The advice of the rose.* Trends Ecol. Evol. 13: 473-474.
419. Mader Elker *Deviance, conflict and power in Shuar-achuar society.* http://www.univie.ac.at/voelkerkunde/theoretical-anthropology/mader.html
420. Maier Richard 1998 Comparative Animal Behavior: An evolutionary and ecological approach Allyn and Bacon, Boston.
421. Maier Walter 1986 Aserah : Extrabiblical Evidence, Scholars Press, Atlanta.
422. Majerus Michael 2003 Genes, bacteria and biased sex ratios. Princetion University Press.
423. Malamat, Abraham 1984 Mari and the Early Israelite Experience, Oxford Univ. Pr. Oxford.
424. Mallory JP 1989 In Search of the Indo-Europeans Thames and Hudson, London.
425. Mann Barbara 2000 Iroquoian Women: the Gantowisas Peter Lang, NY.
426. Marchington DR, Scott Brown MS, Lamb VK, van Golde RJ, Kremer JA, Tuerlings JH, Mariman EC, Balen AH, Poulton J.2002 *No evidence for paternal mtDNA transmission to offspring or extra-embryonic tissues after ICSI.* Mol Hum Reprod. Nov;8(11):1046-9. See also: Marchington, D.R. Scott-Brown, M. Balen, A.H. Lamb,V. Poulton J. *Paternal mtDNA is readily detectable in normal placenta* University of Oxford, Department of Paediatrics.
427. Margulis L., Sagan D. 1995 What is Life? Simon & Schuster, New York.
428. Margulis L., Schwartz K. 1982 Five Kingdoms. WH Freeman & Co.,N.Y.
429. Marks Jonathan 2002 What it Means to be 98% Chimpanzee: Apes, People and their Genes, Univ. Cal. Press, Berkeley.
430. Marlowe, F. 2002. *Why the Hadza are still hunter-gatherers.* In S. Kent (Ed.) Ethnicity, Hunter-gatherers, and the "Other": Association or Assimilation in Africa . Smithsonian Institution Press, Washington D.C. 247-275. http://www.fas.harvard.edu/~hbe-lab/
431. Marshack A 1972 The Roots of Civilization McGraw-Hill, NY
432. Marshall Lorna 1959 *Marriage among the !Kung bushmen* Africa 29 335-364.
433. Marshall Lorna 1976 The !Kung of Nyae Nyae Harvard Univ. Pr. Cambridge, Mass.
434. Marshall, W.F. and Rosenbaum, J.L. 1999. *Cell division: The renaissance of the centriole.* Curr. Biol. 9: R218–R220.
435. Marshall, W.F. and Rosenbaum, J.L. 2000. *Are there nucleic acids in the centrosome?* Curr. Top. Dev. Biol. 49: 187–205.
436. Martin Kay, Voohries Barbara 1975 Female of the Species Columbia Univ. Pr. NY.

437. Mason Betsy 2003 Biggest not always the daddy in mating game New Scientist 2 Aug.
438. Masters William, Johnson Virginia, Kolodny Robert1995 Human Sexuality 5 ed Harper-Collins.
439. Matthews Robert 1998 *Don't get even, get mad* New Scientist, 10 Oct 26-31.
440. Mazur, A. and Booth, A. 1997 *Testosterone and dominance in men.* Behavioural and Brain Sciences, 21, 353-386.
441. McCarter, P. Kyle, Jr. 1987. *Aspects of the Religion of the Israelite Monarchy: Biblical and Epigraphic Data*, 137-155, in Ancient Israelite Religion, ed. P.D. Miller, Jr., P.D. Hanson, and S.D. McBride. Philadelphia: Fortress.
442. McClintock Martha 1971 *Menstrual synchrony and suppression* Nature 229, 244.
443. McClintock Martha 1984 *Estrous synchrony: Modulation of ovarian cycle length by female pheromones* Physiology & Behavior 32, 701-5.
444. McComb Karen 2005 Proc. Royal. Soc. B DOI:10.1098/rsbl.2005.0366.
445. McDougall I., Brown F. H. & Fleagle J. G. 2005 Nature 433 733-73.
446. McElvaine, Robert 2001 Eve's Seed: Biology, the Sexes and the Course of History McGraw-Hill NY
447. McGinnis W., Kuziora M. 1994 *The molecular architects of body design* Scientific American Feb 36-43.
448. McGrath, J. and Solter, D. 1984. *Completion of mouse embryogenesis requires both maternal and paternal genomes.* Cell 37: 179-183.
449. McKenna Terrence 1992 Food of the Gods Rider, London.
450. McKenzie Constanze 2005 Environmental Health Perspectives DOI:10.1289.ehp.8479
451. McVean GT, Hurst LD. 1997 *Evidence for a selectively favourable reduction in the mutation rate of the X chromosome.* Nature Mar 27; **386**(6623):388-92
452. McWhorter John 2001 The Power of Babel Henry Holt, NY.
453. Mead Margaret 1968 Male and Female Laurel NY (1949 Morrow NY.)
454. Meadows, Robin 1995 *Sex and the Spotted Hyena* http://nationalzoo.si.edu/Publications/Zoo-Goer/1995/3/sexandthespottedhyena.cfm
455. Mekel-Bobrov,N; Gilbert, S; Evans,P; Vallender,E; Anderson,J; Hudson, R; Tishkoff,S Lahn B *Ongoing Adaptive Evolution of ASPM, a Brain Size Determinant in Homo sapiens* Science 309 1720-2
456. Mellaart, James 1967 Catal Huyuk, Thames & Hudson, London.
457. Menaker W, Menaker A.1959 *Lunar periodicity in human reproduction: A likely unit of biological time* Am. J. Obstetrics & Gynecology 77:905-14.
458. Merchant, Carolyn 1980 The Death of Nature, Wildwood House, London.
459. Mesnick S.L. 1997 *Sexual alliances: evidence and evolutionary implications* in Gowarty P (ed.) Feminism and Evolutionary Biology: Boundaries, Intersections and Frontiers Chapmann and Hall, N.Y.
460. Meyers Carol 1988 Discovering Eve Oxford Univ. Pr. Oxford.
461. Mi, S. and eleven others. 2000. *Syncytin is a captive retroviral envelope protein involved in human placental morphogenesis.* Nature 403: 785-789.
462. Migeon Barbara, Lee C, Chowdhury A, Carp H 2002 *Species Differences in TSIX/Tsix Reveal the Roles of These Genes in X-Chromosome Inactivation* Am. J. Hum. Genet. 71 286-293
463. Miles, Jack 1995 God, Simon & Schuster, London.
464. Miller, Geoffrey 2000 The Mating Mind Doubleday NY.
465. Mizutani H., Mikuni H., Takahasi M., Noda H. *Study of the photochemical reaction of HCN and its polymer products relating to primary chemical evolution* Origins of Life **6**, (1975), 513.
466. Moffitt Terrie 2002 Science 297 851.
467. Mohen Jean-Pierre 2002 Prehistoric Art: The Mythical Birth of Humanity Pierre Terrail. Paris.
468. Monteiro, Joanita, D., Vlietinck C, R. Kohn, N Lesser, M Gregersen P. 1998 *Commitment to X Inactivation Precedes the Twinning Event in Monochorionic MZ Twins* Am. J. Hum. Genet., 63:339-346.
469. Mookerjee, Ajit 1988 Kali The Feminine Force, Destiny Books , N.Y.
470. Moomjy Maureen, Colombero L, Veeck L., Rosenwaks Z. Palermo G. 1999 Sperm integrity is critical for normal mitotic division and early embryonic development Molecular Human Reproduction, Vol. 5, No. 9, 836-844, September.
471. Morgan Elaine 1982 The Aquatic Ape
472. Morgan Elaine 1986 The Descent of Woman
473. Morgan Elaine 2005 *Father Nature* New Scientist 27 Aug 38-41.
474. Morgan Lewis 1877 Ancient Society, or Researches in the Lines of Human Progress from Savagery, through Barbarism to Civilization Bharati Library Calcutta.
475. Morris, Desmond 1967 The Naked Ape McGraw-Hill, New York.
476. Morris, Desmond 1995 The Human Animal BBC/Discovery Channel, .
477. Morris, Desmond 1997 The Human Sexes: A natural history of man and woman Network, Lond.
478. Morris Desmond 2004 The Naked Woman: A study of the human body Jonathan Cape, Lond.

479. Morwood M. J., et al. 2004 Nature 431 1087-1091.
480. Motluk Alison 2001 *Read my mind* New Scientist 27 Jan 22
481. Motz Lotte 1997 Faces of the Goddess Oxford Univ. Press, Oxford.
482. Moyzis Robert 2005 Proc. of the Nat. Acad. Sci. DOI: 10.1073/pnas.0509691102)
483. Mukerjee Madhusree 1994 *Global Aid Wars* Scientific American November
484. Murphy Yolanda and Michael 1985 Women of the Forest Columbia University Pr., NY.
485. Mylonas, George 1961 Eleusis and the Eleusinian Mysteries, Princeton Univ. Pr., Princeton NJ.
486. Nachman MW, Crowell SL. 2000 *Estimate of the mutation rate per nucleotide in humans.* Genetics 156(1):297-304
487. Nakamura et al., 1997 *Telomerase Catalytic Subunit Homologs from Fission Yeast and Human,* Science 277 955-959.
488. Nedelcu, Victoria 2005 Proceedings of the Royal Society B, DOI: 10.1098/rspb.2005.3151
489. Negev, Abraham 1986 Nabatean Archaeology Today, NY Univ. Pr., New York.
490. Nelson Laura 2004 *Chimp chromosome creates puzzles: First sequence is unexpectedly different from human equivalent* Nature News 27 May.
491. Nielsen R et. al. 2005 Public Library of Science Biology v3, issue 6.
492. Nisbett R, Cohen D 1996 Culture of Honour: The Psychology of Violence in the South Harper-Collins NY.
493. Norberg Karen 2004 *Baby sex link to domestic status* BBC 20 Oct, 02:06 GMT (see Proceedings of The Royal Society).
494. Nordfjäll Katarina et. al. 2005 Proc. Nat. Acad. Sci. DOI: 10.1073/pnas.0501724102.
495. Nowak Martin A., May Robert M. Sigmund Karl, 1995 *The Arithmetic of Mutual Help*, Scientific American, 272/, 50-55.
496. Nowak Martin, Krakauer D. 1999 *The evolutionary language game* J. Theor. Biol. 200 147-62.
497. Nowak Martin, Krakauer D. 1999 *The evolution of language* PNAS 96 8028-33
498. Nowak Martin, Komarova N. 2001 *The evolution of universal grammar* Science 291 114-8.
499. Nowak M., Sigmund K. 2004 *Evolutionary dynamics of biological games* Science 303 793.
500. Occhiogrosso, Peter 1996 The Joy of Sects, Doubleday, NY.
501. O'Flaherty, Wendy 1981 The Rig Veda, Penguin, Harmondsworth.
502. O'Grady, Kathleen 1999 *Contraception and religion* in Young, Serinity The Encyclopedia of Women in World Religion Macmillan, NY.
503. O'Prey, Paul 1982 In Broken Images, Graves Letters, Hutchinson, London.
504. O'Prey, Paul 1984 Between Moon and Moon, Graves Letters 1946-1972, Hutchinson, London.
505. Ortner Sherry 1979 *Is female to male as nature is to culture?* in Rosaldo M and Lamphere L Woman, Culture and Society Stanford Univ. Pr. Stanford 67-88.
506. Ortner, Sherry 1996 Making gender: the politics and erotics of gender Beacon Press Boston.
507. Osborne Lawrence 1997 The women warriors: for decades, scholars have searched for ancient matriarches. Will they ever find one? Lingua Franca Inc. http://www.icubed.com/~ljg/wwarriors.html
508. Osborne Lawrence 2005 Letter from New Guinea New Yorker Apr 18 124-41
509. Ostermeier G, Miller D, .Huntriss J, Diamond M, Krawetz S (2004) Delivering spermatozoan RNA to the oocyte Nature 429, 154.
510. Otto, Walter 1965 Dionysus Myth and Cult, Spring Pubs., Dallas.
511. Pagels, Elaine 1979 The Gnostic Gospels, Random House, N.Y.
512. Pagels, Elaine 1988 Adam Eve and the Serpent, Random House, N.Y.
513. Pagels, Elaine 1995 The Origin of Satan, Random House, N.Y.
514. Pagels, Elaine 2003 Beyond Belief: The Secret Gospel of Thomas, Random House, N.Y.
515. Pagels Heinz 1988 The Dreams of Reason: The Computer and the Rise of the Sciences of Complexity Simon and Schuster.
516. Panchanathan Karthik, Boyd Robert 2004 *Indirect reciprocity can stabilize cooperation without the second-order free rider problem* Nature 432 499-502.
517. Pasternak, Ember C, Ember M 1997 Sex, Gender and Kinship - A Cross Cultural Perspective, Prentice Hall, New Jersey.
518. Pattanaik Devdutt 2003 Indian Mythology Tales, Symbols and Rituals from the Heart of the Subcontinent Inner Traditions, Rochester VT.
519. Pearsall Paul 1994 Sexual Healing : Using the Power of an Intimate, Loving Relationship to Heal Your Body and Soul Crown.
520. Peitgen Heinz-Otto, Jürgens H, Saupe D 2004 Chaos and fractals : new frontiers of science Springer NY.
521. Peitgen Heinz, Saupe D, Barnsley M 1988 The Science of fractal images Springer-Verlag NY.
522. Pellegrini Anthony, Long Jeffrey 2003 *A sexual selection theory longitudinal analysis of sexual segregation and integration in early adolescence* J. Exp. Child Psychology 85 257–278.
523. Penrose R. 1989 The Emperor's New Mind, Oxford University Press.
524. Penrose, R. 1994 Shadows of the Mind. Oxford : Oxford University Press.
525. Peplow Mark 2004 *Giant virus qualifies as 'living organism'* Nature news 14 October 2004 doi:10.1038/
526. Phillips Helen, Singer Emily 2003 *Hungry for love* New Scientist 22 Nov 18

527. Phillips, Kim 2003 Medieval maidens : young women and gender in England, 1270-1540 Manchester Univ. Press NY
528. Pierce Fred 2002 *Population Crash?* New Scientist 20 July.
529. Pierson Roger et. al. 2003 Fertility and Sterility 80 116.
530. Pilcher Helen 2004 *Could we defeat the menopause?* Nature News 1 Jul.
531. Pinker, Steven (1994) The Language Instinct : How the Mind Creates Language, Penguin.
532. Pinker, Steven (2002) The Blank Slate Penguin Viking, N.Y.
533. Pinker, Steven (2003) *Language as an adaption to the cognitive niche* in Christiansen Morten, Kirby Simon (ed.) 2003 Language Evolution, Oxford University Press 16-37.
534. Pipes, Daniel 1999 *Lessons from the Prophet Muhammad's Diplomacy Midde East Quarterly* 6/3
535. Pizzari Tommaso et. al. Current Biology (vol 15 p 1222)
536. Pizzari Tommaso et. al. Nature (vol 426, p 70).
537. Porrit, Jonathan 1991 Save the Earth, Harper-Collins, London.
538. Power Camilla, Watts Ian 1996 *Female strategies and collective behavior* in The archaeology of human ancestry : power, sex, and tradition ed. Steele J. and Shennan S. Routledge.
539. Preti, G., W.B. Cutler, A.Kreiger, G. Huggins, C.R. Garcia and H.J. Lawley 1986 *Human Axillary Secretions Influence Women's Menstrual Cycles:The role of donor extract from women.* Hormones and Behavior 20 474-482.
540. Pribram, Karl (ed.) 1993 Rethinking neural networks : quantum fields and biological data Erlbaum, Hillsdale, N.J.
541. Prigogine Ilya 1997 The end of certainty : time, chaos, and the new laws of nature Free Press NY.
542. Pritchard, James ed. 1974 Solomon and Sheba, Phaidon, N.Y.
543. Prusinkiewicz P., Lindenmayer 1990 The Algorithmic Beauty of Plants Springer-Verlag.
544. Puck JM, Stewart CC, Nussbaum RL 1992 *Maximum-likelihood analysis of human T-cell X chromosome inactivation patterns: normal women versus carriers of X-linked severe combined immunodeficiency.* Am J Hum Genet. Apr;50(4):742-8.
545. Purohit, Shree Swami 1935 The Geeta, Faber, London.
546. Purohit, Shree Swami 1938 Bhagwan Shree Patanjali Aphorisms of Yoga, Faber, London.
547. Purohit, Shree Swami, Yeats W..B. 1937 The Ten Principal Upanishads, Faber, London.
548. Pusey, Anne 2001 *Of genes and apes: chimpanzee social organization and reproduction* in de Waal Frans (ed.) Tree of Origin, Harvard Univ. Pr. Camb. MA.
549. Rafiqul-Haqq M., Newton P. 1996 The Place of Women in Pure Islam http://debate.domini.org/newton/womeng.html
550. Rahman, Qazi 2005 Behavioral Neuroscience 119 311.
551. Ranke-Heinmann, Uta 1988 Eunuchs for Heaven, Andre Deutsch, Hamburg.
552. Ranke-Heinmann, Uta 1992 Putting Away Childish Things, Harper, San Francisco.
553. Raoult D., et al. 2004 Science, doi:10.1126/science.1101485
554. Rawson, Philip 1973 Tantra The Indian cult of Ecstasy Thames and Hudson, London.
555. Rawson P., Legeza L. 1973 Tao The Chinese Philosophy of Time and Change, Thames and Hudson, London.
556. Reichel-Dolmatoff Gerardo 1971 Amazonian Cosmos: The sexual and religious symbolism of the Tukano Indians Univ. Chicago Press, Chicago.
557. Reichel-Dolmatoff Gerardo 1978 Beyond the milky way: Hallucinatory imagery of the Tukano indians UCLA Latin American Center Pubs. LA.
558. Reinach, Salomon 1931 Orpheus, George Routledge & Sons. London.
559. Reiter, R.J. 1972 *The role of the pineal in reproduction.* In: Balin, H. and S. Glass (eds.) Reproductive Biology. Excerpta Medica, New York.
560. Reno P, Meindl R, McCollum M, Lovejoy Owen 2003 *Sexual dimorphism in Australopithecus afarensis was similar to that of modern humans* PNAS 100/16 9404–9409.
561. Reynolds Wanda 1995 Proc. Nat. Acad. of Sci 92, 8229
562. Rice Willian 1996 *Sexually antagonistic male adaption triggered by experimental arrest of female evolution* Nature 381 232-4.
563. Rice W and Holland *The enemies within: intergenomic conflict, interlocus contest evolution (ICE), and the intraspecific Red Queen.*
564. Ridley, Matt 1993 The Red Queen, Penguin, London
565. Ridley, Matt 1996 The Origins of Virtue, Penguin Viking
566. Ridley, Matt 1999 Genome: An autobiography of a species in 23 chapters. Fourth Estate, London.
567. Ridley, Matt 2003 Nature via Nurture Fourth Estate GB, Harper-Collins NY.
568. Riedlinger, Thomas.ed. 1990 The Sacred Mushroom Seeker Diascorides Press, Portland, Or.
569. Riedlinger, Thomas 1996 *Pentecostal Elements in RG Wasson's accounts of the Mazatec mushroom velada,* Shaman's Drum, 43, 26-35.
570. Rilling James, Gutman D, Zeh T, Pagnoni G, Berns Gregory, Kilts C 2004 *A Neural Basis for Social Cooperation* Neuron, 35 395-405.
571. Rizzolatti G, Fadiga L, Fogassi L, Gallese V. 1996 *Premotor cortex and the recognition of*

motor actions. Cogn. Brain Res. 3:131–41
572. Rizzolatti Giacomo, Arbib Michael 1998 *Language within our grasp* Trends in Neuroscience 21/5, 188-94.
573. Rizzolatti Giacomo, Craighero Laila 2004 *The mirror neuron system* Annual Rev. Neurosci. 2004. 27:169-92.
574. Roberts Jani Farrell. 2000 <u>Seven Days: Tales of Magic, Sex and Gender</u> http://www.macha.f9.co.uk/7_Days_intro.html
575. Robbins L et. al. 2005 Current Anthropology, vol 46, p 671.
576. Robinson, James ed. 1990 <u>The Nag Hammadi Library</u>, Harper, S.F.
577. Rohde D. L. T, Olson S. & Chang J. T. 2004 *Modelling the recent common ancestry of all living humans* Nature, 431, 562- 565.
578. Ross, Mark et.al. 2005 The DNA sequence of the human X chromosome Nature 434. 325 - 337.
579. Rothenberg, Beno 1972 <u>Timna: Valley of the Biblical Copper Mines</u>, Thames & Hudson, London.
580. Roughgarden Joan 2004 <u>Evolution's Rainbow: Diversity, gender and sexuality in nature and people</u> Univ. California Press.
581. Rouse G. W., Goffredi S. K., Vrijenhoek R. C. 2004 Science, 305. 668 - 671.
582. Rozen S, Skaletsky H, Marszalek J, Minx P, Cordum H, Waterston R, Wilson R, Page D 2003 *Abundant gene conversion between arms of palindromes in human and ape Y chromosomes* Nature 423, 873 - 876.
583. Rozzi Fernando, Bermudez de Castro Jose 2004 *Surprisingly rapid growth in Neanderthals* Nature 428 936.
584. Rudgley, Richard 1993 <u>The Alchemy of Culture</u>, British Museum Press, London.
585. Ruether, Rosemary Radford 1992 <u>Gaia and God</u> Harper Collins San Francisco.
586. Ruether, Rosemary Radford 2000 <u>Christianity and the Making of the Modern Family</u> Beacon Press Boston.
587. Rushdie, Salman 1988 <u>The Satanic Verses</u>, Penguin, London.
588. Rushton Philipe 2004 DOI:10.1098/rspb.2004.2941
589. Russell, Bertrand 1902 <u>Free Man's Worship in Mysticism and Logic</u> Anchor Books NY 1957.
590. Ruthen, R. 1993 *Adapting to Complexity* Scientific American, 268, 110-117.
591. Sachedina, Abdulaziz 1981 <u>Islamic Messianism</u>, State Univ. N.Y. Pr., Albany.
592. Sachs Jeffery 2003 *No place for piety* New Scientist 8 Nov 19.
593. Sado T, Wang Z, Sasaki H Li E 2001 *Regulation of imprinted X-chromosome inactivation in mice by Tsix Development* 128/8 1275-1286
594. Sampson Geoffrey 1997 <u>Educating Eve</u> Cassel, London.
595. Samuel E. 2001 *Seeing the seeds of cancer* New Scientist 24 Mar 42-45.
596. Sanday, Peggy Reeves 1981 <u>Female Power and Male Dominance: On the Origins of Sexual Inequality</u> Cambridge Univ. Pr., Cambridge.
597. Sanday, Peggy Reeves 2002 <u>Women at the Center : Life in a Modern Matriarchy</u>. Cornell University Press Ithaca, NY.
598. Sapolsky Robert, Share Lisa 2004 Plos Biology.
599. Sathananthan, AH Ratnam, SS Ng SC, Tarin JJ , Gianaroli L.and Trounson A 1996 The sperm centriole: its inheritance, replication and perpetuation in early human embryo Human Reproduction, Vol 11, 345-356.
600. Savage-Rumbaugh, S. Shanker, S.G. Taylor, T.J. (1998). <u>Apes, Language, and the Human Mind</u>. Oxford University Press. New York.
601. Savic I. et. al. 2005 Proc. Nat. Acad. of Sci. DOI: 10.1073/pnas.0407998102.
602. Schmid C. 1998 *Does SINE evolution preclude Alu function?* Nucleic Acids Research 26 4541-4550.
603. Schneebaum Tobias 1969 <u>Keep the River on Your Right</u> Abacus.
604. Schneebaum, T. 1988 <u>Where the spirits dwell: An odyssey in the New Guinea jungle</u>, Grove Weidenfeld, New York.
605. Schneider Jutta M. Lubin Yael 1998 *Intersexual conflict in spiders* OIKOS 83: 496-506. Copenhagen.
606. Schneider Jutta M. Herberstein M., de Crespigny D. Ramamurthy S, Elgar Mark 2000 *Sperm competition and small size advantage for males of the golden orb-web spider* Nephila edulis J . Evol . B iol. 13 939-46.
607. Schneider Jutta M Elgar Mark 2002 *Sexual cannibalism in Nephila plumipes as a consequence of female life history strategies* J . Evol . B iol. 15 84-91.
608. Schneider Jutta M Elgar Mark 2001 *Sexual cannibalism and sperm competition in the golden orb-web spider Nephila plumipes (Araneoidea): female and male perspectives* Behavioral Ecology 12/5: 547–52.
609. Scholem, Gershom 1962, 1991 <u>On the Mystical Shape of the Godhead</u>, Schoken Books NY.
610. Schonfield, Hugh 1965 <u>The Passover plot : new light on the history of Jesus</u>, Hutchinson, Lond.
611. Schroeder Manfred 1991 <u>Fractals, chaos, power laws: minutes from an infinite paradise</u> W.H.

Freeman NY.

612. Schultes Richard Evans, Hofmann Albert 1979 Plants of the Gods, McGraw Hill, N.Y., Reprint Alfred Van Der Marck.

613. Schultes R. E., Hofmann A. 1980 Botany and Chemistry of the Hallucinogens, Charles Thomas, Springfield IL.

614. Schultes R.É. and Raffauf R. 1989 Vine of the Soul Synergetic Press, Oracle AZ.

615. Schuster H.J. 1986 Deterministic Chaos Springer-Verlag Berlin.

616. Schwartz, Regina 1996 The Curse of Cain: The Violent Legacy of Monotheism, University of Chicago Press, Chicago.

617. Schwenk Theodor 1962 Sensitive Chaos, Rudolf Steiner Press, London.

618. Segal J.B. 1963 The Sabian Mysteries in Vanished Civilizations ed. Edward Bacon, Thames & Hudson, London.

619. Segal J.B.1970 Edessa'The Blessed City', Clarendon Press, Oxford.

620. Seielstad M, Minch E, Cavalli-Sforza L 1998 Genetic evidence for a higher female migration rate in humans Nature Genetics 20/3 278-80.

621. Shad, Abdul 1986 From Adam to Muhammad, Noor Publishing, Delhi.

622. Shah, Idries 1968 The Way of the Sufi, Jonathan Cap, London.

623. Shaywitz, B. A. and S.E. Pugh K, Constable R Skudlarski P Fulbrght R Bronen R, Fletcher J Shankweller D, Katz L Gore J 1995, Sex differences in the functional organization of the brain for language. Nature 373, 607-609.

624. Sherfey Mary 1966 The Nature and Evolution of Female Sexuality Vintage / Random House, NY.

625. Shlain Leonard 2003 Sex, Time and Power: How women's sexuality shaped evolution, Penguin Viking NY

626. Shostak, Marjorie 1981 Nisa, Harvard Univ. Pr., Boston.

627. Shostak, Marjorie 2000 Return to Nisa, Harvard Univ. Pr., Boston.

628. Shreeve James 1995 The Neanderthal Enigma: Solving the Mystery of Modern Human Origins, Vol. 1. Morrow,William & Co.

629. Silver, Lee 1999 Remaking Eden: Cloning and Beyond in a Brave New World, Avon Books, Phoenix, London.

630. Simmons Leigh, Kilgallon Sarah 2005 Biology Letters doi:10.1098/rsbl.2005.0324

631. Singer T, Seymour B, O'Doherty J, Stephan K, Dolan R, Frith C 2006 Empathic neural responses are modulated by the perceived fairness of others Nature doi:10.1038/nature04271.

632. Skaletsky H, Kuroda-Kawaguchi T, Minx P, Cordum H, Hillier L, Brown L, Repping S, Pynktikova T, Ali J, Bier T, Chinwalla A, Delehaunty K, Di H, Fewell G, Fulton L, Fulton R, Graves T, Hou S, Latrielle P, Leonard S, Mardis E, Maupin R, McPherson J, Miner T, Nash W, Nguyen C, Ozersky P, Pepin K, Rock S, Rohlfng T, Scott K, Schultz B, Strong C, Tin-Wollam A, Yang S, Waterston R, Wilson R, Rozen S, Page D 2003 The male-specific region of the human Y chromosome is a mosaic of discrete sequence classes Nature 423, 825 - 837.

633. Skarda C.J., Freeman W.J., (1987), How brains make chaos in order to make sense of the world, Behavioral and Brain Sciences 10, 161-195.

634. Small Meredith 1999 A Woman's Curse? The Sciences Jan/Feb 24-29.

635. Smith, W. Robinson 1888 , 1972 The Religion of the Semites, Schoken Books, N.Y.

636. Smolin, Lee 1997 The Life of the Cosmos, Oxford University Press, N.Y.

637. Smuts, Barbara 1992. Male aggression against women. Human Nature 3: 1-44.

638. Smuts, Barbara 1995. The Evolutionary Origins of Patriarchy. Human Nature 6 1-32.

639. Snow L. S. E. & Andrade M. C. B. 2005 Proc R. Soc. Lond. B, doi:10.1098/rspb.2005.3088.

640. Soros George 1997 The Capitalist Threat The Atlantic Monthly; 279/2 Feb 45-58.

641. Sparks John 1999 Battle of the Sexes: The Natural History of Sex TV Books LLC NY.

642. Spector et. al. 2005 Biology Letters, DOI: 10.1098/rsbl.2005.0308

643. Sperling, Susan. 1991. Baboons with Briefcases Vs. Langurs in Lipstick. In Micaela di Leonardo, ed., Gender at the Crossroads of Knowledge: Feminist Antbropology in the Postmodern Era, Berkeley: University of California Press, 204-234.

644. Spong, John 1992 Born of a Woman Harper, San Francisco.

645. Spong, John 1994 Resurrection Myth or reality? Harper Collins San Francisco.

646. Stamets, Paul 1983 The Mushroom Cultivator, Agaricon Press, Olympia, WA.

647. Stamets, Paul 1996 Psilocybe Mushrooms of the World, Ten Speed Press, Berkeley.

648. Starbird, Margaret 1993 The Woman with the Alabaster Jar, Bear & Co., Santa Fe, New Mexico.

649. Starbird, Margaret 1998 The Goddess in the Gospels, Bear & Company, Santa Fe, New Mexico.

650. Steele J. and Shennan S. ed. 1996 The archaeology of human ancestry : power, sex, and tradition ed. Routledge.

651. Steinmann, Jean1964 Saint John the Baptist, Harpers & Bros., New York.

652. Stewart, Desmond 1980 Mecca, Newsweek N.Y.

653. Stoehr, Taylor 1979 Free Love in America AMS Press N.Y.

654. Stone, Linda 1997 Kinship and Gender, Westview Press, Harper-Collins, Boulder

528

655. Storey A, Walsh C, Quinton R, Wynne-Edwards k 2005 *Hormonal correlates of paternal responsiveness in new and expectant fathers* Evolution and Human Behavior 21 79–95.
656. Strate J.M. 1982 An Evolutionary View of Political Culture Ph.D. Univ. Michigan
657. Strassmann Beverly 1993 *Menstrual hut vsits by Dogon Women: A hormonal test distinguishes deceit from honest signalling.* Behavioral Ecology 7/3 304-15.
658. Strassmann Beverly 1997 *Polygyny as a risk factor for child mortality among the Dogon* Current Anthropology 38 688-95.
659. Strassmann Beverly , Warner John 1998 *Predictors of fecundability and conception among the Dogon of Mali* American Journal of Physical Anthropology 105 167-84.
660. Strier Karen 2001 *Beyond the apes: Reasons to consider the entre primate order* in de Waal Frans (ed.) Tree of Órigin, Harvard Univ. Pr. Camb. MA.
661. Surani, M. A. H., Barton, S. C. and Norris, M. L. 1984. *Development of reconstituted mouse eggs suggests imprinting of the genome during gametogenesis.* Nature 308: 548-550.
662. Swaab D, Fliers E. 1985 *A sexually dimorphic nucleus in the human brain.* Science 228 1112–5.
663. Swami Anilantha 2002 *Till death us do part* New Scientist 29 Jun.
664. Sykes Bryan 2002 The Seven Daughters of Eve W W Norton, NY.
665. Symons, Donald. 1979. The Evolution of Human Sexuality. New York: Oxford University Press.
666. Szalavitz Mala 2003 *Hungry for love* New Scientist 22 nov 18
667. Szalavitz Mala 2002 *Love is the drug* New Scientist 23 Nov
668. Tatz Mark, Kent Jody 1977 Rebirth Anchor Press, Doubleday NY.
669. Taylor, Anne Christine *The Gender of the Prey* http://lhomme.revues.org/document35.html
670. Taylor, Timothy 1996 The Prehistory of Sex: Four million years of human sexual culture Bantam, NY.
671. Tchénio T., Casella J-F, Heidmann T., 2000 *Members of the SRY family regulate LINE retrotransposons* Nuc. Acid Res. 28/2 411-425.
672. Ten Raa E. 1969 *The moon as a symbol of lif and fertility in Sandaawe thought* Africa 29 24-53.
673. Thom Rene 1972 Structural Stability and Morphogenesis W.A. Benjamin, Teading, Mass.
674. Thomson, J. A. and Solter, D. 1989. *The developmental fate of androgenetic, parthenogenetic, and gynogenetic cells in chimeric gastrulating mouse embryos.* Genes Dev. 2: 1344-1351.
675. Thompson, William Irwin 1981 The Time Falling Bodies Take to Light, St. Martin's Press, NY.
676. Thornhill, Randy, and N. Thornhill. 1983. *Human Rape: An Evolutionary Analysis.* Ethnology and Sociobiology 4: 137.
677. Thornhill Randy and Palmer Craig 2000 A Natural History of Rape: Biological Bases for Sexual Coercion MIT Press Cambridge Mass.
678. Tidwell John 2004 *The wilder side of sex* http://nationalzoo.si.edu/Publications/ZooGoer/2004/2/wildersideofsex.cfm
679. Tishkoff Sarah, Verrelli Brian 2003 *Patterns of Human Genetic Diversity: Implications for Human Evolutionary History and Disease* Annu. Rev. Genomics Hum. Genet. 4:293–340.
680. Tobias, P. 1971. The Brain in Hominid Evolution. Columbia University Press. New York.
681. Traunmüller Hartmut 2003 *Clicks and the idea of a human protolanguage* http://www.ling.umu.se/fonetik2003/
682. Travis Cheryl Brown (ed.) 2003 Evolution, Gender and Rape Ed MIT Press Cambridge, Mass.
683. Treloar, A.E., R.E. Boynton, D.G. Behn and B.W. Brown 1967 *Variations of the human menstrual cycle through reproductive life.* Int. J. Fertil. 12:777-126
684. Treloar, A.E. 1981 *Menstrual cyclicity and the premenopause.* Maturitas. 3:249-264.
685. Trelogan Stephanie, Martin Sandra 1995 *Tightly regulated developmentally specific expression of the first open reading frame from LINE-1 during mouse embryogenesis* Proc Nat Acad Sci 92 1520 .
686. Trevett, Christine 1996 Montanism, Cambridge Univ. Pr., Cambridge.
687. Tribble, Phyllis 1973 Eve and Adam, Genesis 2-3 reread. Anover Newton Quarterly 13, 251.
688. Tribble, Phyllis 1978 God and the Rhetoric of Sexuality, Fortress Press, Philadelphia.
689. Trivers, Robert 1971 *The evolution of reciprocal altruism* Quart. Rev. Biol. 46/4 35-57.
690. Trivers, Robert 1972 *Parental investment and sexual selection* in Sexual Selection and the Descent of man - 1871-1981 (ed. B Campbell) Aldine Chcago 136-79.
691. Trivers R, Willard D. 1973 *Natural selection of parentalability to vary the sex ratio of offspring* Science 179, 90-2.
692. True H. L., Berlin I. & Lindquist S. L. Nature, 430, doi:10.1038/nature02885 (2004).
693. Turchin Peter 2005 War & Peace & War : The Life Cycles of Imperial Nations Pi Press.
694. Turnbull, C. M. (1961). The forest people. New York: Simon & Schuster.
695. Turnbull, C. M. (1983). The Mbuti pygmies: Change and adaptation. New York: CBS College Publishing.
696. Turner, Gillian 1996 *Intelligence and the X-chromosome*, Lancet 347 1814.
697. Underhill P, Shen P, LinA, Jin L, PassarinoG, Yang W, Kauffman E, Bonné-Tamir B, Bertranpetit J, Francalacci P, Ibrahim M, Jenkins T, Kidd J, Mehdi S, Seielstad M, Wells R. Spencer ,

Piazza A, Davis R, Feldman M, Cavalli-Sforza L, Oefner P 2000 *Y chromosome sequence variation and the history of human populations* nature genetics 26 361.
698. Underhill P, Passarino G, LinA, Shen P, Mirazo M, Lahr N, Foley R, Oefner P, Cavalli-Sforza L, 2001 *The phylogeography of Y chromosome binary haplotypes and the origins of modern human populations* Ann. Hum. Genet., 65, 43-62
699. United Nations Development Programme 2000, 1999, 1998 Human Development Report Oxford University Press New York.
700. Up De Graff F. 1925 Head hunters of the Amazon: Seven Years of Exploration and Adventure, Garden City, New York:
701. van der Post, Laurens and Taylor, Jane Testament to the Bushmen Penguin Books, UK.
702. Van Valen, L. 1973. *A new evolutionary law.* Evol. Theory 1: 1-30.
703. Vollman, R.F. 1968 *The length of premenstrual phase by age of women.* in: Proceedings of the Fifth World Congress on Fertility and Sterility, Stockholm, Amsterdam, Excerpta Medica International Congress Series No.133 pp.1171-1175
704. Vollman, R.F. 1970 *Conception rates by days of the menstrual cycles, BBT, and outcome of pregnancy.* Sixth World Congress of Gynecology and Obstetrics of the International Federation of Gynecology and Obstetrics, New York, Abstracts, Williams and Wilkins, Baltimore No.112
705. Vollman R.F. 1977 *The Menstrual Cycle.* In: Major Problems of Obstetrics and Gynecology. W.B. Saunders, Philadelphia.
706. Waite, A.E. 1992 The Holy Kabbalah Carol Publishing Group, NY.
707. Waldrop Mitchell 1993 Complexity Penguin
708. Walker, Barbara 1983 The Woman's Encyclopedia of Myths and Secrets, Harper & Row, SF.
709. Walker Barbara 1986 The I-Ching of the Goddess Harper & Row NY.
710. Walker, Benjamin 1983 Gnosticism: Its History and Influence, The Aquarian Press, Wellingsborough UK.
711. Walker, E.H. 1977 *Quan tum mechanical tunneling in synaptic and ephaptic transmission* In t. J. Quan t. Chem. 11 ,103–127.
712. Walther, Wiebke 1981 Women in Islam, Marcus Wiener, Princeton.
713. Warner, Rex (fwd)1975 Encyclopedia of World Mythology Octopus, London.
714. Warren W. 1998 *MR Imaging contrast enhancement based on intermolecular zero quantum coherences* Science 281 247.
715. Washburn Sherwood and DeVoire Irven 1961 *Socal behavior of baboons and early man* in Washburn S. (ed.) The Social Life of Early Man Aldine, Chicago.
716. Wasson, Gordon 1972 *The Divine Mushroom of Immortality* in Furst P. Flesh of the Gods Ed. Praeger N.Y.
717. Wasson, Gordon 1972 *What was the Soma of the Aryans?* in Furst P. Flesh ofthe Gods Ed. Praeger N.Y.
718. Wasson, Gordon 1986 Persephone's Quest: Entheogens and the Origins of Religion, Yale Univ. Pr., New Haven CT
719. Watanabe H. and the International Chimpanzee Chromosome 22 Consortium 2004 *DNA sequence and comparative analysis of chimpanzee chromosome 22* Nature 429 382-388.
720. Watson J, Hopkin N, Roberts J, Steitz J, Weiner A 1987 Molecular Biology of the Gene Benjamin/Cummings Menlo Park CA 4th Ed.
721. Watson, Lyall 1995 Dark Nature, Hodder and Stoughton, London. 47, 51, 96.
722. Watt,W Montgomery 1953 Muhammad at Mecca, Clarendon Pr., Oxford.
723. Weil, Gunther, Metzner Ralph, Leary Timothy 1965 The Psychedelic Reader, University Books, NY.
724. Westphal Sylvia P. 2003 *Embryonic stem cells turned into eggs* New Scientist 1 may.
725. Westphal Sylvia P 2004 *The rush to pick a perfect embryo* New Scientist 12 Jul 6-7.
726. White J. 1990 *Viral and cellular membrane fusion proteins.* Annu Rev Physiol 52, 675-97.
727. White Lynn Jr 1967 *The Historical Roots of Our Ecolgic Crisis,* Science 155 10 Mar 1203.
728. Whiten Andrew, Byrne Richard 1988 *Tactical deception in primates* Behavioral and Brain Sciences 11: 233-44.
729. Whiten Andrew, Byrne Richard eds. 1997 Machiavellian Intelligence II Cambridge University Press, Cambridge.
730. Whiting John and Beatrice 1975 *Aloofness and intimacy of husbands and wives* Ethos 3 183-207.
731. Wilde, Oscar 1915 Salome, John Lane Coy. N.Y.
732. Wilhelm, Richard (trans) 1951 I Ching, or Book of Changes Routledge & Kegan Paul, London.
733. Wilhelm, Richard (trans) 1931 The Secret of the Golden Flower, Routledge & Kegan Paul, Lond.
734. Willis R. Ed. 1993 World Mythology RD Press Australia
735. Wills, Christopher 1999 Children of Promethius Perseus Publishing.
736. Wilson, Edmund 1969 The Dead Sea Scrolls, 1947-1969, W. H. Allen, London.
737. Wilson, Edward O. 1981 *The relation of science to theology,* Zygon 15, 425-34.
738. Wilson, Edward O. 1980 Sociobiology: The New Synthesis, Harvard Univ. Pr., Cambridge,

MA.
739. Wilson, Edward O. 1992 <u>The Diversity of Life</u>, Penguin Books London.
740. Wilson, Edward O. 1981 *The relation of science to theology*, Zygon 15, 425-34.
741. Wilson, Ian 1996 <u>Jesus The Evidence</u>, Weddenfield and Nicholson.
742. Witzel Michael, <u>The Home of the Aryans</u> Harvard Boston.
743. Wolfe, Stephen L. 1972 <u>Biology of the Cell</u>,Wadsworth Pub. Coy. Belmont CA.
744. Wolfsberg TG, Bazan JF, Blobel CP, Myles DG, Primakoff P, White JM. 1993. *The precursor region of a protein active in sperm-egg fusion contains a metalloprotease and disintegrin domain.* Proc Natl Acad Sci 90 : 10783-10787.
745. Wolfram, Stephen 2002 <u>A new kind of science</u> Wolfram Media Champaign, IL.
746. Wolfson Richard, Pasachoff Jay 1987 <u>Physics</u> Little Brown & Co.Boston.
747. Wolkenstein, D., Kramer S. 1987 <u>Inanna Queen of Heaven and Earth</u>, Harper & Row, N.Y.
748. Woolley, Sir Leonard 1938 <u>Ur of the Chaldees</u>, Pelican Books, London.
749. Woolley, Sir Leonard 1954 <u>Excavations at Ur</u>, Ernest Benn, Ltd., London.
750. Wrangham R; Peterson D 1996 <u>Demonic Males: Apes and the Evolution of Human Aggresson</u> , Houghton Mifflin, Boston.
751. Wrangham Richard 2001 *Out of the fryng pan into the fire: How our ancestors evolution depended on what they ate* in de Waal Frans (ed.) <u>Tree of Origin</u>, Harvard Univ. Pr. Camb. MA.
752. Wright Lawrence (2004) *The Kingdom of Silence* New Yorker 5 Jan 48-73.
753. Wright Robert 1994 <u>The Moral Animal</u> Pantheon N.Y.
754. Wright Robert 1995 *The Biology of Violence* New Yorker Mar 13.
755. Wright Robert 1996 *Science and Original Sin*, Time Nov 4.
756. Wyckoff G. Lahn B et. al. 2004 Nature Genetics, DOI: 10.1038/ng1471.
757. Xiong Y., Eickbush T.H. (1990) *Origin and evolution of retroelements based upon their reverse transcriptase sequences* EMBO J. **9/10** 3353-62.
758. Young Serinity 1993 <u>An Anthology of Sacred Texts by and about Women</u>, Harper Collins, N.Y.
759. Zechner, U; Wilda, M; Kehrer-Sawatzki,H; Vogel, W; Fundele R; Hameister H 2001 *X-linked genes for general cognitive ability:a run-away process shaping human evolution?* Trends Genet. 17, 697–70
760. Zehren, Eric 1961 <u>The Crescent and the Bull</u>, Sidgwick & Jackson, London.
761. Zeki S. (1992) *The visual image in mind and brain* Sci. Am. **Sep** 43-50.
762. Zhang B., Cech T (1997) *Peptide formation by in-vitro selected ribozymes* Nature **390** 96-100.
763. Zhang B., Cech T (1998) *Peptidyl transferase ribozymes: trans reactons, structural character- ization and ribosomal RNA-like structures* Chemistry and Biology **5** 539-553.
764. Zhivotovsky, L., Rosenberg N, Feldman M 2003 *Features of Evolution and Expansion of Modern Humans, Inferred from Genomewide Microsatellite Markers* Am. J. Human Genetics May.
765. Zhou J, Hofman MA, Gooren L, Swaab D 1995 *A sex difference in the human brain and its relation to transsexuality.* Nature 378 68-70.
766. Zihlman Adrienne 1981 *Women as shapers of the human adaption* in Dahlberg F. (ed.) <u>Woman the Gatherer</u> Yale Univ. Pr., New Haven CT.
767. Zukav Larry 1979 <u>The Dancing Wu-Li Masters</u>, Hutchinson & Co., London.
768. Zurek W., 1991 *Decoherence and the Transition from Quantum to Classical* Physics Today Oct.
769. Zweig, Paul 1968 <u>The Heresy of Self-Love: A Study of Subversive Individualism</u>, Princeton University Press, Princeton.

Etymologies of Key Words

Sex L. *sexus* prob. orig. 'division'. **Contradiction** L. *contra-* against *dicere* speak
Paradox Gk. *paradoxos - para-* 'beyond' (contrary to) *doxa* 'opinion'.
Coitus L. *coitio co-* together, *-ire* go. **Couple, Copulate** L. *copula* a link, bond.
Concupiscence *com-* thoroughly *-cupere* desire.
Primordial, Primeval L. *primus-* 'first' *-ordiri* 'begin a web' *-aevum* 'age'.
Chaos Gk. *kaos* abyss - to 'yawn' or 'gape'. **Cosmos** Gk. *kosmos* order.
Universe L. *universus* - 'turned into one' - *uni-* 'one' *-versere* 'turned'.
Religion L. *re-* 'again' *-ligio* to 'bind' or 'link' - to bind again **Heresy** Gk. *hariesthai* 'choose'.
Dominion L. *dominium - dominus* lord **Apocalypse** Gk. *apo-* from *-kalyptein* cover - unveiling
Patriarchy Gk. *patriarches* head of a family *patria-* family, clan *-archein* to rule.
Matriarchy derived from patriarch by substitution. **Marriage** L. *maritus* a husband **Wed** OE. *weddian* pledge.
Sacred L. *sacer* 'holy' **Holy** OE *halig* 'whole'.
Matrimony L. *matrimonium* marriage - from *mater, matris* mother.
Patrimony L. *patrimonium* an endowment or inheritance - from *pater, patris* father.
Tragedy Gk. *tragōida - tragos-* 'goat' *-ōide* a song (Dionysus' severed goat's head. Death).
Comedy Gk.. *kōmos-* 'revel' *-aeidein* 'sing') - to rejoice. Chaos, Life.

Index

548

Authors

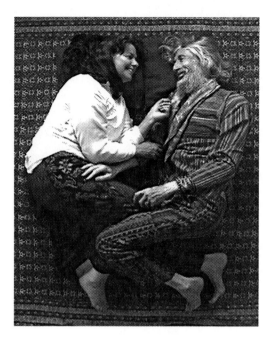

Christine Fielder is a mother and social researcher with an interest in literature, art and culture, the way biology interacts with behavior, and issues affecting the status of women and reproduction. She has had a key role in raising several children in a cooperative conservation community and spent time as a teacher in a remote area school. She has also spent time in South East Asia, China, Europe and America.

christine@sexualparadox.org

Chris King is a father and cosmologist, with an interest in edge of chaos dynamics, quantum reality and their applications to the neurodynamics of consciousness. He also has an interest in how cultural traditions relate to impacts on biodiversity, and how the sexual relationship effects these attitudes. He has travelled widely in South East Asia, China, India, the Middle East, Europe, the US and Central and South America including biodiveristy studies in the Amazon basin. He hosted a millennial rite of passage for sexual reunion on the Mount of Olives for Millennium Eve. He is currently a member of the Mathematics Department at the University of Auckland NZ.

chris@sexualparadox.org

Printed in the United Kingdom
by Lightning Source UK Ltd.
133763UK00001B/45/A